Skeletal Anchorage in Orthodontic Treatment of Class II Malocclusion

Contemporary applications of orthodontic implants, miniscrew implants and miniplates

Dedication

This book is dedicated to my wife Despina, for her unfailing love, understanding, and full support over the years, and to my two sons, Apostolos and Harry, with the wish to serve as an inspiration for their future professional endeavors.

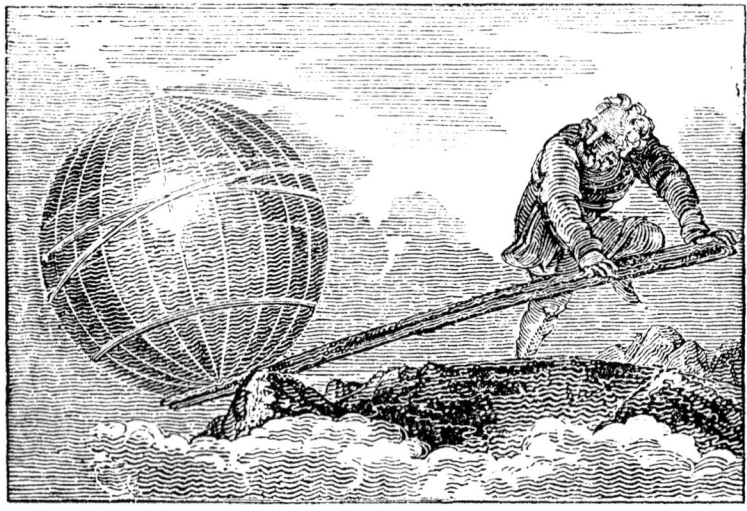

"Give me a place to stand on, and I will move the earth."
Archimedes (287 BC – 212 BC)

The engraving is from Mechanic's Magazine
(cover of bound Volume II, Knight & Lacey, London, 1824)
Courtesy of the Annenberg Rare Book & Manuscript Library,
University of Pennsylvania, Philadelphia, USA

For Elsevier
Content Strategist: Alison Taylor
Content Development Specialist: Barbara Simmons/Carole McMurray
Project Manager: Andrew Riley
Designer/Design Direction: Christian Bilbow
Illustration Manager: Karen Giacomucci
Illustrator: Electronic Publishing Services Inc., NYC

Skeletal Anchorage in Orthodontic Treatment of Class II Malocclusion

Contemporary applications of orthodontic implants, miniscrew implants and miniplates

Edited by

MOSCHOS A. PAPADOPOULOS, DDS, DR MED DENT

Professor, Chairman & Program Director
Department of Orthodontics
School of Dentistry
Aristotle University of Thessaloniki
Thessaloniki, Greece

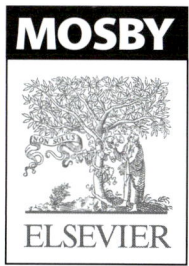

MOSBY

ELSEVIER

Edinburgh   London   New York   Oxford   Philadelphia   St Louis   Sydney   Toronto 2015

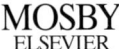

MOSBY
ELSEVIER

Parts of the text and images in Chapter 9 have been previously published in Papadopoulos MA, Tarawneh F. The use of miniscrew implants for temporary skeletal anchorage in orthodontics: a comprehensive review. Oral Surg Oral Med Oral Pathol Oral Radiol Endod 2007;103:e6–15 as per references.

ISBN 9780723436492

British Library Cataloguing in Publication Data
A catalogue record for this book is available from the British Library

Library of Congress Cataloging in Publication Data
A catalog record for this book is available from the Library of Congress

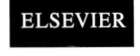

ELSEVIER your source for books, journals and multimedia in the health sciences
www.elsevierhealth.com

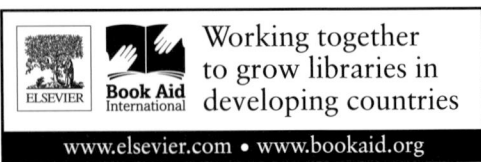

Working together to grow libraries in developing countries

www.elsevier.com • www.bookaid.org

The publisher's policy is to use paper manufactured from sustainable forests

Printed in China

Foreword

In our millennium we are acutely aware of the many challenges that confront us in diverse fields. The field of orthodontics has seen no cataclysmic events – financial or economic quicksand – but only steady progress based on extensive research around the world. Commercial firms provide the armamentarium we need and technical developments have kept pace with scientific progress. Long-term evidence-based assessment of treatment results is now available. The question as to what we can do and what are the borderline situations can be answered in biological, biomechanical and risk-management terms. There are many roads to Rome: many appliances that can accomplish similar results but only one set of fundamental tissue-related principles.

Orthodontics itself has seen a fundamental change (paradigm shift) in direction and treatment emphasis, with greater attention being given to the problem of stationary anchorage without a requirement for patient compliance. This is achieved by using implants instead of extraoral anchorage. This non-compliance approach enables intraoral extradental stationary anchorage without the side effect of anchorage loss. The use of stationary anchorage with implants has been improved our success in reaching the "achievable optimum," the goal of the treatment.

Since the introduction of implants in orthodontics, much information has been generated, mostly disorganized and contradictory with anecdotal case presentations. Dr. Papadopoulos has assembled world-class experts from all over the world to cover all aspects of skeletal anchorage using contemporary application of various orthodontic implants and miniplates. Dr. Papadopoulos is an innovative, enthusiastic pioneer with a holistic approach in his research.

This book is a comprehensive publication, presenting methods and views of 96 authors from 20 countries in 52 chapters. It is a unique work in the orthodontic literature; it is the most extensive compendium of the new millennium. All the available skeletal anchorage devices are presented and discussed by experts in the specific areas. The presented results are evidence based with a combination of internal evidence (individualized clinical expertise and knowledge of the clinicians) and external evidence (randomized controlled clinical studies, systemic reviews) to conclude on what is scientifically recognized therapy.

Admittedly, reading this book for the first time may confuse some novice orthodontic students, but like a sacred text, it must be read again and again. The book provides an exact description of techniques, their biomechanical justifications and examples of their potential for correcting orthodontic problems if the technique is handled properly. The criteria for successful treatment are stability, tissue health and esthetic achievement.

The book discusses all aspects of a more efficient use of skeletal anchorage devices and also biological and biomechanical considerations, biomaterial properties and radiological evaluation. Within the book, all the available methods are described, such as the Strauman Orthosystem, the Graz Implant-Supported Pendulum, the Aarhus Anchorage System, the Spider Screw anchorage, the Advanced Molar Distalization Appliance, the TopJet Distalizer, and many others. Utilizing implants in lingual orthodontics is described in two chapters, The book is completed by an in-depth discussion of complications and risk management.

This unique book makes a deep impression on the reader and shows that the nature of orthodontics does not permit a limited narrow view; it deserves understanding of conflicting opinions and evidence.

Thomas Rakosi, DDS, MD, MSD, PhD
Professor Emeritus and Former Chairman
Department of Orthodontics, University of Freiburg, Germany

Acknowledgements

The editor is most grateful to all colleagues involved in the preparation of the different chapters included in this book for their excellent scientific contributions.

Dr. Jane Ward, Medical Editorial Consultant, is given particular thanks for her invaluable input into the rewriting of many of the contributions.

Finally, Ms Alison Taylor, Senior Content Strategist, and all other Elsevier staff members are also acknowledged for their excellent cooperation during the preparation and publication of this volume. Elsevier Ltd is acknowledged for the high quality of the published Work.

Class II malocclusion is considered the most frequent treatment problem in orthodontic practice. Conventional treatment approaches require patient cooperation to be effective, while non-compliance approaches used to avoid the necessity for patient cooperation have a number of side effects. Most of these side effects are related to anchorage loss, and therefore, they can be avoided by the use of skeletal anchorage devices.

Anchorage is defined as the resistance to unwanted tooth movements and is considered as a prerequisite for the orthodontic treatment of dental and skeletal malocclusions. In addition to conventional orthodontic implants, which have been used for anchorage purposes for some years, miniplates and miniscrew implants have been recently utilized as intraoral extradental temporary anchorage devices for the treatment of various orthodontic problems, including Class II malocclusions. All these modalities may provide temporary stationary anchorage to support orthodontic movements in the desired direction, without the need for patient compliance in anchorage preservation, thus reducing the occurrence of side effects and the total treatment time.

The main remit of this book was to address the clinical use of all the available skeletal anchorage devices, including orthodontic implants, miniplates and miniscrew implants, that can be utilized to support orthodontic treatment of patients presenting with Class II malocclusion. The book provides a comprehensive and critical review of the principles and techniques as well as emphasizing the scientific evidence available regarding the contemporary applications and the clinical efficacy of these treatment modalities.

The book is divided into nine sections, starting from an introduction to orthodontic treatment of Class II malocclusion (Section I) and an introduction to skeletal anchorage in orthodontics (Section II). After a detailed presentation of the clinical and surgical considerations of the use of skeletal anchorage devices in orthodontics (Sections III and IV, respectively), the book continuous with sections devoted on the treatment of Class II malocclusion with the various skeletal anchorage devices, such as orthodontic implants (Section V), miniplates (Section VI) and miniscrew implants (Section VII). A further section is devoted to the treatment of Class II malocclusion with various temporary anchorage devices (Section VIII). Finally, the last section discusses the currently available evidence related to the clinical efficiency as well as the risk management of the skeletal anchorage devices used for orthodontic purposes (Section IX).

The editor invited colleagues who are experts in specific areas related to orthodontic anchorage to contribute with chapters. Most of the authors have either developed or introduced sophisticated devices or approaches, or they have been actively involved in their clinical evaluation. In total, 96 colleagues from 20 different countries participated in this exciting project.

The detailed discussion by a large number of experts of a variety of issues related to skeletal anchorage may be considered as a breakthrough feature not previously seen in this form in orthodontic texts. At present, there is no other book dealing with all possible anchorage reinforcement approaches (including orthodontic implants, miniplates and miniscrew implants) used for the treatment of patients with Class II malocclusion.

It is the hope of the editor that this textbook will provide all the necessary background information for the better understanding and more efficient use of the currently available skeletal anchorage devices to reinforce anchorage during orthodontic treatment of patients presenting Class II malocclusion, and that it will be used as a comprehensive reference by orthodontic practitioners, undergraduate and postgraduate students, and researchers for the clinical management of these patients.

Prof. M. A. Papadopoulos

Contributors

YOUSSEF S. AL JABBARI
Associate Professor, Dental Biomaterials Research and Development Chair, College of Dentistry, King Saud University, Riyadh, Saudi Arabia

GEORGE ANKA
Orthodontist in private practice, Tama-shi, Tokyo, Japan

AYÇA ARMAN ÖZÇIRPICI
Associate Professor and Head, Department of Orthodontics, Faculty of Dentistry, Başkent University, Ankara, Turkey

KARLIEN ASSCHERICKX
Researcher and Lecturer, Vrije Universiteit Brussel, Dental Clinic, Department of Orthodontics, Brussels, Belgium; orthodontist in private practice, Antwerp, Belgium

MUSTAFA B. ATES
Assistant Professor, Department of Orthodontics, Faculty of Dentistry, Marmara University, Istanbul, Turkey

UGO BACILIERO
Director, Department of Maxillofacial Surgery, Regional Hospital of Vicenza, Vicenza, Italy

MARTIN BAXMANN
Visiting Professor, Department of Orthodontics and Pediatric Dentistry, University of Seville, Seville, Spain: Orthodontist in private practice, Kempen & Geldern, Germany

THOMAS BERNHART
Professor, Division of Oral Surgery, Bernhard Gottlieb University Clinic of Dentistry, Medical University of Vienna, Austria

MICHAEL BERTL
Lecturer, Division of Orthodontics, Bernhard Gottlieb University Clinic of Dentistry, Medical University of Vienna, Austria

LARS BONDEMARK
Professor and Head, Department of Orthodontics; Dean, Faculty of Odontology, Malmö University, Malmö, Sweden

S. JAY BOWMAN
Adjunct Associate Professor, Saint Louis University; Instructor, University of Michigan; Assistant Clinical Professor, Case Western Reserve University; orthodontist in private practice, Portage, Michigan, USA

FRIEDRICH K. BYLOFF
Former Clinical Instructor, Department of Orthodontics, School of Dentistry, University of Geneva, Switzerland; orthodontist in private practice, Graz, Austria

VITTORIO CACCIAFESTA
Orthodontist in private practice, Milan, Italy

LESLIE YEN-PENG CHEN
Orthodontist in private practice, Taipei, Taiwan

ADITYA CHHIBBER
Resident, Division of Orthodontics, Department of Craniofacial Sciences, School of Dental Medicine, University of Connecticut, Farmington, CT, USA

HYERAN CHOO
Director of Craniofacial Orthodontics at The Children's Hospital of Philadelphia; Clinical Associate, Department of Orthodontics, University of Pennsylvania, Philadelphia, PA, USA

KYU-RHIM CHUNG
Professor and Chairman, Division of Orthodontics, Ajou University, School of Medicine, Suwon, South Korea

MARIE A. CORNELIS
Assistant Professor, Department of Orthodontics, School of Dentistry, University of Geneva, Switzerland

MAURO COZZANI
Professor of Orthodontics and Gnathology, School of Dental Medicine University of Cagliari, Italy

ADRIANO CRISMANI
Professor and Head, Clinic of Orthodontics, Medical University of Innsbruck, Austria

MICHEL DALSTRA
Associate Professor, Department of Orthodontics, School of Dentistry, University of Aarhus, Denmark

HUGO DE CLERCK
Adjunct Professor, Department of Orthodontics, School of Dentistry, University of North Carolina, Chapel Hill, NC, USA; orthodontist in private practice, Brussels, Belgium

GLADYS C. DOMINGUEZ
Associate Professor, Department of Orthodontics, Faculty of Dentistry, University of Sao Paulo, Brazil

GEORGE ELIADES
Professor and Director, Department of Biomaterials, School of Dentistry, University of Athens, Greece

THEODORE ELIADES
Professor and Head, Department of Orthodontics and Paediatric Dentistry, Center of Dental Medicine, University of Zurich, Switzerland

NEJAT ERVERDI
Professor, Department of Orthodontics, Faculty of Dentistry, Marmara University, Istanbul, Turkey

INGALILL FELDMANN
Senior consultant, PhD, Orthodontic Clinic, Public Dental Helth Service, Gävle and Centre for research and Development, Uppsala University/ County Council of Gävleborg, Gävle, Sweden

MATTIA FONTANA
Orthodontist in private practice, La Spezia, Italy

TADASHI FUJITA

Assistant Professor, Department of Orthodontics and Craniofacial Developmental Biology, Hiroshima University Graduate School of Biomedical Sciences, Hiroshima, Japan

NARAYAN H. GANDEDKAR

Former Assistant Professor, Department of Orthodontics and Dentofacial Orthopedics, SDM College of Dental Sciences and Hospital, Dharwad, India; Dental Officer Specialist and Clinical Researcher, Cleft and Craniofacial Dentistry Unit, Division of Plastic, Reconstructive and Aesthetic Surgery, K.K. Women's and Children's Hospital, Singapore

COSTANTINO GIAGNORIO

Orthodontist in private practice, SanNicandro Garganico (FG), Italy

BETTINA GLASL

Orthodontist in private practice, Traben-Trarbach, Germany

ANTONIO GRACCO

Assistant Professor, Department of Neurosciences, Section of Dentistry, University of Padua, Italy

HIDEHARU HIBI

Associate Professor, Department of Oral and Maxillofacial Surgery, Graduate School of Medicine, Nagoya University, Nagoya, Japan

RYOON-KI HONG

Chairman, Department of Orthodontics, Chong-A Dental Hospital, Seoul; Clinical Professor, Department of Orthodontics, School of Dentistry, Seoul National University, Seoul, South Korea

MASATO KAKU

Assistant Professor, Department of Orthodontics and Craniofacial Developmental Biology, Hiroshima University Graduate School of Biomedical Sciences, Hiroshima, Japan

HANS KÄRCHER

Professor and Head, Department of Maxillo-Facial Surgery, School of Dentistry, University of Graz, Austria

HASSAN E. KASSEM

Assistant Lecturer, Department of Orthodontics, School of Dentistry, Alexandria University, Alexandria, Egypt

BURÇAK KAYA

Assistant Professor, Department of Orthodontics, Faculty of Dentistry, Başkent University, Ankara, Turkey

HYEWON KIM

Orthodontist in private practice, Seoul, South Korea

SEONG-HUN KIM

Associate Professor, Department of Orthodontics, School of Dentistry, Kyung Hee University, Seoul, South Korea

TAE-WOO KIM

Professor, Department of Orthodontics, School of Dentistry, Seoul National University, Seoul, South Korea

GERO KINZINGER

Professor, Department of Orthodontics, University of Saarland, Homburg/Saar; private practice, Toenisvorst, Germany

BEYZA HANCIOGLU KIRCELLI

Former Associate Professor, Department of Orthodontics, University of Baskent; orthodontist in private practice, Adana, Turkey

NAZAN KUCUKKELES

Professor and Head, Department of Orthodontics, Faculty of Dentistry, Marmara University, Istanbul, Turkey

KEE-JOON LEE

Associate Professor, Department of Orthodontics, College of Dentistry, Yonsei University, Seoul, South Korea

GARY LEONARD

Oral surgeon in private practice, Dublin, Republic of Ireland

SEUNG-MIN LIM

Clinical Professor, Department of Orthodontics, Kangnam Sacred Heart Hospital, Hallym University; orthodontist in private practice, Seoul, South Korea

JAMES CHENG-YI LIN

Clinical Assistant Professor, School of Dentistry, National Defense Medical University; Consultant Orthodontist, Department of Orthodontics and Craniofacial Dentistry, Chang Gung Memorial Hospital; private practice of orthodontics and implantology, Taipei, Taiwan

ERIC JEIN-WEIN LIOU

Chairman, Faculty of Dentistry, Chang Gung Memorial Hospital; Associate Professor, Department of Orthodontics and Craniofacial Dentistry, Chang Gung Memorial Hospital, Taipei, Taiwan

GUDRUN LÜBBERINK

Assistant Clinical Professor, Department of Orthodontics, School of Dentistry, University of Duesseldorf, Germany

BJÖRN LUDWIG

Scientific collaborator, Department of Orthodontics, University of Saarland, Homburg/Saar; orthodontist in private practice, Traben-Trarbach, Germany

CESARE LUZI

Orthodontist in private practice, Rome, Italy

B. GIULIANO MAINO

Visiting Professor of Orthodontics at Ferrara University and Insubria University; orthodontist in private practice, Vicenza, Italy

FRASER MCDONALD

Professor and Head, Department of Orthodontics, King's College London Dental Institute, London, UK

BIRTE MELSEN

Professor and Head, Department of Orthodontics, School of Dentistry, University of Aarhus, Denmark

ANNA MENINI

Orthodontist in private practice, Monterosso al Mare (SP), Italy

CAMILLO MOREA

Postdoctoral Researcher, Department of Orthodontics, Faculty of Dentistry, University of Sao Paulo, Brazil

MELIH MOTRO
Assistant Professor, Department of Orthodontics, Faculty of Dentistry, Marmara University, Istanbul, Turkey

RAVINDRA NANDA
Professor and Head, Division of Orthodontics, Department of Craniofacial Sciences, School of Dental Medicine, University of Connecticut, Farmington, CT, USA

CATHERINE NYSSEN-BEHETS
Professor, Pole of Morphology, Institute of Clinical and Experimental Research, Catholic University of Louvain, Brussels, Belgium

JUNJI OHTANI
Assistant Professor, Department of Orthodontics and Craniofacial Developmental Biology, Hiroshima University Graduate School of Biomedical Sciences, Hiroshima, Japan

PAOLO PAGIN
Orthodontist in private practice, Bologna, Italy

MOSCHOS A. PAPADOPOULOS
Professor, Chairman and Program Director, Department of Orthodontics, School of Dentistry, Aristotle University of Thessaloniki, Greece

SPYRIDON N. PAPAGEORGIOU
Resident, Department of Orthodontics; Doctoral fellow, Department of Oral Technology, School of Dentistry, University of Bonn, Germany

YOUNG-CHEL PARK
President, World Implant Orthodontic Association; Professor, Department of Orthodontics, College of Dentistry, Yonsei University, Seoul, South Korea

MARCO PASINI
Orthodontist in private practice, Massa, Italy

ZAFER OZGUR PEKTAS
Associate Professor, Department of Orthodontics, University of Baskent, Department of Oral and Maxillofacial Surgery, Ankara, Turkey

BEN PILLER
Scientific collaborator, Department of Orthodontics, The Maurice and Gabriela Goldschleger School of Dental Medicine, Tel Aviv University, Israel

IOANNIS POLYZOIS
Lecturer/Consultant in Periodontology, Dublin Dental University Hospital, Trinity College Dublin, Republic of Ireland

ROBERT RITUCCI
Orthodontist in private practice, Plymouth, MA, USA

KIYOSHI SAKAI
Postdoctoral Researcher, Department of Oral and Maxillofacial Surgery, Graduate School of Medicine, Nagoya University, Nagoya, Japan

MASARU SAKAI
Orthodontist in private practice, Nagoya, Japan

ÇAĞLA ŞAR
Assistant Professor, Department of Orthodontics, Faculty of Dentistry, Başkent University, Ankara, Turkey

MICHAEL SCHAUSEIL
Research Assistant, Department of Orthodontics, School of Dentistry, University of Marburg, Germany

GIUSEPPE SICILIANI
Professor and Head, Department of Orthodontics, School of Dentistry, University of Ferrara, Italy

HIROKO SUNAGAWA
Clinical Associate, Department of Orthodontics and Craniofacial Developmental Biology, Hiroshima University Graduate School of Biomedical Sciences, Hiroshima, Japan

PHILIPPOS SYNODINOS
Orthodontist in private practice, Athens, Greece

KYOTO TAKEMOTO
Orthodontist in private practice, Tokyo, Japan

KAZUO TANNE
Professor and Head, Department of Orthodontics and Craniofacial Developmental Biology, Hiroshima University Graduate School of Biomedical Sciences, Hiroshima, Japan

FADI TARAWNEH
Research Associate, Department of Orthodontics, School of Dentistry, Aristotle University of Thessaloniki, Greece

HILDE TIMMERMAN
Orthodontist in private practice, Brussels, Belgium

STEPHEN TRACEY
Orthodontist in private practice, Upland, CA, USA

SINA UÇKAN
Professor, Department of Oral and Maxillofacial Surgery, Faculty of Dentistry, Başkent University, Ankara, Turkey

MINORU UEDA
Professor, Department of Oral and Maxillofacial Surgery, Graduate School of Medicine, Nagoya University, Nagoya, Japan

MADHUR UPADHYAY
Assistant Professor and Program Director (Orthodontic Fellowship Program), Division of Orthodontics, Department of Craniofacial Sciences, School of Dental Medicine, University of Connecticut, Farmington, CT, USA

FLAVIO URIBE
Associate Professor and Program Director, Division of Orthodontics, Department of Craniofacial Sciences, School of Dental Medicine, University of Connecticut, Farmington, CT, USA

HEINER WEHRBEIN
Professor and Head, Department of Orthodontics, Johannes Gutenberg University Hospital, Mainz, Germany

BENEDICT WILMES
Professor, Department of Orthodontics, University of Duesseldorf, Germany

HEINZ WINSAUER

Orthodontist in private practice, Bregenz, Austria

SUMIT YADAV

Assistant Professor, Division of Orthodontics, Department of Craniofacial Sciences, School of Dental Medicine, University of Connecticut, Farmington, CT, USA

ABBAS R. ZAHER

Professor, Department of Orthodontics, School of Dentistry, Alexandria University, Alexandria, Egypt

FRANCESCO ZALLIO

Orthodontist in private practice, Sestri Levante (GE), Italy

SPIROS ZINELIS

Assistant Professor, Department of Biomaterials, School of Dentistry, University of Athens, Greece; Dental Biomaterials Research and Development Chair, King Saud University, Riyadh, Saudi Arabia

IOANNIS P. ZOGAKIS

Resident, Department of Orthodontics, School of Dentistry, University of Jerusalem, Israel

VASILEIOS F. ZYMPERDIKAS

Military Dentist, 71st Airmobile Medical Company, 71st Airmobile Brigade, Nea Santa, Greece

Contents

Section VIII: Treatment of Class II malocclusion with different temporary anchorage devices

Section IX: Efficiency of skeletal anchorage and risk management

Diagnostic considerations and conventional strategies for treatment of Class II malocclusion

1

Abbas R. Zaher and Hassan E. Kassem

INTRODUCTION

Treatment of Class II malocclusion in the adolescent period is based on whether there is still growth potential; if so, correction can be attempted by stimulating differential growth of the maxilla and mandible.[1,2] This has been classically done with headgear or functional appliances.

Where there is a mild or moderate Class II malocclusion in an adult, or an adolescent who is too old for growth modification, camouflage by tooth movements can be used: (a) moving maxillary molars distally, followed by the entire maxillary arch; (b) extraction of premolars and retraction of maxillary anterior teeth into the extraction spaces; or (c) a combination of retraction of the maxillary arch and forward movement of the mandibular arch. Surgical correction is reserved for adults with severe Class II malocclusion and no further growth potential.

Because of individual variation in skeletal, dental and soft tissue morphology, treatment plans must be tailored to each patient's diagnosis, needs and goals, including treatment approach, appliance design and choice, and biomechanics.

DIAGNOSTIC CONSIDERATIONS

From the early 2000s, orthodontic treatment has focused on facial soft tissue appearance rather than skeletal and dental relations. Facial proportions can be evaluated clinically using photographs and cephalometric radiographs. Accordingly, diagnostic considerations for the Class II patient should focus upon the effect of treatment on the patient's facial esthetics.

THE POSITION OF THE UPPER LIP

Several cephalometric lines, distances and angles have been proposed to assess the anteroposterior maxillary lip position, of which the E-line is the most popular.[3] The distance of the most prominent point of the upper lip to a line dropped from subnasale perpendicular to the Frankfurt horizontal is used to assess variation in nose and chin positions and size. The accepted norm for males is 4–5 mm and for females 2–3 mm. There is no good predictor of the precise upper lip response to orthodontic treatment[4] and response may vary from 40% to 70% of maxillary incisor movement.[5] Any lip changes that do occur will be in the direction of movement of the maxillary anterior teeth.[6] A protrusive upper lip can be adjusted by distal movement of the maxillary incisors and molars, or by tooth extraction.

THE CHIN

The chin point is an important issue and 85–90% of young patients with Class II malocclusion who present with mandibular deficiency.[7] Various cephalometric lines have been proposed for spatial evaluation of the chin position, including the perpendicular to the Frankfurt horizontal from subnasale and the distance from the pogonion (the most prominent point of the soft tissue chin) to the subnasale. If a patient with Class II malocclusion presents with a deficient chin, the treatment plan should involve a change of chin position. In adults, the chin point can only be consistently brought forward by surgical procedures.[8] There is no evidence that functional appliances increase mandibular growth beyond that which would be normally achieved.[9,10] Growth acceleration does occur, which could be misinterpreted for true additional growth. However, several studies have investigated the use of functional appliance treatment to increase mandibular length in adults[11–13] and in growing and adult subjects with a specific genetic make-up.[14,15]

CROWDING

Crowding in either jaw is always a complicating factor in Class II treatment. In the maxilla, the objective is to retract the maxillary incisors and reduce overjet. However, space provided by distal movement of molars or premolar extraction is likely to be taken up by resolving the crowding, leaving little space for incisor retraction.

In the mandible, treatment aims to maintain the mandibular incisors in their position or to advance them slightly to help to correct the dental discrepancy in the sagittal plane. There is general agreement that mandibular incisor advancement should not exceed 2 mm or 3° as beyond this, reduced stability and periodontal problems can arise.

Hence, crowding of more than 4 mm warrants extraction in the mandible and subsequently in the maxilla. Treatment should be prudent to resolve crowding without retracting the mandibular incisors, as any inadvertent retraction necessitates additional retraction of the maxillary incisors, making overjet reduction more difficult to achieve and having effects on facial esthetics.

GROWTH POTENTIAL

When some growth potential exists, the sensible approach is to attempt growth modification. Patients in late adolescence with little growth left for successful modification can be treated with camouflage tooth movements with reasonable facial esthetics unless there is very severe Class II malocclusion. The remaining vertical growth will offset any further extrusion and will reduce the possibility of backward rotation of the mandible, which would increase facial profile convexity. In adults, camouflage treatment is difficult because there will be no more vertical facial growth. Excellent vertical control is essential for adults receiving camouflage treatment. In one study, greater molar extrusion occurred in growing patients (4.7 mm) than in adults; however, the orginal mandibular plane angle did not change appreciatively during treatment in the adolescents, while adults failed to maintain the original angle despite minimal molar extrusion (1.3 mm).[16] Recent skeletal anchorage-based treatments have proven very beneficial in this aspect.

OTHER FACTORS

The significance of the axial inclinations of the posterior teeth is not often mentioned in the Class II literature. Mesially tipped first molars would lend themselves more readily to distal tipping, correcting a Class II relation. In contrast, premolars and molars may be tipped distally. In such a case, if a straight wire is used for leveling and alignment, it will move all these teeth forward, thus worsening the Class II condition. Therefore, it can be advised to bond the brackets at an angle in relation to the axis of these teeth.

TREATMENT STRATEGIES

GROWTH MODIFICATION: HEADGEARS AND FUNCTIONAL APPLIANCES

Four randomized controlled trials have clearly shown that headgears and functional appliances can successfully be used to correct a Class II discrepancy with no appreciable difference between the two modalities.[17–20] However, the debate centers on how the correction is achieved.

Is the short-term increase in mandibular length achieved with functional appliances clinically significant? Several studies have concluded that it is unlikely to be of clinical significance[21,22] and can be explained by the observation that the mandible moves downwards rather than forwards as it increases in size.[23]

The Herbst appliance and the Mandibular Anterior Repositioning Appliance (MARA) are considered to be the only true fixed functional appliances as they function by dislocating the condyles (believed to increase mandibular length).[1,24] An evaluation of the relative skeletal and dental changes produced by the crown or banded Herbst appliance in growing patients with Class II division 1 malocclusion concluded that dental changes had more correcting effect than skeletal changes.[25]

The effectiveness of the Herbst appliance compared with a removable functional appliance (Twin Block) has been assessed in several studies, none of which found a significant difference in skeletal, soft tissue or dental changes as well as in final treatment outcome.[26–28] One study did note that while treatment time was the same with the two approaches, significantly more appointments were needed for repair of the Herbst appliance.[26] A comparison of the soft tissue effects found that both appliances effectively reduced the soft tissue profile convexity but there was greater advancement of mandibular soft tissues in the Twin Block group.[28] The Herbst appliance may have an advantage in terms of increased patient compliance[26] and is also compatible with multibracket therapy, which may reduce total treatment time in adolescents.

EXTRACTION TREATMENT

The objective of extraction in Class II malocclusion is to compensate the position of the dentition to mask the underlying skeletal discrepancy.

The most popular extraction pattern is the extraction of maxillary first premolars to provide space to correct the canine relationship from Class II to Class I and to correct the incisor overjet. The molars remain in Class II intercuspation. Maximum maxillary posterior anchorage is necessary to minimize mesial movement of the maxillary molars and second premolars while retracting the anterior segment.

Extraction of mandibular second premolars is considered if there is significant mandibular incisor crowding or labial inclination, in order to provide space for the retraction of the mandibular canines to align the mandibular incisor. However, in Class II malocclusion, the mandibular canine is already distal to the maxillary canine and so even further retraction of the maxillary canines is required, stressing maxillary posterior anchorage even more. In addition, maximum mandibular anterior anchorage is necessary to avoid excessive retraction of the mandibular incisors, which would increase the convexity of the profile.

An alternative is to extract two maxillary premolars and one mandibular incisor. This provides 5–6 mm of space to correct the alignment and axial inclination of the mandibular incisors; however, it may lead to a residual excess overjet or a slight Class III canine relation.

Uncommonly, maxillary second molars can be extracted instead of first premolars. Success depends on the third molar eruption path and timing, both of which are not readily predictable for a particular patient. However, such an approach requires retracting the entire maxillary dentition without reciprocal protrusion of the incisors.

Maxillary Posterior Anchorage

Different strategies have been described for maximizing maxillary posterior anchorage.

Tweed–Merrifield approach

This uses J-hook headgears to conserve anchorage by delivering force directly to the anterior segment, sparing the posterior anchor unit. It requires extractions and relies heavily on patient compliance in wearing the appliance full-time to ensure efficient tooth movement. In late adolescents or adults, compliance will be an issue.

Class II elastics and similar non-compliance fixed interarch appliances

These use the mandibular arch to balance the maxillary retraction forces. There are side effects of Class II traction while the use of Class II elastics still relies on patient compliance.

Palatal appliances

These include transpalatal arches, the Nance holding arch and, less frequently, palatal removable retainers.

Balancing retraction forces against posterior unit

Increasing the anchorage value of the posterior segment can be achieved by balancing the retraction forces of the anterior segment against the posterior anchorage unit, including the maxillary first molars, second molars and second premolars.

Two-stage space closure

First the canine is retracted to avoid stressing the anchor unit and then the canine is added to the posterior segment to increase its anchorage value during incisor retraction.

Segmented arch mechanics

Precise differential moments are used to maximize posterior anchorage; in this case the posterior anchorage is not affected by the friction that is encountered with sliding mechanics.[29]

Classical Begg technique

Anchorage preservation uses distal tipping of the maxillary anterior segment followed by uprighting. The contemporary appliance using this technique is the Tip-Edge system.[30]

Mandibular Anterior Anchorage

To reinforce mandibular anterior anchorage, several strategies have been suggested:

- subdividing the protraction of the posterior segment: the mandibular incisors and canines combined into a single unit to anchor the mesial movement of the posterior teeth one by one

- balancing the protraction of the mandibular posterior segment against the maxillary arch using Class II elastics and similar appliances.
- utilizing differential moments: the segmented arch technique uses an asymmetric V-bend to place a large clockwise moment on the anterior segment;[29] the bidimensional technique uses lingual root torque applied to mandibular incisors and distal root tip to the mandibular canines to provide stationary anchorage by balancing the bodily movement of the anterior segment against the forward movement of the posterior segment.[23]
- utilizing differential tooth movement: the Tip-Edge technique tips the posterior teeth followed by uprighting to avoid stressing the anterior anchorage.[30]

The Effects of Extraction of Premolars on Dentofacial Structures

The position of the upper and lower lips after treatment is influenced by the patient's pretreatment profile as well as by tooth size–arch length discrepancy. A study of patients with Class II malocclusion compared patients with extraction of the four first premolars with patients who did not have extractions.[31] The extraction group had more protrusive upper and lower lips relative to the esthetic plane prior to treatment; hence the extraction decision had been influenced by the patient's pretreatment profile as well as tooth size–arch length discrepancy. Following treatment, the extraction group tended to have more retrusive lips, straighter faces and more upright incisors compared with the non-extraction group. However, the average soft tissue and skeletal measurements for both groups were close to the corresponding averages from the Iowa normative standards.

Similarly, discriminate analysis scores based on crowding and protrusion were used to create an extraction and a non-extraction group.[32] Premolar extraction produced greater reduction in hard and soft tissue protrusion but long-term follow-up indicated slightly more protrusion in the extraction group. This was attributed to the greater initial crowding and protrusion in the extraction group. This finding refuted the influential belief that premolar extraction frequently causes dished-in profiles.

A recent study determined predictive factors for a good long-term outcome after fixed appliance treatment of Class II division 1 malocclusion. The only treatment variable predictive of a favorable peer assessment rating (PAR) at recall was the extraction pattern.[33] The patients who had extraction of either maxillary first premolars or both maxillary first and mandibular second premolars were more likely to have ideal soft tissue outcome as judged by the Holdaway angle. The outcome was less favorable when the extraction pattern included the first molars and, to a lesser extent, the mandibular first premolars.

NON-EXTRACTION TREATMENT

Maxillary Molar Distalization

Maxillary molar distalization is an integral part of most non-extraction treatment philosophies for Class II malocclusion.[34] Extraoral traction using a facebow headgear is the traditional approach. However, headgear such as the facebow may be used not only for molar distalization but for growth modification as well.[23] The two treatment effects are not mutually exclusive and depend to a degree on the intention of treatment. Yet, it is not always possible to discriminate one effect from the other during treatment.

Here the use of the headgear is discussed in the context of strategies to move maxillary molars distally to a Class I position in 6 months or less and to open space in the maxillary arch for the retraction of the remainder teeth of the arch. Once a Class I molar has been achieved, no further

orthopedic correction is allowed. Hence, studies reporting posterior positioning of point A or distal movement of the entire dentition might not reflect the use of headgear purely for molar distalization since a growth modification effect might be involved. For this reason, studies that apply headgear forces directly to the first molar are preferred when considering the success of headgear use for molar distalization.

A study of the use of cervical pull headgear plus implants on the craniofacial complex compared the effect of adjusting the outer bow of the headgear 20° upwards to 20° downwards relative to the occlusal plane.[35] In the first group, only slight distal molar movement occurred, yet the entire maxillary complex moved downwards and backwards relative to the anterior cranial base. In the second group, more tooth movement was observed, particularly a distal tipping to the first molar. Tilting the outer bow upwards was considered to be appropriate for patients with true maxillary prognathism, while tilting the outer bow downwards may be more suitable for patients with mesially migrated and/or tipped maxillary first molars.

The presence of maxillary second molars is an important consideration in distal molar movement. Maxillary molars move distally more readily before the eruption of second molars.[18] However, if treatment is initiated before the eruption of the second molar, it is advisable to evaluate the relative position of the unerupted second molars to the roots of the first molars to avoid impactions. An optimal relationship exists when the crowns of the second permanent molars have erupted beyond the apical third of the roots of the first molars as depicted in periapical radiographs.[36]

Non-compliance Maxillary Molar Distalization

The Pendulum and the Jones Jig appliances were the early non-compliance distalization appliances. These appliances can be classified based on the source of their intramaxillary anchorage:[37]

- flexible palatally positioned distalization force systems, e.g. the Pendulum appliance,[38] the Keles Slider[39] and the Molar Distalizer.[40]
- flexible buccally positioned distalization force systems, e.g. the Jones Jig,[41] Lokar Molar Distalizer,[42] Ni-Ti coil springs[43] and Magneforce.[44]
- flexible palatally and buccally positioned distalization force systems, e.g. the Greenfield Molar Distalizer.[45]
- rigid palatally positioned distalization force systems, e.g. Veltri Distalizer.[46]
- hybrid appliances with rigid buccal and flexible palatal component, e.g. the First Class Appliance.[47]
- transpalatal arches for molar rotation and/or distalization used as an initial phase in Class II treatment.

Papadopoulos has reviewed the different molar distalization appliances and their management in Class II malocclusion orthodontic treatment.[37]

Antonarakis and Kiliaridis have reviewed published data on distal molar movement in addition to anchorage loss in premolars and incisors when using non-compliance intramaxillary appliances with conventional anchorage designs.[48] First molars demonstrated a mean of 2.9 mm distal movement with 5.4° of distal tipping. Incisors showed a mean of 1.8 mm mesial movement with 3.6° of mesial tipping. Palatal appliances produced less distal molar tipping (3.6° versus 8.3°) and less mesial incisor tipping (2.9° versus 5°). Friction-free appliances (e.g. pendulum appliances) were associated with a large amount of distal molar movement and concomitant substantial tipping when no therapeutic uprighting activation was applied.

Fixed Interarch Appliances

Fixed interarch appliances are used in the non-extraction treatment of Class II malocclusion with retraction of the maxillary teeth and forward movement of the mandibular teeth. They can be viewed as the fixed alternative of Class II elastics. A common indication for these appliances is Class II dental occlusion with retroclined mandibular incisors and deep overbite.[49] Some have claimed that these appliances have an orthopedic effect,[50,51] while others failed to observe this.[52] Proffit et al. have maintained that these "flexible correctors" have little growth effect because they do not displace the condyles far enough for an orthopedic response.[1]

The fixed interarch appliances are classified into three groups.

1. *Extension springs*. These are the fixed replica of Class II elastics. The classic example is the Saif spring (severable adjustable intermaxillary force) but this is no longer commercially available.
2. *Curvilinear leaf springs*. These springs use a push force rather the more common pull force of Class II elastics, avoiding the undesirable extrusion of maxillary anterior and mandibular posterior teeth, backward rotation of the mandible (worsening the Class II profile), increase of the anterior face height and excessive gingival display. The forerunner of this group is the Jasper Jumper,[53] which is considered the most successful and widely used system. Other examples include the Klapper Superspring II[54] and the Forsus Nitinol Flat Spring.[55]
3. *Interarch compression springs*. The Eureka Spring was the first system introduced in the market.[56] These appliances are the most rapidly expanding Class II non-compliance systems because of the promise of fewer breakages, which plagued the Jasper Jumper. The Twin Force,[57] Forsus[58] and Sabbagh Universal Spring[59] followed.

Papadopoulos gives a more comprehensive review of these appliances.[60]

CONCLUSIONS

The patient with a Class II malocclusion represents a large part of the workload of any orthodontic practice. Generating a problem list and treatment objectives for such a patient requires careful consideration of a plethora of factors either involving the malocclusion itself or affecting treatment outcome. Careful evaluation of the available evidence is crucial to provide each patient with the most suitable treatment strategy within reasonable expectations. Practitioners need to update their knowledge of new appliances continuously and become familiar with their use.

REFERENCES

1. Proffit WR, Fields HW, Sarver DM. Orthodontic treatment planning: limitations, controversies and special problems. In: Proffit WR, Fields HW, Sarver DM, editors. Contemporary orthodontics. 4th ed. St. Louis, MO: Elsevier-Mosby; 2007. p. 234–67.
2. Alexander RG. The Alexander discipline: The 20 principles of the Alexander discipline. Hanover Park, IL: Quintessence; 2008.
3. Ricketts R. Planning treatment on the basis of the facial pattern and estimate of its growth. Angle Orthod 1957;27:14–37.
4. Lai J, Ghosh J, Nanda R. Effects of orthodontic therapy on the facial profile in long and short vertical facial patterns. Am J Orthod Dentofacial Orthop 2000;118:505–13.
5. Proffit WR, White RP, Sarver DM. Contemporary treatment of dentofacial deformities. St Louis, MO: Elsevier-Mosby; 2002. p. 215.
6. Kocadereli I. Changes in soft tissue profile after orthodontic treatment with and without extractions. Am J Orthod Dentofacial Orthop 2002;118:67–72.
7. McNamara JA Jr. Components of Class II malocclusion in children 8–10 years of age. Angle Orthod 1981;51:117–210.
8. Talebzadeh N, Porgel MA. Long-term hard and soft tissue relapse after genioplasty. Oral Surg Oral Med Oral Pathol Oral Radiol Endod 2001;91:153–6.
9. Papadopoulos MA, Gkiaouris I. A critical evaluation of meta-analyses in orthodontics. Am J Orthod Dentofacial Orthop 2007;131:589–99.
10. Huang G. Ask Us – Functional appliances and long term effects on mandibular growth. Am J Orthod Dentofacial Orthop 2005;128:271–2.
11. Ruf S, Pancherz H. Orthognathic surgery and dentofacial orthopedics in adult Class II, division 1 treatment: Mandibular sagittal split osteotomy versus Herbst appliance. Am J Orthod Dentofacial Orthop 2004;126:140–52.
12. Ruf S, Pancherz H. Herbst/multibracket appliance treatment of Class II, division 1 malocclusions in early and late adulthood: a prospective cephalometric study of consecutively treated subjects. Eur J Orthod 2006;28:352–60.
13. Pancherz H. The Herbst appliance: a paradigm shift in Class II treatment. World J Orthod 2005;6(Suppl.):8–10.
14. Purkayastha SK, Rabie AB, Wong R. Treatment of skeletal class II malocclusion in adult patients: Stepwise vs. single-step advancement with the Herbst appliance. World J Orthod 2008;9:233–43.
15. Chaiyongsirisern A, Rabie AB, Wong RW. Stepwise Herbst advancement versus mandibular sagittal split osteotomy: Treatment effects and long-term stability of adult Class II patients. Angle Orthod 2009;79:1084–94.
16. McDowell EH, Baker IM. The skeletodental adaptations in deep bite corrections. Am J Orthod Dentofacial Orthop 1991;100:370–5.
17. Ghafari J, Shofer FS, Jacobsson-Hunt U, et al. Headgear versus function regulator in the early treatment of Class II, division 1 malocclusion: a randomized clinical trial. Am J Orthod Dentofacial Orthop 1998;113:51–61.
18. Wheeler TT, McGorray SP, Dolce C, et al. Effectiveness of early treatment of Class II malocclusion. Am J Orthod Dentofacial Orthop 2002;121:9–17.
19. Tulloch JF, Proffit WR, Phillips C. Outcomes in a 2-phase randomized clinical trial of early Class II treatment. Am J Orthod Dentofacial Orthop 2004;125:657–67.
20. O'Brien K, Wright J, Conboy F, et al. Early treatment of Class II, division 1 malocclusion with the Twin-block appliance: a multi-center, randomized, controlled, clinical trial. Am J Orthod Dentofacial Orthop 2009;135:573–9.
21. Marsico E, Gatto E, Burrascano M, et al. Effectiveness of orthodontic treatment with functional appliances on mandibular growth in the short term. Am J Orthod Dentofacial Orthop 2011;139:24–36.
22. Creekmore TD, Radney LJ. Frankel appliance therapy: orthopedic or orthodontic? Am J Orthod 1993;83:89–108.
23. Gianelly AA, Bednar J, Cociani S, et al. Bidimensional technique theory and practice. Bohemia, NY: GAC International; 2000, pp. 172–81.
24. De Vincenzo JP. Treatment options for sagittal corrections in noncompliant patients. In: Graber TM, Vanarsdall RL, Vig KWL, editors. Orthodontics: current principles and techniques. St Louis, MO: Elsevier-Mosby; 2005.
25. Barnett GA, Higgins DW, Major PW, et al. Immediate skeletal and dental effects of the crown- or banded type Herbst appliance on Class II, division 1 malocclusion. Angle Orthod 2008;78:361–9.
26. O'Brien K, Wright J, Conboy F, et al. Effectiveness of treatment of Class II malocclusion with the Herbst or twin-block appliances: a randomized, controlled trial. Am J Orthod Dentofacial Orthop 2003;124:128–37.
27. Schaefer AT, McNamara JA Jr, Franchi L, et al. Cephalometric comparison of treatment with the Twin-block and stainless steel crown Herbst appliances followed by fixed appliance therapy. Am J Orthod Dentofacial Orthop 2004;126:7–15.
28. Baysal A, Uysal T. Soft tissue effect of Twin block and Herbst appliance in patients with Class II division 1 retrognathy. Eur J Orthod 2013;35:71–81.
29. Nanda R, Kuhlberg A, Uribe F. Biomechanics of extraction space closure. In: Nanda R, editor. Biomechanics and esthetic strategies in clinical orthodontics. St Louis, MO: Elsevier-Mosby; 2005.
30. Parkhouse R. Tip-Edge orthodontics and the Plus bracket. St Louis, MO: Elsevier-Mosby; 2009. p. 9–12.
31. Bishara SE, Cummins DM, Jakobsen JR, et al. Dentofacial and soft tissue changes in Class II, division 1 cases treated with or without extractions. Am J Orthod Dentofacial Orthop 1995;107:28–37.
32. Luppapornlap S, Johnson LE. The effects of premolar extraction: a long-term comparison of outcomes in "clear-cut" extraction and nonextraction Class II patients. Angle Orthod 1993;63:257–72.
33. McGuinness NJ, Burden DJ, Hunt OT, et al. Long-term occlusal and soft-tissue profile outcomes after treatment of Class II, division 1 malocclusion with fixed appliances. Am J Orthod Dentofacial Orthop 2011;139:362–8.
34. Celtin NM, Spena R, Vanarsdall RL Jr. Non extraction treatment. In: Graber TM, Vanarsdall RL Jr, Vig KWL, editors. Orthodontics: current principles and techniques. St Louis, MO: Elsevier-Mosby; 2005.
35. Melsen B, Enemark H. Effect of cervical anchorage studied by the implant method. Trans Eur Orthod Soc 1969;45:435–47.
36. Bishara SE. Class II malocclusion: diagnosis and clinical considerations with and without treatment. Semin Orthod 2006;12:11–24.
37. Papadopoulos M. Non-compliance distalization: a monograph of the clinical management and effectiveness of a jig assembly in Class II malocclusion orthodontic treatment. Thessaloniki, Greece: Phototypotiki Publications; 2005. p. 5–12.
38. Hilgers JJ. The pendulum appliance for Class II non-compliance therapy. J Clin Orthod 1992;26:706–14.
39. Keles A, Sayinsu K. A new approach in maxillary molar distalization. Intraoral bodily molar distalizer. Am J Orthod Dentofacial Orthop 2000;117:39–48.
40. Keles A. Maxillary unilateral molar distalization with sliding mechanics: a preliminary investigation. Eur J Orthod 2001;23:507–15.
41. Jones RD, White JM. Rapid Class II molar correction with an open-coil. J Clin Orthod 1992;10:661–4.
42. Scott MW. Molar distalization: More ammunition for your operatory. Clin Impressions 1996;33:16–27.
43. Gianelly AA, Bednar J, Dietz VS. Japanese NiTi coils used to move molars distally. Am J Orthod Dentofacial Orthop 1991;99:564–6.

44. Blechman AM, Alexander C. New miniaturized magnets for molar distalization. Clin Impressions 1995;4:14–19.
45. Greenfield RL. Fixed piston appliance for rapid Class II correction. J Clin Orthod 1995;29:174–83.
46. Veltri N, Baldini A. Slow sagittal and bilateral expansion for the treatment of Class II malocclusions. Leone Boll Int 2001;3:5–9.
47. Fortini A, Luopoli M, Parri M. The First Class Appliance for rapid molar distalization. J Clin Orthod 1999;33:322–8.
48. Antonarakis GS, Kiliaridis S. Maxillary molar distalization with noncompliance intramaxillary appliances in Class II malocclusion: a systematic review. Angle Orthod 2008;78:1133–40.
49. McSherry PF, Bradley H. Class II correction reducing patient compliance: a review of the available techniques. J Orthod 2000;27:219–25.
50. Weiland FJ, Ingervall B, Bantleon HP, et al. Initial effects of treatment of Class II malocclusion with the Herren activator, activator-headgear combination and Jasper Jumper. Am J Orthod Dentofacial Orthop 1997;112:19–27.
51. Stucki N, Ingervall B. The use of the Jasper Jumper for the correction of Class II malocclusion in the young permanent dentition. Eur J Orthod 1998;20:271–81.
52. Cope JB, Buschang PH, Cope DD, et al. Quantitative evaluation of craniofacial changes with Jasper Jumper therapy. Angle Orthod 1994;64:113–22.
53. Jasper JJ. The Jasper Jumper: a fixed functional appliance. Sheybogan, WI: American Orthodontics; 1987.
54. Klapper L. The SUPERspring II: a new appliance for non-compliant Class II patients. J Clin Orthod 1999;33:50–4.
55. Vogt W. A new fixed interarch device for Class II correction. J Clin Orthod 2003;37:36–41.
56. De Vincenzo JP. The Eureka Spring: a new interarch delivery system. J Clin Orthod 1997;31:454–67.
57. Rothenberg J, Campell ES, Nanda R. Class II correction with Twin Force Bite Corrector. J Clin Orthod 2004;38:232–40.
58. Vogt W. The Forsus Fatigue Resistant Device. J Clin Orthod 2006;40:368–77.
59. Sabbagh A. The Sabbagh Universal Spring. In: Papadopoulos M, editor. Orthodontic treatment of the Class II non-compliant patient: current principles and techniques. Edinburgh: Elsevier-Mosby; 2006. p. 203–16.
60. Papadopoulos M. Orthodontic treatment of the Class II non-compliant patient: current principles and techniques. Edinburgh: Elsevier-Mosby; 2006.

2

Non-compliance approaches for management of Class II malocclusion

Moschos A. Papadopoulos

INTRODUCTION

Class II malocclusion is considered the most frequent problem presenting in the orthodontic practice, affecting 37% of school children in Europe and occurring in 33% of all orthodontic patients in the USA.[1] Class II malocclusion may also involve craniofacial discrepancies, which can be adjusted when patients are adolescent. The usual treatment options in growing patients include extraoral headgears, functional appliances and full fixed appliances with intermaxillary elastics and/or teeth extractions. In adults, moderate Class II malocclusion can be corrected with fixed appliances in combination with intermaxillary elastics and/or teeth extractions, and severe malocclusion with fixed appliances and orthognathic surgery. While the efficiency of these conventional treatment modalities has improved, particularly in growing patients,[2] most require patient cooperation in order to be effective, which is often a major problem.[3]

THE PROBLEM OF COMPLIANCE

In general, orthodontic appliances interfere with daily life, causing unpleasant sensations and impeding speech. It is difficult to ensure appliance use by children or adolescents, particularly as treatment can take several years and is likely to occur at a time of complex social and developmental changes. As orthodontic correction of a malocclusion is an elective treatment, non-compliance usually has no vital consequences for the patient.[3]

Reasons for non-compliance do not just relate to the discomfort and appearance of wearing for example the headgear; there is also a risk of injury, such as eye and facial tissue damage,[4] and unwanted effects of the elastic cervical strap on the cervical spine, muscles and skin. Cephalometric evaluations have indicated that extraoral appliances almost always have skeletal effects in addition to the desired dentoalveolar effects.[5] This could be a problem where only molar distalization is needed to gain the appropriate space for teeth alignment with no restriction of maxillary growth, such as in Class I malocclusion with maxillary crowding. The use of headgears in Class II caused by maxillary crowding can produce unwanted edge-to-edge incisor relationships or even anterior crossbite situations.[6]

Finally, orthodontic treatment in patients with limited compliance can, among other effects, result in longer treatment times, destruction of the teeth and periodontium, extraction of additional teeth, frustration for the patient and additional stress for clinicians and family.

Consequently, much effort has been directed to develop efficient approaches for the non-compliance patient with Class II malocclusion, particularly when non-extraction protocols have to be utilized.

CHARACTERISTICS AND CLASSIFICATION OF THE NON-COMPLIANCE APPLIANCES

Almost all of the non-compliance appliances used for Class II correction have the following characteristics:

- forces either to advance the mandible to a more forward position or to move molars distally are produced by means of fixed auxiliaries, either intra- or intermaxillary

- the appliances almost always require the use of dental and/or palatal anchorage, such as fixed appliances, lingual or transpalatal arches or modified palatal buttons
- most appliances use resilient wires, particularly those for molar distalization, e.g. superelastic nickel–titanium (Ni-Ti) and titanium–molybdenum (TMA) alloys.

All these appliances can be classified into two groups based on their mode of action and type of anchorage: intermaxillary and intramaxillary.[7]

INTERMAXILLARY NON-COMPLIANCE APPLIANCES

Intermaxillary non-compliance appliances have intermaxillary anchorage and act in both maxilla and mandible in order to advance the mandible to a more forward position (e.g. the Herbst appliance, the Jasper Jumper, the Adjustable Bite Corrector and the Eureka Spring). These appliances can be further classified based on the force system used to advance the mandible:

- rigid
- flexible
- hybrid of rigid and flexible
- substituting for elastics.

Rigid Intermaxillary Appliances

In addition to the popular Herbst appliance (Dentaurum, Ispringen, Germany), several other modifications have been proposed.

The Herbst appliance

The Herbst appliance functions like an artificial joint between the maxilla and the mandible (Fig. 2.1). The original design had a bilateral telescopic mechanism attached to orthodontic bands on the maxillary first permanent molars and on mandibular first premolars (or canines); this maintained the mandible in a continuous protruded position – a continuous anterior jumped position. Bands are also usually placed on maxillary first premolars and mandibular first permanent molars, while a horseshoe-type lingual arch is used to connect the premolars with the molars on each dental arch.[8]

Each telescopic mechanism has a tube and a plunger, which fit together, two pivots and two locking screws.[8,9] The pivot for the tube is soldered to the maxillary first molar band and the pivot for the plunger to the mandibular first premolar band. The tubes and plungers are attached to the pivots with locking screws and can easily rotate around their point of attachment. Special attention should be given to the length of the tube and the plunger. If the plunger is too short, it may slip out of the tube if the patient's mouth is opened wide and could then jam on the opening of the tube.[10] If the plunger is much longer than the tube, it will extend behind the tube distally to the maxillary first molar and could wound the buccal mucosa.[10]

The appliance permits large opening and small lateral movements of the mandible, mainly because of the loose fit of the tube and plunger at their sites of attachment. These lateral movements can be increased by widening the pivot openings of the tubes and plungers.[9] If larger lateral movements

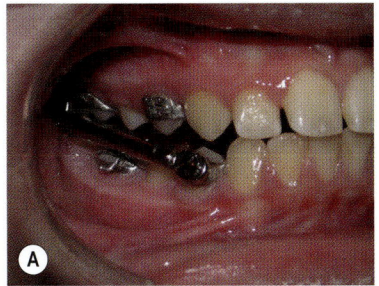 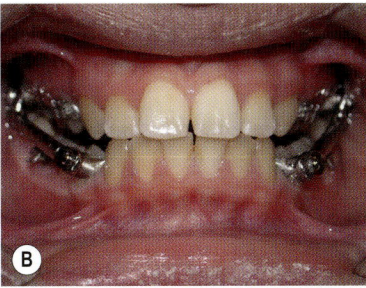 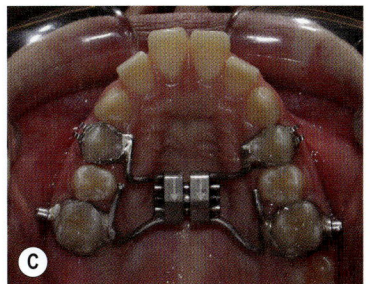 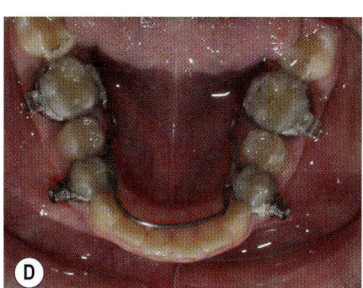

Fig. 2.1 The Herbst appliance (banded Herbst design).

are desired, the Herbst telescope with balls can be utilized, which provides greater freedom of lateral movements.

There are several design variations depending on how the telescopic mechanisms are attached: banded (usual), cast splint,[8] stainless steel (SS) crowns or acrylic resin splints. In addition to these four basic designs, other variations include space-closing, cantilevered and expansion designs.[9,11]

The anchorage teeth can be stabilized with partial or total anchorage.[9] In maxillary partial anchorage, the bands of the first permanent molars and first premolars are connected with a half-round (1.5 mm × 0.75 mm) lingual and/or buccal sectional archwire on each side. In the mandible, the bands of the first premolars are connected with a half-round (1.5 mm × 0.75 mm) or a round (1 mm) lingual archwire touching the lingual surfaces of the anterior teeth.[8,10] When partial anchorage is considered to be inadequate, the incorporation of supplementary dental units is advised, thus creating total anchorage.[8,10] In maxillary total anchorage, a labial archwire is ligated to brackets on the first premolars, canines and incisors. In addition, a transpalatal arch can be attached on the first molar bands. In mandibular total anchorage, bands are cemented on the first molars and connected to the lingual archwire, which is extended distally. In addition, a premolar-to-premolar labial rectangular archwire attached to brackets on the anterior teeth can be used.[12] When maxillary expansion is required, a rapid palatal expansion screw can be soldered to the premolar and molar bands or to the cast splint (Fig. 2.1C).[8,10] Maxillary expansion can be accomplished simultaneously[10,11,13] or prior to Herbst appliance fitment.[14] The Herbst appliance can also be used in combination with a headgear when banded[15] or splinted.[16]

The telescopic mechanism exerts a posteriorly directed force on the maxilla and its dentition and an anterior force on the mandible and its dentition.[17,18] Mandibular length is increased through stimulation of condylar growth and remodeling in the articular fossa, which can be attributed to the anterior shift in the position of the mandible.[17] The amount of mandibular protrusion is determined by the length of the tube, which sets plunger length. In most cases, the mandible is advanced to an initial edge-to-edge incisal position at the start of the treatment, and the dental arches are placed in a Class I or overcorrected Class I relationship.[13,19–21] In some cases, a step-by-step advancement procedure is followed (usually by adding shims over the mandibular plungers) until an edge-to-edge incisal relationship is established.[16]

Treatment with the banded Herbst appliance usually lasts 6–8 months.[10,13,22] However, a longer treatment period of 9–15 months may give better outcomes.[10]

Following treatment, a retention phase is required to avoid any relapse of the dental relationships from undesirable growth patterns or lip–tongue dysfunction habits.[10,22] In patients with mixed dentition and an unstable cuspal interdigitation,[10,17] this phase may last 1 to 2 years or until stable occlusal relationships are established when the permanent teeth have erupted.[23] The retention phase uses removable functional appliances or positioners. When a second phase with fixed appliances follows, retention

is required for 8–12 months to maintain stable occlusal relationships.[10,13,17,22] Class II elastics can also be used.[24]

The Herbst appliance is indicated for

- non-compliance treatment of Class II skeletal discrepancies, mainly in young patients, to influence mandibular and maxillary growth efficiently
- patients with a high-angle vertical growth pattern caused by increased sagittal condylar growth
- patients with deep anterior overbite
- patients with mandibular midline deviation
- patients who are mouth breathers, as Herbst does not interfere with breathing
- patients with anterior disk displacement.

It is also most suitable for treatment of Class II malocclusion in patients with retrognathic mandibles and retroclined maxillary incisors.[10,13] Other indications for use of the Herbst appliance are outlined later in the chapter under "Indications and contraindications for non-compliance appliances", including its use in obstructive sleep apnea[25,26] and as an alternative to orthognathic surgery in young adults.[13,20,27]

The main advantages of the Herbst appliance include:

- short and standardized treatment duration
- lack of reliance on patient compliance to attain the desired treatment
- easy acceptance by the patient
- patient tolerance.

The Herbst appliance is fixed to the teeth and so is functioning 24 hours a day and treatment duration is relatively short (6–15 months) rather than 2–4 years with removable functional appliances. In addition, the distalizing effect on the maxillary first molars contributes to the avoidance of extractions in Class II malocclusions with maxillary crowding.[28] Other advantages include the improvement in the patient's profile immediately after appliance placement, the maintenance of good oral hygiene, the possiblity of simultaneous use of fixed appliances and the ability to modify the appliance for various clinical applications.

There are also some disadvantages. The main ones are anchorage loss of the maxillary (spaces between the maxillary canines and first premolars) and mandibular (proclination of the mandibular incisors) teeth during treatment, chewing problems during the first week of the treatment and soft tissue impingement. There can also be appliance dysfunction.[29]

Numerous modifications of the Herbst appliance have been proposed, including Goodman's Modified Herbst Appliance,[30] the upper SS crowns and lower acrylic resin Herbst design,[31] the Mandibular Advancement Locking Unit,[32] the Magnetic Telescopic Device,[33] the Flip-Lock Herbst Appliance,[34] the Hanks Telescoping Herbst Appliance,[35] the Ventral Telescope,[36] the Universal Bite Jumper,[37] the Open-Bite Intrusion Herbst,[38] the Intraoral Snoring Therapy Appliance,[36] the Cantilever Bite Jumper,[39] the

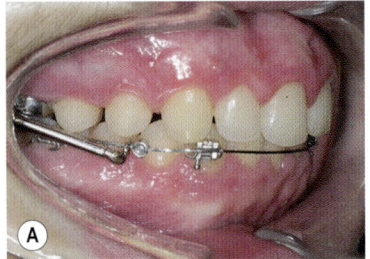
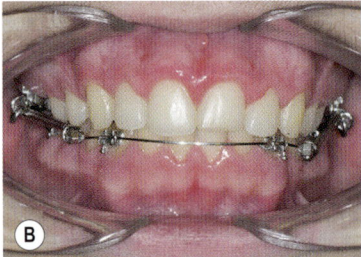

Fig. 2.2 The Ritto appliance. (With permission from Papadopoulos.[2])

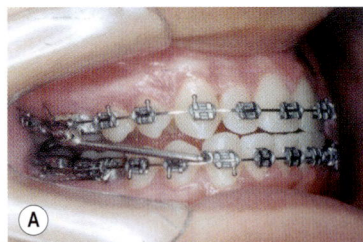
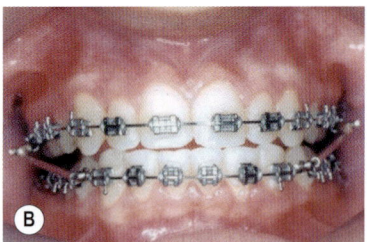

Fig. 2.3 The Mandibular Protraction appliance. (With permission from Papadopoulos.[2])

Molar-Moving Bite Jumper,[40] the Mandibular Advancing Repositioning Splint[41] and the Mandibular Corrector Appliance.[42]

The Ritto appliance

The Ritto appliance is a miniaturized telescopic device with simplified intraoral application and activation (Fig. 2.2).[2] It is a one-piece device with telescopic action that is fabricated in a single form to be used bilaterally, attached to upper and lower archwires. A steel ball-pin and a lock-controlled sliding brake are used as fixing components. Two maxillary and two mandibular bands and brackets on the mandibular arch can support the appliance adequately. The appliance is activated by sliding the lock around the mandibular arch distally and fixing it against the appliance. The activation is performed in two steps, an initial adjustment activation of 2–3 mm and a subsequent activation of 1–2 mm 1 week later, while further activations of 4–5 mm can be performed after 3 weeks.

The Mandibular Protraction appliance

The Mandibular Protraction appliance was introduced for the correction of Class II malocclusion (Fig. 2.3). It has been continuously developed since its initial introduction and four different types have been proposed.[2,43]

The latest version (MPA IV) consists of a T-tube, a maxillary molar locking pin, a mandibular rod and a rigid mandibular SS archwire with two circular loops distal to the canine.[44] The mandibular rod is inserted into the longer section of the T-tube and the molar locking pin is inserted into the smaller section. To place the appliance, the mandibular rod is inserted into the circular loop of the mandibular archwire; the mandible is protruded to an edge-to-edge position and the molar locking pin is inserted into the maxillary molar tube from the distal and bent mesial for stabilization. Thus, the maxillary extremity of the appliance can slide around the pin wire. The appliance can also be inserted from the mesial. If activation is necessary, it can be performed by inserting a piece of Ni-Ti open coil spring between the mandibular rod and the telescopic tube.[43]

The Mandibular Anterior Repositioning Appliance

The Mandibular Anterior Repositioning Appliance (MARA; AOA/Pro Orthodontic Appliances, Sturtevant, WI, USA) keeps the mandible in a continuous protruded position.[44] It can be considered as a fixed Twin Block because it incorporates two opposing vertical surfaces placed in such a way as to keep the mandible in a forward position (Fig. 2.4).

The MARA consists of four SS crowns (or rigid bands) attached to the first permanent molars. Each mandibular molar crown incorporates a double tube soldered on, consisting of a 0.045 inch tube and a 0.022 × 0.028 inch tube for the maxillary and mandibular archwires. A 0.059 inch arm is also soldered to each mandibular crown, projecting perpendicular to its buccal surface and engaging the elbows on the maxillary molar. For stabilization, the mandibular crowns can be connected through a soldered lingual arch, particularly if no braces are used. A lingual arch is also recommended to prevent crowding of the second premolars

Fig. 2.4 The Mandibular Anterior Repositioning Appliance. (With permission from Papadopoulos.[2])

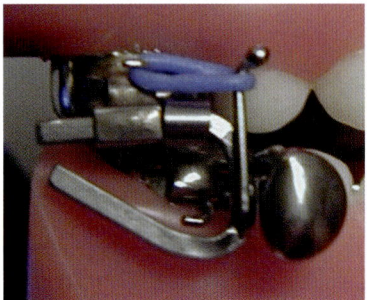

and mesiolingual rotation of the mandibular first molars.[44–46] Each maxillary molar crown also incorporates the same double tube as the mandibular crown. In addition, square tubes (0.062 inch) are soldered to each of the maxillary crowns, into which slide the corresponding square upper elbows (0.060 inch). These upper elbows are inserted in the upper square tubes while guiding the patient into an advanced forward position, and are hung vertically. The elbows are tied in by ligatures or elastics after placement of the device. The buccal position of the upper elbows is controlled by torquing them with a simple tool, while their anteroposterior position is controlled by shims. Occlusal rests can be used on the maxillary and mandibular second molars or premolars. These rests are used in order to prevent intrusion and tip-back of the maxillary first molars and extrusion of the maxillary second molars.[46] Brackets on the maxillary second premolars should not be used to avoid interfering with the elbow during its insertion and removal. The appliance can be combined with maxillary and mandibular expanders, transpalatal arches, adjustments loops, fixed orthodontic appliances and maxillary molar distalization appliances.[44–46]

Before placement of the appliance, the maxillary incisors should be aligned, properly torqued and intruded if required so as not to interfere with mandibular advancement, while the maxillary arch should be wide enough to allow the elbows to hang buccally to the mandibular crowns. The mandible is usually advanced, either in one step or in gradual increments, into an overcorrected Class I relationship to counteract the expected small relapse usually observed during the post-treatment period.[44–46] When 4–5 mm of mandibular advancement is required, the mandible is advanced to an edge-to-edge incisor position. When 8–9 mm correction is needed, the advancement is performed in two steps to avoid excessive strain on the temporomandibular joint or appliance breakage. The mandible is advanced initially 4–5 mm and maintained in that position for about 6 months; it is then advanced in an edge-to-edge position for an additional period of 6 months. Alternatively, the advancement can be performed in gradual increments of 2–3 mm every 8–12 weeks, by adding shims on the elbows.[44–46]

After insertion of the MARA, the patient should be informed that it will take 4–10 days to be comfortable with the new, advanced mandibular position, during which period some chewing difficulties may occur. If the patient is a mouth breather or suffers from bruxism, vertical elastics can be placed during sleeping to keep the mouth closed. The posterior open bite, which may be observed after appliance placement, is reduced while the posterior teeth erupt normally without interference with the appliance.

Treatment duration depends on the severity of the Class II malocclusion and the patient's age, but usually lasts 12–15 months.[44–46] The patient is monitored at intervals of 12 to 16 weeks for further adjustments or reactivations.

After treatment is completed and the dental arches are brought into a Class I relationship, the appliance is removed and fixed appliances can be used to further adjust the occlusion. If the mandible is not advanced in an overcorrected position, Class II elastics can be used for approximately 6 months after appliance removal.

The Functional Mandibular Advancer

The Functional Mandibular Advancer was developed as an alternative to the Herbst appliance for the correction of Class II malocclusions.[47] It is a rigid intermaxillary appliance based on the principle of the inclined plane. It is similar to the MARA but with some fundamental differences. It consists of cast splints, crowns or bands on which the main parts of the appliance, the guide pins and inclined planes, are laser welded buccally. The bite-jumping mechanism of the appliance is attached at a 60° angle to the horizontal, thus actively guiding the mandible in a forward position while closing, which provides unrestricted mandibular motion and increases patient adaptation. The anterior shape of the bite-jumping device and the active components of the abutments are designed to allow mandibular guidance even in partial jaw closure, thus ensuring its effectiveness even in patients with habitual open mouth posture. The appliance is reactivated by adjusting the threaded insert supports over a length of 2 mm, using guide pins of different widths or by fitting the sliding surfaces of the inclined planes with spacers of different thicknesses. Mandibular advancement is accomplished using a step-by-step procedure, which provides better patient adaptation, particularly for adults.[47]

Flexible Intermaxillary Appliances

The main flexible intermaxillary appliance is the Jasper Jumper. Similar appliances are the Flex Developer, the Adjustable Bite Corrector, the Bite Fixer, the Churro Jumper and the Forsus Nitinol Flat Spring.

The Jasper Jumper

The Jasper Jumper (American Orthodontics, Sheboygan, WI) is a flexible intermaxillary appliance introduced to address the restriction of mandibular lateral movements that occurs with the Herbst appliance.[48] It consists of a flexible force module, an SS coil spring, enclosed in a polyurethane cover and attached at both ends to SS endcaps with holes to facilitate anchoring (Fig. 2.5).[48] The modules differ for the right and left sides and are supplied in seven lengths, ranging from 26 to 38 mm in 2 mm increments. Ball-pins, small plastic Teflon friction balls or Lexan beads and auxiliary sectional archwires are the anchors that are used to attach the appliance on the maxillary and mandibular fixed appliances.

The appropriate size of Jasper Jumper is determined by guiding the mandible in centric relation and measuring the distance between the mesial of the maxillary first molar headgear tube and the point of insertion to the mandibular arch at the distal of the small plastic beads, adding 12 mm.[49]

The appliance is attached after placement of conventional fixed appliances and alignment of the teeth in both arches.[48] The force module is anchored to the upper headgear tube with a ball-pin passing through the upper hole of the Jumper and through the distal end of the headgear tube. Then, the mesial extension of the pin is bent back over the tube to keep it in position.[49] The attachment of the force module to the mandibular archwire can be performed in two ways. In the first, offsets are placed in the

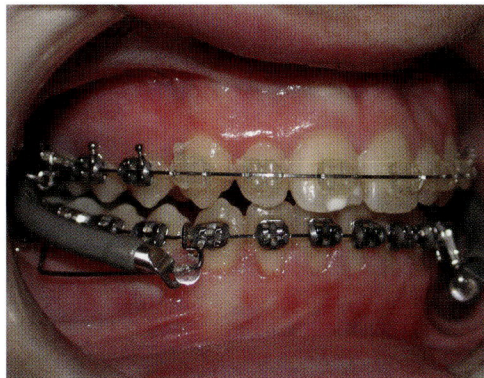

Fig. 2.5 The Jasper Jumper.

fully engaged mandibular archwires distal to the canine brackets and the first (or the first and second) premolar bracket is removed. A small plastic bead is put on to the archwire to provide an anterior stop, followed by the lower end of the jumper; the arch is then ligated in place (Fig. 2.5).[48] However, the most effective method uses an auxiliary tube on the mandibular first molar and sectional archwires (0.017 × 0.025 inch). The distal end of the sectional archwire, which incorporates an out-set bayonet bent mesial to the mandibular molar's auxiliary tube, is inserted into this tube, while the mesial end is looped over the main archwire between the first premolar and the canine. Thus, there is no need to remove the premolar brackets and the patient has a greater range of jaw movements.[48,49] In patients with mixed dentition, the maxillary attachment is similar to that described above, while the mandibular attachment is achieved through an archwire extending between the mandibular first molar bands and lateral incisor brackets, thus avoiding the primary canine and molar areas.[48] However, in these patients, a transpalatal arch and a fixed lingual arch must always be used to prevent undesirable effects.[48]

Prior to appliance placement, heavy rectangular archwires should be placed in the maxillary and mandibular arches.[49] In addition, a lingual arch can be used in the mandibular arch in order to increase lower anchorage, unless extractions are used, and brackets with −5° lingual torque should be bonded to the mandibular anterior teeth for the same reason.[49] In the maxillary arch, a transpalatal bar should be used to enhance lateral anchorage. However, when maxillary molar distalization is needed, the use of transpalatal bars and cinching or tying back the maxillary archwire should be avoided. The Jasper Jumper can also be combined with rapid palatal expanders if maxillary expansion is needed.[50]

The Jasper Jumper exerts a light, continuous force and can deliver functional, bite-jumping, headgear-like forces, activator-like forces, elastic-like forces or a combination of these.[49] When the force module is straight, it is in passive condition. It is activated when the teeth come into occlusion, thus compressing the spring. A compression of 4 mm can deliver about 250 g of force. The appliance delivers sagittally directed forces with a posterior direction to the maxilla and its dentition and reciprocal anteriorly directed forces on the mandible and its dentition, intrusive forces on the maxillary posterior teeth and the mandibular anterior teeth, as well as buccal forces on the maxillary arch that tend to expand it.[51,52]

Reactivation of the appliance can take place 2–3 months after initial activation by shortening the ball-pin attached to the maxillary first molar bands or by adding crimpable stops mesial to the ball on the mandibular archwire. Treatment with the Jasper Jumper usually lasts 3–9 months, after which the appliance can be left passively in place for 3–4 months for retention, and then finishing procedures can follow.[49]

The Flex Developer

The Flex Developer (LPI Ormco, Ludwig Pittermann, Maria Anzbach, Austria) is similar to the Jasper Jumper but is supplied as a kit to be assembled by the clinician.[53] The force module is an elastic minirod made of polyamide, while additional components include an anterior hooklet module, a posterior attachment module, a preformed auxiliary bypass arch, a securing mini-disk and a ball-pin. The anterior locking module is relockable, thus permitting easy insertion and removal (Fig. 2.6). The appliance is used in combination with conventional fixed appliances and is attached to the headgear tubes of maxillary first molar bands and to a mandibular bypass arch.

The length of the elastic minirod is determined by measuring the distance between the entrance of the maxillary headgear tube and the labial end of the bypass arch using a specially designed gauge. After adjusting the length of the minirod, ensuring that the posterior attachment module and the anterior hooklet are parallel, and following placement of the ball-pin into the headgear tube from the distal, the patient protrudes the mandible into the desired position and the anterior hooklet is secured on the bypass archwire.[53] To reactivate the appliance, the ball-pin can be shortened to the mesial or the bypass arch can be shortened distally, thus pushing back the sliding arch and bending its end upwards. Alternatively, the sliding section of the arch can be shortened by adding an acrylic resin ball at its mesial end.

The Flex Developer delivers a continuous force of 50–1000 g between the maxilla and the mandible, which can be adjusted by thinning the minirod's diameter; the length of the minirod can also be reduced to allow proper fit of the appliance.[53] Lip bumpers, headgears or reversed headgears can also be used in combination with the Flex Developer.

Hybrid Appliances

Among the hybrid intermaxillary appliances that use a combination of rigid and flexible force systems, the Eureka Spring is the most common for non-compliance Class II orthodontic treatment. Others include the Sabbagh Universal Spring, the Forsus Fatigue Resistant Device and the Twin Force Bite Corrector.

The Eureka Spring

The Eureka Spring (Eureka Orthodontics, San Luis Obispo, CA, USA) is a hybrid appliance consisting of an open coil spring encased in a plunger,

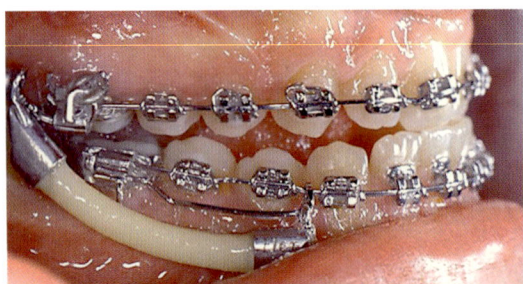

Fig. 2.6 The Flex Developer. (With permission from Papadopoulos.[2])

flexible ball-and-socket attachments and a shaft for guiding the spring (Fig. 2.7A).[54] The appliance is used with full-bracketed maxillary and mandibular dental arches. The open coil spring is attached directly to the upper or lower archwire with a closed or open ring clamp. The plunger has a 0.002 inch tolerance in the cylinder, and a triple telescopic action allows mouth opening to 60 mm, beyond which the appliance is disengaged; however, it can be easily reassembled by the patient. The cylinder is connected to the molar tube with a 0.032 inch wire annealed at its anterior end, and a 0.036 inch ball at the posterior end functioning as a universal joint, thus allowing lateral and vertical movements of the cylinder.[54]

The advantages of the Eureka Spring include lack of reliance on patient compliance, esthetic appearance, resistance to breakage, maintenance of good oral hygiene, prevention of tissue irritation, rapid tooth movement, optimal force direction, 24-hour continuous force application even when the mouth is opened up to 20 mm, functional acceptability, easy installation, low cost and minimal inventory requirements.[54]

The Sabbagh Universal Spring

The Sabbagh Universal Spring (Dentaurum, Ispringen, Germany) is another hybrid appliance; it consists of a telescopic element, a U-loop anteriorly and a telescope rod with a U-loop posteriorly (Fig. 2.7B).[55] The telescopic unit consists of an inner spring over an inner tube, a guide tube and a middle telescopic tube. Before insertion of the appliance, alignment, leveling and decompensation of the dental arches should be completed, while brackets with fully engaged SS archwires (i.e. at least 0.016 × 0.022 inch) in both arches should be used. The appliance is attached to the maxillary molar headgear tube and to the mandibular archwire. To fit the appliance, a 0.25 inch ball retainer clasp is placed from the distal through the loop in the headgear tube and is bent mesially on the tube. After bending of the tube inwards, the telescopic rod with U-loop is inserted into the maxillary fixed telescopic element, and the U-loop is attached to the lower SS archwire between the first premolar and the canine bracket.

The size of the spring can be adjusted by inserting or unscrewing the inner telescopic tube or by presetting the length of the inner tube with an activation key. When skeletal effects are required, the spring force should be minimized, whereas the spring force should be maximized when dentoalveolar effect is mostly needed. The spring can be activated by inserting or unscrewing the inner telescope tube manually or with an activation key, by extending or shortening the distal distance of the ball-pin in the headgear tube, by inserting activation springs or by placing the U-loop between the mandibular incisor and canine bracket.[55]

The Forsus Fatigue Resistant Device

The Forsus Fatigue Resistant Device (3M Unitek, Monrovia, CA, USA) is a hybrid appliance designed to address the problem of fatigue failure and consists of a three-piece telescopic spring device. The appliance is attached to the maxillary first molar headgear tube with an L-shaped

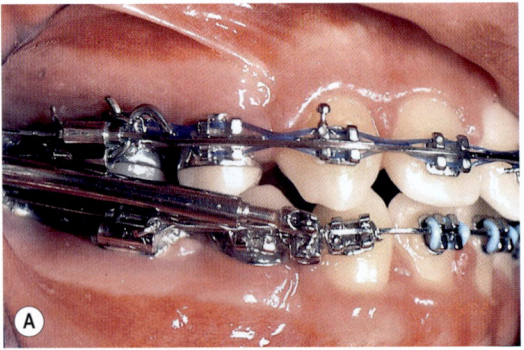
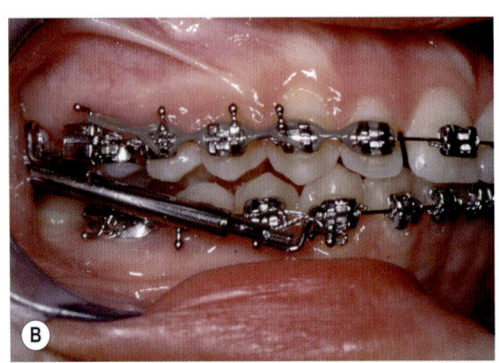
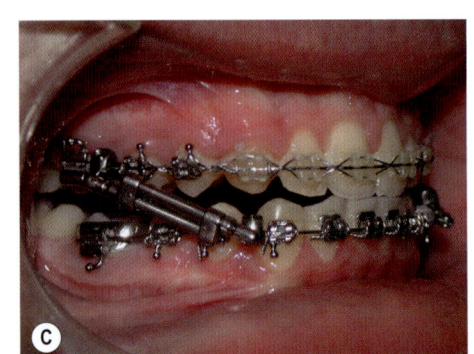

Fig. 2.7 Hybrid appliances. (A) The Eureka Spring. (B) The Sabbagh Universal Spring. (C) The Twin Force Bite Corrector. (With permission from Papadopoulos.[2])

ball-pin and to the mandibular archwire through a bypass archwire. The appropriate length of the rod is selected to allow full spring compression without advancing the mandible when advancement is not required. To simplify the insertion, a direct push rod is incorporated in the device, which permits direct attachment to the mandibular archwire. Ligating the mandibular canine to the first molar using brackets is advised to avoid creating space distal to the canine.[56] To reactivate the spring, ring bushings can be added distal on the stop of the distal rod, thus compressing the spring 2–3 mm, or a longer rod can be used to maintain engagement. Patients should be told not to open their mouth widely because there is a risk of disengagement.

The Twin Force Bite Corrector

The Twin Force Bite Corrector (Ortho Organizers, San Marcos, CA, USA) is also a hybrid appliance, which is used with conventional full fixed appliances. It consists of dual plungers containing Ni-Ti springs with ball-and-socket joints in their ends, an anchor wire and an archwire clamp (Fig. 2.7C).[57,58] To eliminate the need for a headgear tube, a double lock was developed. The appliance is attached to the lower archwire between the canine and the first premolar with a ball-and-socket wire clamp and to the maxillary molar headgear tube with the anchor wire, which has a ball-and-socket adjustable joint. Before appliance placement, palatal expansion and alignment of the maxillary and mandibular dental arches should be completed.[57,58] Bands with double buccal tubes should also be placed on the maxillary first molars and lingual sheaths in order to facilitate the use of transpalatal arches. In addition, the mandibular arch should be leveled, the overbite should be opened and mandibular and maxillary archwires (cross-section 0.017 or 0.018 × 0.025 inch) should be engaged. A lingual lower arch can also be used to enhance anchorage. To avoid mandibular incisor proclination, an elastic chain or a figure-of-eight wire tie can be used from the right to the left molar, cinching back bends at the distal ends of the archwire.

The appliance exerts a continuous light force of 100–200 g and does not require reactivation, while it permits lateral movements and a wide range of motion because of its ball joints. After appliance placement, the patient should be seen a week later and then monitored once a month.[57,58] After the desired occlusion has been achieved, the appliance is maintained in place for 2–3 months. On its removal, Class II elastics are used to stabilize cuspal interdigitation. Retention appliances can be used to maintain the mandibular position.

Appliances Acting as Substitutes for Elastics

Three devices act as substitutes for elastics: the Calibrated Force Module, the Alpern Class II Closers and the Saif Springs.

INTRAMAXILLARY NON-COMPLIANCE DISTALIZATION APPLIANCES

Intramaxillary non-compliance appliances have intramaxillary or absolute anchorage and act only in the maxilla in order to move molars distally (e.g. the Pendulum appliance, the Distal Jet, the Jones Jig, the Sectional Jig assembly, palatal implants and miniscrew implants). These devices can also be classified based on the force system used to distalize the maxillary molars:

- flexible force system positioned palatally or buccally, or both palatally and buccally
- rigid force system positioned palatally
- hybrid appliances combining a rigid force system buccally and a flexible one palatally.

Appliances with a Flexible Distalization Force System Palatally Positioned

The Pendulum appliances and the Distal Jet are the most common non-compliance appliances that use a flexible molar distalization force system positioned palatally. Other appliances include the Intraoral Bodily Molar Distalizer, the Simplified Molar Distalizer, the Keles Slider, Nance Appliances in conjunction with Ni-Ti open coil springs and the Fast Back Appliance.

The Pendulum appliance

The Pendulum appliance consists of a large acrylic resin Nance button that covers the mid-portion of the palate for anchorage, and two 0.032 inch TMA springs (e.g. Ormco, Orange, CA, USA), which are the active elements for molar distalization and delivering a light, continuous and pendulum-like force from the midline of the palate to the maxillary molars (Fig. 2.8A).[59] The Nance button usually extends from the maxillary first molars anteriorly to just posterior of the lingual papilla and is stabilized with four retaining wires that extend bilaterally and are bonded as occlusal rests to the maxillary first and second premolars (or to the first and second primary molars).[60] Alternatively, the two posterior wires can be soldered to first premolars or first primary molar bands, thus adding to the stability of the appliance. Each of the two TMA springs consists of a recurved molar insertion wire, a small horizontal adjustment loop, a closed helix and a loop for retention in the acrylic resin button.[59] These springs are mounted as close as possible to the center and distal aspects of the Nance button and when in a passive state they extend posteriorly, almost parallel to the midpalatal suture.

When activated, each of the springs is inserted into a lingual sheath (0.036 inch) on bands cemented on the maxillary first molars; this produces

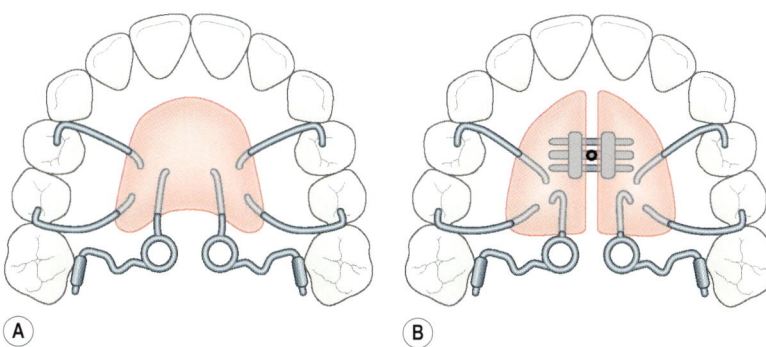
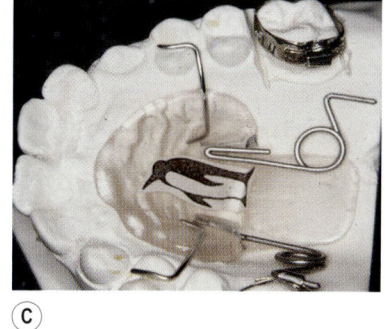
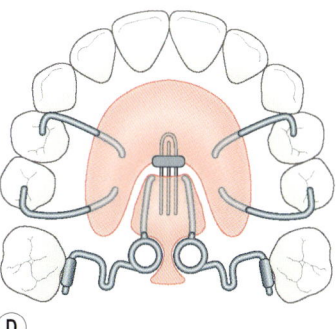

Fig. 2.8 Pendulum appliances. (A) The basic appliance. (B) The Pendex appliance. (C) The Penguin Pendulum appliance. (D) The K-Pendulum appliance. (With permission from Papadopoulos.[2])

almost 60° of activation and delivers a distalizing force of approximately 230 g, which moves the molars distally and medially.[59,61] After the initial activation of the springs, the patients should be seen, usually every 3–4 weeks, in order to check the spring pressure and to perform appropriate adjustments if needed. According to Hilgers, approximately 5 mm of distal molar movement can be achieved in a period of 3–4 months.[59]

Following the introduction of the Pendulum appliance, a number of modifications have been presented, such as the Pendex appliance,[62,63] the Penguin Pendulum appliance,[64] the K-Pendulum appliance[65] and the Bi-Pendulum and Quad Pendulum appliances (Fig. 2.8).[66]

The Intraoral Bodily Molar Distalizer

The Intraoral Bodily Molar Distalizer consists of an anchorage unit with a wide acrylic resin Nance button and an active unit with square-sectioned TMA distalizing springs (0.032 × 0.032 inch) to achieve improved control in the transverse plane.[67] In addition, bands are placed on the maxillary first molars and premolars, SS retaining wires (0.045 inch) are attached to the premolar bands and the slot size (0.032 × 0.032 inch) cap palatal attachments are welded on the palatal side of the first molar bands.

The springs consist of two sections, the distalizing section that exerts a crown-tipping force and an uprighting section that applies a root-uprighting force to the first molars.[67] In contrast to the Pendulum appliances, the springs distalize the maxillary first molars towards the direction in which the springs are inactive, exerting a distalizing force of approximately 230 g. The Nance button is very wide, covering the palatal surfaces of the incisors as much as possible in order to obtain support from a wider palatal tissue and increase anterior anchorage. Thus, it functions as an anterior bite plane in order to improve deep bite correction as well as enhance molar distalization by discluding the posterior teeth.[67]

Class I molar relationships can be accomplished in approximately 7.5 months. Then, the molars are stabilized for almost 2 months with a conventional Nance appliance attached to the hinge caps, thus providing easy removal of the appliance for cleaning and if there is soft tissue irritation. Following the stabilization period, full fixed appliances are used as the second phase of the overall treatment.[67]

The Distal Jet

The Distal Jet appliance (American Orthodontics, Sheboygan, WI, USA) consists of two bayonet wires inserted in two bilateral tubes embedded in a modified acrylic resin Nance button (see Fig. 31.1).[68] The Nance button acts as an anchorage unit, while the active part of the appliance consists of a telescopic unit incorporating two Ni-Ti or SS springs with screw clamps, sliding through two tubes (internal diameter 0.036 inch) attached bilaterally to the Nance button.[68] A wire ending in a bayonet bend is inserted in the lingual sheath of the first molar band and the free end is inserted like a piston into the bilateral tubes.[68,69] The telescopic unit and presumably the line of action of the Distal Jet should be parallel to the occlusal plane and located approximately 4–5 mm apical from the maxillary molar centroid (midpoint on root axis) so that the force produced passes as close as possible to the center of resistance (CR) of the molars.[68,69]

In the standard design of the Distal Jet, the Nance button is as large as possible to increase stability, extending about 5 mm from the teeth.[68] Usually, the Nance button is retained with wires extending bilaterally and soldered to bands on the first premolars, the second premolars or the second primary molars. Alternatively, the retaining wires can be bonded as occlusal rests to the maxillary first or second premolars.[68,70]

To activate the appliance, the screw clamp is moved distally, thus compressing the coil spring and creating a distalization force, which is applied to the molar band for 3–10.5 months until correction of Class II malocclusion or a super-Class I relationship has been achieved. During this

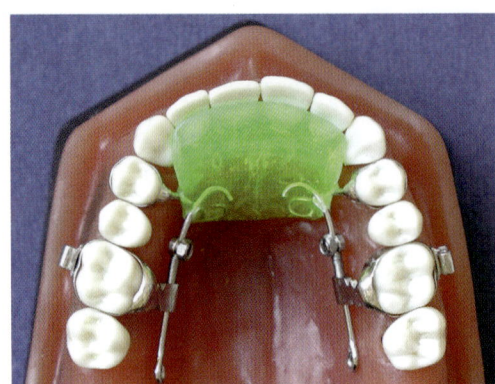

Fig. 2.9 The Keles Slider. (With permission from Papadopoulos.[2])

period, the patient should be monitored every 4–6 weeks for further adjustments.

The Keles Slider

The Keles Slider was developed for unilateral or bilateral molar distalization. The design is intended to apply a consistent distal force at the CR of the first molar, thus producing a more bodily distal molar movement.[71] The device consists of a Nance button with an anterior bite plane, tubes soldered palatally to the maxillary first molars, wire rods (0.036 inch) for sliding of the first molars, heavy Ni-Ti open coil springs (0.036 inch) and screws to activate the springs (Fig. 2.9).[71]

The anchorage unit consists of a wide Nance button to minimize anchorage loss, including an anterior bite plane to disclude the posterior teeth, enhance the distal molar movement and correct the anterior deep bite. The acrylic resin Nance button is usually stabilized with retaining wires attached to bands on the maxillary first premolars, allowing the second premolars to drift distally under the influence of the transeptal fibers.[71] The active unit of the appliance has several parts. Tubes 0.275 inch (1.1 mm) in diameter are soldered palatally on the first molar bands, and an SS wire 0.9 mm in length is inserted in the acrylic resin about 5 mm apical to the first molar gingival margin, passing through the tube and parallel to the occlusal plane. A helix is placed at the distal end of the steel rod to control the amount of distal molar movement and prevent any disconnection of the tube from the rod. The Ni-Ti coil springs are positioned between the screw on the wire and the tube in full compression, thus producing approximately 200 g of distalizing force to the molars. To deactivate the appliance before cementing it, another screw is placed at the distal side of the tube. This screw is removed to activate the appliance. After placement of the appliance, the patient is monitored once a month and the screws can be reactivated if necessary.

Nance appliance with coil springs

A Nance appliance in conjunction with Ni-Ti coil springs can be used for unilateral maxillary molar distalization[72] or for bilateral distalization of both first and second molars.[73]

The appliance for unilateral maxillary molar distalization is a modification of the traditional Nance holding arch and consists of an active Class II side, where molar distalization takes place, and an inactive Class I side. The inactive Class I side has an SS wire framework (0.036 inch) ending in an anteriorly projecting arm like that of a Quad helix to resist the horizontal moment that can cause distal molar rotation and expansion in the premolar area. The active Class II side consists also of an arm bend like the Quad helix with the anterior end soldered to the first premolar band. An omega loop is soldered to the anterior end of the framework to allow distal sliding of the loop when it is opened for activation. A 10 mm long open coil spring (0.036 inch) is positioned between the omega loop and

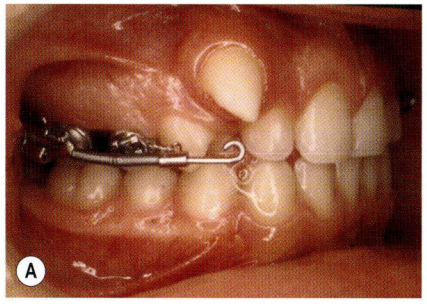 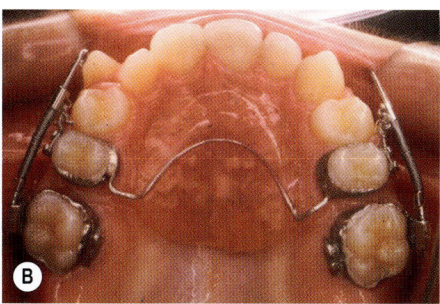

Fig. 2.10 The Jones Jig. Lateral (A) and occlusal view (B) of the appliance after cementation and initial maxillary molar distalization.

the first molar band assembly. A 0.045 inch tube is soldered on the lingual side of the first molar band and connected to the wire arm with the framework moving through the tube, thus allowing sliding of the band assembly. Following appliance cementing, the omega loop is opened to compress the coil spring to a length of 7 mm, which delivers a distalization force of approximately 150 g. The patient is monitored every 2 weeks for further adjustments and reactivations until Class I molar relationship has been achieved.

The intra-arch Ni-Ti coil appliance for bilateral distalization of both first and second molars also has an anchorage unit and an active unit.[73] The anchorage unit includes a modified Nance appliance and a 0.9 mm lingual archwire soldered to bands on the maxillary second premolars. This lingual archwire has two distal pistons that pass through the palatal tubes of the first molars, which are parallel to the pistons both occlusally and sagittally. The active unit consists of a Ni-Ti coil spring of length 10–14 mm, diameter 0.012 inch and lumen 0.045 inch, which is inserted into the distal piston (GAC International, Islandia, NY, USA). The spring is compressed to half its length when the tube of the molar band is adapted to the distal piston of the lingual archwire, thus activating the spring and producing an initial distalization force of approximately 200 g; this reduces to 180 g as the molars are distalized. No further activation is required during the distalization phase of the treatment.

The Fast Back Appliance

The Fast Back Appliance (Leone, Florence, Italy) consists of a Nance button for anchorage, two palatally positioned sagittal screws and superelastic open Memoria coil springs.[74] The Nance button is stabilized with extension wires soldered on the first premolar bands and includes also the mesial parts of the screws. Each screw incorporates two wire arms. The mesial one is soldered on the first premolars, while the distal one passes through the palatal first molar tube and incorporates also an open Memoria coil spring that delivers a distalization force of approximately 200–300 g on the maxillary first molars. A self-locking terminal stop with a hole is added at the distal end of this arm for safety reasons. After the first molars are distalized 1.5–2 mm, the screws can be activated to compress the coil springs, thus maintaining the distalization force. Once the required distalization has been accomplished, the first molars can be maintained in position by tying an SS ligature between the molar tubes and the hole of the self-locking terminal stop.

Appliances with a Flexible Distalization Force System Buccally Positioned

The Jones Jig is one of the most commonly used flexible buccally positioned distalization force appliances for non-compliance Class II orthodontic treatment. Modifications of the Jones Jig include the Lokar Molar Distalizing Appliance and the Sectional Jig Assembly. These appliances use Ni-Ti coil springs in conjunction mainly with Nance buttons, repelling magnets and Ni-Ti wires. Other appliances of this type use various

distalizing arches, including the Bimetric Distalizing Arch, the Molar Distalization Bow, and the Acrylic Distalization Splints.

The Jones Jig

The Jones Jig (American Orthodontics, Sheboygan, WI, USA) has an active unit positioned buccally that consists of active arms or jig assemblies incorporating Ni-Ti open coil springs and an anchorage unit consisting of a modified Nance button (Fig. 2.10).[75]

The modified Nance button is stabilized with SS wires (0.036 inch) that extend bilaterally and are soldered to bands on the maxillary first or second premolars or to primary second molars.[75,76] The jig assembly consists of a 0.036 inch wire that holds the Ni-Ti open coil spring and a sliding eyelet tube. An additional stabilizing wire is attached along with a hook to the distal portion of the main wire. Thus, the jig assembly includes two arms in its distal end, which are used to stabilize the appliance.[76]

After cementation of the modified Nance appliance, the main arm of the Jones Jig is inserted into the headgear tube and the stabilizing arm is inserted into the archwire slot of the maxillary first molar buccal attachment.[76] The distal hook is tied with an SS ligature to the hook of the buccal molar tube to further increase stability. The appliance is activated by tying back the sliding hook to the anchor teeth (first or second premolars) with an SS ligature, thus compressing the open coil spring 1–5 mm. The activated open coil spring can produce approximately 70–75 g of continuous distalizing force to the maxillary first molars for 2.5–9 months depending on the severity of the initial malocclusion. The patient is monitored every 4–5 weeks for further adjustments and the maxillary molars are shifted distally until a Class I relationship has been achieved.[75,76]

The Sectional Jig assembly

The Sectional Jig assembly is a modification of the Jones Jig consisting also of an active and an anchorage unit (Fig. 2.11).[76,77] The anchorage unit is a modified Nance button attached with a 0.032 inch SS wire to the maxillary second premolar bands. Thus, all teeth mesial to the molars are indirectly utilized. Bands with headgear tubes and hooks placed gingivally are cemented to the first molars. The active unit consists of an active arm that is fabricated from a 0.028 inch round SS wire 30–35 mm in length). A 3 mm long open loop constructed at a distance of 8 mm from the wire end divides the wire arm into two sections, a small distal and a larger mesial one. A Ni-Ti open coil spring (25–30 mm long, with a wire cross-section of 0.010 inch and a helix diameter of 0.030 inch) is inserted through the mesial end of the sectional wire. Two sliding tubes are used for positional stabilization of the spring. The distal tube is placed close to the loop of the sectional wire and stabilizes the coil spring, preventing its sliding into the loop. The mesial tube is provided with a hook and is placed close to the mesial end of the sectional wire, which is subsequently bent gingivally. This bend prevents the coil spring from sliding away from the wire and ensures that there is no soft tissue impingement.[76,77]

After cementing the modified Nance button and the first maxillary molar bands, the distal end of the Sectional Jig assembly is inserted into the

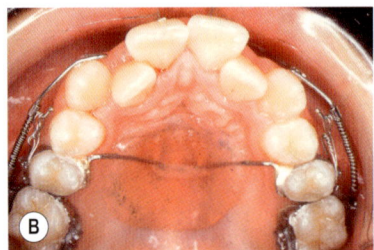 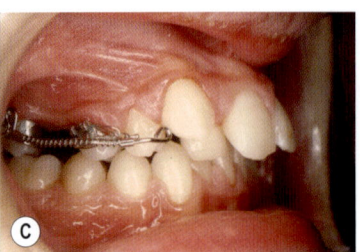 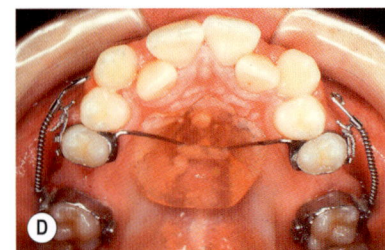

Fig. 2.11 The Sectional Jig assembly. Lateral (A) and occlusal (B) views of the appliance immediately after insertion. Lateral (C) and occlusal (D) views of the appliance after maxillary molar distalization.

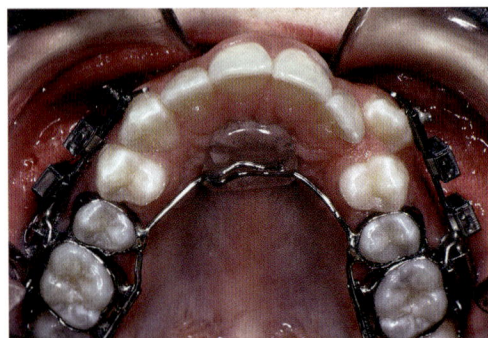

Fig. 2.12 A magnetic distalization appliance. (With permission from Papadopoulos.[2])

headgear tube of the first molar band. An SS ligature is then tied between the open loop of the active arm and the gingival hook of the molar band, thus adding stability to the system and preventing rotation of the sectional archwire. The spring is activated by ligating the hook of the second (mesial) sliding tube to the bracket of the second premolar band. Optimal activation of the coil spring will deliver 80 g per side. The patient is monitored every month for further adjustments and reactivation of the appliance.[76,77]

Magnets Used for Molar Distalization

The development of rare metal permanent magnets has allowed the clinical application of magnetic forces in orthodontics, since there had been speculation on the possible biological effects of static magnetic fields on the mechanism of orthodontic tooth movement.[78,79] Blechman was the first to develop an intraoral magnetic appliance in conjunction with fixed appliances and sectional archwires to distalize the maxillary first molars.[80] Later, the Molar Distalizing System (Medical Magnetics, Ramsey, NJ, USA)[81] and a prefabricated magnetic device (Modular Magnetic, New City, USA) were introduced to distalize maxillary molars.[82]

To reinforce anchorage, a modified Nance button is used and stabilized to the maxillary first or second premolar bands or maxillary first primary molar bands (Fig. 2.12).[73,81,83] Bondemark et al. suggested the incorporation of an anterior bite plane to the Nance button to disclude the posterior teeth.[84] The active unit consists of a pair of repelling magnets attached to a sectional wire, the surfaces of which are brought into contact to deliver a distalization force. The mesial magnet is mounted so that it can move freely along the sectional wire.[83,84]

To activate the appliance, the repelling surfaces of the magnets are brought into contact by passing a 0.014 inch ligature wire through the loop on the auxiliary wire and then tying back a washer anterior to the magnets, producing a continuous distalization force of 200–225 g. As the distance between the magnets increases to 1–1.5 mm, this force decreases to a minimum of 60–100 g, below which the magnets should be reactivated, approximately every 1–4 weeks.[83,84]

Distalizing Arches, Acrylic Resin Distalization Splints and the Carriere Distalizer

Several other appliances have been proposed for maxillary molar distalization, including

- distalizing arches, e.g. the Bimetric Distalizing Arch (RMO, Denver, CO, USA),[85] the Multi-Distalizing Arch (Ortho Organizers, San Marcos, CA, USA), the Molar Distalization Bow[86] and the Korn Lip Bumper (American Orthodontics, Sheboygan, WI, USA)
- acrylic resin distalization splints, e.g. the acrylic resin splint with Ni-Ti coils[87] and the Removable Molar Distalization Splint[88]
- the Carriere Distalizer (ClassOne Orthodontics, Lubbock, TX, USA).[89]

However, almost all of these devices require some form of patient cooperation either because they are removable or because they have to be used in conjunction with intermaxillary elastics.

Appliances with a Double Flexible Distalization Force System Positioned Both Palatally and Buccally

Two appliances have a double flexible distalization force system positioned both palatally and buccally: the Piston appliance (i.e. the Greenfield Molar Distalizer) and a Nance appliance in conjunction with Ni-Ti open coil springs and an edgewise appliance.

The Piston appliance (Greenfield Molar Distalizer)

The Piston appliance (Nx Orthodontic Services, Coral Springs, FL, USA) has an active unit positioned both palatally and buccally consisting of superelastic Ni-Ti open coil springs and an anchorage unit incorporating an enlarged modified Nance button.[90] The modified Nance acrylic resin palatal button is stabilized with SS wires (0.040 inch), which are soldered to the first premolar bands. The active unit consists of superelastic Ni-Ti open coil springs (0.055 inch) positioned around the piston assemblies. The piston assemblies are fabricated with SS wires (0.030 inch) soldered buccally and palatally to the first molar bands and tubes (0.036 inch) soldered on the maxillary first premolar bands. To activate the appliance, 2 mm ring stops are added to the mesial of the buccal and palatal tubes in each piston every 6–8 weeks, thus delivering 25 g of distalizing force to each piston assembly, and subsequently 50 g of distalization force for each molar. The molars are distalized with a monthly rate of 1 mm.

Appliances with a Rigid Distalization Force System Palatally Positioned

The Veltri Distalizer and the New Distalizer are the most common appliances using expansion screws as a rigid distalization force system positioned palatally.

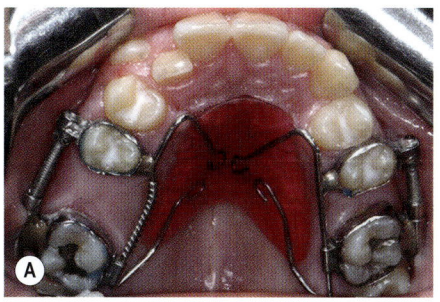 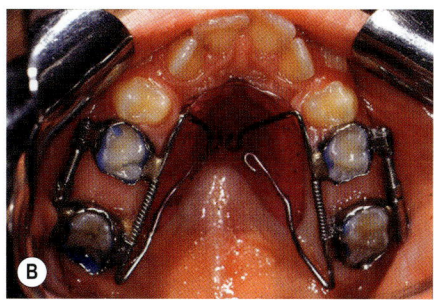

Fig. 2.13 Bilateral maxillary molar distalization with the First Class Appliance in a patient with permanent dentition (A) and one with mixed dentition (B).

Veltri Distalizer

The Veltri Distalizer (Leone, Florence, Italy) consists of a Veltri sagittal expansion screw palatally positioned and incorporating four extension arms, which are soldered bilaterally to the first and second maxillary molar bands in a similar way to the Hyrax expansion screw.[91] The appliance is used for maxillary second molar distalization incorporating as anchorage all the teeth anterior to the second molars, including the first molars. The appliance is activated by turning the screw half a turn twice every week until the second molars are completely distalized. Then, distalization of the first molars follows by means of the Ni-Ti coil springs. To reinforce anchorage during the distalization of the first molars, a palatal bar with Nance button attached to the second molars, full fixed appliances incorporating an archwire with stops mesial to the second premolars and Class II elastics can be used. Consequently, some form of patient compliance is required during this phase of treatment. When the first maxillary molars are in Class I relationship, the retraction of the anterior teeth can be initiated.

The New Distalizer

The New Distalizer (Leone, Florence, Italy) can be regarded as a modification of the Veltri Distalizer.[92] The appliance consists of a Veltri palatal sagittal screw for bilateral molar distalization that is soldered by means of extension arms to bands on the maxillary first molars and second premolars (or second primary molars). A Nance button connected to the body of the screw by means of two soldered extension wires adds to the anchorage. The appliance is activated at a rate of two-quarters of a turn every week. When distalization of the maxillary first molars has been accomplished, the screw is blocked and the arms connecting the screw with the second premolar bands are cut off. Thus, the first molar position can be maintained and a second phase of treatment with full fixed appliances can follow.

Hybrid Appliances

The only hybrid appliance that uses a combination of a rigid distalization force system, which is buccally positioned, and a flexible one, which is palatally positioned, is the First Class Appliance.

First Class Appliance

The First Class Appliance (Leone, Florence, Italy) consists of a vestibular framework, a palatal framework and four bands (Fig. 2.13).[93,94] The active unit of the appliance includes bilateral screws, buccally positioned, and a spring, palatally positioned. On the buccal side of the first molar bands, 10 mm long vestibular screws are soldered occlusally to the single tubes (0.022×0.028 inch) in which the base arches can be positioned after molar distalization. The vestibular screws are seated into closed rings that are welded to the bands of the second primary molars or the second premolars. Each vestibular screw is activated by a quarter turn once per day

for bilateral distalization. The anchorage unit of the appliance consists of a large palatal Nance button having a "butterfly" shape with wires (0.045 inch) embedded in the acrylic resin. Anteriorly, these extension wires are soldered lingual to the second primary molar or premolar bands; posteriorly they are inserted into tubes (0.045 inch) welded to the palatal sides of the first molar bands.[93,94] The molar tubes act as a guide during distalization to enhance bodily tooth movement. Between the solder joint on the second primary molar or premolar band and the tube on the molar band, 10 mm long Ni-Ti open coil springs are positioned in full compression. The continuous force produced by the springs compensates the action of the vestibular screws so that the distal molar movement takes place in a "double-track" system, preventing rotations or the development of posterior crossbites.[94] The First Class Appliance can be used in patients presenting with either permanent (Fig. 2.13A)[94] or mixed (Fig. 2.13B) dentition.[95]

Transpalatal Arches for Molar Rotation and/or Distalization

Transpalatal arches can be an effective adjunct for gaining space in the maxillary dental arch in terms of molar derotation or distalization. They are particularly useful when the need for derotation is the same on both sides of the dental arch. Since the introduction of the transpalatal bar, several designs, soldered (fixed) or removable, have become available. These include:

- prefabricated transpalatal arch for maxillary molar derotation (GAC International, Islandia, NY, USA)[96]
- Zachrisson-type transpalatal bar[97,98]
- Palatal Rotation Arch[99]
- Nitanium Molar Rotator 2 and Nitanium Palatal Expander 2 (Ortho Organizers, San Marcos, CA, USA)[100]
- 3D (Wilson) Palatal Appliance (RMO, Denver, CO, USA)[101]
- TMA transpalatal arch[102]
- Distalix, which is based on the Quad helix appliance, using the four helices as well as a distalization pendulum spring[103]
- Keles transpalatal arch.[104]

MODE OF ACTION OF THE NON-COMPLIANCE APPLIANCES

INTERMAXILLARY NON-COMPLIANCE APPLIANCES

There are some distinct differences between using intermaxillary non-compliance appliances or intermaxillary elastics to correct a Class II malocclusion. Class II elastics are oriented in a posterior–inferior to anterior–superior direction, exercising a pulling type force in a forward and upward direction to the mandibular dentition and in a backward and downward direction to the maxillary dentition (Fig. 2.14A). Analyzing

Fig. 2.14 Biomechanics of mandibular advancement with intermaxillary Class II elastics in sagittal view. (A) Original forces. (B) Horizontal and vertical force components and moments generated by the elastics. Although there is a vertical component to the force, the anteroposterior components are greater. This pulling configuration on the maxillary arch results in extrusion and retrusion of the anterior teeth, while on the mandibular arch it results in a forward reposition of the mandible as well as extrusion of the posterior teeth.

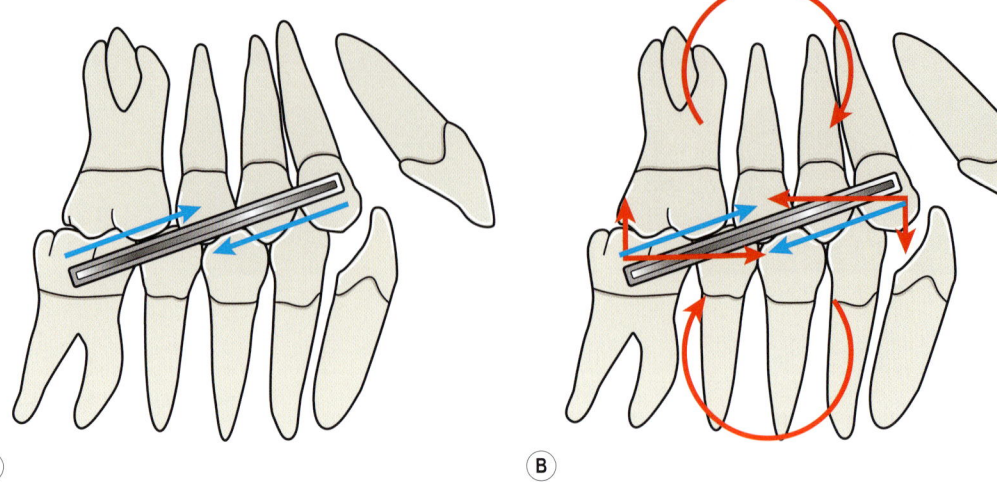

Fig. 2.15 Biomechanics of mandibular advancement with intermaxillary non-compliance appliances in sagittal view. (A) Original forces at treatment start. (B) Horizontal and vertical force components and moments generated by the appliance. Although there is a vertical component to the force, the anteroposterior components are greater. This pushing configuration on the maxillary arch results in distalization and intrusion of the posterior teeth and retrusion of the anterior teeth, while on the mandibular arch it results in a forward reposition of the mandible as well as in intrusion and proclination of the anterior teeth.

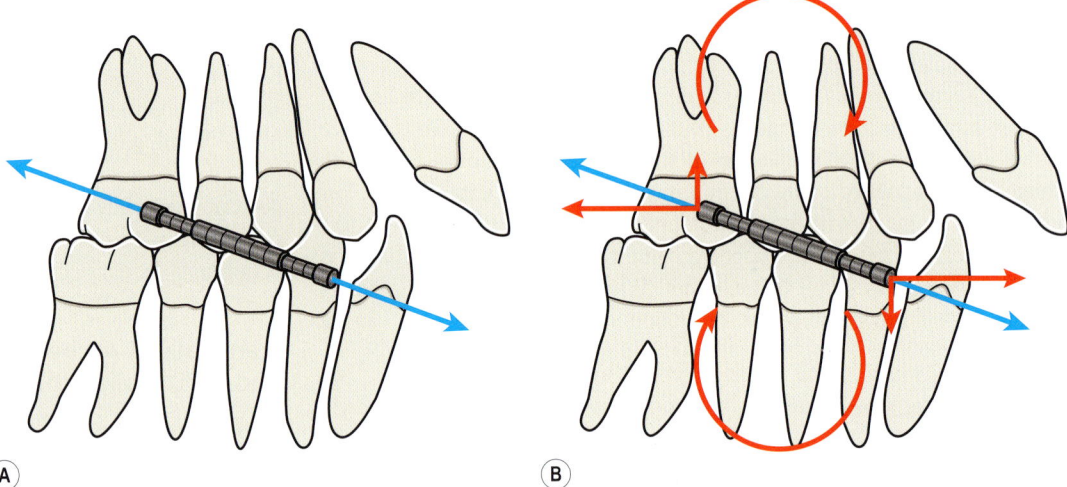

these forces in their horizontal and vertical components and taking also into consideration the CR of the maxillary and mandibular dentition, it becomes obvious that this pulling configuration results in Fig. 2.14B:

- retrusion and extrusion of the anterior teeth of the maxillary arch
- a more forward reposition of the mandible, as well as in extrusion of the posterior teeth of the mandibular arch.

There is also the tendency for a downward tilt of the occlusal plane because of the moments applied to the maxillary and mandibular dentition. The effect on the proclination of the mandibular anterior teeth is much smaller than that seen with the pushing type device (i.e. intermaxillary non-compliance appliances), while there is also the same tendency for a downward tilt of the occlusal plane because of the similar moments applied to the maxillary and mandibular dentition. Therefore, Class II intermaxillary elastics are not indicated in Class II malocclusions with deep bite and/or with proclination of the mandibular anterior teeth.

In contrast, the intermaxillary non-compliance appliances used to advance the mandible are oriented in a posterior–superior to anterior–inferior direction. This positioning results in a pushing type of force in a forward and downward direction to the mandibular dentition and in a backward and upward direction to the maxillary dentition (Fig. 2.15A). Analyzing the applied forces in their horizontal and vertical components and taking into consideration the CR of the maxillary and mandibular dentition, this pushing configuration results in Fig. 2.15B:

- distalization and intrusion of the posterior teeth and retrusion of the anterior teeth of the maxillary arch

- a forward reposition of the mandible, as well as in intrusion and proclination of the anterior teeth of the mandibular arch.

The effect on the proclination of the mandibular anterior teeth is greater than that seen with the pulling type device (i.e. intermaxillary elastics). There is also a similar tendency as with intermaxillary elastics for a downward tilt of the occlusal plane because of the moments applied to the maxillary and mandibular dentition. Consequently, intermaxillary non-compliance appliances, such as the Herbst appliance, are not indicated in Class II malocclusions with open bite or/and with proclination of the mandibular anterior teeth.

Based on this analysis, it becomes obvious that the desired effects produced by the use of intermaxillary appliances include:

- mandibular advancement in a more forward position
- maxillary molar distalization or retrusion of the maxillary dentition.

However, there are some side effects with this type of appliance, including:

- intrusion
- protrusion or proclination of the mandibular anterior teeth.

In addition, treatment with the Herbst appliance may induce anchorage loss of the maxillary teeth in terms of spacing between the maxillary canines and first premolars. These effects may take place in various degrees during mandibular advancement using intermaxillary non-compliance devices in Class II malocclusion. They represent a very important negative aspect of their application and must be seriously considered before initiating treatment with these appliances.

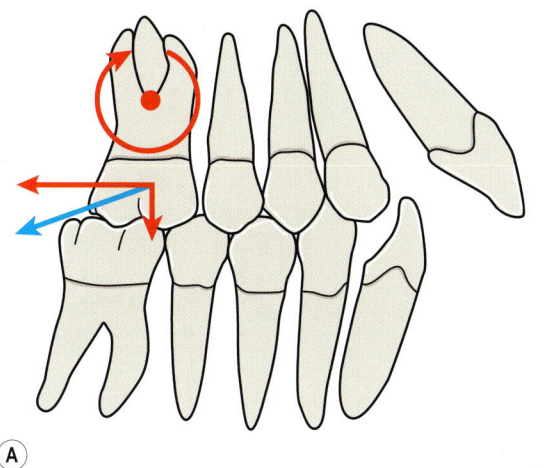
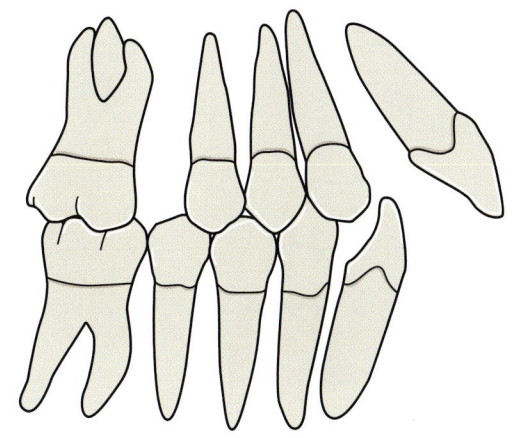

Fig. 2.16 Biomechanics of maxillary molar distalization with cervical headgear in sagittal view. (A) Original forces along with the corresponding horizontal and vertical components, and moments generated by the appliance at treatment start. (B) Situation after molar distalization: distal crown tipping and extrusion can be observed as side effects.

(A)

(B)

INTRAMAXILLARY NON-COMPLIANCE DISTALIZATION APPLIANCES

During maxillary molar distalization, either with conventional extraoral headgear or with non-compliance distalization appliances, a number of unwanted effects always takes place diminishing their clinical effectiveness. These side effects of intramaxillary devices may vary with the type of distalization appliance, but they always accompany molar distalization and can be posterior (distal molar crown tipping, distal crown rotation and occasionally molar extrusion) or anterior (forward movement and proclination of the maxillary anterior teeth) anchorage loss. They result from the biomechanics involved and thus the orthodontist should always consider where the CR of the teeth to be moved is located and the relationship of this to the point of force application.

For example, when moving maxillary molars distally with cervical headgears, taking into consideration that in sagittal view the CR is located at the bifurcation of their roots, the point of force application is located more occlusally and thus the resulting movement will not be a pure bodily distal movement but will have some distal molar crown tipping and extrusion (Fig. 2.16). In addition, in occlusal view, the point of force application is located buccally in relation to the CR of the molars (Fig. 2.17A) and so a distal rotation of the molar crowns is also observed. Distal tipping, distal rotation and extrusion of the molars are considered as anchorage loss, since additional force systems have to be applied to counteract these unwanted side effects.

There will also be side effects on other areas of the body. Newton's third law of motion states that when one body exerts a force on another the second body will simultaneously exert a force equal in magnitude and opposite in direction to that of the first. As use of headgears will apply such a reaction force to the patient's neck, this can put a strain on the cervical spine and the neck muscles.

Finally, lingual tipping of the maxillary incisors often takes place when using headgears to distalize maxillary molars; it occurs from pulling of transeptal fibers (drifting) and from restriction of maxillary growth. The later effect will, occasionally, be unwanted, for example in Class II malocclusion with maxillary crowding, where space has to be created for teeth alignment and there is no need for maxillary growth restriction.

Intramaxillary non-compliance distalization appliances have similar problems to those discussed above for cervical headgear: the CR of the maxillary molars is at the bifurcation of their roots but the point of force application is located more occlusally. Hence, the resulting movement is again accompanied by distal molar crown tipping and extrusion (Fig. 2.18). In addition, in occlusal view, the point of force application of many of these appliances (e.g. the Sectional Jig assembly) is located buccally in relation to the CR and so distal rotation of the molar crowns is also

observed (Fig. 2.17B). In some other distalization appliances, such as the Pendulum appliances, the point of force application is located palatally to the CR of the molars and this leads to a distal rotation of the maxillary molars in almost every case (Fig. 2.17C). This rotation is significantly more pronounced with the Pendulum appliances because the arc type of movement not only rotates the molars distally but also moves them towards the midline, producing a posterior maxillary arch constriction and a crossbite tendency. Distal tipping, distal rotation and extrusion of the molars are considered as posterior anchorage loss, since measures have to be taken to counteract them.

Non-compliance distalization appliances usually utilize the first or second premolars for their anchorage and so the reaction forces produced by the various coil springs are applied indirectly to the anterior dental unit: premolars, canines and incisors. The CR of this dental unit is located somewhere between the root apices of the premolars; consequently, the premolars and canines are moving forward with mesial inclination, the incisors are proclined and the overjet is usually increased (Fig. 2.18). These effects are considered as anterior anchorage loss.

These side effects are observed in various degrees when examining the clinical efficacy of all non-compliance devices,[105] including the Sectional Jig assembly used for simultaneous distalization of maxillary first and second molars,[77] similar devices with Ni-Ti coil springs and the First Class Appliance.[95] However, there is still lack of high-quality evidence-based studies investigating not only the appliances and approaches used for non-compliance molar distalization but also many other issues related to clinical orthodontics that could impact on the use of these modalities.[106]

After molar distalization has been accomplished using a non-compliance distalization appliance, the appliance is usually removed and the first molars are retained in position usually by a new modified Nance holding arch for a "stabilization period" of approximately 2 months. This allows for a spontaneous distal drift of the first and second premolars through the pull of the transeptal fibers. Alternatively, a transpalatal arch or a utility archwire or an archwire with stops mesial to the molar tubes can be used to maintain the position of the maxillary first molars. However, some non-compliance distalization devices, such as the Distal Jet, do not need to be removed after molar distalization is accomplished. These appliances can be converted to a passive appliance (in other words to a modified Nance holding arch) to retain the maxillary molars in their new positions. The conversion steps are usually quite simple.

Finally, in order to complete the correction of Class II malocclusion after this stabilization period, a second phase of comprehensive orthodontic treatment with full fixed appliances should follow, including retraction of the anterior teeth and leveling and alignment of the dental arches. A variety of methods mechanics is available to complete these tasks, such as typical orthodontic biomechanics with preadjusted appliances and Class II

Fig. 2.17 Biomechanics of maxillary molar distalization in occlusal view. (A) Forces and moments generated by cervical headgear. (B) Forces and moments generated by non-compliance distalization appliances, such as the Sectional Jig assembly, with a force system buccally positioned. (C) Forces and moments generated by non-compliance distalization appliances, such as the Pendulum appliance, with a force system palatally positioned.

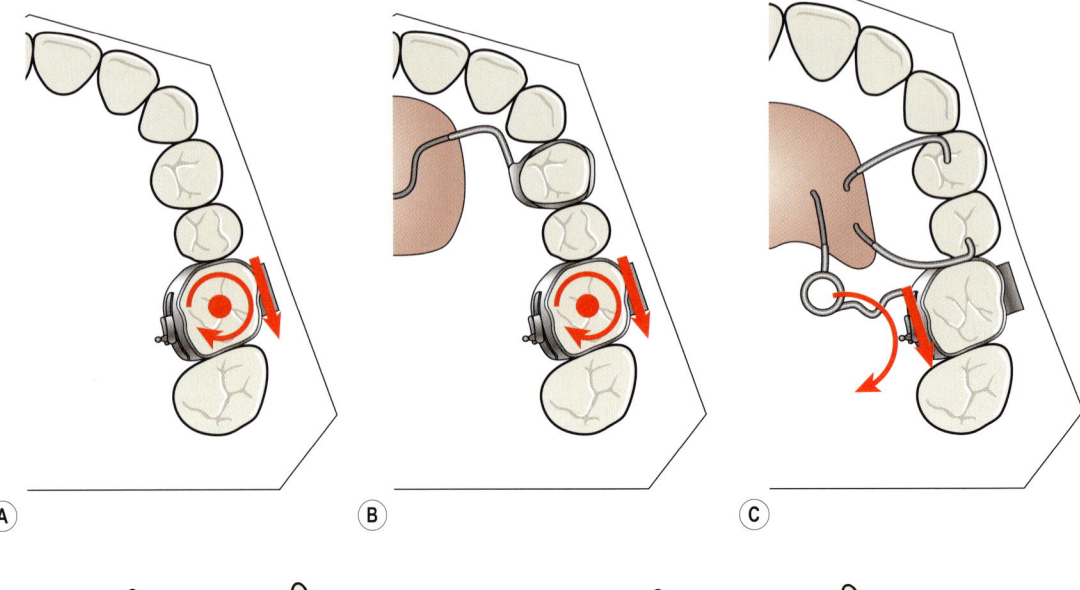

Fig. 2.18 Biomechanics of maxillary molar distalization with non-compliance distalization appliances on the sagittal view. (A) Forces and moments generated by the appliance at treatment start. (B) Situation after maxillary molar distalization: distal crown tipping and extrusion can be observed as side effects, as well as anchorage loss in terms of incisor proclination and mesial movement and inclination of the premolars and canines.

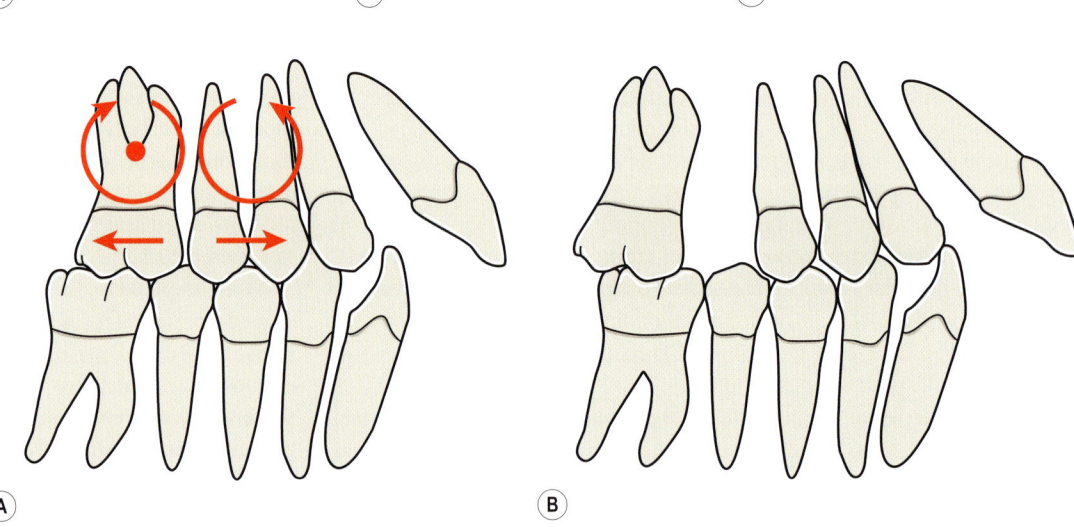

elastics. However, compliance with elastic wear may be a serious problem and this can have a negative effect on the posterior anchorage that needs to be maintained in a maximum state during anterior teeth retraction. Furthermore, if the patient does not cooperate, the gains from molar distalization may even be jeopardized during this phase, with mesial movement of the molars that have just been distalized. In these instances, the combined use of fixed functional appliances, such as the Jasper Jumper, Sabbagh Spring or Eureka Spring, may support the mesial forces applied to the maxillary molars. The fixed functional appliances serve in these situations much like a cervical headgear, without the need for compliance, to support maxillary molar position during active retraction of anterior teeth.

In summary, when non-compliance distalization appliances are used, three problems mainly occur:

- anchorage loss of the anterior dental unit, in terms of mesial movement and proclination of the anterior teeth, both taking place during molar distalization
- distal tipping of the molars, taking place during molar distalization
- anchorage loss of the posterior dental unit in forward direction that takes place after distalization and during the stage of anterior teeth retraction and final alignment of the dental arches.

Consequently, clinically efficient maxillary molar distalization using intramaxillary non-compliance distalization devices must provide a biomechanical force system that will not also cause the unwanted distal crown tipping, rotation and extrusion of the maxillary molars. It is also crucial

to reinforce anchorage both during distalization, in order to avoid mesial movement and proclination of the anterior teeth serving as a dental anchorage unit, as well as following distalization for the subsequent retraction of the anterior teeth. This anchorage reinforcement can be achieved by skeletal anchorage using orthodontic implants, miniplates or miniscrew implants.

INDICATIONS AND CONTRAINDICATIONS FOR NON-COMPLIANCE APPLIANCES

INTERMAXILLARY NON-COMPLIANCE APPLIANCES

Compared with removable functional appliances, the intermaxillary non-compliance appliances are fixed to the teeth directly or indirectly and are, therefore, able to work 24 hours a day. In addition, the duration of treatment is relatively short (6–15 months for the Herbst appliance, 3–4 months for the rest), compared with 2–4 years for the removable functional appliances. This makes these appliances suitable for postpubertal patients while the Herbst appliance may also be suitable for young adults.

The non-compliance intermaxillary appliances used for mandibular advancement have similar indications and contraindications. There is, however, one significant difference. In contrast to the Herbst appliance, almost all of the other non-compliance appliances produce mainly dentoalveolar effects and they are, therefore, indicated only for the correction of dentoalveolar Class II molar relationships and not for treatment of Class

II skeletal discrepancies. In moderate or dentoalveolar Class II, full fixed appliances and intermaxillary Class II elastics can be applied but in Class II skeletal or severe dentoalveolar discrepancies, the Herbst appliance is preferred. When the use of Class II elastics is not indicated or is not efficient, or when there is no patient cooperation, the use of intermaxillary non-compliance appliances, such as the Jasper Jumper, the Eureka Spring, the Sabbagh Spring, or the Twin Force Bite Corrector can be used in combination with the fixed appliances, since they are more easily applied at this stage of treatment than the Herbst appliance.

The Herbst appliance is indicated for the non-compliance treatment of Class II skeletal discrepancies, deep anterior overbite and mandibular midline deviation, as well as in mouth breathers and in patients with anterior disk displacement. It is also suitable for the treatment of Class II malocclusion in patients with retrognathic mandibles and retroclined maxillary incisors. The removable acrylic resin Herbst appliance can be used in patients suffering from obstructive sleep apnea, in order to improve the clinical symptoms.[25,26]

Choosing the correct time to initiate treatment with a Herbst appliance is considered critical for success. Treatment before the pubertal peak of growth can lead to normal skeletal and soft tissue morphology at a young age, providing a foundation for normal growth of these structures. However, while this is the most suitable age to initiate treatment, this early approach requires retention of the treatment device until the eruption of all the permanent teeth into a stable cuspal interdigitation, and so the possibility of occlusal relapse is greater. By initiating treatment in the permanent dentition at or just after the pubertal growth peak, the increase in condylar growth and the shorter retention phase required could lead to a more stable occlusion and reduced post-treatment relapse. Herbst treatment can also be effective in patients in late adolescence who still have some residual growth.[10,13,18,20] It can be used in young adults as an alternative to orthognathic surgery because it has shown favorable results for intermaxillary jaw base relationships and skeletal profile convexity, as well as being of lower cost and risk for the patient.[13,20,27]

The prognosis for Herbst treatment is best in subjects with a brachyfacial growth pattern and it is contraindicated in autistic children, patients with severe bruxism,[29] vertical growth pattern, skeletal or dental open bites, and proclined mandibular anterior teeth. Unfavorable growth, unstable occlusal conditions and oral habits that persist after treatment are potential risk factors for occlusal relapse.[9]

INTRAMAXILLARY NON-COMPLIANCE DISTALIZATION APPLIANCES

Maxillary molar distalization using headgears is typically indicated in patients presenting with bilateral Class II molar relationships and overjet, while the intramaxillary non-compliance distalization devices are indicated in young children with mixed dentition, as well as in adolescents or adults with permanent dentition and Class II malocclusion presenting minimal cooperation when either a bilateral or a unilateral distalization of the maxillary molars is required. Non-compliance distalization is also particularly indicated in patients with dentoalveolar Class II malocclusion or a tendency towards skeletal Class I or Class III relationships. It is also used when there is crowding in the maxillary arch and space has to be created for teeth alignment; here there is a need only for molar distalization while no restriction of maxillary growth is desirable.

Whether distalization of first maxillary molars is affected by second molars is a matter of controversy. Some authors have reported that the presence and the position of second molars do not influence the amount and the type of maxillary first molar distal movement. In contrast, other authors suggest that the presence of second molars increases the duration of treatment time, produces more tipping and more anchorage loss. It has

been suggested that the eruption stages of the second molar have a basic qualitative and quantitative impact on the distalization of the first molars because a tooth bud may act as a fulcrum on the mesial neighboring tooth. It has also been shown that tipping of the first molars is much more pronounced when the second molars are still at the budding stage, and that tipping of the second molars is greater when a third molar bud is located in the direction of movement.[107] For this reason, germectomy of wisdom teeth is recommended in order to achieve bodily distalization of both molars even when the second molars are not banded.

Intraoral non-compliance distalization appliances are not solely indicated in patients with minimal compliance and can also be useful in compliant patients, particularly when non-extraction treatment protocols have to be utilized. They can be used, for example, during the early phase of permanent dentition in patients with almost completed pre-pubertal growth, as well as when the second maxillary molars have already erupted and treatment with headgears would be difficult, requiring almost 24 hours a day wear in order to be effective.[77]

Nevertheless, the use of non-compliance distalization appliances has some contraindications. These include the crowding or spacing conditions of the maxillary dental arch and the growth pattern of the craniofacial complex, as well as the anatomical characteristics of the palatal vault. Severe crowding or spacing in the maxillary dental arch can lead to disproportionate anchorage loss of the anterior dental unit. In addition, patients with insufficient seating of the Nance button because of a reduced palatal vault inclination may be unsuitable for molar distalization with these appliances. Further, non-compliance molar distalization is also contraindicated in patients with vertical growth pattern and the presence of, or a tendency towards, an anterior open bite, because of the extrusive component of the distal molar movement, as well as in patients with severe protrusive profiles.

Consequently, selecting the right patients for the individual treatment modality is a very important factor for a successful outcome and it is strongly recommended that this is a major consideration before initiating a non-compliance maxillary molar distalization.

ADVANTAGES AND DISADVANTAGES OF THE NON-COMPLIANCE APPLIANCES

INTERMAXILLARY NON-COMPLIANCE APPLIANCES

The main advantages of the intermaxillary non-compliance appliances include the short and standardized treatment duration, the lack of reliance on patient compliance to attain the desired treatment effects, the easy acceptance and patient tolerance. In addition, the distalizing effect on the maxillary first molars contributes to the avoidance of extractions in Class II malocclusions with maxillary crowding. Other advantages include the improvement in the patient's profile immediately after appliance placement, the maintenance of good oral hygiene, the simultaneous use of fixed appliances and the ability to modify the appliances for various clinical applications.

However, there also some disadvantages, such as chewing problems during the first week of treatment, soft tissue impingement, breakage or distortion of the appliances, bent rods, loose or broken bands, loose brackets, and in some cases broken or loose screws.

INTRAMAXILLARY NON-COMPLIANCE DISTALIZATION APPLIANCES

The main advantages of the intramaxillary non-compliance distalization appliances include producing rapid maxillary molar distalization, requiring minimal patient cooperation, easy acceptance by patients, requiring minimal chair-time for reactivations, unilateral or bilateral use, distalizing both first and second molars simultaneously (or in some cases consecutively) and creating space for the alignment of the maxillary dental arch without extractions in dentoalveolar Class II discrepancies (or even in patients with a tendency for skeletal Class I or Class III relationships) with maxillary crowding.

However, although these appliances can produce rapid distalization of the maxillary molars, they present some disadvantages, such as anchorage loss of the anterior dental unit (in terms of forward movement of the premolars and canines, incisor proclination and/or increased overjet) and distal tipping of the molars. Therefore, the mesial movement and slight protrusion of the anterior dental anchorage unit during distalization have to be considered seriously when applying these non-compliance approaches and, again, selecting the right patients for the treatment modality and careful treatment planning is vital. Anchorage loss of the posterior dental unit (in terms of mesial movement of the distalized maxillary molars) that takes place during the subsequent phase of the anterior teeth retraction is another major disadvantage that has to be taken also into consideration before initiation of treatment.

REFERENCES

1. Proffit WR. Contemporary orthodontics. St. Louis, MO: Mosby; 2000.
2. Papadopoulos MA, editor. Orthodontic treatment for the Class II non-compliant patient: current principles and techniques. Edinburgh: Elsevier-Mosby; 2006.
3. Zentner A. The problem of compliance in orthodontics. In: Papadopoulos MA, editor. Orthodontic treatment for the Class II non-compliant patient: current principles and techniques. Edinburgh: Elsevier-Mosby; 2006. p. 3–7.
4. Samuels RH, Brezniak N. Orthodontic facebows: Safety issues and current management. J Orthod 2002;29:101–7.
5. Papadopoulos MA, Rakosi T. Results of a comparative study of skeletal Class II cases after activator, headgear and combined headgear-activator treatment. Hell Stomatol Ann 1990;34:87–96.
6. Papadopoulos MA. Non-compliance distalization: a monograph on the clinical management and effectiveness of a jig assembly in Class II malocclusion orthodontic treatment. Thessaloniki: Phototypotiki; 2005.
7. Papadopoulos MA. Classification of the non-compliance appliances used for Class II correction. In: Papadopoulos MA, editor. Orthodontic treatment for the Class II non-compliant patient: current principles and techniques. Edinburgh: Elsevier-Mosby; 2006. p. 9–17.
8. Pancherz H. The modern Herbst appliance. In: Graber TM, Rakosi T, Petrovic AG, editors. Dentofacial orthopedics with functional appliances. 2nd ed. St. Louis, MO: Mosby-Year Book; 1997. p. 336–66.
9. Pancherz H. The Herbst appliance: its biologic effects and clinical use. Am J Orthod 1985;87:1–20.
10. White LW. Current Herbst appliance therapy. J Clin Orthod 1994;28:296–309.
11. Rogers MB. Herbst appliance variations. J Clin Orthod 2003;37:156–9.
12. Pancherz H, Hansen K. Mandibular anchorage in Herbst treatment. Eur J Orthod 1988;10:149–64.
13. Pancherz H, Ruf S. The Herbst appliance: research-based updated clinical possibilities. World J Orthod 2000;1:17–31.
14. McNamara JA Jr, Brudon WL, Buckhardt DR, et al. The Herbst appliance. In: McNamara JA Jr, Brudon WL, editors. Orthodontics and dentofacial orthopedics. Ann Arbor, MI: Needham Press; 2001. p. 285–318.
15. Wieslander L. Intensive treatment of severe Class II malocclusions with a headgear-Herbst appliance in the early mixed dentition. Am J Orthod 1984;86:1–13.
16. Hagg U, Du X, Rabie AB. Initial and late treatment effects of headgear-Herbst appliance with mandibular step-by-step advancement. Am J Orthod Dentofacial Orthop 2002;122:477–85.
17. Pancherz H, Hansen K. Occlusal changes during and after Herbst treatment: a cephalometric investigation. Eur J Orthod 1986;8:215–28.
18. Konik M, Pancherz H, Hansen K. The mechanism of Class II correction in late Herbst treatment. Am J Orthod Dentofacial Orthop 1997;112:87–91.
19. Pancherz H, Ruf S, Thomalske-Faubert C. Mandibular articular disk position changes during Herbst treatment: a prospective longitudinal MRI study. Am J Orthod Dentofacial Orthop 1999;116:207–14.
20. Ruf S, Pancherz H. Dentoskeletal effects and facial profile changes in young adults treated with the Herbst appliance. Angle Orthod 1999;69:239–46.
21. O'Brien K, Wright J, Conboy F, et al. Effectiveness of treatment for Class II malocclusion with the Herbst or twin-block appliances: a randomized controlled trial. Am J Orthod Dentofacial Orthop 2003;124:128–37.
22. Pancherz H. The nature of Class II relapse after Herbst appliance treatment: a cephalometric long-term investigation. Am J Orthod Dentofacial Orthop 1991;100:220–33.
23. Pancherz H. The effects, limitations, and long-term dentofacial adaptations to treatment with the Herbst appliance. Semin Orthod 1997;3:232–43.
24. Eberhard H, Hirschfelder U. Treatment of Class II, division 2 in the late growth period. J Orofac Orthop 1998;59:352–61.
25. Bloch KE, Iseli A, Zhang JN, et al. A randomized, controlled crossover trial of two oral appliances for sleep apnea treatment. Am J Respir Crit Care Med 2000;162:246–51.
26. Shadaba A, Battagel JM, Owa A, et al. Evaluation of the Herbst Mandibular Advancement Splint in the management of patients with sleep-related breathing disorders. Clin Otolaryngol 2000;25:404–12.
27. Paulsen HU, Thomsen JS, Hougen HP, et al. A histomorphometric and scanning electron microscopy study of human condylar cartilage and bone tissue changes in relation to age. Clin Orthod Res 1999;2:67–78.
28. Rogers MB. Troubleshooting the Herbst appliance. J Clin Orthod 2002;36:268–74.
29. Pancherz H, Anehus-Pancherz M. The headgear effect of the Herbst appliance: a cephalometric long-term study. Am J Orthod Dentofacial Orthop 1993;103:510–20.
30. Goodman P, McKenna P. Modified Herbst appliance for the mixed dentition. J Clin Orthod 1985;19:811–14.
31. Valant JR, Sinclair PM. Treatment effects of the Herbst appliance. Am J Orthod Dentofacial Orthop 1989;95:138–47.
32. Schiavoni R, Bonapace C, Grenga V. Modified edgewise-Herbst appliance. J Clin Orthod 1996;30:681–7.
33. Ritto AK. Tratamento das Classes II divisão 1 com a BielaMagnética. Dissertation Thesis; 1997.
34. Miller RA. The flip-lock Herbst appliance. J Clin Orthod 1996;30:552–8.
35. Hanks SD. Herbst therapy: trying to get out of the 20th century. Good Pract Newsletter Am Orthod 2003;4:2–4.
36. Ritto AK. Fixed functional appliances: an updated classification. Orthod CYBERJ 2012 <http://orthocj.com/2001/06/fixed-functional-appliances-a-classification-updated/>; [accessed 27 Ocotober 2013].
37. Calvez X. The universal bite jumper. J Clin Orthod 1998;32:493–9.
38. Dischinger TG. Open-bite intrusion Herbst. AOA Orthod Appliances 2001;5:1–4. <www.aoalab.com/learning/publications/aoaVol/ aoaVol5No2.pdf>; [accessed 27 Ocotober 2013].
39. Faulkner J. An interview with Dr. Joe Mayes on the Cantilever Bite Jumper. Orthod CYBERJ 1997 <http://orthocj.com/archive/issue3/p0000077.htm>; [accessed 27 Ocotober 2013].
40. Mayes JH. The molar-moving bite jumper (MMBJ). Clin Impressions 1998;7:16–19.
41. Clements RM Jr, Jacobson A. The MARS appliance: report of a case. Am J Orthod 1982;82:445–55.
42. Jones M. Mandibular corrector. J Clin Orthod 1985;19:362–8.
43. Coelho Filho CM. Mandibular protraction appliance IV. J Clin Orthod 2001;35:18–24.
44. Eckhart JE. The MARA Appliance. AOA Orthod Appliances 1997;1:1–2.
45. Eckhart JE, White LW. Class II therapy with the Mandibular Anterior Repositioning Appliance. World J Orthod 2003;4:135–44.
46. Eckhart JE. MARA provides effective adult treatment. Clin Impressions 2001;10:16–17.
47. Kinzinger G, Ostheimer J, Forster F, et al. Development of a new fixed functional appliance for treatment of skeletal Class II malocclusion: first report. J Orofac Orthop 2002;63:384–99.
48. McNamara JA Jr, Brudon WL. The Jasper Jumper. In: McNamara JA Jr, Brudon WL, editors. Orthodontics and dentofacial orthopedics. Ann Arbor, MI: Needham Press; 2001. p. 333–42.
49. Blackwood HO 3rd. Clinical management of the Jasper Jumper. J Clin Orthod 1991;25:755–60.
50. Mills CM, McCulloch KJ. Case report: modified use of the Jasper Jumper appliance in a skeletal Class II mixed dentition case requiring palatal expansion. Angle Orthod 1997;67:277–82.
51. Covell DA Jr, Trammell DW, Boero RP, et al. A cephalometric study of Class II, division 1 malocclusions treated with the Jasper Jumper appliance. Angle Orthod 1999;69:311–20.
52. Stucki N, Ingervall B. The use of the Jasper Jumper for the correction of Class II malocclusion in the young permanent dentition. Eur J Orthod 1998;20:271–81.
53. Winsauer H. Flex Developer. Adjustable power developer: Variable length and force. Maria Anzbach, Austria: LPI-Ormco; 2002 <www.flexdeveloper.com>; [accessed 27 Ocotober 2013].
54. DeVincenzo J. The Eureka Spring: a new interarch force delivery system. J Clin Orthod 1997;31:454–67.
55. Sabbagh A. The Sabbagh Universal Spring (SUS). In: Papadopoulos MA, editor. Orthodontic treatment for the Class II non-compliant patient: current principles and techniques. Edinburgh: Elsevier-Mosby; 2006. p. 203–16.
56. Dionne DG. Clinical trial report: Forsus Fatigue Resistant Device. Orthod Perspect 2002;IX:11–12.
57. Corbett MC, Molina FG. Twin Force Bite Corrector: light force and patient friendly. Syllabus. San Marcos, CA: Ortho Organizers; 2001.
58. Uribe F, Rothenberg J, Nanda R. The twin force bite corrector in the correction of Class II malocclusion in adolescent patients. In: Papadopoulos MA, editor.

Orthodontic treatment for the Class II non-compliant patient: current principles and techniques. Edinburgh: Elsevier-Mosby; 2006. p. 181–202.

59. Hilgers JJ. The pendulum appliance for Class II noncompliance therapy. J Clin Orthod 1992;26:706–14.
60. Hilgers JJ. The pendulum appliance: an update. Clin Impressions 1993;2:15–17.
61. Bussick TJ, McNamara JA Jr. Dentoalveolar and skeletal changes associated with the pendulum appliance. Am J Orthod Dentofacial Orthop 2000;117:333–43.
62. Byloff FK, Darendeliler MA. Distal molar movement using the pendulum appliance. Part 1: clinical and radiological evaluation. Angle Orthod 1997;67:249–60.
63. Byloff FK, Darendeliler MA, Clar E, et al. Distal molar movement using the pendulum appliance. Part 2: The effects of maxillary molar root uprighting bands. Angle Orthod 1997;67:261–70.
64. Mayes JH. The Texas Penguin: a new approach to pendulum therapy. AOA Orthod Appliances 1999;3:1–2.
65. Kinzinger G, Fuhrmann R, Gross U, et al. Modified pendulum appliance including distal screw and uprighting activation for noncompliance therapy of Class II malocclusion in children and adolescents. J Orofac Orthop 2000;61:175–90.
66. Kinzinger G, Fritz U, Diedrich P. Bipendulum and quad pendulum for noncompliance molar distalization in adult patients. J Orofac Orthop 2002;63:154–62.
67. Keles A, Sayinsu K. A new approach in maxillary molar distalization: Intraoral bodily molar distalizer. Am J Orthod Dentofacial Orthop 2000;117:39–48.
68. Carano A, Testa M. The distal jet for upper molar distalization. J Clin Orthod 1996;30:374–80.
69. Carano A, Bowman SJ. Noncompliance Class II treatment with the Distal Jet. In: Papadopoulos MA, editor. Orthodontic treatment for the Class II non-compliant patient: current principles and techniques. Edinburgh: Elsevier-Mosby; 2006. p. 249–71.
70. Bolla E, Muratore F, Carano A, et al. Evaluation of maxillary molar distalization with the distal jet: a comparison with other contemporary methods. Angle Orthod 2002;72:481–94.
71. Keles A. The Keles Slider Appliance for bilateral and unilateral maxillary moral Distalization. In: Papadopoulos MA, editor. Orthodontic treatment for the Class II non-compliant patient: current principles and techniques. Edinburgh: Elsevier-Mosby; 2006. p. 273–81.
72. Reiner TJ. Modified Nance appliance for unilateral molar distalization. J Clin Orthod 1992;26:402–4.
73. Bondemark L. A comparative analysis of distal maxillary molar movement produced by a new lingual intra-arch NiTi coil appliance and a magnetic appliance. Eur J Orthod 2000;22:683–95.
74. Lanteri C, Francolini F, Lanteri V. Distalization using the Fast Back. Leone Boll Int 2002;4:1–3.
75. Jones RD, White MJ. Rapid Class II molar correction with an open-coil jig. J Clin Orthod 1992;26:661–4.
76. Papadopoulos MA. The Jones Jig and modifications. In: Papadopoulos MA, editor. Orthodontic treatment for the Class II non-compliant patient: current principles and techniques. Edinburgh: Elsevier-Mosby; 2006. p. 283–95.
77. Mavropoulos A, Karamouzos A, Kiliaridis S, et al. Efficiency of non-compliance simultaneous first and second upper molar distalization: a 3D tooth movement analysis. Angle Orthod 2005;75:468–75.
78. Papadopoulos MA. Clinical applications of magnets in orthodontics. Hell Orthod Rev 1999;1:31–42.
79. Papadopoulos MA. Biological aspects of the use of permanent magnets and static magnetic fields in orthodontics. Hell Orthod Rev 1998;1:145–57.
80. Blechman AM. Magnetic force systems in orthodontics: clinical results of a pilot study. Am J Orthod 1985;87:201–10.
81. Gianelly AA, Vaitas AS, Thomas WM. The use of magnets to move molars distally. Am J Orthod Dentofacial Orthop 1989;96:161–7.
82. Bondemark L, Kurol J, Bernhold M. Repelling magnets versus superelastic nickel–titanium coils in simultaneous distal movement of maxillary first and second molars. Angle Orthod 1994;64:189–98.
83. Bondemark L. The use of magnets for maxillary molar distalization. In: Papadopoulos MA, editor. Orthodontic treatment for the Class II non-compliant patient: current principles and techniques. Edinburgh: Elsevier-Mosby; 2006. p. 297–307.
84. Bondemark L, Kurol J, Bernhold M. Repelling magnets versus superelastic nickel–titanium coils in simultaneous distal movement of maxillary first and second molars. Angle Orthod 1994;64:189–98.
85. Wilson WL. Modular orthodontic systems. Part 2. J Clin Orthod 1978;12:358–75.
86. Jeckel N, Rakosi T. Molar distalization by intra-oral force application. Eur J Orthod 1991;3:43–6.
87. Manhartsberger C. Headgear-free molar distalization. Fortschr Kieferorthop 1994;55:330–6.
88. Ritto AK. Removable distalization splint. Orthodontic CYBERJ 1997;2.
89. Carrière L. A new Class II distalizer. J Clin Orthod 2004;38:224–31.
90. Greenfield RL. Fixed piston appliance for rapid Class II correction. J Clin Orthod 1995;29:174–83.
91. Veltri N, Baldini A. Slow sagittal and bilateral palatal expansion for the treatment of Class II malocclusions. Leone Boll Int 2001;3:5–9.
92. Baccetti T, Franchi L. A new appliance for molar distalization. Leone Boll Int 2000;2:3–7.
93. Fortini A, Lupoli M, Parri M. The First Class Appliance for rapid molar distalization. J Clin Orthod 1999;33:322–8.
94. Fortini A, Franchi L. The First Class Appliance. In: Papadopoulos MA, editor. Orthodontic treatment for the Class II non-compliant patient: current principles and techniques. Edinburgh: Elsevier-Mosby; 2006. p. 309–29.
95. Papadopoulos MA, Melkos A, Athanasiou AE. Noncompliance maxillary molar distalization by means of the First Class Appliance: a randomized controlled trial. Am J Orthod Dentofacial Orthop 2010;137:586.
96. Dahlquist A, Gebauer U, Ingervall B. The effect of a transpalatal arch for the correction of first molar rotation. Eur J Orthod 1996;18:257–67.
97. Gunduz E, Zachrisson BU, Honigl KD, et al. An improved transpalatal bar design. Part I. Comparison of moments and forces delivered by two bar designs for symmetrical molar derotation. Angle Orthod 2003;73:239–43.
98. Gunduz E, Crismani AG, Bantleon HP, et al. An improved transpalatal bar design. Part II. Clinical upper molar derotation: case report. Angle Orthod 2003;73:244–8.
99. Cooke MS, Wreakes G. Molar derotation with a modified palatal arch: an improved technique. Br J Orthod 1978;5:201–3.
100. Corbett MC. Slow and continuous maxillary expansion, molar rotation, and molar distalization. J Clin Orthod 1997;31:253–63.
101. Young DR. Orthodontic products update. Removable quad helices and transpalatal arches. Br J Orthod 1997;24:248–56.
102. Mandurino M, Balducci L. Asymmetric distalization with a TMA transpalatal arch. J Clin Orthod 2001;35:174–8.
103. Langlade M. Clinical distalization with the Distalix. World J Orthod 2003;4:215–28.
104. Keles A. An effective and precise method for rapid molar derotation: Keles TPA. In: Papadopoulos MA, editor. Orthodontic treatment for the Class II non-compliant patient: current principles and techniques. Edinburgh: Elsevier-Mosby; 2006. p. 331–7.
105. Papadopoulos MA. Clinical efficacy of the noncompliance appliances used for Class II orthodontic correction. In: Papadopoulos MA, editor. Orthodontic treatment for the Class II non-compliant patient: current principles and techniques. Edinburgh: Elsevier-Mosby; 2006. p. 367–87.
106. Papadopoulos MA, Gkiaouris I. A critical evaluation of meta-analyses in orthodontics. Am J Orthod Dentofacial Orthop 2007;131:589–99.
107. Kinzinger GS, Fritz UB, Sander FG, et al. Efficiency of a pendulum appliance for molar distalization related to second and third molar eruption stage. Am J Orthod Dentofacial Orthop 2004;125:8–23.

3 The significance of anchorage in orthodontics

Ingalill Feldmann and Lars Bondemark

INTRODUCTION

Anchorage preparation is decisive in achieving successful orthodontic treatment. Often anchorage in an orthodontic appliance attempts to dissipate the reaction forces over as many teeth as possible and thus keep pressure in the periodontal ligaments of the anchor teeth to a minimum.[1] Theoretically, anchor values for teeth can be estimated from their root surface areas, but this is not always reliable since anchorage capacity is also influenced by attachment level, density and structure of the alveolar bone, periodontal reactivity, muscular activity, occlusal forces, craniofacial morphology and friction within the appliance resulting from tooth movement.[2]

Use of an extraoral appliance such as headgear to reinforce anchorage is effective in that the reactive forces that normally create anchorage loss do not affect the dentition. However, these techniques require unconditional compliance; consequently, various intraoral appliances have been developed with minimal compliance demands. The need for maximal anchorage control in these intraoral appliances has also led to increased use of implants.

ANCHORAGE IN ORTHODONTICS

SKELETAL ANCHORAGE

Methods to reinforce anchorage use a selection of devices temporarily anchored in bone. The devices can be fixed to bone, osseointegrated or non-osseointegrated, and they can be located subperiosteally or endosteally.[3–11]

When direct skeletal anchorage is used, the forces needed for the desired tooth movements are applied directly to the device. This usually requires a more detailed biomechanical treatment plan than with indirect skeletal anchorage, where the teeth that act as reactive units are indirectly stabilized by the skeletal device via a wire or transpalatal arch. With indirect anchorage, the stability of the anchoring teeth also depends on the rigidity of the connecting units.

OSSEOINTEGRATED ANCHORAGE SYSTEMS

Dental implants are now routinely used for complex prosthetic restorations. The bone–implant contact is sufficiently stable to withstand the occlusal and the much lower orthodontic forces.[12] Conventional implants, however, require space in the dental arch and are most useful when combined orthodontic and prosthodontic treatment is required.[13] When patients have complete dentitions, alternative placements and designs for implantable devices to reinforce anchorage are needed, and various modifications have been designed. The Orthosystem implant (Institut Straumann, Basel, Switzerland) is one of the most documented (Fig. 3.1).[4,14,15] The Orthosystem implant is an endosseous titanium screw-type implant with a sandblasted, large-grit, acid-etched surface; the implant is usually placed in the palate or the retromolar area (see Figs. 7.2 and 7.3B).

The Onplant System (Nobel Biocare, Göteborg, Sweden)[3] is an osseointegrated anchorage system that is placed subperiosteally in the palate when vertical bone height is limited (Fig. 3.2). The Onplant is a titanium disc coated with a thin layer of hydroxyapatite to facilitate osseointegration (Fig. 3.3). Surgical placement and removal of an Onplant involves a larger area of the palate compared with an implant, and second-stage surgery is required to uncover it. All temporary osseointegrated anchorage devices need a healing period, usually 10–12 weeks, although a shorter healing period (e.g. 6 weeks) for palatal implants is possible.[16]

NON-OSSEOINTEGRATED ANCHORAGE SYSTEMS

Ideally, an implanted anchorage device should be easy to insert and remove, be inexpensive and preferably should be insertable by an orthodontist. Orthodontic miniscrew implants are derived from maxillofacial fixation techniques and rely on mechanical retention for anchorage, but their heads are specifically modified to engage orthodontic auxiliaries.[5,6] Osseointegration per se requires a healing period of 10–12 weeks, but studies with early loading have indicated that the presence of intermediate fibrous tissue does not compromise the clinical stability of the implant during treatment.[6,17] This has led to the use of miniscrew implants, which are easy to insert and remove by the orthodontist, are immediately loadable and are inexpensive compared with osseointegrated orthodontic implants or onplants. The Aarhus Anchorage System,[17] the Spider Screw,[8] the Abso-Anchor Micro Implant[7] and the IMTEC Ortho Implant[18] are some commercial examples. Their small diameter makes insertion between the roots of teeth fairly easy (Fig. 3.4); however, a sufficient diameter is more important than implant length for mechanical interlocking in bone. The complications of miniscrew implants are predominately the potential risk for iatrogenic root lesions and poor soft tissue response.

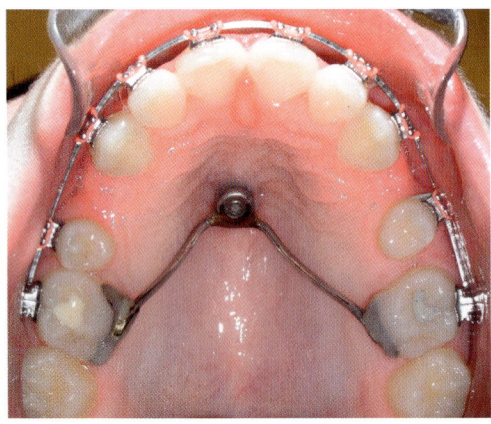

Fig. 3.1 The Orthosystem implant connected to the molars via a transpalatal bar (1.2 mm SS).

Fig. 3.2 The Onplant System connected to the molars via a transpalatal bar (1.3 mm SS).

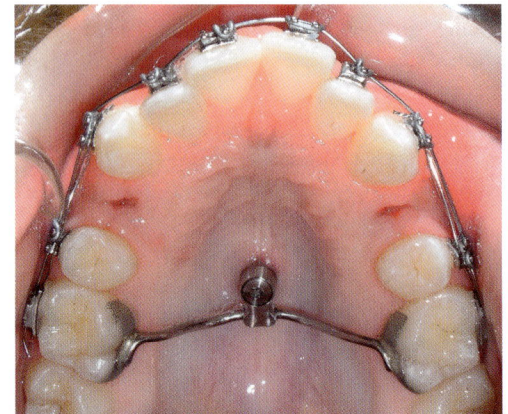

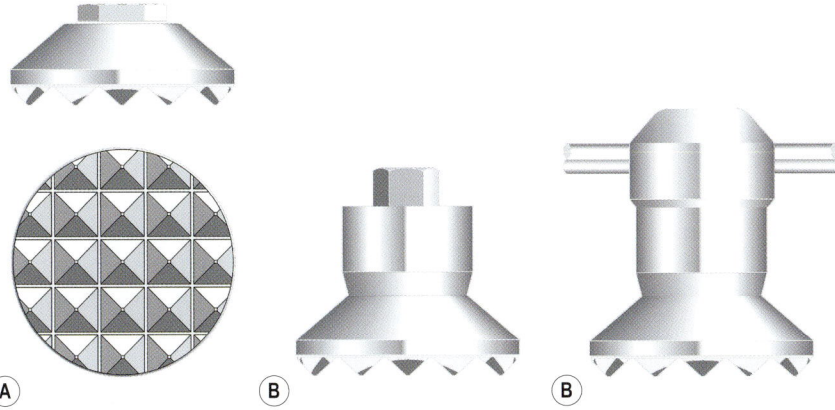

Fig. 3.3 (A) The Onplant disk with a diameter of 7.7 mm; (B) After a second-stage surgery where the disk is uncovered, an abutment is placed on top of the Onplant; (C) The suprastructure with a connecting transpalatal bar in place.

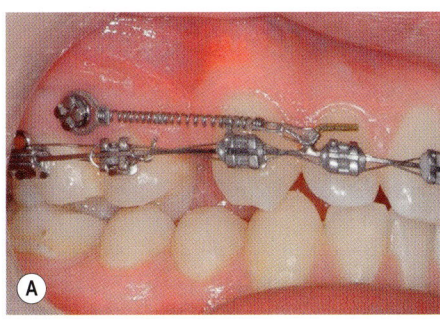
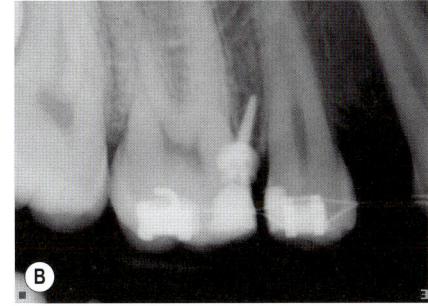

Fig. 3.4 The Spider Screw miniscrew implant. (A) Placement to reinforce anchorage during space closure after premolar extractions. (B) Radiograph showing placement between roots of maxillary first molar and second premolar.

In 1999, Umemori et al. introduced an orthodontic titanium miniplate system, the Skeletal Anchorage System,[9] for stable anchorage with immediate loading. Since then, other designs such as the OrthoAnchor System[10] (see Fig. 45.2D,E) and the Zygoma Anchorage System[11] (see Fig. 22.1) have been introduced. The advantage of these plates is that they are located away from the dentition and do not interfere with tooth movements (see Fig. 22.2C). However, placement of miniplates is far more invasive than placement of miniscrew implants, and infections can occur (see Chapter 13).[19]

OSSEOINTEGRATED VERSUS NON-OSSEOINTEGRATED SYSTEMS

Several studies have demonstrated that both the osseointegrated Ortho-system and Onplant systems are successful and suitable as absolute anchorage during space closure after premolar extractions.[15,20,21] Recent research has also demonstrated that both mini-implants and miniplates can withstand orthodontic forces and serve as anchorage in situations where anchorage is crucial.[22,23] Failure rates are, however, still higher than with osseointegrated implants and this must be taken into account when comparing studies that do not use an intention-to-treat approach.[24] Osseointegrated anchorage systems have the additional advantage of being stable in all three dimensions. Costs have not been considered in any comparative studies published but are certainly important since osseointegrated devices are more expensive to purchase and require surgical referrals. However, when treating patients with significant anchorage problems, the secure or absolute anchorage of the osseointegrated device is invaluable and may have benefits in terms of time efficiency for patients, parents and orthodontists. Osseointegrated implants also require a healing period, which delays application of orthodontic forces and increases the overall treatment time.

At present, there is no published study that compares osseointegrated implants with non-osseointegrated miniscrew implants or miniplates.

CONVENTIONAL ANCHORAGE

Headgear

One of the most traditionally used systems to reinforce anchorage is the headgear, which also has the advantage of being an active distalizing unit (Fig. 3.5). Patient compliance is essential and girls are known to cooperate better than boys.[21,25] Several studies comparing skeletal anchorage (both osseointegrated and non-osseointegrated) and headgear for molar anchorage during space closure after premolar extractions have found significantly larger anchorage loss with headgear.[20–23] Patients had a tendency to cooperate well with headgear during the first phase (leveling/aligning) but compliance decreased over time[21] and some patients do not cooperate at all.[21] Consequently, a treatment plan that involves headgear as an anchorage unit during the entire treatment must consider the possibility of anchorage loss.

In clinical trials, there is also the risk of the Hawthorne effect (positive bias), which means that subjects are more compliant because they know that they are a part of a trial and real life results may be less good. Consequently, headgear cannot be considered as suitable for orthodontic anchorage purposes where there are maximum needs for reinforced anchorage.

Transpalatal Bars and Arches

The transpalatal bar, which theoretically produces anchorage by blocking the maxillary first molars with a stable bar in combination with the pressure from the tongue, has been widely used in clinical orthodontics. Despite this, surprisingly few studies have examined its anchorage effect. The transpalatal bar is usually passive and so is fabricated as rigidly as possible. However, transpalatal arches can also be active and less rigid (Goshgarian design),[26,27] thus enabling tooth movements, for example derotation of teeth, correction of crossbites and torquing of the maxillary molars (Fig. 3.6).

Fig. 3.5 Headgear anchorage. (A) Occlusal and (B) lateral view of a headgear with a force of about 400 g and a direction corresponding to medium pull.

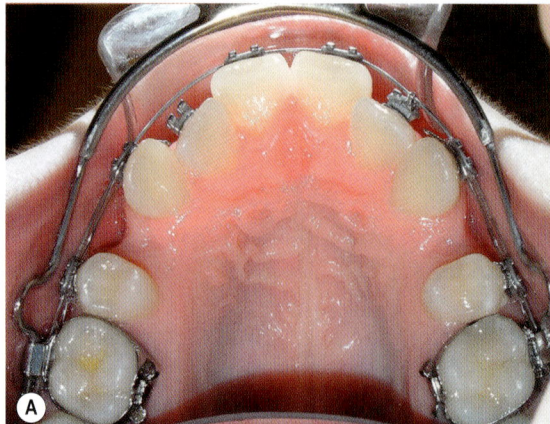
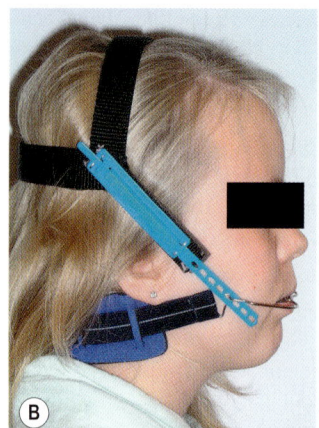

Fig. 3.6 Occlusal view of transpalatal bars. (A) A passive bar. (B) An active transpalatal arch with Goshgarian design.

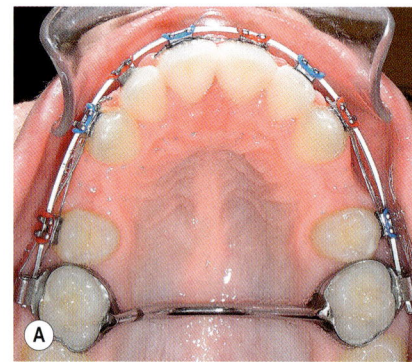
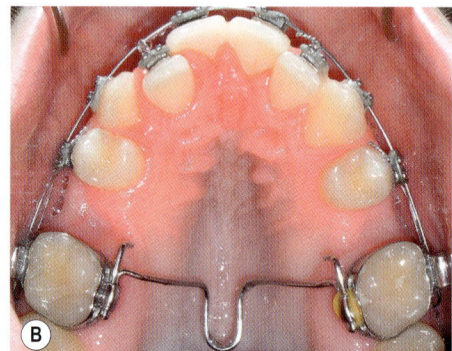

A randomized controlled trial (RCT) compared the anchorage capacity of a transpalatal bar with osseointegrated skeletal anchorage with the Orthosystem implant or the Onplant System. Both the osseointegrated systems were stable during treatment but the transpalatal bar demonstrated large anchorage loss along with mesial molar tipping.[21] The transpalatal bar was a passive soldered bar (1.0 cm × 2.0 cm) positioned 2 mm from the palatal mucosa at the midpalatal surface of the maxillary first molars. The ratio of anchorage loss to active movement was 0.54 for the total observation period. Similar results have been presented in studies when canines were retracted after premolar extractions, but bar designs and dimensions were all different. Comparison with other studies without reinforced anchorage on the molars indicates that the transpalatal bar had some anchoring effects, although substantially less than expected. A retrospective study concluded that a transpalatal arch (Goshgarian design) had no anchoring effect in anteroposterior direction;[28] a finite element analysis of stress-related molar response to a transpalatal bar concluded that the bar decreased molar rotation, had no effect on molar tipping and was insufficient as a sagittal anchorage device.[29]

In addition, a study of tongue pressure on the loop of a transpalatal arch during deglutition revealed that the pressure was highest if the transpalatal bar was positioned further back at the level of the second molars and was 4–6 mm from the palatal mucosa.[27] This suggests that an alternative design for the bar might increase its anchorage capacity.

Based on these studies, the use of transpalatal bars or arches should be restricted to situations where there are moderate to minimum needs of anchorage reinforcement.

Fig. 3.7 Maxillary molar distalization with an Onplant bar.

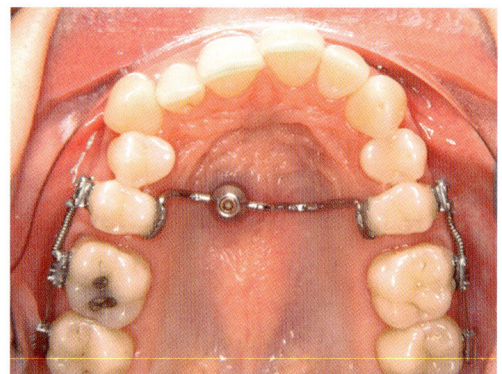

anchorage loss in the molar region. Both approaches require anchorage and for both implants may be useful.

Although extraoral devices, such as the headgear, are most commonly used to reinforce anchorage in Class II treatment or to distalize the molars to a Class I molar relationship, the problem of patient compliance has led to the development of a number of non-compliance appliances, for example the Jones Jig, Distal Jet, Pendulum appliances, Keles Slider, repelling magnets and compressed coil springs.[30–32] These methods, however, have side effects that reduce their clinical effectiveness, such as anchorage loss in terms of mesial movement and proclination of the maxillary anterior teeth. Consequently, skeletal anchorage is considered useful as anchorage when molars are distalized (Fig. 3.7).

ANCHORAGE IN CLASS II TREATMENT

A Class II malocclusion is commonly corrected by either a non-extraction approach with molar distalization to establish a Class I molar relationship, premolar extraction followed by space closure, with potential risk for

EVIDENCE-BASED DECISIONS

The RCT is the gold standard study design for evaluation in an evidence-based approach; this is followed by controlled trials, trials without controls, case series, case reports and, finally, expert opinions. Randomization ensures that confounders and both known and unknown determinants of outcome are evenly distributed between groups. Differences in estimated magnitude of treatment effects are common when RCTs are compared with non-randomized prospective studies.[33–35] However, the RCT is not appropriate to answer all questions and ethical issues can arise, particularly if untreated controls with malocclusions are used over a long period. Consequently, well-designed prospective and retrospective studies can provide valuable evidence although careful analysis of their results is required.

Systematic reviews are helpful tools providing a comprehensive summary of the available evidence from scientific studies for practitioners. Often a quality analysis of the methodological soundness of the selected studies is included in the review.[36]

Evidence-based decision making combines the best available scientific evidence with clinical experience and can minimize the risk of ineffective treatment methods and variation in treatment care and outcome. However, patient preferences must be given full consideration, and this is often neglected in comparative studies.

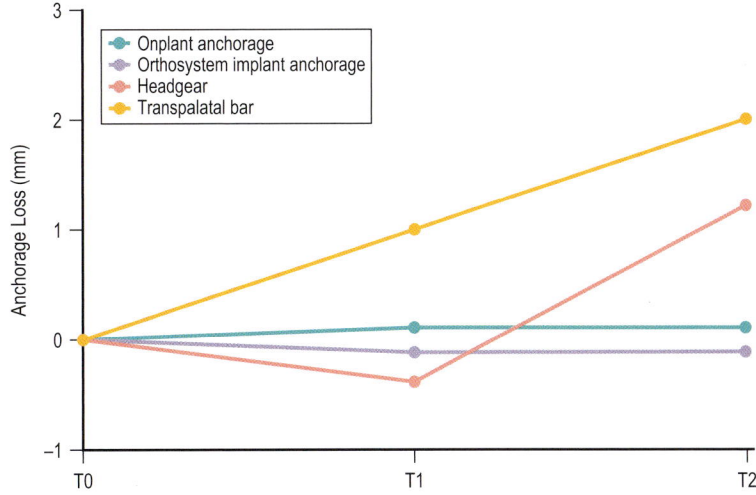

Fig. 3.8 Maxillary first molar movements (anchorage loss) from baseline (T0) during leveling/aligning (T1, mean 8.2 months) and space closure (T2, mean 17.4 months) after premolar extraction using four different anchorage systems.

EVIDENCE AND ANCHORAGE

To date several studies have been published concerning different anchorage systems dealing with application, function or effectiveness issues. In evaluating results and clinical relevance, a critical approach to the evidence is recommended.

A systematic review[37,38] examined orthodontic anchorage systems/application for the effectiveness of anchorage and the quality of the evidence for conclusions. The review surveyed papers in the Medline database and the Cochrane Collaboration Oral Health Group Database of Clinical Trials for the period from January 1966 to July 2007. The search identified 751 articles, but retained only 25 as meriting final evaluation; these included RCTs and prospective and retrospective studies with a control group. Quality assessment used a modification of the method described by Antcak et al.[33] and Jadad et al.[39] that assessed studies as being low, medium or high quality based on a point system. Only RCTs could be categorized as high-quality studies according to this system.

Since July 2007, several new articles have been published about anchorage and this systematic review has been updated for the purpose of this chapter to December 2010, but only to include RCTs. Two main anchorage situations were investigated in the original articles of the review: (a) anchorage of molars during space closure after premolar extractions and (b) anchorage in the incisor/premolar region during molar distalization. Both are applicable for Class II treatment. Summarized data from the original and updated review resulted in nine RCTs. Five of them evaluated anchorage loss during space closure after premolar extraction (Table 3.1),[20–22,40,41] and four evaluated molar distalization (Table 3.2).[32,34,42,43]

ANCHORAGE OF MOLARS DURING SPACE CLOSURE

Table 3.1 summarizes the results from the five relevant RCTs.[20–22,40,41] Two compared anchorage of molars during leveling/aligning with or without laceback ligatures and presented conflicting results. Usmani et al.[40] demonstrated no difference in anchorage loss of molars during leveling the maxillary dental arch with or without laceback ligatures while Irvine et al.[41] demonstrated a significant larger anchorage loss when laceback ligatures were used for leveling the mandibular dental arch.

Three studies compared skeletal anchorage with conventional anchorage (Table 3.1). Benson et al.[20] found no significant difference in anchorage loss of molars from treatment start to the end of space closure between Orthosystem implant anchorage and headgear. In contrast, Feldmann and Bondemark[21] found that the Onplant and Orthosystem were significantly superior to headgear or transpalatal bar (Fig. 3.8). Upadhyay et al.[22]

reported significantly less anchorage loss with mini-implants compared with conventional anchorage, such as headgear, transpalatal bars, banding of the second molars and application of differential moments. These studies suggest that skeletal anchorage is superior to conventional anchorage; however, other factors, such as failure rates, load deflection of the connecting units and cost-effectiveness, must be considered when making recommendations.

ANCHORAGE DURING DISTAL MOVEMENT OF MOLARS

Four RCTs assessed anchorage loss measured at premolars or incisors, which varied between 0.2 mm and 1.6 mm (Table 3.2).[32,34,42,43] In two RCTs,[34,42] intraoral appliances were compared with headgear and both showed a gain in anchorage in the headgear groups during the observation period. The third RCT compared the First Class Appliance with an untreated control group[43] and revealed some forward movement of the incisors in the control group although the observation period was short. As most orthodontic studies are performed on growing patients, anchorage loss can also be influenced by growth effects and, therefore, use of matched control groups becomes essential. The fourth RCT compared a removable plate with a Jones Jig/Nance appliance and showed no significant difference in anchorage capacity.[32] None of these four studies evaluated any skeletal anchorage.

Conclusions

The systematic review was based on 1408 papers from 1966 to December 2010. Only RCTs were considered for assessment, in total nine studies, all published since 2002, covering the two main anchorage approaches discussed above. The main weaknesses were small sample sizes, inadequate selection description plus a lack of blinding during measurements. It is clear that there is still a need for well-conducted RCTs with sufficient sample sizes in order to provide clear recommendations for anchorage preparation.

EVIDENCE COMPARING SKELETAL AND CONVENTIONAL ANCHORAGE

While it is generally accepted that osseointegration of implants is sufficiently stable to withstand both occlusal and orthodontic forces, it is

Table 3.1 Randomized controlled trials of anchorage loss during space closure after premolar extraction[a]

Study	Participants	Treatment time	Active unit	Anchorage unit	Outcome	Anchorage loss/active movement	Conclusions
Usmani et al. (2002)[40]	22 girls, 13 boys (13.7 ± 1.8 years) I: 16 II: 19	Unknown	I: leveling with laceback ligatures II: leveling without laceback ligatures		Analysis of upper molar and incisor position measured on study casts before and after leveling	I: 0.49 mm/0.5 mm II: 0.5 mm/−0.36 mm	No significant difference in anchorage loss with or without lacebacks
Irvine et al. (2004)[41]	13.7 years I: 18 girls, 12 boys II: 18 girls, 14 boys	6 months	I: leveling with laceback ligature II: leveling without laceback ligature	No auxiliary anchorage unit present	Cephalometric analysis of molar and incisor position before and after leveling	I: 0.75 mm/0.53 mm II: −0.08 mm/0.44 mm	Significantly larger anchorage loss with lacebacks
Benson et al. (2007)[20]	I: 18 girls, 7 boys (14.8 years) II: 20 girls, 6 boys (15.7 years)	Unknown	Lacebacks and Ni-Ti closing springs	I: midpalatal implant with a transpalatal bar II: headgear	Cephalometric analysis of maxillary molar and incisor position before treatment and after space closure	I: 1.5 mm/2.1 mm II: 3.0 mm/0.7 mm	No significant difference between midpalatal implant anchorage and headgear
Feldmann and Bondemark (2008)[21]	I: 14 girls, 15 boys (14.0 years) II: 15 girls, 15 boys (14.6 years) III: 15 girls, 15 boys (14.0 years) IV: 15 girls, 14 boys (14.4 years)	I: 17.1 months II: 16.6 months III: 17.3 months IV: 18.8 months	I, II: lacebacks and tiebacks	I: Onplant anchorage II: Orthosystem anchorage III: headgear IV: transpalatal bar	Cephalometric analysis of maxillary molar and incisor position before treatment and after space closure	I: 0.1 mm/3.9 mm II: −0.1 mm/4.7 mm III: 1.2 mm/4.8 mm IV: 2.0 mm/3.3 mm	Stable anchorage was provided with the Onplant and Orthosystem implant compared with headgear and transpalatal bar
Upadhyay et al. (2008)[22]	I: 18 (17.6 years) II: 18 (17.3 years)	I: 8.6 months II: 9.9 months	I,II: Ni-Ti closing springs	I: mini-implants II: conventional anchorage	Cephalometric analysis of maxillary molar and incisor position before and after space closure	I: −0.78 mm/7.22 mm II: 3.22 mm/6.33 mm	Mini-implants provided absolute anchorage

[a]All five studies were assessed as high quality.

Table 3.2 Randomized controlled trials of anchorage loss during molar distalization[a]

Study	Participants	Treatment time	Active unit/ anchorage unit	Outcome measurement	Anchorage loss/ active movement	Conclusions
Paul et al. (2002)[32]	16 girls, 7 boys I: 12 individuals (13.5 years) II: 11 individuals (14.8 years)	6 months	I: upper removable appliance II: Jones Jig /Nance appliance	Analysis of upper premolar and first molar position measured on study casts	I: 0.18 mm/1.3 mm II: 0.18 mm/1.17 mm	No significant difference in anchorage loss between the two groups
Bondemark and Karlsson (2005)[42]	I: 10 girls, 10 boys (11.4 years) II: 10 girls, 10 boys (11.5 years)	I: 5.2 months II: 6.4 months	I: intraoral appliance II: headgear	Cephalometric analysis of maxillary first molars and incisor position	I: 1.6 mm/2.2 mm II: −0.3 mm/1.0 mm	Intraoral appliance more effective to distalize molars but with anchorage loss
Papadopoulos et al. (2010)[43]	I: 7 girls, 8 boys (7.6–10.8 years) II: 6 girls, 5 boys (7.1–11.9 years)	I: 17.2 weeks II: 22 weeks	I: First Class Appliance II: Untreated control group	Cephalometric analysis of maxillary first molar, premolar and incisor position; analysis of upper first molar, premolar and incisor position measured on study casts	I: 1.6 mm/4.0 mm II: 0.28 mm/−0.04 mm	First Class Appliance efficient to distalize molars in mixed dentition but associated with anchorage loss
Acar et al. (2010)[34]	I: 7 girls, 8 boys (15.0 years) II: 10 girls, 5 boys (14.2 years)	I,II: 12 weeks	I: Pendulum appliance K-loop combination II: headgear	Cephalometric analysis of maxillary first molars and incisor position	I: 0.33 mm/4.53 mm II: −1.57 mm/2.23 mm	Anchorage loss with a Pendulum appliance K-loop combination was significantly decreased

[a]The studies by Paul et al.[32] and Acar et al.[34] were assessed as medium quality and the other two as high quality.

important to demonstrate that the benefits of skeletal anchorage are made use of in a clinical situation. There will always be implants that fail to osseointegrate or become loose later during treatment, and in an intention-to-treat approach these will be presented as anchorage loss. In studies where implants are used as indirect anchorage (e.g. connection via a trans-palatal bar), it is also important to remember that success rates depend on the rigidity and stability of the bar as well as on implant stability. An in vitro study on permanent deformation of transpalatal arches connected with palatal implants concluded that stainless steel arches with dimensions from 0.8 mm × 0.8 mm to 1.2 mm × 1.2 mm underwent deformation at a force of 500 cN.[44] Moreover, it is important to recognize that deflection of the bar rises in proportion to increased force application and that anchorage needs should determine bar dimensions.

Nevertheless, a recent meta-analysis evaluating the clinical effectiveness of miniscrew implants for anchorage reinforcement compared with conventional orthodontic means showed a mean difference in anchorage loss between the implant and conventional groups of 2.4 mm (95% confidence interval, 2.9–1.8; $p = 0.000$), indicating that MIs were more effective as anchorage supporting devices since they significantly decreased or negated loss of anchorage.[45]

When new methods or techniques are introduced, it is important to compare them with conventional procedures using a clear definition of ideal anchorage; for example, an ideal anchorage could be described as: simple to use, providing clinically equivalent or superior results when compared with traditionally anchorage systems, inexpensive and without the need for patient compliance.

PAIN AND DISCOMFORT

For all new treatment methods, particularly if surgical procedures are involved, it is necessary to explore acceptability to the patients and issues such as pain. Pain has been reported to be patients' major concern during orthodontic treatment, and studies on adults and adolescents reveal that 95% of patients reported pain experiences during such treatment.[46] Pain perception is subjective and not merely related to the strength of the pain stimulus, perception being also influenced by emotional, cognitive, environmental, and cultural factors. It has, for example, been shown that elevated anxiety levels increase pain reports while high motivation for orthodontic treatment reduces pain reports.[47]

One study has examined patients' experience of surgical placement of an Onplant or an Orthosystem implant compared with experiences of premolar extraction.[48] Since orthodontic treatment often combines these, the comparison is particularly valuable. The conclusions in terms of pain intensity were that the Onplant installation was comparable to premolar extraction but installation of the Orthosystem implant was better tolerated. Indications for the two osseointegrated anchorage systems are the same, and both surgical procedures are simple and take about 10 minutes to perform. One explanation for the higher pain intensity and discomfort reported in the Onplant group is that Onplant installation involves a larger surgical area than the Orthosystem implant. This agrees with a comparative study of surgical placement of miniscrew implants and miniplates, where patients complained more about pain and discomfort after procedures involving mucoperiosteal incision or flap surgery than about procedures that did not.[19] Overall, the surgical placement of the osseointegrated devices was well tolerated by patients.[49]

It is also important to assess patients' experience of skeletal anchorage devices throughout the whole treatment period, from baseline to the end of treatment, and compare it with conventional anchorage systems. In a recent study, perception of pain, discomfort and jaw function impairment were compared between patients with osseointegrated anchorage systems (Orthosystem implant and Onplant) and patients treated with conventional anchorage (headgear or transpalatal bars).[50] The conclusion was that there were very few significant differences between patients' perceptions of skeletal and conventional anchorage systems. All four anchorage systems were connected to the maxillary molars, which were the sites with the second highest levels of pain over time. There was significantly less pain intensity the first 4 days in treatment for the skeletal anchorage groups compared with the transpalatal bar group, but with no significant difference compared with the headgear group. Consequently, skeletal anchorage is well accepted by patients in a long time perspective, and can, therefore, be recommended.

REFERENCES

1. Proffit WR, Fields HWJ. Reorganisation of the periodontal and gingival tissues. In: Proffit WR, Fields HW Jr, Sarver DM, editors. Contemporary Orthodontics. 4th ed. St. Louis, MO: Mosby; 2007. p. 618–19.
2. Ren Y, Maltha JC, Kuijpers-Jagtman AM. Optimum force magnitude for orthodontic tooth movement: a systematic literature review. Angle Orthod 2003;73:86–92.
3. Block MS, Hoffman DR. A new device for absolute anchorage for orthodontics. Am J Orthod Dentofacial Orthop 1995;107:251–8.
4. Wehrbein H, Glatzmaier J, Mundwiller U, et al. The Orthosystem: a new implant system for orthodontic anchorage in the palate. J Orofac Orthop 1996;57:142–53.
5. Kanomi R. Mini-implant for orthodontic anchorage. J Clin Orthod 1997;31:763–7.
6. Costa A, Raffainl M, Melsen B. Miniscrews as orthodontic anchorage: a preliminary report. Int J Adult Orthodon Orthognath Surg 1998;13:201–9.
7. Kyung HM, Park HS, Bae SM, et al. Development of orthodontic micro-implants for intraoral anchorage. J Clin Orthod 2003;37:321–8, quiz 314.
8. Maino BG, Bednar J, Pagin P, et al. The Spider Screw for skeletal anchorage. J Clin Orthod 2003;37:90–7.
9. Umemori M, Sugawara J, Mitani H, et al. Skeletal anchorage system for open-bite correction. Am J Orthod Dentofacial Orthop 1999;115:166–74.
10. Chung KR, Kim YS, Linton JL, et al. The miniplate with tube for skeletal anchorage. J Clin Orthod 2002;36:407–12.
11. De Clerck H, Geerinckx V, Siciliano S. The Zygoma Anchorage System. J Clin Orthod 2002;36:455–9.
12. Odman J, Lekholm U, Jemt T, et al. Osseointegrated implants as orthodontic anchorage in the treatment of partially edentulous adult patients. Eur J Orthod 1994;16:187–201.
13. Huang LH, Shotwell JL, Wang HL. Dental implants for orthodontic anchorage. Am J Orthod Dentofacial Orthop 2005;127:713–22.
14. Wehrbein H, Merz BR, Diedrich P, et al. The use of palatal implants for orthodontic anchorage. Design and clinical application of the Orthosystem. Clin Oral Implants Res 1996;7:410–16.
15. Wehrbein H, Feifel H, Diedrich P. Palatal implant anchorage reinforcement of posterior teeth: a prospective study. Am J Orthod Dentofacial Orthop 1999;116:678–86.
16. Crismani AG, Bernhart T, Schwarz K, et al. Ninety percent success in palatal implants loaded 1 week after placement: a clinical evaluation by resonance frequency analysis. Clin Oral Implants Res 2006;17:445–50.
17. Melsen B, Verna C. A rational approach to orthodontic anchorage. Prog Orthod 1999;1:10–22.
18. Herman RJ, Currier GF, Miyake A. Mini-implant anchorage for maxillary canine retraction: a pilot study. Am J Orthod Dentofacial Orthop 2006;130:228–35.
19. Kuroda S, Sugawara Y, Deguchi T, et al. Clinical use of miniscrew implants as orthodontic anchorage: success rates and postoperative discomfort. Am J Orthod Dentofacial Orthop 2007;131:9–15.
20. Benson PE, Tinsley D, O'Dwyer JJ, et al. Midpalatal implants vs. headgear for orthodontic anchorage: a randomized clinical trial: cephalometric results. Am J Orthod Dentofacial Orthop 2007;132:606–15.
21. Feldmann I, Bondemark L. Anchorage capacity of osseointegrated and conventional anchorage systems: a randomized controlled trial. Am J Orthod Dentofacial Orthop 2008;133:339.
22. Upadhyay M, Yadav S, Patil S. Mini-implant anchorage for en-masse retraction of maxillary anterior teeth: a clinical cephalometric study. Am J Orthod Dentofacial Orthop 2008;134:803–10.
23. Ma J, Wang L, Zhang W, et al. Comparative evaluation of micro-implant and headgear anchorage used with a pre-adjusted appliance system. Eur J Orthod 2008;30:283–7.
24. Wehrbein H, Gollner P. Miniscrews or palatal implants for skeletal anchorage in the maxilla: comparative aspects for decision making. World J Orthod 2008;9:63–73.
25. Cucalon A 3rd, Smith RJ. Relationship between compliance by adolescent orthodontic patients and performance on psychological tests. Angle Orthod 1990;60:107–14.
26. Baldini G, Luder HU. Influence of arch shape on the transverse effects of transpalatal arches of the Goshgarian type during application of buccal root torque. Am J Orthod 1982;81:202–8.

27. Chiba Y, Motoyoshi M, Namura S. Tongue pressure on loop of transpalatal arch during deglutition. Am J Orthod Dentofacial Orthop 2003;123:29–34.

28. Zablocki HL, McNamara JA Jr, Franchi L, et al. Effect of the transpalatal arch during extraction treatment. Am J Orthod Dentofacial Orthop 2008;133:852–60.

29. Bobak V, Christiansen RL, Hollister SJ, et al. Stress-related molar responses to the transpalatal arch: a finite element analysis. Am J Orthod Dentofacial Orthop 1997;112:512–18.

30. Kinzinger GS, Eren M, Diedrich PR. Treatment effects of intraoral appliances with conventional anchorage designs for non-compliance maxillary molar distalization: a literature review. Eur J Orthod 2008;30:558–71.

31. Patel MP, Janson G, Henriques JF, et al. Comparative distalization effects of Jones Jig and pendulum appliances. Am J Orthod Dentofacial Orthop 2009;135:336–42.

32. Paul LD, O'Brien KD, Mandall NA. Upper removable appliance or Jones Jig for distalizing first molars? A randomized clinical trial. Orthod Craniofac Res 2002;5: 238–42.

33. Antczak AA, Tang J, Chalmers TC. Quality assessment of randomized control trials in dental research. Part I. Methods. J Periodont Res 1986;21:305–14.

34. Acar AG, Gursoy S, Dincer M. Molar distalization with a pendulum appliance K-loop combination. Eur J Orthod 2010;32:459–65.

35. Chalmers TC, Smith H Jr, Blackburn B, et al. A method for assessing the quality of a randomized control trial. Control Clin Trials 1981;2:31–49.

36. Guyatt GH, Sackett DL, Sinclair JC, et al. Users' guides to the medical literature. IX. A method for grading health care recommendations. Evidence-Based Medicine Working Group. JAMA 1995;274:1800–4.

37. Feldmann I, Bondemark L. Orthodontic anchorage: a systematic review. Angle Orthod 2006;76:493–501.

38. Feldmann I. Orthodontic anchorage: evidence-based evaluation of anchorage capacity and patients' perceptions. Swed Dent J Suppl 2007;191:10–86.

39. Jadad AR, Moore RA, Carroll D, et al. Assessing the quality of reports of randomized clinical trials: is blinding necessary? Control Clin Trials 1996;17:1–12.

40. Usmani T, O'Brien KD, Worthington HV, et al. A randomized clinical trial to compare the effectiveness of canine lacebacks with reference to canine tip. J Orthod 2002;29: 281–6, discussion 277.

41. Irvine R, Power S, McDonald F. The effectiveness of laceback ligatures: a randomized controlled clinical trial. J Orthod 2004;31:303–11, discussion 300.

42. Bondemark L, Karlsson I. Extraoral vs. intraoral appliance for distal movement of maxillary first molars: a randomized controlled trial. Angle Orthod 2005;75: 699–706.

43. Papadopoulos MA, Melkos AB, Athanasiou AE. Noncompliance maxillary molar distalization with the first class appliance: a randomized controlled trial. Am J Orthod Dentofacial Orthop 2010;137:586, discussion 586–7.

44. Crismani AG, Celar AG, Burstone CJ, et al. Sagittal and vertical load-deflection and permanent deformation of transpalatal arches connected with palatal implants: an in-vitro study. Am J Orthod Dentofacial Orthop 2007;131:742–52.

45. Papadopoulos MA, Papageorgiou SN, Zogakis IP. Clinical effectiveness of orthodontic miniscrew implants: a meta-analysis. J Dent Res 2011;90:969–76.

46. Krishnan V. Orthodontic pain: from causes to management: a review. Eur J Orthod 2007;29:170–9.

47. Doll GM, Zentner A, Klages U, et al. Relationship between patient discomfort, appliance acceptance and compliance in orthodontic therapy. J Orofac Orthop 2000;61: 398–413.

48. Feldmann I, List T, Feldmann H, et al. Pain intensity and discomfort following surgical placement of orthodontic anchoring units and premolar extraction: a randomized controlled trial. Angle Orthod 2007;77:578–85.

49. Sandler J, Benson PE, Doyle P, et al. Palatal implants are a good alternative to headgear: a randomized trial. Am J Orthod Dentofacial Orthop 2008;133:51–7.

50. Feldmann I, List T, Bondemark L. Orthodontic anchoring techniques and its influence on pain, discomfort, and jaw function: a randomized controlled trial. Eur J Orthod 2012;34:102–8.

Biological principles and biomechanical considerations of implants, miniplates and miniscrew implants

4

Ioannis Polyzois, Gary Leonard and Philippos Synodinos

INTRODUCTION

Early attempts to use implants in dentistry had limited success as the implant surface became encapsulated in a fibrous layer which prevented direct bone–implant contact; as a result, there was a reliance on mechanical undercuts to achieve clinical stability. To overcome this problem biologically inert materials such as titanium and certain calcium phosphate ceramics were used, which allowed osseointegration.[1]

PRINCIPLES OF OSSEOINTEGRATION

Osseointegration involves the incorporation of a non-reactive foreign material into the structure of living bone (Fig. 4.1).[2] Histological analysis of implants, some of which had been in function for up to 5 years, has shown a direct bone–implant contact without intervening epithelium or fibrous tissue bone (Fig. 4.1B) and with extensive remodeling of cortical bone at the bone–implant interface. Within trabecular bone Brånemark described a "capsule-like" arrangement of bone adjacent to the implant in many instances. Where the marrow space bordered the surface of the implant, no inflammatory cells or other signs of tissue reaction were observed.[2] The histology of bone healing around endosseous dental implants is now well documented from prospective *in vivo* animal studies.[2–4]

Retrospective analysis of explanted dental implants removed for reasons other than failure of osseointegration (e.g. implant fracture, psychological causes, postmortem) have shown a similar picture in humans for the mature bone–implant interface.

Two studies examined clinically stable machined surface screw root-shaped (SRS) implants explanted from oral and non-oral sites. A retrospective analysis of 38 SRS implants explanted from 18 patients after functioning for 5–90 months showed sound histological evidence of successful osseointegration with intimate contact between implant and bone at an ultrastructural level.[5] A histological analysis of 30 machined surface SRS implants that had been in clinical function for at least 1 and up to a maximum of 16 years, retrieved from 17 patients, showed an average of 84.9% direct bone–implant contact and 81.8% average bone area in individual threads when measured at the cortical passage.[6] The authors suggested that "osseointegration" corresponds to 60% or more

bony contact and 70% or more bone filling of individual threads in the cortical passage.

A histological analysis of un-decalcified ground sections of explanted implants was performed under light microscopy for a large collection of endosseous root-shaped dental implants explanted from humans over a 30-year period.[7] The implants had all been in clinical function for at least a year and so were surrounded by mature bone and provided a picture of the equilibrium reached at the end of the peri-implant bone healing process. The implants included both SRS and plateau root-shaped (PRS) designs made of commercially pure titanium and a titanium alloy. A subset had a hydroxyapatite (HA) spray coating. While both SRS and PRS implants showed "maturity and load-bearing anatomical characteristics," there were differences in bone structure between the implant designs. Within the cortical bone, the SRS implants showed a narrow (<1 mm) zone of new Haversian bone that continued around the implant perimeter, within the non-cortical alveolar regions, and was backed by trabecular bone of varying density. This was consistent with the corticalization of cancellous bone around SRS implants.[8] In contrast, the PRS implants showed a semi-circular orientated mixed woven-to-Haversian type of bone between the plateaus with a centrally located vascular feature within this bone.[7] For the uncoated titanium PRS implants, the bone extending inside the plateaus did not always extend to the central shaft of the implant. Interestingly, this deficit was not present with the HA-coated PRS implants, which exhibited bone extending into and along the central shaft of the implant. The explanation offered was that calcium phosphates such as HA are avid protein absorbers and they may offer a more secure anchorage surface for the peri-implant blood clot and, as a result, improve osteoconduction.[7]

Based on these structural differences between the SRS and PRS peri-implant bone, Lemons suggested that bone healing and maturation differs for the two types mainly because of variation in the implant fit and shape within the osteotomy. He also suggested that the combination of different healing and structural characteristics could influence the biomechanical aspects of short- and long-term loading capacities of the implants.[7]

Another study examined the most dynamic period of peri-implant bone healing (first 3 months post-placement) in order to observe if bone healing is significantly different for PRS and SRS implants.[9] Development of secondary stability was similar for both designs but there was prominent woven bone (callus) in the bone-healing process around PRS implants (Fig. 4.2), which would make these less suitable for early loading.

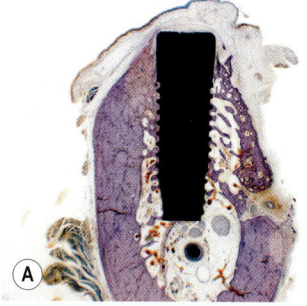
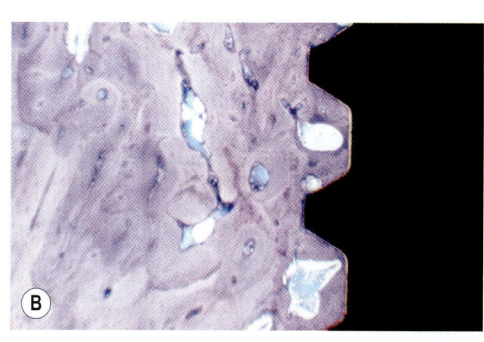

Fig. 4.1 Photomicrograph of a titanium screw root-shaped implant in a dog's mandible after 10 weeks of healing in low (A) and high (B) magnification. The ground section was surface stained with toluidine blue.

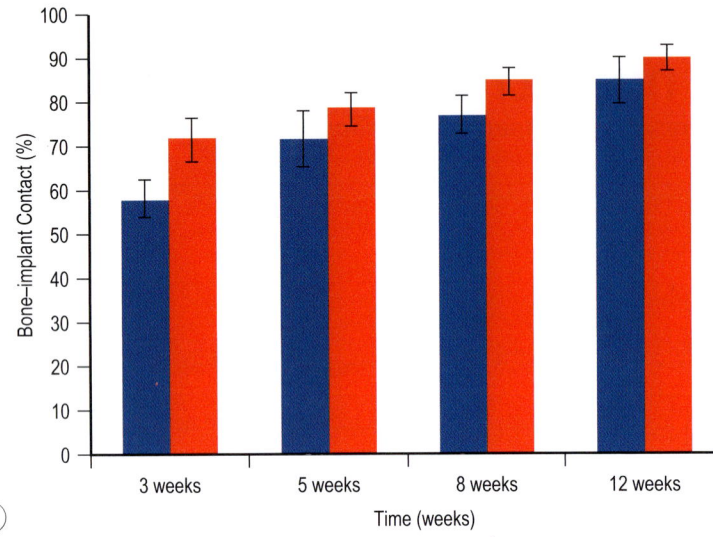

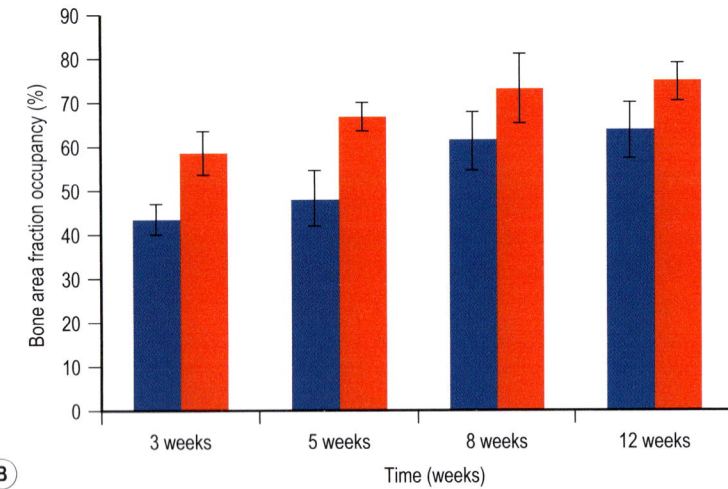

Fig. 4.2 Comparison of screw root-shaped (red) and plateau root-shaped (blue) implants after placement: bone-implant contact (A) and bone area fraction occupancy (B) over time. (Adapted from Leonard et al., 2009[9].)

ULTRASTRUCTURAL ANALYSIS OF PERI-IMPLANT BONE

Use of transmission electron microscopy has allowed a description of the intact bone–implant interface. An "amorphous layer" of ground substance bone–implant adjacent to a stable 10 nm thick titanium oxide layer on the implant surface was described 5–90 months after implant placement.[5] Examination of bone–implant surface in explanted SRS osseointegrated implants which had been in function for 1–16 years also showed that, in areas of direct mineralized bone-titanium contact, mineralized bone reached close to the implant surface but was separated by a non-calcified non-cellular amorphous layer.[10] This 100–400 nm thick amorphous layer was further delineated from the mineralized bone by a 50 nm thick electron-dense "lamina limitans."

The amorphous layer has been described as an extracellular "cement line matrix" consisting of two non-collagenous bone proteins, osteopontin and sialoprotein,[11] which may reflect a continuous process of interface remodeling.[12]

Some authors have suggested that the interface zone at HA-coated implant surface is unique in demonstrating a continuity of the mineral phase of forming bone and may form the basis of what has been described as HA implant–bone bonding.[13] However, scanning electron microscopy indicated that there was a very thin non-mineralized organic bone matrix resembling a reversal line of bone tissue at the implant–bone interface.[14]

In assessing all these ultrastructural studies of the bone–implant interface, it should be taken into consideration that the forces used for specimen cutting or grinding in slide preparation can affect the surface and make it difficult to determine the true nature of the interface.[14]

BONE-HEALING SEQUENCE OF EVENTS AND TIMESCALE

The osseointegration of endosseous dental implants involves a complex mix of both bone modeling (change in shape or size) and bone remodeling (internal turnover or replacement of bone). An understanding of the physiological sequence and timescale of these processes is a necessary starting point in understanding osseointegration.

BONE MODELING

Peri-implant bone modeling occurs through both appositional bone formation and intramembraneous ossification. Appositional bone formation involves the orderly deposition of new lamellar bone directly onto the surface of the old bone lining the osteotomy wall. This occurs at a relatively slow rate of 0.7–1 μm/day.[15] In contrast, intramembraneous ossification gives rise to new bone in a manner similar to bone healing in fractures. Woven bone (callus) forms in the blood clot that fills the gap at the bone–implant interface. The bridging callus of woven bone is formed rapidly, at 30–50 μm/day.[15] It is subsequently strengthened by lamellar bone formation on the porous lattice of woven bone. The intermediary mix of woven and lamellar bone is termed composite bone. The process of lamellar compaction ultimately culminates in the complete substitution of composite bone with load-bearing lamellar bone (bone remodeling). It has been suggested that the less precise bone–implant fit of certain implant designs encourages intramembraneous bone formation due to the larger peri-implant space available for blood clot formation.[16]

Evidence on bone remodeling around an implant has been contradictory. A study in dogs with porous-surfaced intramedullary orthopedic implants indicated that a fracture-healing process was occurring, with rapid cancellous bone ingrowth that could bridge a bone–implant gap of up to 1 mm.[17] However, a study in human knee replacement suggested that bone advanced appositionally at the bone–implant interface at a rate of 1 μm/day and that bone ingrowth did not occur when the bone was over 50 μm from the implant surface.[18] There is a strong body of animal histological evidence that bone modeling by means of fracture healing (woven bone) occurs where a blood clot forms in an osseous defect that is protected from epithelial/fibrous tissue ingrowth. This has also been demonstrated in healing extraction sockets, under membrane-protected bone defects and in large bone–implant interface gaps in dogs.[19,20]

Distance and Contact Osteogenesis

Peri-implant bone modeling has been examined by a number of researchers. Davies has described two different forms of peri-implant bone modeling: appositional bone formation and intramembraneous ossification (as seen in callus/fracture type healing).[11,21] He described the latter as "*de novo*" bone formation, which is dependent upon the initial formation of a hematoma in the gap at the initial bone–implant interface. The hematoma is soon replaced by a collagen-rich matrix. The subsequent recruitment and migration of osteogenic cells through this matrix he described as osteoconduction. Once the migrating osteogenic cells have reached their desired location, they become stationary osteoblasts and secrete an osteoid matrix, which is mineralized to form irregular woven bone.[11,21] This combination of "*osteoconduction*" and "*de novo*" bone formation can culminate in "*contact osteogenesis*": the formation of bone directly on to an implant surface at a distance from the old parent bone lining the osteotomy wall.[11] This theory relies on the assumption that the osteogenic stem cell migrates to the surface of the implant, differentiates into an osteoblast and then deposits bone directly on to the implant surface. The layer of new bone then separates the osteoblast from the implant surface, resulting in a very intimate bone–implant contact.

Surface modeling has also been described as occurring by means of appositional bone formation.[22] This involves the slow and synchronous secretion of more precisely organized lamellar bone on to the surface of old bone lining the osteotomy wall. It does not involve the migration of osteogenic cells across a matrix. Instead, an existing population of already differentiated osteoblasts that line the surface of the old bone secretes new bone that encroaches on the implant. As the polarized osteoblasts secrete bone matrix from their basal side, they passively recede towards the surface of the implant and eventually become trapped between the bone they are forming and the surface of the implant.[22] The authors surmise that the only possible outcome for these cells is death, and they use the term "*distance osteogenesis*" to describe this appositional process, which theoretically results in a less intimate bone–implant contact.[22]

The terminology has slowly become incorporated into the literature, with the terms "*distance osteogenesis*" and "*contact osteogenesis*" being used to describe, respectively, appositional bone formation on parent bone of the osteotomy wall and woven bone formation on the implant surface at a distance from the parent bone. Indirect evidence for contact osteogenesis is provided by ultrastructural studies of explanted implants showing a cement line matrix directly in contact with the implant surface.[5,10] This would be consistent with an osteoblast depositing bone directly on to the implant surface and subsequently becoming separated from the implant surface by the newly formed bone.

Since cortical healing relies predominantly on osteonal remodeling, the concept of bone modeling is more relevant to peri-implant bone healing in trabecular bone, which is capable of de novo bone formation and so would be better adapted to rapid healing than cortical bone.[21] This would be particularly relevant for Class III and Class IV bone. Modifications of implant design to optimize "*de novo*" bone formation could enhance implant stability in this environment, particularly since Class III and IV bone is often associated with insufficient cortex to provide stability.[21]

Two approaches have been used experimentally to facilitate "*de novo*" bone formation: cutting chambers into the implant to increase the contact-free surface available[20] and alteration of the surface design to enhance bone–implant bonding through micromechanical retention of the cement lines with the material surface.[21]

The latter approach is consistent with the move away from machined implant surfaces to macro-roughened (sandblasted and/or acid-etched) ones.[4,13,23] Implant surface technology has also progressed to encompass surface roughness at an ultrastructural level, as with ion beam-assisted deposition of thin-film HA coatings.[24]

In addition to surface topography, surface chemistry has also been assessed as a variable for peri-implant bone modeling. Surface wettability has been shown to enhance the interaction between the implant surface and the implant environment.[25] Storage of sandblasted/acid-etched implants in isotonic sodium chloride appeared to protect the titanium surface from carbonates and other atmospheric contaminants and to enhance surface hydrophilicity and wettability.[26]

Peri-implant Hematoma

The peri-implant blood clot has an important role in stimulating "*de novo*" bone formation. Its formation is affected by implant surface topography. Hemorrhage caused by the implantation process results in formation of a fibrin-rich clot that usually lasts only a few days before being replaced by

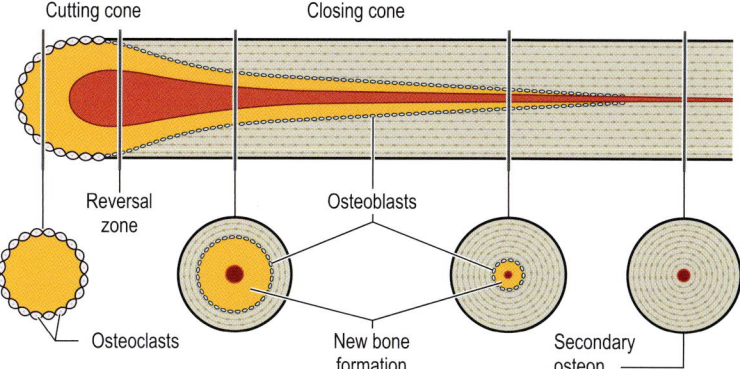

Fig. 4.3 Schematic representation of the evolution and completion of a secondary osteon.

granulation tissue. Platelet degranulation results in the conversion of fibrinogen to fibrin and in the release of cytokines and growth factors that have a stimulating effect on bone regeneration.[11,21,22] Surfaces with a greater microtopography have increased fibrinogen adsorption *in vitro*,[27] and higher forces are required to detach fibrin clots *in vitro* from acid-etched as opposed to machined implant surfaces.[22] Consequently, a roughened fibrin–implant interface may have a greater capacity to withstand the contractile forces generated by both clot retraction and the migration of osteogenic cells across the transitory matrix, thus enhancing "*de novo*" bone formation.

BONE REMODELING

Remodeling is the turnover or restructuring of previously existing bone by a coupled process of bone resorption followed by appositional deposition of ordered lamellar bone. Following implant placement, a 1 mm peri-implant zone of devitalized bone develops quickly around the implant, particularly in the cortical region, as a result of surgical trauma and pressure necrosis.[5] This devitalized interface bone must first be resorbed and then replaced. During this period, there will be a reduction in the primary stability of the implant. Interface remodeling is most pronounced during the initial bone-healing process following implant insertion. Once the peri-implant bone reaches full maturity and the implant persists in function, there is a less pronounced but continuous long-term remodeling process that maintains a necessary dynamic equilibrium of bone turnover.[12]

The basic multicellular unit for remodeling consists of an ordered collection of osteoclasts and osteoblasts. Osteoclasts, which are derived from monocytes in the bone marrow, resorb bone at the rate of 27–39 μm/day and open up a cavity, the cutting-filling cone, of approximately 120–180 μm in diameter and 1300 μm in length (Fig. 4.3). When the resorption cavity is complete, a reversal occurs and osteoclasts are replaced by osteoblasts in a brief quiescent period. Osteoblasts are derived from undifferentiated perivascular connective tissue cells, the pericytes, which slowly form appositional bone at a rate that varies between species (0.7 μm/day for humans). A central vascular supply within each cutting-filling cone persists after new bone apposition is complete. The resulting secondary osteon, a concentric lamellar structure, has a scalloped margin with a cement line that clearly demarcates new bone from old. Trabecular bone also undergoes remodeling but without the cutting-filling cone seen in cortical bone. Instead, the basic multicellular unit rests in a hollow, called a Howship lacuna, on the surface of the trabecular bone within the marrow cavity.

A study of enhanced remodeling at the bone–implant interface and in peri-implant-supporting bone indicated that remodeling is greatest in the bone adjacent to the bone–implant interface (within 1 mm), and that elevated remodeling (turnover >500% a year) is an ongoing and sustained response of bone adjacent to an implant.[12] Although this study had several experimental design weaknesses, including a highly diverse sample and a low number of specimens in certain groups, this histomorphometric pattern was identical in all specimens. The authors suggested that the ongoing process of elevated peri-implant remodeling is necessary to repair local areas of bone microdamage and fatigue-induced microdamage and, as such, it is essential to the successful maintenance of osseointegration.[12]

IMPLANT DESIGN

Ever since the formal acceptance of Brånemark's cylindrical threaded design by the American Dental Association in 1986, the SRS endosseous implant has become the pre-eminent morphology for endosseous dental implants, with published 10- and 15-year performance data.[28,29]

A large number of other implant designs (endosseous and non-endosseous) have been employed over the years. Non-endosseous implants, including subperiosteal, ramus frame and fiber mesh designs, are now largely obsolete. A variety of endosseous designs have been developed with widely varying morphologies, including non-root-shaped designs (e.g. the mandibular staple bone plate and the blade-vent implant systems), root-shaped designs (e.g. the vented hollow cylinder (basket), the combination screw and hollow cylinder, the non-threaded cylinder, the stepped cylinder) and PRS designs.[1,30] With the exception of the PRS design, most if not all of these systems have been surpassed by endosseous SRS implants. One problem with the early data on this wide variety of implants is that implant survival rates were often quoted as success rates.[30,31]

Endosseous dental implants were preceded by subperiosteal implants. These rigid plate-like devices, which were surgically placed on bone beneath the periosteum, were in common use up to the late 1980s.[1] There was a clear drop in outcome over longer assessment periods, with a success rate of only 60% after an average follow-up period of 3.3 years in one study[33] and survival rates at 5, 10 and 15 years of 90%, 60% and 50%, respectively, in another.[32] A comparative review of the literature[30] concluded that subperiosteal implants had "not survived the scrutiny of time and could not be recommended for routine clinical usage."

IMPLANT STABILITY

The precise interference fit between implant and bone is crucial for primary stability of the implant, and several studies have shown superior primary stability for the SRS dental implant.[34,35] As practitioners began to use single-staged procedures or immediate loading techniques, thread shape of the implant became of increasing importance. A study of 72 SRS implants placed into rabbit tibias with three different thread designs – V-shaped, square-shaped and reverse buttress – showed that the square-thread design had significantly greater bone–implant contact and reverse torque test strength at 12 weeks.[36] Unfortunately, implant stability at insertion was not measured as an assessment of baseline primary stability.

The PRS dental implant has reduced primary stability because its contact fit is only where the outer tips of the fins engage the osteotomy wall.[37] Consequenly, while PRS implants can be immediately temporized, the temporary PRS restoration must not be subjected to any immediate occlusal forces.[38] However, there are no published studies providing baseline primary stability values for PRS implants over the initial bone-healing period (1–12 weeks).

STRESS DISTRIBUTION

While SRS implants provide excellent primary stability, their stress distribution qualities have been a subject of debate. It is difficult to directly measure the load-bearing and stress-dissipation properties of dental implants in vivo. The development of computer-based finite element analysis (FEA) modeling has provided a means of analyzing the effects of implant external geometry on stress distribution within surrounding bone.[39] Such analysis showed that variations in the size and profile of the thread have a profound effect on the magnitude and distribution of stresses in the surrounding bone.[40] In particular, a small ratio of top radius of curvature to thread depth (sharp edges) should be avoided. This is consistent with retrieval studies that revealed bone defects mainly located at the thread tips.[30,41]

It has been suggested that PRS implants provide a more functional load-bearing surface for the efficient resistance and distribution of occlusal loads to the supporting bone.[42] An FEA study demonstrated lower compressive stresses around serrated dental implants because of their larger surface areas.[43] Stress concentration and distribution properties of SRS and PRS dental implants assessed by FEA have indicated that the enhanced stress distribution properties of PRS implants, with their greater surface area, rendered them more suitable to serve as free-standing implants.[44]

The principle of achieving better biomechanical stress distribution characteristics through greater surface area has been utilized in the Mark IV Brånemark SRS implants, which possess an increased thread surface area to enhance performance in Class IV bone.[8]

ORTHODONTIC USE OF DENTAL IMPLANTS

The use of conventional dental implants has extended from treatment of partially dentate adults to orthodontic treatments requiring minimal patient compliance. Implant-based anchorage allows unidirectional tooth movement without reciprocal action and it is also effective in treating adults with absent molars who are not compliant with conventional extraoral devices.[45] Performance of conventional implants as anchorage units for orthodontic treatment has been assessed over a number of years and the results suggest that they can remain stable when loaded with forces necessary for orthodontic tooth movement.[45]

Despite their reportedly excellent performance as anchorage devices, conventional implants have a significant diameter and are not always practical if there is a shortage of available bone and space. They also require several surgical stages, a waiting period of about 3 months for osseointegration before an orthodontic load can be applied and they cannot be placed in young growing patients. Furthermore, an additional surgical procedure is required for their removal following orthodontic treatment. To overcome these limitations, several orthodontic implant designs have been developed and tested over the years, with encouraging results.

TEMPORARY SKELETAL ANCHORAGE DEVICES

Temporary skeletal anchorage devices were introduced as an endosseous form of orthodontic anchorage. Although based on the same principles of structural and functional anchorage, there are substantial differences between these and conventional implants. Several designs have been introduced but currently only two are widely used in orthodontic treatment: miniscrew implants and miniplates. Excluding size, there are three main differences between these skeletal devices and conventional implants: temporary skeletal anchorage devices are loaded prior to osseointegration, they are intended to allow removal following completion of orthodontic treatment, and, finally, the forces applied are light and continuous compared with the high, non-continuous forces that are applied to conventional implants. Some concerns have emerged regarding the hard tissue reaction to these continuous forces and whether these can affect osseointegration. A small number of experimental studies have attempted to answer specific questions such as the amount of healing time necessary before loading and how easily these anchorage systems can be removed following orthodontic treatment.

Several animal studies have examined bone remodeling and miniscrew implant stability in implants with and without immediate loading. In one study, comparing loading immediately and at 6 or 12 weeks, 50% of implants failed through lack of primary stability. However, the overall mean osseointegration at 6 months was 74.48% and there were no significant differences between the groups. Additionally, the miniscrew implants could be easily removed after 6 months of loading, which was advantageous for orthodontic applications.[46] Other studies have shown similar results, with one study suggesting that loading may stimulate bone formation at the interface when loading does not not exceed a certain limit.[47] Overall, it appears that immediate loading with light orthodontic forces does not seem to have an adverse effect on osseointegration for both miniscrew implants and miniplates.[48–50]

CONCLUSIONS

The literature contains few well-controlled studies and the ones reported vary greatly in design; the species used; the anchorage devices, with different lengths and/or diameters; as well as in loading forces. This heterogeneity makes it difficult to draw firm conclusions for the best use of implants as anchorage devices in humans.

REFERENCES

1. Balkin BE. Implant dentistry: Historical overview with current perspective. J Dent Educ 1988;52:683–5.
2. Brånemark PI, Breine U, Adell R, et al. Intraosseous anchorage of dental prostheses. I. Experimental studies. Scand J Plast Reconstr Surg 1969;3:81–100.
3. Roberts WE, Smith RK, Zilberman Y, et al. Osseous adaptation to continuous loading of rigid endosseous implants. Am J Orthod 1984;86:95–111.
4. Buser D, Schenk RK, Steinemann S, et al. Influence of surface characteristics on bone integration of titanium implants: a histomorphometric study in miniature pigs. J Biomed Mater Res 1991;25:889–902.
5. Albrektsson T, Brånemark PI, Hansson HA, et al. Osseointegrated titanium implants: requirements for ensuring a long-lasting direct bone-to-implant anchorage in man. Acta Orthop Scand 1981;52:155–70.
6. Albrektsson T, Eriksson AR, Friberg B, et al. Histologic investigations on 33 retrieved Nobelpharma implants. Clin Mat 1993;12:1–9.
7. Lemons JE. Biocompatibility of implant materials. In: Proceedings of the 3rd Annual Indiana Conference. Indianapolis: Indiana School of Dentistry, Medical Education Resource Program; 2002. p. 79 89.
8. Sennerby L. Implant integration and stability. In: Palacci P, Ericsson I, editors. Esthetic implant dentistry. Berlin: Quintessence; 2001. p. 15–31.
9. Leonard G, Coehlo P, Polyzois I, et al. A study of the bone healing kinetics of plateau versus screw root design titanium dental implants. Clin Oral Implants Res 2009;20:232–9.
10. Sennerby L, Thomsen P, Ericson LE, et al. Structure of the bone–titanium interface in retrieved clinical dental implants. Clin Oral Implants Res 1991;2:103–11.
11. Davies JE. Mechanisms of endosseous integration. Int J Prosthodont 1998;11:391–401.
12. Garetto LP, Chen J, Parr JA, et al. Remodelling dynamics of bone supporting rigidly fixed titanium implants: a histomorphometric comparison in four species including humans. Implant Dent 1995;4:235–43.
13. Masuda T, Yliheikkilä PK, Felton DA, et al. Generalizations regarding the process and phenomenon of osseointegration. Part 1: In vivo studies. Int J Oral Maxillofac Implants 1998;13:17–29.
14. Piatelli A, Trisi P, Romasco N, et al. Histologic analysis of a screw implant retrieved from man: influence of early loading and primary stability. J Oral Implantol 1993;19:303–6.
15. Roberts WE, Garetto LP. Bone physiology and metabolism. In: Misch CE, editor. Contemporary implant dentistry. St. Louis, MO: Mosby; 1998. p. 225–39.
16. Lemons JE. Biomaterials, biomechanics, tissue healing and immediate function dental implants. J Oral Implantol 2004;30:318–24.
17. Bobyn JD, Pilliar RM, Cameron HU, et al. Osteogenic phenomena across endosteal bone-implant spaces with porous surfaced intramedullary implants. Acta Orthop Scand 1981;52:145–53.
18. Bloebaum RD, Bachus KN, Momberger NG, et al. Mineral apposition rates of human cancellous bone at the interface of porous coated implants. J Biomed Mat Res 1994;28:537–44.
19. Cardaropoli G, Araujo M, Lindhe J. Dynamics of bone tissue formation in tooth extraction sites: an experimental study in dogs. J Clin Periodontol 2003;30:809–18.
20. Berglundh T, Abrahamsson I, Lang K, et al. De novo alveolar bone formation adjacent to endosseous implants. Clin Oral Implants Res 2003;14:251–62.
21. Davies JE. Understanding peri-implant endosseous healing. J Dent Edu 2005;67:932–49.
22. Davies JE, Hosseini MM. Histodynamics of endosseous wound healing. In: Davies JE, editor. Bone engineering. Toronto: Em squared; 2000. p. 1–14.
23. Cochran DL, Schenk RK, Lussi A, et al. Bone response to unloaded and loaded titanium implants with a sandblasted and acid-etched surface: a histometric study in the canine mandible. J Biomed Mater Res 1998;40:1–11.
24. Coelho PG, Suzuki M. Evaluation of an IBAD thin-film process as an alternative method for surface incorporation of bioceramics on dental implants: a study in dogs. J Appl Oral Sci 2005;13(1):87–92.
25. Kipaldi DV, Lemons JE. Surface energy characterization of unalloyed titanium implants. J Biomed Mater Res 1994;28:1419–25.
26. Steinemann SG. Titanium – the material of choice? Periodontol 2000;17:7–21.
27. Park JY, Davies JE. Red blood cell and platelet interactions with titanium implant surfaces. Clin Oral Implants Res 2000;11:530–9.
28. Brånemark PI, Hansson BO, Adell R, et al. Osseointegrated implants in the treatment of the edentulous jaw: Experience from a 10-year period. Scand J Plast Reconstr Surg 1977;11(Suppl. 16):1–132.
29. Adell R, Lekholm U, Rockler B, et al. A 15 year study of osseointegrated implants in the treatment of the edentulous jaw. Int J Oral Surg 1981;10:387–416.
30. Albrektsson T, Sennerby L. State of the art in oral implants. J Clin Periodontol 1991;18:474–81.
31. Smith DE, Zarb GA. Criteria for success of osseointegrated endosseous implants. J Prosth Dent 1989;62:567–72.
32. Bodine RL, Yanase RT, Bodine A. Forty years of experience with subperiosteal implant dentures in 41 edentulous patients. J Prosthet Dent 1996;75:33–44.
33. Mercier P, Cholewa J, Djokovic S. Mandibular subperiosteal implants: retrospective analysis in light of Harvard consensus. J Can Dent Assoc 1981;47:46–51.
34. Carlsson L, Rostlund T, Albrektsson B, et al. Implant fixation improved by close fit: cylindrical implant-bone interface studied in rabbits. Acta Orthop Scand 1988;59:272–5.
35. Gotfredsen K, Nimb L, Hjörting-Hansen E, et al. Histomorphometric and removal torque analysis for TiO_2-blasted titanium implants: an experimental study on dogs. Clin Oral Implants Res 1992;3:77–84.
36. Steigenga J, Al-Shammari K, Misch C, et al. Effects of implant thread geometry on percentage of osseointegration and resistance to reverse torque in the tibia of rabbits. J Periodontol 2004;75:1233–41.
37. Chess JT. Technique for placement of root form implants of the finned or serrated type. J Am Dent Assoc 1990;121:414–17.
38. Bicon. Surgical manual: step by step techniques. Boston, MA: Bicon Dental Implants; 2010 <http://www.bicon.com/pdf/Bicon_Surgical.pdf>; [accessed 27 Ocotober 2013].
39. Bozkaya D, Muftu S, Muftu D. Evaluation of load transfer characteristics of five different implants in compact bone at different load levels by finite elements analysis. J Pros Dent 2004;92:523–30.
40. Hansson S, Werke M. The implant thread as a retention element in cortical bone: the effect of thread size and thread profile: a finite element study. J Biomech 2003;36:1247–58.
41. Tsuboi N, Tsuboi Y, Sennerby L, et al. Histomorphometric analysis of bone–titanium interface in human retrieved implants. In: Ueda M, editor. Proceedings of the Third International Congress on Tissue Integration in Oral and Maxillofacial Reconstruction. Tokyo: Quintessence; 1996. p. 86–7.
42. Morris HF, Ochi S. Survival and stability (PTVs) of six implant designs from placements to 36 months. Ann Periodontol 2000;5:15–21.
43. Lin S, Shi S, Le Geros RZ, et al. Three-dimensional finite element analyses of four designs of a high-strength silicon nitride implant. Implant Dent 2000;9:53–60.
44. Rieger MR, Fareed K, Adams WK, et al. Bone stress distribution for three endosseous implants. J Prosthet Dent 1989;61:223–8.
45. Janssen KI, Raghoebar M, Vissink A, Sandham A. Skeletal anchorage in orthodontics: a review of various systems in animal and human studies. Int J Oral Maxillofac Implants 2008;23:78–88.
46. van de Vannet B, Sabzevar MM, Wehrbein H, et al. Osseointegration of miniscrews: a histomorphometric evaluation. Eur J Orthod 2007;29:437–42.
47. Büchter A, Wiechmann D, Gaertner C, et al. Load-related bone modelling at the interface of orthodontic micro-implants. Clin Oral Implants Res 2006;17:714–22.
48. Luzi C, Calalberta V, Melsen B. Immediate loading of orthodontic mini-implants: a histomorphometric evaluation of tissue reaction. Eur J Orthod 2009;31:21–9.
49. Woods PW, Buschang PH, Owens SE, et al. The effect of force, timing and location on bone to implant contact of miniscrew implants. Eur J rthod 2009;31:232–40.
50. Cornelis MA, Mahy P, Devogelaer JP, et al. Does orthodontic loading influence bone mineral density around titanium miniplates? An experimental study in dogs. Orthod Craniofac Res 2010;13:21–7.

5 Biomaterial properties of orthodontic miniscrew implants

Spiros Zinelis, Youssef S. Al Jabbari, Moschos A. Papadopoulos, Theodore Eliades and George Eliades

INTRODUCTION

Although miniscrew implants (MIs) have been used in a broad spectrum of applications, few studies have explored their fundamental material properties such as strength, structure and design; surface properties; electrochemical behavior; and ion release.[1,2] Moreover, the clinical impact of these properties on pullout strength,[3] implant stability[4] and nature of the bone–implant interface[5] has not been systematically investigated, apart from some published data regarding failure rates of these devices.[6–8] This chapter reviews current information on the properties of orthodontic MIs discussing their possible clinical implications.

DESIGN PRINCIPLES

Commercially available contemporary MIs have significant differences in the design of the retentive head and the intraosseous components (Fig. 5.1). Although there is no official standard design, manufacturers have adopted various concepts in order to avoid clinical complications and achieve specific clinical goals. Some design principles from conventional dental implants have been retained, for example the need for primary and secondary stability. Primary stability relates to the implant diameter and its intraosseous design,[9–11] and secondary stability to the surface chemical composition and roughness of the implant.[12,13] Implant design is mainly characterized by the head and thread shapes and associated geometrical features, such as shaft type, thread face, helix angle and thread depth.[3]

The button-like head with spheroid or hexagonal shape is most common, although bracket-like and hook designs do occur. The head design is intended for the secure attachment of wires and spring coils while ensuring the best stress transfer distribution to the bone crest.

The intraosseous thread design is either conical with a small tapered end (Dual-Top and AbsoAnchor) or parallel (Spider Screw); there is also a hybrid design with conical and tapered shafts (Vector-TAS) (Fig. 5.1).

The great diversity in designs gives rise to variation in primary stability as assessed by a pullout strength test using artificial bone blocks that simulated osteoporotic and normal cancellous bone (Fig. 5.2).[3] The pullout force increased with higher intraosseous surface area with a weak correlation ($r = 0.54$) for the "osteoporotic" block and medium correlation ($r = 0.79$) for the "normal cancellous bone" block based on re-interpretation of previously published data[3] (Fig. 5.2). The variation in statistical correlation might reflect deviations in linearity or effects of other geometrical features such as thread number or thread face and helix angle, which were not taken into account. As yet, no mathematical model exists to correlate design parameters with the primary stability of MIs. This is an interesting field for further developments.

MATERIALS

Orthodontic MIs are mainly manufactured using commercially pure titanium (cp-Ti) (graded as I–IV, with decreasing purity towards higher grades) and a titanium, aluminum (6%) and vanadium (4%) alloy (Ti-6Al-4V; grade V) (Table 5.1). However, while grade V is the most commonly used form, the corresponding mechanical properties vary, as they are influenced by the content in trace elements and the thermomechanical history. Ti-6Al-4V is extensively used in aerospace (80% of annual production), medical (orthopedic artificial prostheses, 3%), marine and chemical industries because of its tailored properties, which can be adjusted by specific mechanical and heat treatments.[14] The alloy is supplied as Ti-6Al-4V or Ti-6Al-4VELI (extra low interstitials). The latter contains lower trace element content (O and Fe) and has improved ductility, fracture toughness and corrosion resistance. Typically, it is used without aging for maximum toughness.[14] The properties of Ti-6Al-4V are strongly modified by specific thermal treatments. As an alpha–beta alloy,

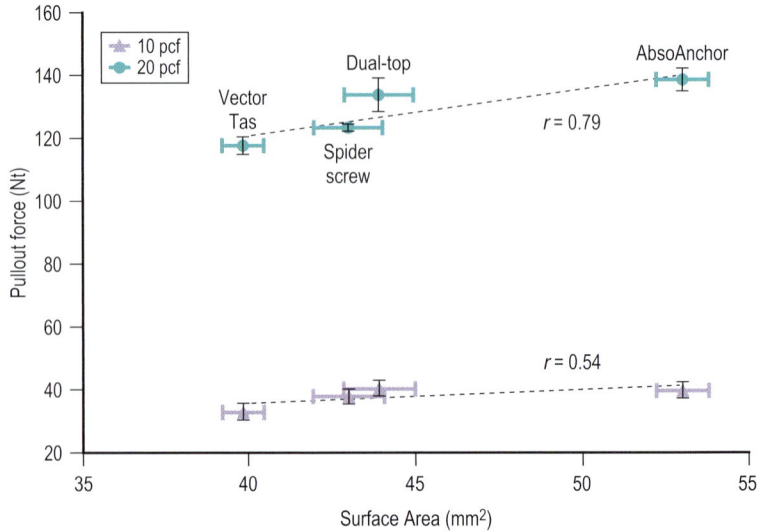

Fig. 5.2 Pullout strength with increasing surface area as measured in artificial bone blocks made of solid rigid polyurethane foam of 10 and 20 pcf (pounds per cubic inch) density, simulating osteoporotic and normal cancellous bone, respectively. The pullout force required increased with higher intraosseous surface area with a weak correlation ($r = 0.54$) for the 10 pcf block and a medium one ($r = 0.79$) for the 20 pcf block. Re-interpretation of published results.[3]

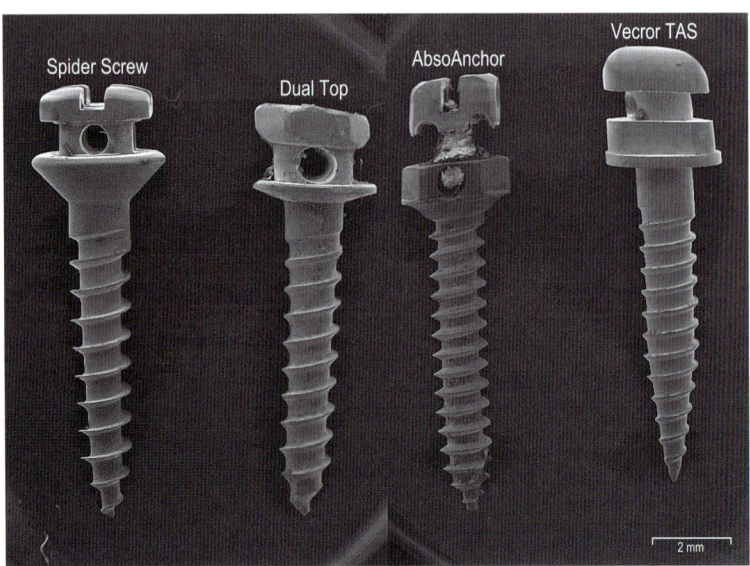

Fig. 5.1 Stereomicroscopic image of contemporary MIs (bar: 2mm).

Table 5.1 Nominal composition and mechanical properties of commercially pure titanium grades I–IV and Ti6-Al4-V alloy[a]

Grade	N	C	H	Fe	O	Ti	Al	V	Young modulus (GPa)	Yield strength (MPa)	Ultimate tensile strength (MPa)	Ultimate strain (%)
I	<0.03	<0.1	<0.015	<0.2	<0.18	Bal			102.7	170	240	24
II	<0.03	<0.1	<0.015	<0.2	<0.25	Bal			102.7	275	345	20
III	<0.05	<0.1	<0.015	<0.2	<0.35	Bal			103.4	380	450	18
IV	<0.05	<0.1	<0.015	<0.2	<0.40	Bal			104.1	485	550	25
V (Ti6-Al4-V)[b]	<0.05	<0.1	<0.015	<0.4	<0.20	Bal	5.5~6.75	3.5~4.5	105~116	711~904	856~911	6~36
Ti6-Al4-V-ELI	<0.05	<0.08	<0.012	<0.025	<0.13	Bal	5.5~6.75	3.5~4.5	114	795	860	10

Bal, balance; ELI, extra low interstitials.
[a]Additional information for small deviations among different standards can be found in the relevant references.[14]
[b]Mechanical properties of Ti-6Al4V are strongly dependent on previous thermomechanical treatment. The ranges shown in this table correspond to the minimum and maximum values the alloy can achieve after different thermomechanical treatments.
Source: from Boyer et al. (1994).[14]

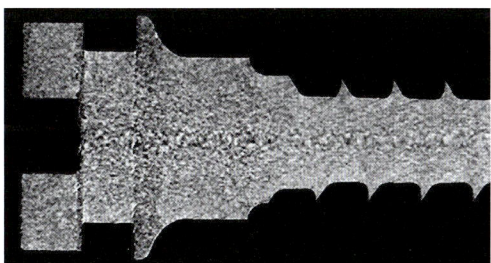

Fig. 5.3 A longitudinal 2D reconstruction obtained from a micro-XCT analysis of an unused MI. The section is free of pores, cracks or other defects.

it may demonstrate different contents of alpha (hexagonal lattice) and beta (face-centered cubic lattice) phases, with great variations in microstructure dependent on particular thermomechanical treatments. The different microstructures are classified as lamellar, equiaxial and bimodal (i.e. a mixture of both). More than seven types of thermomechanical treatments are used to modify the mechanical properties and most are well described in relevant literature.[14] Currently no information exists on the microstructure of MIs.

Apart from the stainless steel (SS) orthodontic MIs, all others are manufactured from cp-Ti grade IV or Ti-6Al-4V alloy.[3] It might be postulated that Ti-6Al-4V is more appropriate than cp-Ti because of its significantly higher mechanical properties, corrosion resistance and fabricability. The removal torque of cp-Ti approaches its yield strength during the removal process,[15] which would increase the risk of bulk fracture. Regarding the internal structure, computerized X ray microtomography (xCT) has shown no internal defects (cracks or pores) in the bulk structure of an unused commercially available MI (Fig. 5.3),[16] findings that were confirmed by cross-sectional analysis.

SURFACE CHARACTERIZATION

Osseointegration of orthodontic MIs is not a demanding task and so MI surface properties have not attracted great interest. Nonetheless, surface roughness and composition are the dominant factors for secondary stability as they influence the postsurgical cellular response. The results for the composition of the near surface region (~1 μm depth) obtained after energy dispersive X-ray microanalysis (EDX) are summarized in Table 5.2, while Fig. 5.4 shows representative EDX spectra obtained from MIs. The presence of Al and V are indicative of the alloy type, which is probably Ti-6Al-4V, while the presence of O should be attributed to surface

Table 5.2 Elemental composition of orthodontic microscrew implants (energy dispersive X-ray microanalysis)

Product	Atomic %					
	N	O	Al	P	Ti	V
AbsoAnchor	11.1	3.9	9.2	ND	73.3	2.4
Dual-Top	12.1	ND	9.0	ND	76.5	2.2
Spider Screw	8.3	4.2	7.5	ND	77.0	2.8
Vector-TAS	2.2	46.1	5.8	0.3	44.5	1.2
Thomas	6.9	6.2	8.5	ND	75.8	2.4
New Anchor Plus	9.9	2.9	9.4	ND	75.2	2.4

ND, not detected.
Source: from Alsamak et al. (2012)[3] and EDX unpublished data.

layer of TiO_2. Interestingly, Vector-TAS had a much higher O content than the other implants, which might be attributed to its much thicker yellow-colored TiO_2 layer. Morphological, compositional and optical surface modifications can be performed by various techniques, such as anodic oxidation,[17] plasma ion implantation,[18] or thermal oxidation.[19] However, the presence of P in this MI, a typical impurity of an anodizing solution, along with the increased O content, indicates that an anodic oxidation technique was used. The presence of N is sometimes reported as a raw material impurity and, along with C, is considered as a surface contaminant associated with the manufacturing procedure, storage and/or sterilization.[14] The presence of these surface contaminants makes the surface less hydrophilic,[20] adversely affecting cell-attachment capacity.[21] Surface analysis with X-ray photoelectron spectroscopy, with a sampling depth of approximately 3 nm, provides information on both elemental composition and the binding state of the elements (Fig. 5.5). Titanium is mainly identified as TiO_2, along with some Ti_2O_3 and metal Ti. Al and V were not identified with XPS analysis denoting that MI are fully covered by Ti oxides as in the case of pure Ti. The presence of C, and traces of Ca, Si and P were considered to be ambient or processing contamination.

Fig. 5.6 shows the surface texture of the treaded part of MIs as imaged in a scanning electron microscope with a backscattered electron detector. Miniscrew implants display parallel striations oriented almost vertically to the longitudinal implant axis, which are attributed to the turning manufacturing process. Differences in manufacturing process may explain difference in the inclination of these striations among the materials tested. This is also seen in the three-dimensional images shown in Fig. 5.7. Studies on several MI threads have disclosed no statistically significant differences in

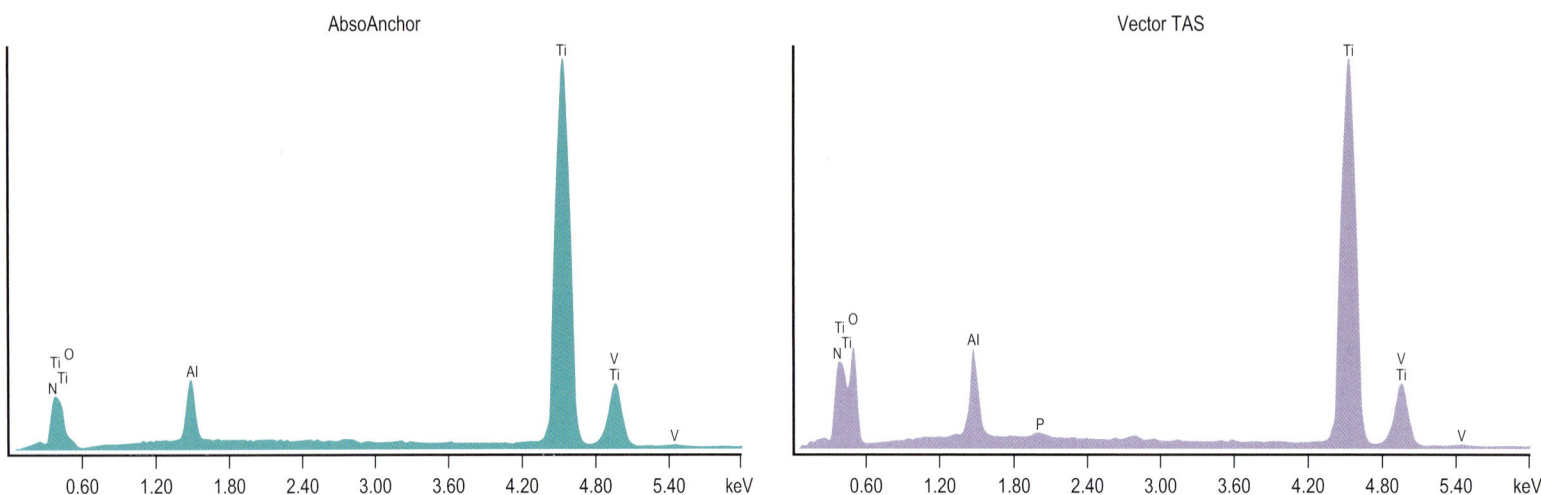

Fig. 5.4 Energy dispersive X-ray microanalysis spectra of two miniscrew implants.

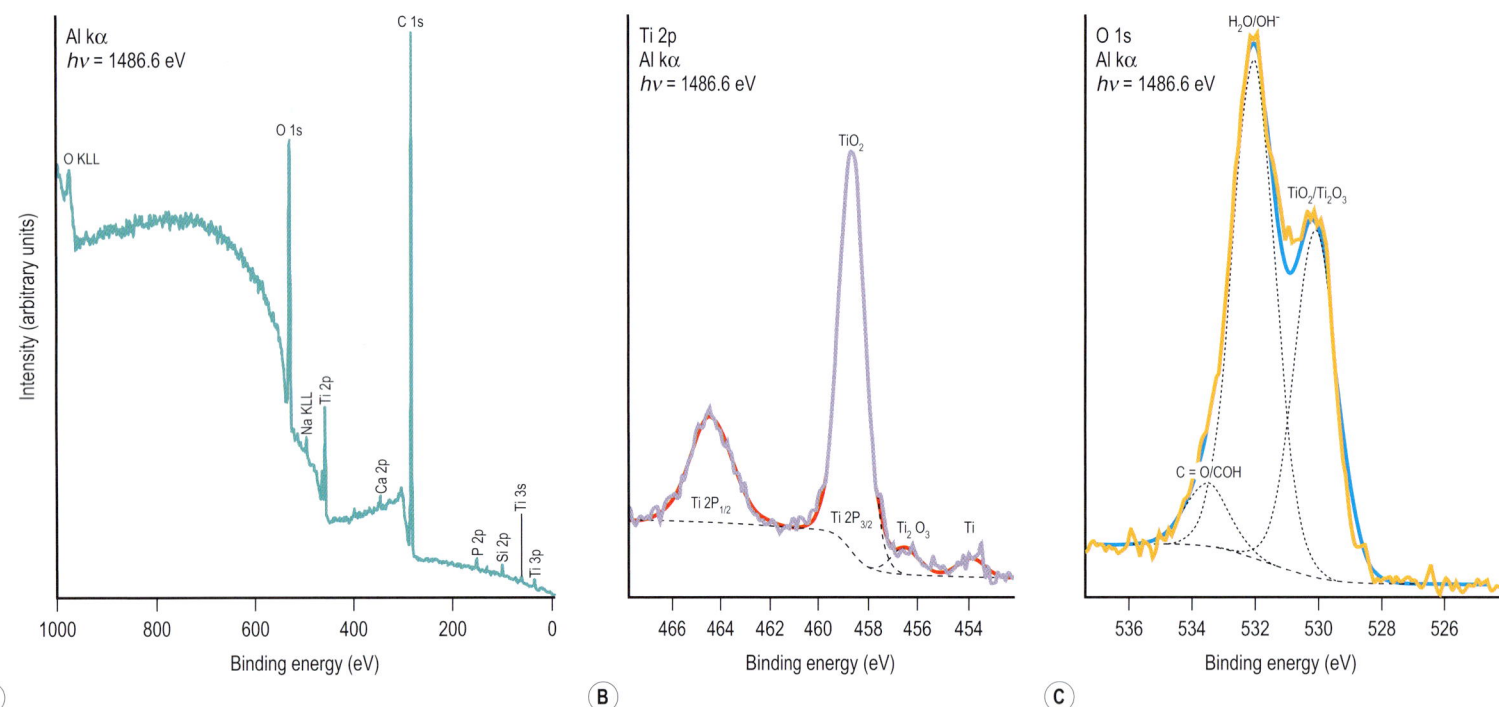

Fig. 5.5 X ray photoelectron spectroscopic analysis of AbsoAnchor minisrew implants. (A) Survey scan revealing the presence of Ti and C, N (ambient contamination), Ca, P and Si (processing contamination). (B,C) High resolution analysis after curve fitting of T12p (B) and O1s (C) peaks, with the corresponding elemental binding states.

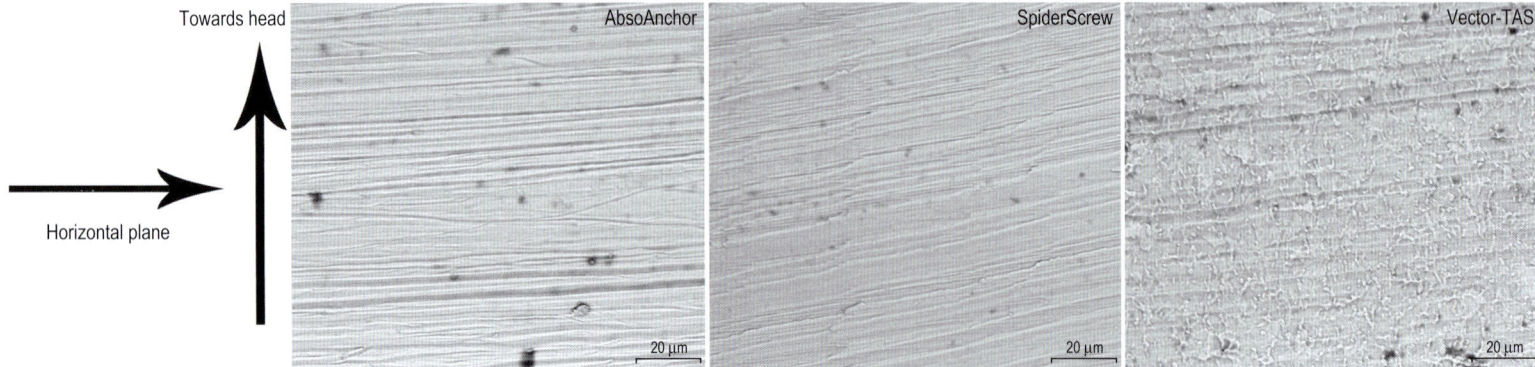

Fig. 5.6 Backscattered electron images of modern orthodontic miniscrew implants. Pictures were taken between two successive threads (nominal magnification ×1000, bar = 20 μm). The small black regions of low mean atomic number represent areas of contamination or manufacturing defects.

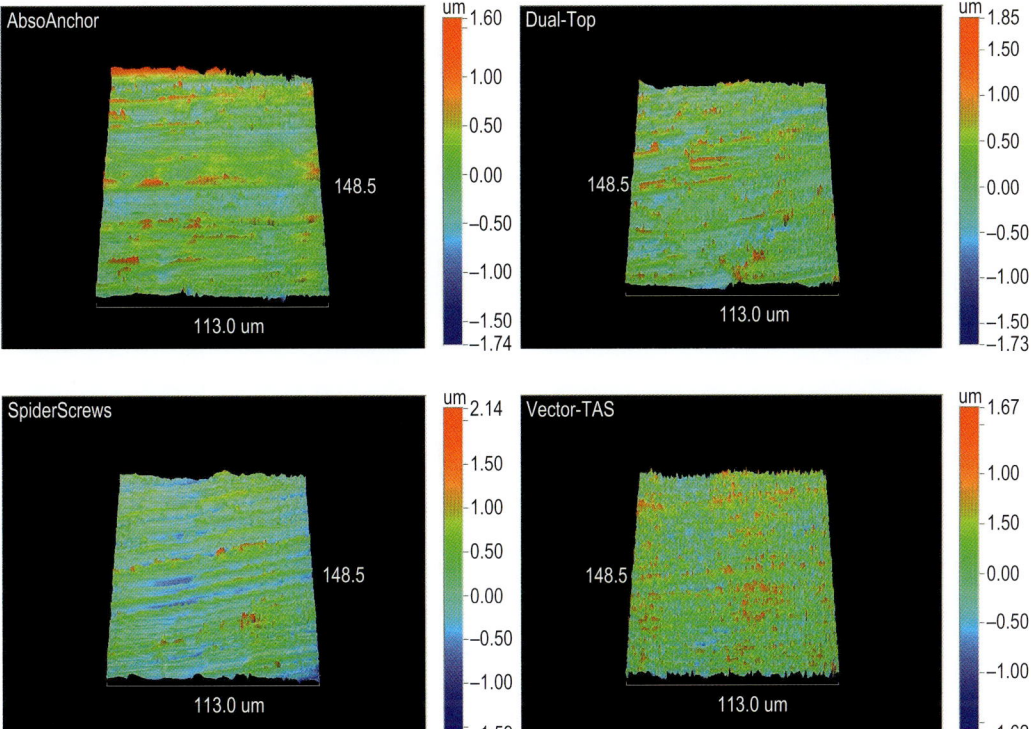

Fig. 5.7 Representative three-dimensional profilometric images from the threaded region of miniscrew implants taken between two successive threads. The orientation is the same as in Figure 5.6. The parallel serrations are profound, although with different inclination to the horizontal plane. (Original magnification ×41, sampling window, 113.0 μm × 148.5 μm.)

Table 5.3 Results of selected surface roughness parameters for microscrew implants using optical interferometric profilometry[3]

Product	S_a (nm)	S_z (μm)	S_{dr} (%)	S_{ds} (μm^{-2})	S_{ci} (%)
AbsoAnchor	258 ± 27	3.4 ± 0.5	8.4 ± 0.5	0.02	1.52 ± 0.03
Dual-Top	270 ± 36	3.3 ± 0.1	19.9 ± 1.4	0.02	1.60 ± 0.02
Spider Screw	330 ± 94	3.3 ± 0.4	19.0 ± 3.7	0.02	1.66 ± 0.08
Vector-TAS	286 ± 9	3.0 ± 0.2	30.7 ± 0.7	0.03	1.69 ± 0.02

S_a, S_z, amplitude parameters; S_{dr}, S_{ds}, hybrid parameters; S_{ci}, functional parameter. Straight lines connect mean values without statistical significant differences.

amplitude parameters (S_a S_z), but significant differences in hybrid (S_{dr}, S_{ds}) and functional (S_{ci}) parameters (Table 5.3). The S_a and S_z values recorded were within the range reported for smooth-machined dental implants, requiring a few months for osseointegration.[22] However, the high S_{dr} and S_{ds} values of Vector-TAS are associated with enhanced bone–implant contact, with a beneficial effect on pullout and torque removal strength.[13,23] The S_{ds} parameter seems to be associated with the development of a more favorable stress pattern at the implant–bone interface, distributing the stresses over a larger area and thus reducing stress concentration. High values of the functional parameter S_{ci} have been shown to exert a positive effect on pullout strength.[24]

Although primary and secondary stability are required for the clinical efficacy of orthodontic MIs, osseointegration is considered as a complication, and thus surface chemistry and morphology must be adjusted accordingly.

ELECTROCHEMICAL PROPERTIES

Placement of any metallic component in the oral cavity gives rise to concerns about the potential adverse consequences of corrosion and ionic release. Apart from the electrochemical properties of metallic materials exposed to a biological environment, the presence of dissimilar metals (a common finding in orthodontic therapy) might trigger galvanic phenomena.

While there are many analytical techniques to define electrochemical properties of metallic materials, experimental results cannot be extrapolated directly to the clinical situation, as intraoral corrosion of metallic biomaterials is not simply based on the contact of the surface with an electrolyte, but it is strongly dependent on the oral biofilms developed in service. Consequently, laboratory results should be considered as indicative, rather than conclusive, for in vivo electrochemical behavior.

Generally, cp-Ti and Ti-6Al-4V have high corrosion resistance, but the presence of Al and V could be problematic in that V has been associated with cytotoxic effects and adverse tissue reactions and Al may be implicated in neurological disorders.[25,26] Because of concerns regarding leakage of these ions,[27] Ti-6Al-4V has been replaced for orthopedic purposes with Ti-6Al-7Nb, using Nb instead of V as the beta stabilizer.[14] The release of ions from Ti-6Al-4V orthodontic MIs has been demonstated in a rabbit model (Fig. 5.8).[2] However, the authors postulated that such results might not be alarming because:

- the released amounts were very low
- orthodontic MIs have a short service life compared with orthopedic devices
- the surface to body weight ratio is much smaller in rabbits (20 : 3), where the study was carried out, compared with adult humans (20 : 70) with four MIs.

Galvanic corrosion could be a potential problem with MIs as they are placed in the oral cavity along with a variety of dissimilar alloys as part

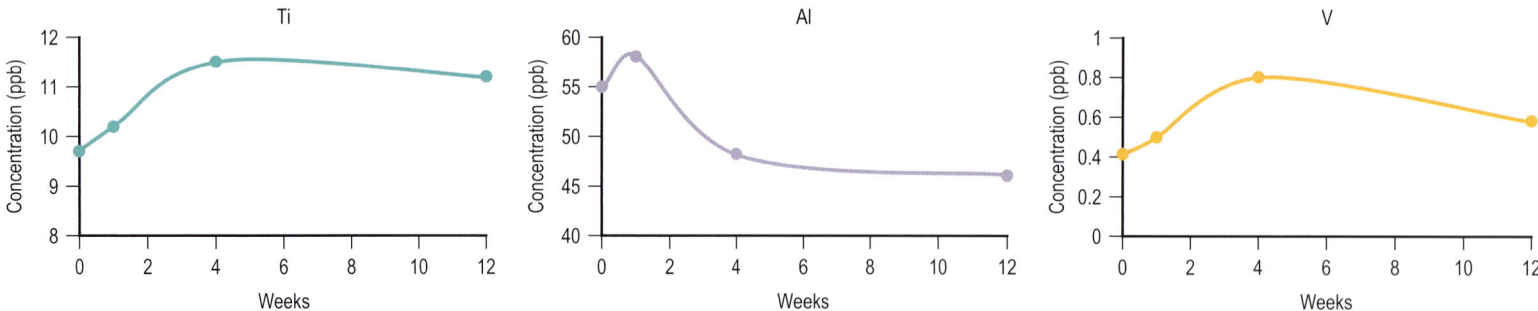

Fig. 5.8 Concentration of Ti, Al and V in rabbit tissues as a function of time after implantation. The pattern was similar for kidneys, livers and lungs. (From De Morais et al., 2009.[2])

of orthodontic treatment, such as different SS grades and Ti alloys used for brackets; precious, semiprecious and base brazing alloys used for joining wing and base bracket components; and a variety of SS and Ti alloys (Ni-Ti and beta phase alloys) for archwires.[28–31] Although galvanic action requires a minimum difference in electrochemical potential greater than 0.2 V, it is not possible to predict what the potential difference will be in the oral cavity while clear evidence of galvanic coupling is rare in orthodontic literature.[30] However, in vitro studies indicate that Ti and Ti alloys undergo galvanic corrosion when coupled with precious alloys (high-Au and low-Au, Ag-alloys, Pd-alloys) and they cause galvanic corrosion to Ni-Cr and Co-Cr alloys.[32–34]

CONCLUSIONS

The material, the surface composition and the geometrical design of orthodontic MIs are important factors in their clinical efficacy. Optimization of their surface chemistry and topography, along with enhancements of their design by modifying geometrical features, may reduce clinical complications such as early failure or later displacement of these devices.

REFERENCES

1. Morais LS, Serra GG, Muller CA, et al. Titanium alloy mini-implants for orthodontic anchorage: immediate loading and metal ion release. Acta Biomater 2007;3:331–9.
2. De Morais LS, Serra GG, Albuquerque Palermo EF, et al. Systemic levels of metallic ions released from orthodontic mini-implants. Am J Orthod Dentofacial Orthop 2009;135:522–9.
3. Alsamak S, Bitsanis E, Makou M, et al. Morphological and structural characteristics of orthodontic mini-implants. J Orofac Orthop 2012;73:58–71.
4. Gedrange T, Hietschold V, Mai R, et al. An evaluation of resonance frequency analysis for the determination of the primary stability of orthodontic palatal implants: a study in human cadavers. Clin Oral Implants Res 2005;16:425–31.
5. Buchter A, Wiechmann D, Gaertner C, et al. Load-related bone modelling at the interface of orthodontic micro-implants. Clin Oral Implants Res 2006;17:714–22.
6. Chen YJ, Chang HH, Huang CY, et al. A retrospective analysis of the failure rate of three different orthodontic skeletal anchorage systems. Clin Oral Implants Res 2007;18:768–75.
7. Chen Y, Shin HI, Kyung HM. Biomechanical and histological comparison of self-drilling and self-tapping orthodontic microimplants in dogs. Am J Orthod Dentofacial Orthop 2008;133:44–50.
8. Crismani AG, Bernhart T, Schwarz K, et al. Ninety percent success in palatal implants loaded 1 week after placement: a clinical evaluation by resonance frequency analysis. Clin Oral Implants Res 2006;17:445–50.
9. Kim YK, Kim YJ, Yun PY, et al. Effects of the taper shape, dual-thread, and length on the mechanical properties of mini-implants. Angle Orthod 2009;79:908–14.
10. Wilmes B, Ottenstreuer S, Su YY, et al. Impact of implant design on primary stability of orthodontic mini-implants. J Orofac Orthop 2008;69:42–50.
11. Wilmes B, Rademacher C, Olthoff G, et al. Parameters affecting primary stability of orthodontic mini-implants. J Orofac Orthop 2006;67:162–74.
12. Larsson C, Thomsen P, Aronsson BO, et al. Bone response to surface-modified titanium implants: studies on the early tissue response to machined and electropolished implants with different oxide thicknesses. Biomaterials 1996;17:605–16.
13. Sul YT, Kang BS, Johansson C, et al. The roles of surface chemistry and topography in the strength and rate of osseointegration of titanium implants in bone. J Biomed Mater Res A 2009;89:942–50.
14. Boyer R, Welsch G, Collings EW, editors. Materials properties handbook: titanium alloys. Materials Park, OH: ASM International; 1994.
15. Motoyoshi M, Hirabayashi M, Uemura M, et al. Recommended placement torque when tightening an orthodontic mini-implant. Clin Oral Implants Res 2006;17:109–14.
16. Eliades T, Zinelis S, Papadopoulos MA, et al. Characterization of retrieved orthodontic miniscrew implants. Am J Orthod Dentofacial Orthop 2009;135:10, discussion 10–11.
17. Liu XY, Chu PK, Ding CX. Surface modification of titanium, titanium alloys, and related materials for biomedical applications. Mater Sci Eng R Rep 2004;47:49–121.
18. Li JL, Sun MR, Ma XX. Structural characterization of titanium oxide layers prepared by plasma based ion implantation with oxygen on Ti6A14V alloy. Appl Surf Sci 2006;252:7503–8.
19. Zhu X, Kim KH, Jeong Y. Anodic oxide films containing Ca and P of titanium biomaterial. Biomaterials 2001;22:2199–206.
20. Serro AP, Saramago B. Influence of sterilization on the mineralization of titanium implants induced by incubation in various biological model fluids. Biomaterials 2003;24:4749–60.
21. Dohan Ehrenfest DM, Coelho PG, Kang BS, et al. Classification of osseointegrated implant surfaces: materials, chemistry and topography. Trends Biotechnol 2009;28:198–206.
22. Coelho PG, Granjeiro JM, Romanos GE, et al. Basic research methods and current trends of dental implant surfaces. J Biomed Mater Res B Appl Biomater 2009;88:579–96.
23. Hallgren C, Reimers H, Chakarov D, et al. An in vivo study of bone response to implants topographically modified by laser micromachining. Biomaterials 2003;24:701–10.
24. Lamolle SF, Monjo M, Lyngstadaas SP, et al. Titanium implant surface modification by cathodic reduction in hydrofluoric acid: surface characterization and in vivo performance. J Biomed Mater Res A 2009;88:581–8.
25. Okazaki Y, Gotoh E, Manabe T, et al. Comparison of metal concentrations in rat tibia tissues with various metallic implants. Biomaterials 2004;25:5913–20.
26. Steinemann SG. Titanium: the material of choice? Periodontol 2000 1998;17:7–21.
27. Gioka C, Bourauel C, Zinelis S, et al. Titanium orthodontic brackets: structure, composition, hardness and ionic release. Dent Mater 2004;20:693–700.
28. Eliades T, Zinelis S, Papadopoulos MA, et al. Nickel content of as-received and retrieved NiTi and stainless steel archwires: assessing the nickel release hypothesis. Angle Orthod 2004;74:151–4.
29. Pelsue BM, Zinelis S, Bradley TG, et al. Structure, composition, and mechanical properties of Australian orthodontic wires. Angle Orthod 2009;79:97–101.
30. Siargos B, Bradley TG, Darabara M, et al. Galvanic corrosion of metal injection molded (MIM) and conventional brackets with nickel–titanium and copper-nickel–titanium archwires. Angle Orthod 2007;77:355–60.
31. Zinelis S, Eliades T, Pandis N, et al. Why do nickel–titanium archwires fracture intraorally? Fractographic analysis and failure mechanism of in-vivo fractured wires. Am J Orthod Dentofacial Orthop 2007;132:84–9.
32. Reclaru L, Meyer JM. Study of corrosion between a titanium implant and dental alloys. J Dent 1994;22:159–68.
33. Grosgogeat B, Reclaru L, Lissac M, et al. Measurement and evaluation of galvanic corrosion between titanium/Ti6A14V implants and dental alloys by electrochemical techniques and auger spectrometry. Biomaterials 1999;20:933–41.
34. Taher NM, Al Jabab AS. Galvanic corrosion behavior of implant suprastructure dental alloys. Dent Mater 2003;19:54–9.

Structure and mechanical properties of orthodontic miniscrew implants

Antonio Gracco, Costantino Giagnorio and Giuseppe Siciliani

6

INTRODUCTION

Miniscrew implants (MIs) are biocompatible, mechanically retentive temporary anchorage devices that can be used in conjunction with osseointegrated plates or miniplates.[1] They were originally designed for fixing bone for orthopedic purposes, but they are now widely employed in orthodontics providing skeletal anchorage. Their increasing popularity is based on a number of advantages over other available anchorage systems:

- ease of insertion and removal
- versatility in that they can be inserted in many anatomical sites
- possibility of immediate loading
- small size so relatively low risk of damaging tooth roots or neurovascular structures near the insertion site
- lower costs.

IMPLANT STRUCTURE

There are many types of MIs on the market, each possessing different design characteristics. However, although structural features may vary, all MIs have a head, neck and shank (Fig. 6.1).

THE HEAD

The head is the most coronal portion of the MI and protrudes from the soft tissues following insertion into bone. The head facilitates the use of a driver for MI insertion and removal, and its shape depends on whether direct or indirect anchorage is used, so that anchorage devices can be bonded, ligated or hooked on to the MI (Fig. 6.2).[1]

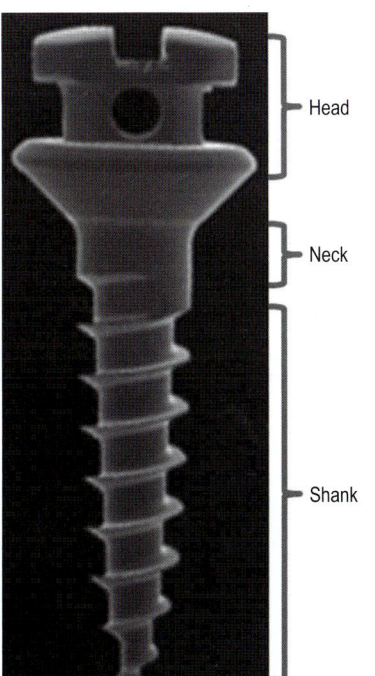

Fig. 6.1 Basic components of a miniscrew implant.

Head

Neck

Shank

Each type of head presents distinct clinical advantages and disadvantages.[2] A spherical head can only carry one or two coil springs, as their angle of insertion needs to be fairly acute with respect to the cortical plate, and only two-dimensional control of dental movement is possible. A head with a hook can house more than two coil springs and there is less risk of detachment as the MI is inserted at a steep angle. Bracket-like heads have a central slot and are small, creating problems for ligating archwires and for three-dimensional control of tooth movement. A head with a rectangular slot can provide optimal housing for archwires and is, therefore, clinically the most useful design.

The driver socket can be external, in which the MI head is inserted into the hollow tip of a driver, or internal, in which the tip of a driver is inserted into the socket on the head of the MI. The internal single or Phillips slots allow acute insertion angles and have little risk of disengagement or bone stripping.[3]

THE NECK

The neck is the portion of the MI between the head and the threaded intraosseous shank (Fig. 6.1). It may vary in length but is usually smooth to prevent tissue irritation, although a rough surface has also been proposed (see below).[4]

THE SHANK

Miniscrew implant shanks are either cylindrical or conical (tapered) and threaded (Fig. 6.3). The thread transforms a rotational movement of the MI into a roto-translation one, facilitating insertion, and acts as a retention mechanism in bone, counteracting the axial and longitudinal forces that might otherwise cause the implant to work out of the bone.

INTRAOSSEOUS RETENTION

Prosthetic implants are intended to be retained in the mouth and so good osseointegration is a vital factor in their success. By comparison, MIs are intended to be removed at the end of treatment and so they need to be stable but have limited osseointegration to facilitate their removal.[1] Retention is provided by mechanical or primary retention derived from the interaction between the MI screw threads and the bone itself (Fig. 6.4). Insertion of the MI also generates controlled compression forces on the surrounding bone that contribute to the stability of the fixture.[5,6] As osseointegration is not required, loading of orthodontic forces can be applied immediately following insertion.[7]

Although immediate loading considerably reduces treatment time, it can be deleterious from a biomechanical perspective, with issues of tipping or displacing occurring. In general, tipping is less of a problem with MIs inserted into thicker cortical bone and in MIs inserted into the maxilla. Migration of the MI can occur after bone resorption triggered by damage to the bone during insertion or after secondary remodeling. Primary stability is best achieved by ensuring that at least three to four MI threads are anchored in cortical bone and by achieving optimal bone–screw locking at the moment of insertion.[6,8]

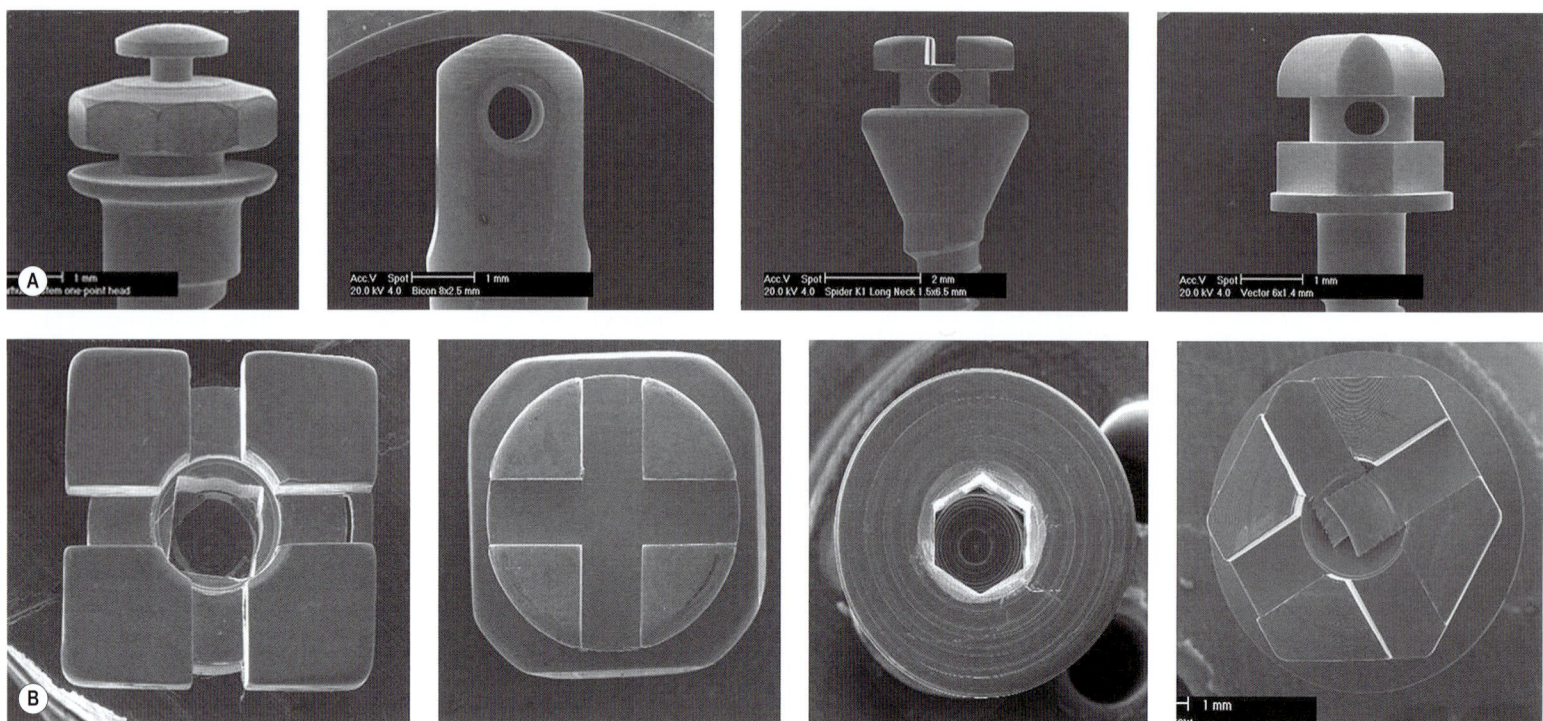

Fig. 6.2 Miniscrew implant heads. Various head designs (A) and surfaces (B).

Fig. 6.3 Conical (A) and cylindrical (B) miniscrew implant shanks.

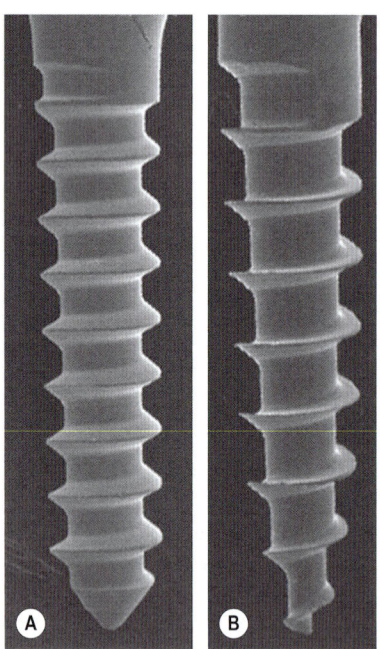

Fig. 6.4 Bone-screw locking condition.

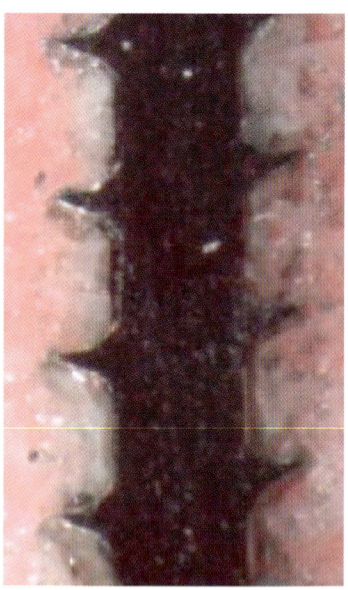

Bone–implant contact, a widely used indicator of osseointegration, is on average 25% in MIs subject to immediate loading and 18.9% in MIs loaded following an appropriate healing period. No association between the length of healing period and MI success rate has been documented.[9]

There has been debate as to the degree of loading force that can be applied to MIs but it appears that MIs are able to withstand loads of up to 500 g, indicating that they are able to function properly in clinical orthodontics.[10]

Because removal of MIs at the end of treatment requires that osseointegration is limited, the vast majority of MIs on the market have a smooth intraosseous portion. Even these will see a degree of osseointegration (~25%) but this still permits their simple removal.[11]

MINISCREW IMPLANT SUCCESS RATES: BIOLOGICAL AND MECHANICAL CONSIDERATIONS

The success rate of MIs is currently very high and may reach a mean value of 93.43%.[12] For successful use as a skeletal anchorage, a MI must be able to withstand the forces applied to it without deformation and/or breakage, particularly during insertion and removal. From a physical perspective, MIs are subjected to three phases of mechanical loading:

- torsion during insertion
- flexion during the period of orthodontic treatment
- torsion during removal.

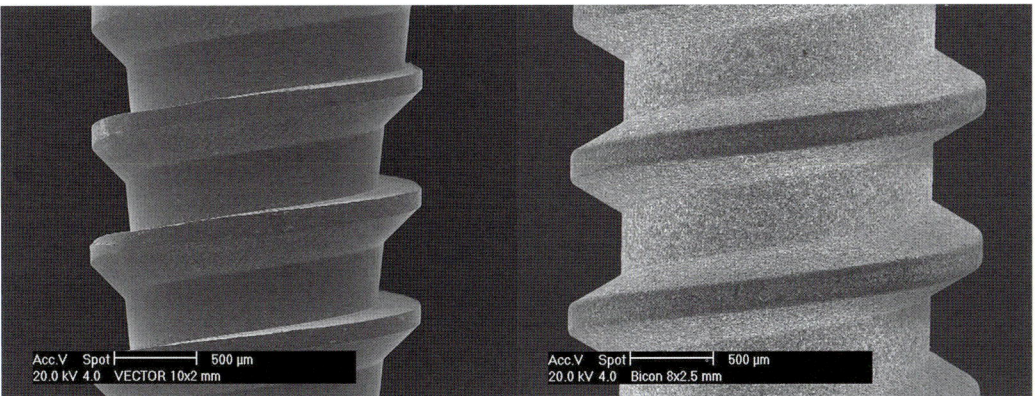

Fig. 6.5 Smooth (left) and rough (right) miniscrew implant surfaces.

Various factors influence the MI success rate:

- biological factors: patient health, age, insertion site, occlusion, skeletal morphology
- factors linked to operator dexterity/experience
- axial inclination of the device
- surgical insertion procedures
- structural and design characteristics of the MI: surface, length, diameter, neck, platform
- post-implantation factors: orthodontic movements, hygiene, smoking.

MINISCREW IMPLANT STRUCTURAL CHARACTERISTICS

Surface Characteristics

The characteristics of the surface of the MI have never been implicated in the failure of MIs subject to immediate loading.[13] Use of acid etching on the coronal portion of MIs increases the surface area at the interface, allowing for very close contact between the bone and the MI (Fig. 6.5). In one study, primary stability was not affected by acid etching but secondary stability was improved even without an intervening healing period. Ease of implant removal was not evaluated.[14]

Length

Although numerous studies have shown better success rates are achieved with longer MIs, some authors do not consider this an important factor in MI success.[1]

Diameter

Diameter has clearly been shown to have an influence on implantation success.[15] The outer diameter is the total diameter to the outer edge of the screw, while the internal, or root, diameter is the diameter of the shaft carrying the screw thread. Manufacturers tend only to give the external diameter and so most studies only refer to this.

Based on success rates, 1.2 mm can be considered the minimum diameter required to achieve adequate implantation success. This may be because it is more difficult to achieve the optimal placement torque of at least 5–10 Ncm for good primary stability with narrower MIs.[7,15] In terms of maximal diameter, microfractures are particularly prevalent when using MIs with a diameter of 2 mm and so diameters of 1.5 mm and 1.6 mm represent a satisfactory compromise between MI resistance and cortical lesioning.[16]

Although there is a need to achieve sufficient torque, this must be balanced by the fact that excessive placement torque can cause microfractures and ischemia in the bone surrounding the implant, thereby undermining bone health and increasing the probability of failure. Hence, it is recommended that insertion torque be limited to 10 Ncm.[17,18] Damage to bone leading to inflammation and bone remodeling is generally limited to 1 mm of surrounding bone but it can spread further and cause device failure.[16]

The degree of cortical damage inflicted by cylindrical MIs does not differ significantly from that caused by conical MIs of the same diameter, indicating that diameter, rather than shape, is the determining factor in bony tissue damage.[16] The insertion site also must be considered (e.g. maxilla or mandible, keratinized or non-keratinized mucosa).[19] Overheating of the bone during drilling can occur where a pilot hole is drilled first, with excessive insertion speed and also with prolonged perforation times. Overheating is more common with MIs inserted in the generally thicker cortical bone of the mandible.[20–22] These considerations, in addition to analysis of implantation success rates, have led to the conclusion that MIs with a diameter greater than 1.4 mm should be used in the mandible.[19]

Neck Characteristics

The neck is the portion of the MI that connects the head to the threaded intraosseous shank. Various lengths are manufactured to allow for adaptation to different thicknesses of mucosa. This prevents the soft tissues from burying the MI head, an event that would undoubtedly lead to MI failure. Greater neck thickness confers greater mechanical resistance, a useful consideration given that this is an area subject to particularly high levels of mechanical stress. In fact, if the neck is too narrow, MI breakage can easily occur, particularly during the removal procedure.[23]

In general, the surface of the neck is smooth as this is thought to cause less damage to soft tissues (see Fig. 10.4).[1] However, a MI neck featuring microgrooves has recently been proposed (Fig. 6.6).[4] The authors reported that the connective tissue fibers of the gingiva adhere in a perpendicular fashion to the rough surface of their sandblasted, large-grit, and acid-etched implant similar to the situation in a natural tooth. In contrast, these fibers are thought to adhere to a smoother surface in a circular fashion, creating a circular peri-implant ligament that runs parallel to the MI surface, which permits epithelial growth and the creation of a pocket capable of harboring microorganisms, a possible cause of device failure.[24] However, studies examining the success rates of this MI have not been performed.

Platform

The platform is a raised area below the head that comes into contact with soft tissues (Fig. 6.7), serving to compress and protect these tissues from the auxiliary devices attached to the MI. The ideal platform should have

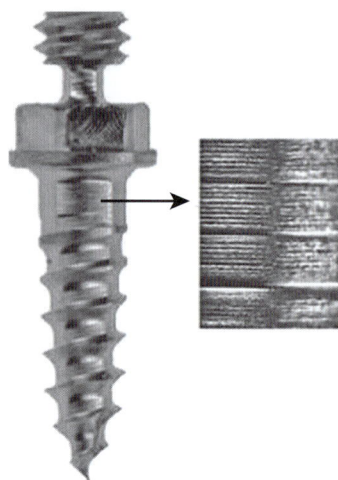

Fig. 6.6 Neck of a miniscrew implant featuring microgrooves. (With permission of Kim et al.[4])

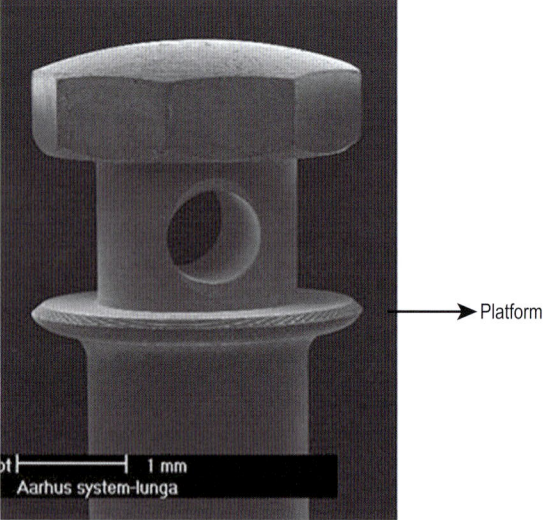

Platform

1 mm
Aarhus system-Iunga

Fig. 6.7 Miniscrew implant platform.

a smooth surface to reduce tissue irritation and to promote healing of the insertion wound. The platform should be 1–2 mm thicker than the soft tissues upon which it is positioned to prevent tissue growth around the neck of the MI. Direct contact between this structure and the underlying anatomical planes is thought to confer greater stability to the device.[2]

PRIMARY STABILITY OF MINISCREW IMPLANTS

Primary stability is indispensable for the clinical application of MIs as anchorage. Optimal primary stability is particularly important if MIs are to be subject to immediate loading as stability reduces the potential for micromovement. This effect favors tissue healing at the insertion site, a necessary condition for long-term stability.[6] From a mechanical perspective, the ultimate goal of MI placement is to create maximum interdigitation between the bony tissue and the threads of the MI and to generate controlled compression forces in the bone.[6] Both of these properties are fundamental for achieving primary stability.

There are no good data regarding the acceptable level of micromovement that still allows primary stability for osseointegrated devices; prosthetic implants should have a range limited to 50–150 μm upon insertion[25] but lower values are more likely for MIs of smaller dimensions.

Stability deteriorates progressively during the 3 weeks following insertion and then increases over the fourth and fifth week;[26] the initial decrease is probably caused by bone remodeling and it is more evident in sites with unattached mucosa.

Primary stability depends on a number of factors:

- device features: length, diameter, thread type, thread shape, thread pitch, thread design, cutting flute, construction material
- operator/surgical technique-related factors: cortical predrilling insertion angle
- patient characteristics: cortical bone thickness.

The following discussion examines the effect of MI design on primary stability.

DESIGN AND STRUCTURAL CHARACTERISTICS

Length

Length generally refers to the threaded portion of the MI rather than the entire head-to-tip length and can vary from 4 to 15 mm. An increase in MI length results in an increase in maximum insertion torque, removal torque and pullout resistance. In particular, a longer-threaded portion confers a greater resistance to pullout with axial loads, although it does not influence the resistance to lateral loads applied at 20 or 40°. However, primary stability does not increase significantly beyond MI lengths of 5 mm because these greater lengths will be entering medullary bone.

The selection of MI length must also take into account the thickness of the soft tissues at the insertion site, bearing in mind that the MI must be supported by 5–6 mm of bone. For example, the palatal mucosa is an average of 4 mm thick and so a MI of at least 10 mm is required for 6 mm to be held in bone.

From a strictly biomechanical perspective, the ideal length of a MI is 9 mm, as this is thought to cause less stress on the surrounding bone than shorter MIs and has less risk of damage to neighboring anatomical structures than longer MIs.[27] From a clinical standpoint, a MI of 4–6 mm can be inserted into the majority of intraoral sites.[28] When choosing a MI, therefore, it is necessary to strike a balance between the ideal length with respect to the biomechanics and the best clinical option.

Hong et al.[29] have designed two MIs to be positioned above the dental roots, thereby avoiding potentially damaging radicular contact (Fig. 6.8). There are two versions: N1, which is cylindrical, has a diameter of 4.1 mm and length of 2.6 mm; and N2, which is conical, 2 mm in length and 3 mm in diameter. The reduced lengths were inspired by a cone beam CT study analyzing the cortex above the roots at labial anatomical sites, which revealed a mean cortical thickness of 2.3 mm. However, N1 required excessive insertion torques (15.6 Ncm), which could lead to considerable bone damage and so N2 was devised with a reduced diameter and a conical shape. Mechanical tests performed on the N2 appear to confirm its superior performance with respect to control MIs in terms of both placement torque and lateral displacement.[29]

Diameter

The primary stability of a MI is directly proportional to its diameter, as the forces applied are distributed over a larger surface area when MIs of larger diameters are used, resulting in a reduction in pressure on the bone at the insertion site.[30] It is diameter rather than length that is most influential with respect to biomechanical yield,[31] implantation success[32] and resistance to fracture.[33] Furthermore, to obtain optimal biomechanical yield from a device, a good relationship between its external and internal diameters is required.[34]

The external diameter has a large and directly proportional influence on placement torque, pullout resistance and removal torque. These properties, in turn, affect primary stability, particularly in conical rather than cylindrical MIs.[35] This latter difference between the MI types is because the tensile

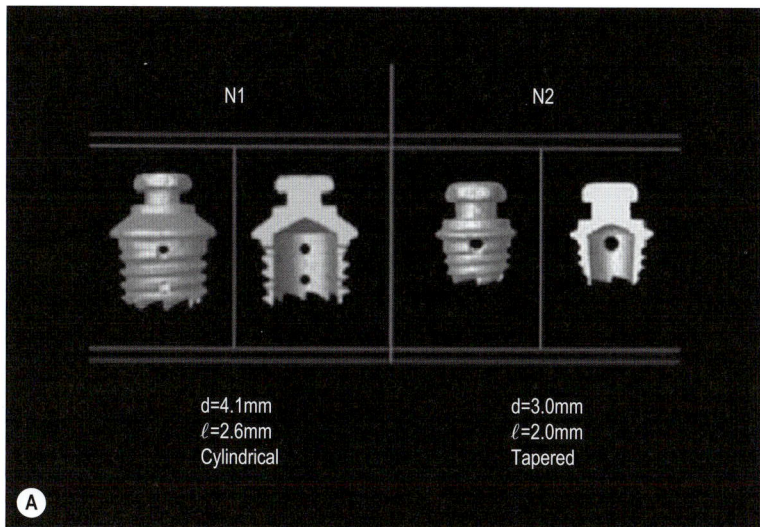
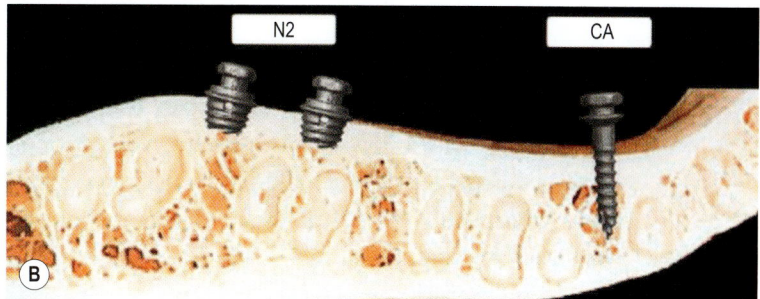

Fig. 6.8 The N1 and N2 miniscrew implants (A) Structural differences. (B) Supraradicular cortical placement of N2 miniscrew implants compared with inter-radicular traditional commercially available (CA) miniscrew implants. (With permission of Hong et al.[29])

resistance corresponds to the cube of the greatest diameter of the MI. The external diameter also influences clinical use because MIs with smaller diameters can be positioned in smaller interdental spaces.[1]

Internal diameter has no statistically significant influence on stability, although it has been suggested that a smaller internal diameter allows greater thread depth and thus increases the flank overlap area (the area of the bone in contact with the MI threads), leading to larger bony bridges between the threads, particularly near the tip of the MI.[36]

The external diameter of the MIs must be greater than 1 mm; purchase varies with diameters ranging from 1 mm to 1.5 mm but appears stable for those with diameters of 1.5–2.3 mm in both jaws. A significant loss of anchorage has been observed when using MIs with external diameters of less than 1.2 mm.[2] The ideal external diameter is probably between 1.3 and 1.5 mm, a compromise between primary stability, mechanical resistance and clinical versatility. The mean inter-radicular space is generally between 2.5 mm and 3.5 mm, so there is a risk of unwanted root contact when MIs of diameters greater than 2 mm are used.[2]

The space necessary to accommodate a MI and so reduce the risk of damage to neighboring structures can be calculated from the MI diameter, its mean displacement (equal to its diameter), the thickness of the periodontal ligament of the adjacent teeth and the inter-radicular distance necessary to house the MI without anatomical damage (average, 0.25 mm).

A success rate of 88.6% has been reported for MIs with a 1.3 mm diameter, which is not particularly high but needs to be weighed against the lesser risk of iatrogenic damage.[37] Miniscrew implants of even smaller diameter, however, are less resistant to loading perpendicular to their long axis.[38] Those with a diameter of less than 1.2 mm tend to possess poor mechanical resistance and are prone to fracture, particularly in highly mineralized tissues.[32,39] A reduction in MI diameter of 0.2 mm leads to a reduction of approximately 50% in the resistance of the device.[40]

The choice of MI diameter may also be influenced by the thickness of the cortical layer at the insertion site. In the palate, for example, the use of MIs with a diameter of at least 1.5 mm is recommended. In the mandible, however, diameters of at least 2 mm are preferable.

Miniscrew Implant Type

Miniscrew implants can be pretapped, self-tapping or self-drilling. Early MIs were pretapped and required an initial pilot hole to be drilled through the entire thickness of the cortical layer. A suitable bur was then used to create another pilot hole in the medullary bone to house the entire length of the MI. "Threads" in the medullary bone to engage the threads of the MI were then created with a tapping drill.

Self-tapping devices rapidly followed and had a blunt tip, a cylindrical shank and asymmetrical sharp (cutting) threads. Sometimes there was a cutting flute in the terminal part of the threaded portion. The surface of the threads in these MIs is nearly perpendicular to the direction of the pullout force, allowing for maximum load transmission. Moreover, some self-tapping MIs possess a "thread-forming" or "thread-cutting" feature. The former compress the surrounding bone during their insertion, forming threads in the bone by plastic deformation and, therefore, produce no osseous debris. The latter cut into bone to form threads as they are inserted, pushing some of the small debris created along the shank to the surface during the implantation procedure. The remainder of the debris is compressed between the MI and the surrounding bone.

Self-tapping devices also require a pilot hole to be made through the cortical layer and into the spongy bone but only one drill is required and there is no tapping procedure.[41]

The self-drilling implant was designed to be inserted through the mucosa directly into the bone using a manual driver or handpiece,[41] thus avoiding any predrilling. Self-drilling devices are similar to bottle-openers in that they are equipped with a cutting tip that is able to perforate the bony cortex and a hollow cutting flute on the terminal portion of the thread (Fig. 6.9A,B). These cut into the bone and facilitate insertion, but also transport the bony debris produced during the procedure to the surface so that it is not compressed against the walls of the hole (Fig. 6.9C).[42,43]

Although pretapped MIs are more time consuming to insert than the self-drilling versions, they are still used. They should not be used in areas where the cortical layer is thin or where the spongy bone is particularly sparse (e.g. the midfacial area), as the tapping drill can easily cause stripping, leading to a loss of MI purchase on the bone.[42] Moreover, pretapped MI threads tend not to engage tightly with those created in the bone, and a loss of stability is more likely. Nonetheless, this type of device can be employed successfully in anatomical areas featuring a thick cortical layer or when inserted through the spongy bone into the underlying cortical layer (bicortical implantation).

Self-tapping MIs have a number of advantages over their pretapped counterparts, including better purchase in thin cortical layers,[43] simplified insertion procedures and the consequent need for fewer tools and less chair-side time. They also decrease the risk of placement torque and bone damage, and reduce the heat generated during the insertion.

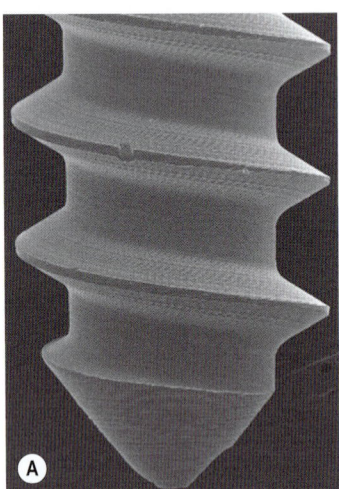
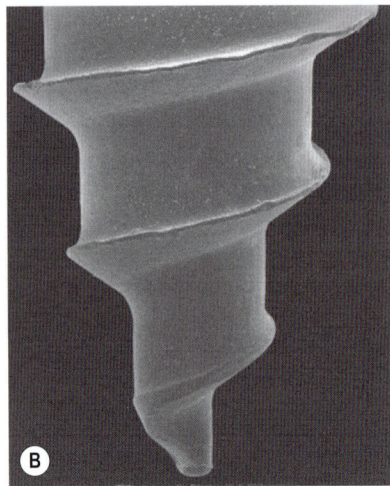

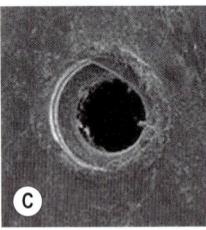
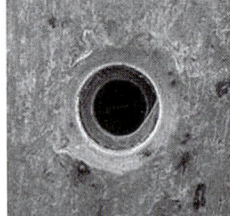
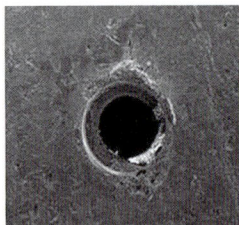

Fig. 6.9 (A) Self-tapping miniscrew implant with a round tip. (B) Self-drilling miniscrew implant with a crock-screw tip. (C) Implant insertion/pilot holes in bone.

Placement torque is greatly influenced by the diameter of a pilot hole. Although torque increases with a smaller diameter of pilot hole, fracture is more likely with MIs of small diameter.[44,45] The ideal pilot hole diameter is 0.2–0.5 mm smaller than that of the MI.[46] Pretapped systems have the advantage of a 40% reduction in placement torque compared with self-tapping MIs and they also allow bone debris to be easily removed before device placement.

The predrilling phase adds time to a procedure and there is a risk of excessive perforation and damage to the nerves, roots and tooth buds plus the possibility of drill tip breakage and thermal necrosis of the bone.[42] Whenever a MI is inserted into bone, the Haversian canal system (the supporting structure of the bone) is interrupted, and the tissue responds. Predrilling can aggravate this type of damage by generating more heat in the bone. Furthermore, bone fracture and atrophy are more likely with pretapped and self-tapping MIs as they both create a radial displacement of bone at the MI tip, which can result in compression damage.[43]

The bone–MI interface is better with self-tapping MIs than with pre-tapped MIs: complete contact has been demonstrated in 65.8% of samples of self-tapping MIs compared with a mere 3.7% of pretapped MIs.[47] Reduced contact between the bone and the MI translates into less mechanical stability. Moreover, pretapped devices have been shown to create more bone damage and so there is a greater degree of bone remodeling and tissue formation. At the end of a healing period, greater contact is achieved at the bone–MI interface with drill-free insertion than for self-tapping devices. The drilling process for pretapped devices removes the spicules of bone it creates during perforation, creating gaps in the trabecular bone, whereas self-drilling systems tend to compress these bone fragments into the trabecular gaps. The disadvantages of self-drilling are the risk of damage to neighboring anatomical structures, overheating of the surrounding tissues, and loosening of any pilot hole during MI insertion. All may lead to a reduction in primary stability.

The pullout resistance of pretapped and self-tapping MIs is comparable.[48] However, some clinicians consider that self-tapping MIs are easier to grip while others consider there is no significant difference between the two types.

Although the self-drilling systems require only a single-step insertion procedure, some authors recommend predrilling a pilot hole with a diameter of 0.3 mm and a depth of 2–3 mm at sites with a cortical thickness 2 mm or greater to reduce the risk of damage to the MI tip.[1,2] Although self-drilling MI placement is far less invasive than placement of self-tapping MIs, the pressure exerted on the bone during perforation of the cortical layer and the greater placement torque required for insertion creates more stress on bone and MI, leading to a greater risk of fracture for both.[42,49]

Placement of self-drilling MIs requires a high peak insertion torque, the maximum force of the clockwise movement required for complete insertion of the device, in both the maxilla and mandible. High torques indicate a greater degree of contact between the MI and bone (in particular the cortex) and thus a better grip force, resistance to MI failure and stability under orthodontic loads.[47] However, the high peak insertion torque with self-drilling MIs means that care must be taken when they are inserted into particularly compact bone as this will increase the probability of fracture during the placement.[50]

In contrast, the peak removal torque appears to be similar for self-drilling and self-tapping devices.[49]

Of the three types of MI, the self-drilling versions appear to possess a greater primary stability and a superior bone–implant contact, which can be considered an indicator of both stability and reduced bone damage.[43] The presence of numerous bony fragments in contact with the threads of self-drilling MIs can also be interpreted as proof of the lack of damage to the surrounding bone, as this indicates that the bone is incised rather than compressed.[43]

The self-drilling MIs possess great stability but generate more friction upon their contact with the bone; they also possess a lower grip capacity in vitro than self-tapping MIs.[43] However, numerous authors maintain that self-drilling MIs permit a greater degree of contact between the MI and the bone, provoke less damage and have a greater success rate than other systems.[34,41,49,51]

The choice between self-drilling or self-tapping MIs should not be made based only on the morphological characteristics of the device; the material the MI is made of must also be taken into consideration. Indeed, commercially pure titanium MIs require a predrilling phase to reduce subsequent insertion stress on the device, whereas MIs made of titanium alloys have been purpose-designed to avoid a need for predrilling (see Chapter 5).[2]

Whatever the choice of material, it should be noted that all MIs are subject to micromovements at loading and during the period of orthodontic force application. These movements will increase the longer the MI is subject to orthodontic forces but will not necessarily lead to clinical instability or device failure.[52]

Shaft Shape

Shafts can be conical or cylindrical and the shape has biomechanical and clinical effects. From a biomechanical perspective, conical shafts with their tapered shape promote increased placement torque,[6,41,53,54] particularly during insertion of the coronal portion of the device, and provide a greater surface for interface with the surrounding bone.[55] They are also easier to insert into cortical bone and permit better mechanical cohesion between the MI threads and the surrounding bony tissue.[56] Combined with the progressive compression of the surrounding bone that occurs during their insertion, this leads to the greater stability of conical over cylindrical MIs.[36,57]

When comparing conical and cylindrical MIs of the same length, the maximum insertion torque is generally higher in the former; it increases with length of the cylindrical MI but remains the same for conical MIs of increasing shaft length. Cylindrical MIs do not require greater torque with thicker cortical bone whereas conical MIs do.[18,58]

Another fundamental characteristic of cylindrical MIs is their improved grip on the resistant layer of spongy bone underlying the cortical bone. This is a consequence of the greater diameter of cylindrical MIs and guarantees tight contact at the MI–spongy bone interface. In contrast, slight loosening of a conical implant, for any reason, is accompanied by a relatively large reduction in grip.[59] Aside from loss of purchase, conical MIs have the added drawback of increased insertion speed.[18]

The shape also influences pullout resistance, with conical MIs being more resistant to transverse loads at 20 or 40°.[41,54] However, the reduced thread depth at the coronal portion of a conical MI would decrease resistance to pullout.[35] Hence, the pullout resistance of conical MIs is a compromise between that obtained by compacting the bone and that lost through decreased thread depth.[35]

A conical shaft also increases the removal torque.[58] The maximum removal torque and torque loss (difference between insertion and removal torque) are greater for conical than for cylindrical MIs.[58]

One undisputed advantage of conical MIs is that they possess a greater resistance to fatigue and breakage than their cylindrical counterparts.[35] This mechanical resistance is thought to derive from their smaller diameter at the junction between the threaded area and the neck, the region most susceptible to stress.[60]

By comparison with biomechanical features, several studies have examined clinical differences between conical and cylindrical MIs. A study by Kim et al.[58] concluded that conical MIs offered no actual clinical benefit apart from elevated primary stability, with no significant differences in bone–implant contact, bone area and success rates. This can be ascribed to the fact that conical MIs have 20–30% less surface area than cylindrical devices,[61] and that the greater placement torque required for their insertion is more likely to provoke adverse effects in the surrounding tissues.[58] To counteract this, it is advisable to predrill the cortical layer at the insertion site.

A further study indicated that while primary stability is greater with conical MIs, after 12 weeks there are no differences in terms of bone–implant contact or removal torque.[62] However, while the bone–implant contact of conical MIs is excellent even immediately after insertion, it is necessary to allow a healing period of at least 8 weeks to obtain a comparable level of contact as seen with cylindrical MIs.[63]

Thread Pitch

Miniscrew implant threads come in different shapes and pitches, the pitch being the distance between the peaks of two adjacent threads (Fig. 6.10). A reduction in pitch and the consequent increase in tips per unit length increase the stability of an implant. Reduced pitch has been shown to increase resistance to pullout in porous materials,[40] although pullout force

increases between pitches of 0.75 and 1 mm but does not increase between pitches of 1 and 1.25 mm.[40]

A smaller pitch (0.5 mm or less) is also thought to decrease the amount of bone penetration per turn, thereby reducing the concentration of stress on the bone and creating greater compression on the surrounding tissue. However, it also appears that the pitch has a greater influence on the stability of MIs with a diameter of 2 mm than on the stability of smaller versions.

When choosing the most appropriate MI, it is important to bear in mind that those with very small pitch are able to engage with very little solid material, particularly in less compact bone. These MIs engage with only a few fragments of bone, which do not contribute to pullout resistance or the stability of the device.[36]

Indeed, a more useful indicator of MI suitability is its thread shape factor, the relationship between the thread depth and pitch. In fact, it is necessary to increase a MI's thread shape factor by increasing the pitch and reducing the thread depth, or vice versa, to increase its pullout resistance.

Thread Design

Miniscrew implant threads come in different shapes, which can influence their primary stability.[34] The best thread shape in terms of mechanical performance appears to be asymmetric and features a leading angle of 45° (Fig. 6.11) at the lower edge of the thread and a trailing angle of 90° at the upper edge of the thread. This design is thought to aid insertion and resistance to removal[55] by increasing the pullout resistance.[64] The design also provides maximal load transmission, particularly if the thread is attached by means of a "sharp" angle rather than a rounded joint.[42]

Orthopedic studies have found no difference in the pullout force between buttress and disk-shaped threads.[65] In contrast, Gracco et al. (unpublished data) found that reverse buttress, trapezoidal, rounded reverse buttress and reverse buttress with 75° thread joint shank shapes provide superior pullout resistance to those of the buttress design when inserted into a homogeneous support (Fig. 6.12).

A double-threaded conical MI increased the cortical bone–implant contact area and provided a better purchase in terms of greater removal torque when compared with single-threaded conical MIs and single- and double-threaded cylindrical MIs (Fig. 6.13).[66] However, Kim et al.[67] showed lower maximum insertion torque for a so-called dual-thread design, with one series of threads at double the number of thread tips per inch than the single-threaded version. In contrast, the double-threaded MI proposed by Hong et al. featured two series of threads, each with the same number of tips per inch as the single-threaded version used as a control (Fig. 6.13).[66]

Cutting Flute

The cutting flute is a helical groove in the apical portion of self-tapping and self-drilling implants (see Fig. 6.12) to allow the MI to cut into the

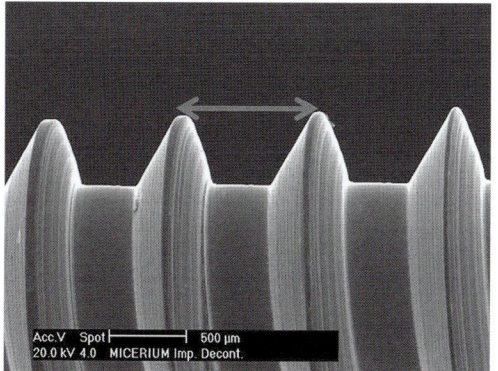

Fig. 6.10 Miniscrew implant thread pitch.

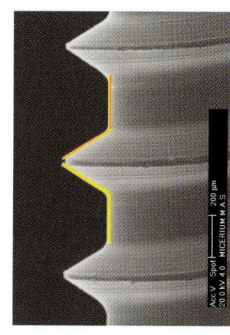
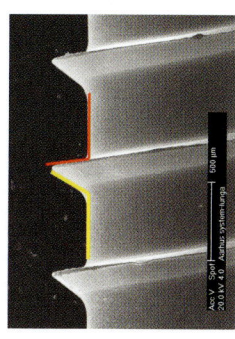

Fig. 6.11 Cutting flute with a 115° trailing angle (orange), a 90° trailing angle (red) and a 45° leading angle (yellow).

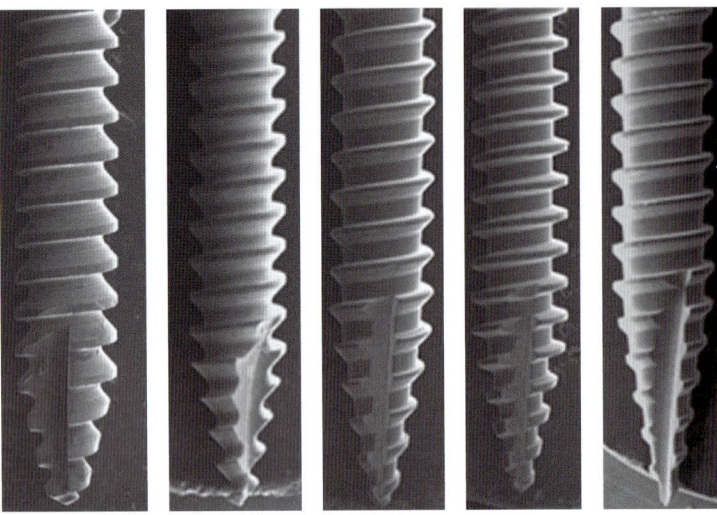

Fig. 6.12 Various miniscrew implant thread designs. From left: buttress, reverse buttress with 75° thread joint, rounded reverse buttress, trapezoidal, reverse buttress with 90° thread joint.

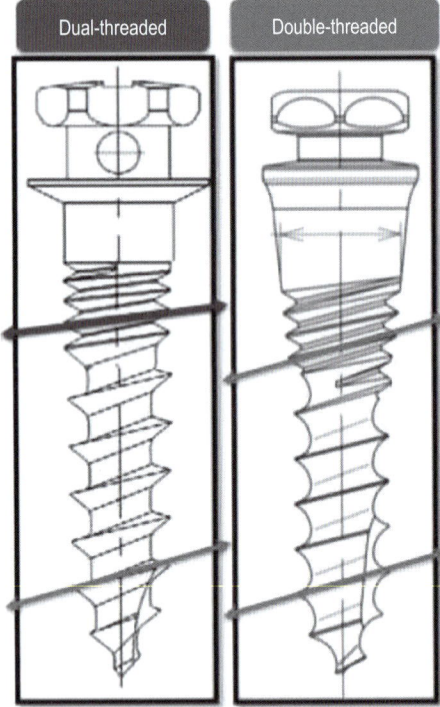

Fig. 6.13 "Dual-thread" and "double-thread" threads. (With permission of Hong et al.[66])

bone and to contain the bone fragments accumulated during the insertion procedure. Some fragments are compressed radially against the bone by the MI tip, and others are brought to the surface by the MI threads. Although the flute aids insertion, it also leads to a loss of local grip of approximately 30%.

Orthopedic literature has shown that the cutting capacity of self-tapping implants is also affected by the cutting thread relief, the chamfer position, the cutting depth and the incision angle.[68,69] The only orthodontic study published reported that MIs with a cutting flute had higher placement torque and pullout resistance than those without.[70] The increased placement torque is presumably because of the compression of bone fragments against the walls of the insertion chamber, resulting in greater friction and insertion resistance. The increased pullout resistance may be explained by the flute interrupting the thread and making it more flexible and thus allowing the overall rigidity of the MI to approach that of the surrounding bone.

The deformation potentials of the two systems are matched and their combined resistance is increased.

Material

It is also important to consider the material used to construct MIs as this influences not only the clinical procedures used for their insertion and removal[2,70] but also their mechanical resistance under orthodontic loads. This topic is covered in detail in Chapter 5.

REFERENCES

1. Papadopoulos MA, Tarawneh F. The use of miniscrew implants for temporary skeletal anchorage in orthodontics: a comprehensive review. Oral Surg Oral Med Oral Pathol Oral Radiol 2007;103:e6–15.
2. Lin JCY, Liou EJW, Yeh CL, et al. A comparative evaluation of current orthodontic miniscrew system. World J Orthod 2007;8:136–44.
3. Spencer KR, Ferguson JW, Smith AC, et al. Screw head design: an experimental study to assess the influence of design on performance. J Oral Maxillofac Surg 2004;62:473–8.
4. Kim TW, Baek SH, Kim JW, et al. Effects of microgrooves on the success rate and soft tissue adaptation of orthodontic miniscrews. Angle Orthod 2008;78:1057–64.
5. Brettin BT. Bicortical vs monocortical orthodontic skeletal anchorage. Am J Orthod Dentofacial Orthop 2008;134:625–35.
6. Cha JY, Kil JK, Yoon TM, et al. Miniscrew stability evaluated with computerized tomography scanning. Am J Orthod Dentofacial Orthop 2010;137:73–9.
7. Park HS, Jeong SH, Kwon OW. Factors affecting the clinical success of screw implants used as orthodontic anchorage. Am J Orthod Dentofacial Orthop 2006;130:18–25.
8. Deguchi T, Nasu M, Murakami K, et al. Quantitative evaluation of cortical bone thickness with computed tomographic scanning for orthodontic implants. Am J Orthod Dentofacial Orthop 2006;129:721.e7–12.
9. Cheng SJ, Tseng IY, Lee JJ, et al. A prospective study of the risk factors associated with failure of mini-implants used for orthodontic anchorage. Int J Oral Maxillofac Implants 2004;19:100–6.
10. Ohashi E, Pecho OE, Moron M, et al. Implant vs screw loading protocols in orthodontics. A systematic review. Angle Orthod 2006;76:721–7.
11. Cornelis MA, Scheffler NR, De Clerck HJ, et al. Systematic review of the experimental use of temporary skeletal anchorage devices in orthodontics. Am J Orthod Dentofacial Orthop 2007;131(Suppl. 4):52–8.
12. Antoszewska J, Papadopoulos MA, Park HS, et al. Five-year experience with orthodontic miniscrew implants: a retrospective investigation of factors influencing success rates. Am J Orthod Dentofacial Orthop 2009;136:158.e1–10.
13. Chaddad K, Ferreira AFH, Geurs N, et al. Influence of surface characteristics on survival rates of mini-implants. Angle Orthod 2008;78:107–13.
14. Ikeda H, Rossouw PE, Campbell PM, et al. Three-dimensional analysis of peri-bone-implant contact of rough-surface miniscrew implants. Am J Orthod Dentofacial Orthop 2011;139:e153–63.
15. Wiechmann D, Meyer U, Büchter A. Success rate of mini- and micro-implants used for orthodontic anchorage: a prospective clinical study. Clin Oral Implants Res 2007;18:263–7.
16. Lee NK, Baek SH. Effects of the diameter and shape of orthodontic mini-implants on micro-damage to the cortical bone. Am J Orthod Dentofacial Orthop 2010;138:e1–8.
17. Motoyoshi M, Hirabayashi M, Uemura M, et al. Recommended placement torque when tightening an orthodontic mini-implant. Clin Oral Implants Res 2006;17:109–14.
18. Lim SA, Cha JY, Hwang CJ. Insertion torque of orthodontic miniscrews according to changes in shape, diameter and length. Angle Orthod 2008;78:234–40.
19. Wu TY, Kuang SH, Wu CH. Factors associated with the stability of mini-implants for orthodontic anchorage: a study of 414 samples in Taiwan. J Oral Maxillofac Surg 2009;67:1595–9.
20. Reingewirtz Y, Szmukler-Moncler S, Semger B. Influence of different parameters on bone heating and drilling time in implantology. Clin Oral Res 1997;8:189–97.
21. Sharawy M, Misch CE, Weller N, et al. Heat generation during implant drilling: The significance of motor speed. J Oral Maxillofac Surg 2002;60:1160–9.
22. Brisman DL. The effect of speed, pressure, and time on bone temperature during the drilling of implant sites. Int J Oral Maxillofac Implants 1996;11:35–7.
23. Costa A, Pasta G, Bergamaschi G. Intraoral hard and soft tissue depths for temporary anchorage devices. Semin Orthod 2005;11:10–15.
24. Schierano G, Ramieri G, Cortese M, et al. Organization of the connective tissue barrier around long-term loaded implant abutments in man. Clin Oral Implants Res 2002;13:460–4.
25. Szmukler-Moncler S, Salama H, Reingewirtz Y, et al. Timing of loading and effect of micromotion on bone–dental implant interface: review of experimental literature. J Biomed Mater Res 1998;43:192–203.

26. Ure AD, Oliver DR, Kim KB, et al. Stability changes of miniscrew implants over time: a pilot resonance frequency analysis. Angle Orthod 2011;81:994–1000.

27. Gracco A, Cirignaco A, Cozzani M, et al. Numerical/experimental analysis of the stress field around miniscrews for orthodontic anchorage. Eur J Orthod 2009;31:12–20.

28. Costa A, Pasta G, Bergamaschi G. Intraoral hard and soft tissue depths for temporary anchorage devices. Semin Orthod 2005;11:10–15.

29. Hong C, Truong P, Song HN, et al. Mechanical stability assessment of novel orthodontic mini-implant designs: Part 2. Angle Orthod 2011;81:1001–9.

30. Kim YH, Yang SM, Kim S, et al. Midpalatal miniscrews for orthodontic anchorage: factors affecting clinical success. Am J Orthod Dentofacial Orthop 2010;137:66–72.

31. Brown GA, McCarthey T, Bourgeault A, et al. Mechanical performance of standard and cannulated 4.0 mm cancellous bone screws. J Orthop Res 2000;18:307–12.

32. Lim JW, Kim WS, Son CY, et al. Three dimensional finite element method for stress distribution on the length and diameter of orthodontic miniscrew and cortical bone thickness. Korean J Orthod 2003;33:11–20.

33. Johansson CB, Han CH, Wennerberg A, et al. A quantitative comparison of machined commercially pure titanium and titanium-aluminium-vanadium implants in rabbit bone. Int J Oral Maxillofac Implants 1998;13:315–21.

34. Wilmes B, Rademacher C, Olthoff G, et al. Parameters affecting primary stability of orthodontic mini-implants. J Orofac Orthop 2006;67:162–74.

35. Chao CK, Hsu CC, Wang JL, et al. Increasing bending strength and pullout strength and pullout strength in conical pedicle screws: biomechanical tests and finite element analyses. J Spinal Disord Tech 2008;21:130–8.

36. Krenn MH, Piotrowski WP, Penzkofer R, et al. Influence of thread design on pedicle screw fixation. Laboratory investigation. J Neurosurg Spine 2008;9:90–5.

37. Kuroda S, Sugawara Y, Deguchi T, et al. Clinical use of miniscrew implants as orthodontic anchorage: success rates and postoperative discomfort. Am J Orthod Dentofacial Orthop 2007;131:9–15.

38. Morarend C, Qian F, Marshall SD, et al. Effect of screw diameter on orthodontic skeletal anchorage. Am J Orthod Dentofacial Orthop 2009;136:224–9.

39. Mah J, Bergstrand F. Temporary anchorage devices: a status report. J Clin Orthod 2005;39:132–6.

40. De Coster TA, Heetderks DB, Downey DJ, et al. Optimizing bone screw pullout force. J Orthop Trauma 1990;4:169–74.

41. Mischkowski RA, Kneuertz P, Florvaag B, et al. Biomechanical comparison of four different miniscrew types for skeletal anchorage in the mandibulomaxillary area. Int J Oral Maxillofac Surg 2008;37:948–54.

42. Heidemann W, Gerlach K, Gröbel L, et al. Drill free screws: a new form of osteosynthesis screw. J Cranimaxillofac Surg 1998;26:163–8.

43. Heidemann W, Terheyden H, Gerlach KL. Analysis of the osseous/metal interface of drill free screws and self-tapping screws. J Craniomaxillofac Surg 2001;29:69–74.

44. Sakoh J, Wahlmann U, Stender E, et al. Primary stability of a conical implant and a hybrid, cylindric screw-type implant in vitro. Int J Oral Maxillofac Implants 2006;21:560–6.

45. Öktenoğlu BT, Ferrara LA, Andalkar N, et al. Effects of hole preparation on screw pullout resistance and insertional torque: a biomechanical study. J Neurosurgery Spine 2001;94:91–6.

46. Chen Y, Kyung HM, Zhao WT, et al. Critical factors for the success of orthodontic mini-implants: a systematic review. Am J Orthod Dentofacial Orthop 2009;135:284–91.

47. Bähr W. Pretapped and self-tapping screws in the human midface. Torque measurements and bone screw interface. Int J Oral Maxillofac Surg 1990;19:51–3.

48. Vangsness CT Jr, Carter DR, Frankel VH. In vitro evaluation of the loosening characteristics of self-tapped and non-self-tapped cortical bone screws. Clin Orthop Relat Res 1981;157:279–86.

49. Chen Y, Shin HI, Kyung HM. Biomechanical and histological comparison of self-tapping and self-drilling microimplants in dogs. Am J Orthod Dentofacial Orthop 2008;133:44–50.

50. Ellis JA Jr, Laskin DM. Analysis of seating and fracturing torque of bicortical screws. J Oral Maxillofac Surg 1994;52:483–7.

51. Kim JW, Ahn SJ, Chang YI. Histomorphometric and mechanical analysis of the drill-free screw as orthodontic anchorage. Am J Orthod Dentofacial Orthop 2005;128:190–4.

52. Wang YC, Liou EJ. Comparison of the loading behavior of self-drilling and predrilled miniscrews throughout orthodontic loading. Am J Orthod Dentofacial Orthop 2008;133:38–43.

53. Song Y, Cha J, Hwang C. Evaluation of insertion torque and pullout strength of miniscrews according to different thickness of artificial bone. Korean J Orthod 2007;37:5–15.

54. Florvaag B, Kneuert P, Lazar F, et al. Biomechanical properties of orthodontic miniscrews: an in-vitro study. J Orofac Orthop 2010;71:53–67.

55. Carano A, Lonardo P, Velo S, et al. Mechanical properties of three different commercially available miniscrews for skeletal anchorage. Prog Orthod 2005;6:82–97.

56. Glauser R, Portmann M, Ruhstaller P, et al. Initial implant stability using different implant designs and surgical techniques. A comparative clinical study using insertion torque and resonance frequency analysis. Appl Osseointegr Res 2001;2:6–8.

57. Abshire BB, McLain RF, Valdevit A, et al. Characteristics of pullout failure in conical and cylindrical pedicle screws after full insertion and back-out. Spine J 2001;1:408–14.

58. Kim JW, Baek SH, Kim TW, et al. Comparison of stability between cylindrical and conical type mini-implants. Angle Orthod 2008;78:692–8.

59. Lill CA, Schlegel U, Wahl D, et al. Comparison of the in vitro holding strengths of conical and cylindrical pedicle screws in a fully inserted setting and backed out 180 degrees. J Spinal Disord 2000;13:259–66.

60. Lill CA, Schneider E, Goldhahn J, et al. Mechanical performance of cylindircal and dual core pedicle screw in calf and human vertebrae. Arch Orthop Trauma Surg 2006;126:686–94.

61. Drago CJ, Del Castillo RA. A retrospective analysis of osseotite NT implants in clinical practice: 1-year follow-up. Int J Periodontics Restorative Dent 2006;26:337–45.

62. Cha JY, Takano-Yamamoto T, Hwang CJ. The effect of miniscrew taper morphology on insertion and removal torque in dogs. Int J Oral Maxillofac Implants 2010;25:777–83.

63. Yano S, Motoyoshi M, Uemura M, et al. Tapered orthodontic miniscrews induce bone screw cohesion following immediate loading. Eur J Orthod 2006;28:541–6.

64. Tencer AF, Asnis E, Harrington RM, et al. Biomechanics of cannulated and noncannulated screws. In: Asnis SE, Kyle RF, editors. Cannulated screw fixation: principles and operative techniques. New York: Springer; 1996. p. 15–40.

65. Halsey D, Fleming B, Pope MH, et al. External fixator pin design. Clin Orthop 1992;278:305–12.

66. Hong C, Lee H, Webster R, et al. Stability comparison between commercially available mini-implants and a novel design: part 1. Angle Orthod 2011;81:692–9.

67. Kim YK, Kim YJ, Yun PY, et al. Effects of the taper shape, dual-thread, and length on the mechanical properties of mini-implants. Angle Orthod 2009;79:908–14.

68. Yerby S, Scott CC, Evans NJ, et al. Effects of cutting flute design on cortical bone screw insertion torque and pullout strength. J Orthop Trauma 2001;15:216–21.

69. Brinley CL, Behrents R, Kim KB, et al. Pitch and longitudinal fluting effects on the primary stability of miniscrew implants. Angle Orthod 2009;79:1156–61.

70. Baumgart FW, Cordey J, Morikawa K, et al. AO/ASIF self-tapping screws (STS). Injury 1993;24:1–7.

71. Carano A, Velo S, Leone P, et al. Clinical applications of the miniscrew anchorage system. J Clin Orthod 2005;19:19–24.

7 The use of implants as skeletal anchorage in orthodontics

Karlien Asscherickx

INTRODUCTION

When no ankylosed tooth is present and dental elements lack either quantity or quality, or when compliance during treatment is unlikely, implants are an excellent alternative to traditional orthodontic anchorage methods. They have a high success rate and there is a lot of expertise and evidence-based research on their use in dentistry.

Skeletal anchorage with implants requires osseointegration, which is clinically manifest as an absence of mobility. To ensure sufficient resistance to continuous loading, such as conventional orthodontic forces, an osseointegration of at least 10% should be present between the implant surface and the surrounding bone.[1] However, implants also have to be removed at the end of orthodontic treatment, requiring another minor surgical procedure, and ease of removal will also be affected by the degree of osseointegration.

The major advantages of implants include positional stability, intraoral placement (invisible) and independence from compliance. Furthermore, when inserted in the palate for orthodontic anchorage, one implant can be sufficient, instead of two miniscrew implants (MIs) or two miniplates.

An implant can be used for different purposes in orthodontics:

- *orthodontic–prosthetic implant anchorage*: the implant is first used to provide orthodontic anchorage control, and then it is used to support a crown or bridgework[2]
- *pure orthodontic implant anchorage*: the implant is used solely for orthodontic purposes and is removed at the end of treatment[3]
- *orthopedic anchorage*: skeletal anchorage is used to expand or move bones in a certain direction, with the implant being removed at the end of treatment.[4]

Where implants are removed after they have served orthodontic purposes, they are referred to as temporary anchorage devices.[2]

This chapter provides an overview of the different types of implants that can be used for skeletal anchorage in orthodontics, with a special focus on palatal implants.

IMPLANT TYPES

Implants can be placed conventionally in the alveolar ridge or within the palate. An important precondition for successful implant osseointegration is a satisfactory bone base, with both bone height and bone mineral density being factors affecting the success of implant osseointegration.

The main feature of conventional titanium endosseous dental implants is osseointegration to provide rigid three-dimensional anchorage control. The implants can only be inserted in edentulous areas with adequate bone support. Since the implants behave like ankylosed teeth, they do not erupt like normal teeth and the vertical development of the alveolar process is restricted. Therefore, their indication is limited to partially edentulous and full-grown patients in order to avoid infra-occlusion of the implant during the normal eruption of neighbouring teeth in growing patients.[5] The indications are rather limited and they are rarely used for the treatment of Class II malocclusion.

An alternative site for implantation of osseointegrated implants is the palate. Clear benefits include the facts that the palatal bone is of good quality and there is no interference with the roots of teeth, and so maxillary posterior teeth can be easily distalized without interference with the implant. Design of an implant must be suitable to fit the palatal region, which has a decreased bone height compared with the alveolar ridge. The length of the implants is decreased while the diameter can be augmented since no root interference will occur. This allows an enlarged implant surface in direct contact with bone.

The midline of the palatine bone is of particular anatomic interest. The vertical height of the bone in the midsagittal area was found to be at least 2 mm higher than apparent on cephalometric radiographs.[6] In the broad median suture zone, the bone is relatively dense compared with the more paramedian region and consequently this should be the area of choice for the placement of palatal orthodontic implants in adults.

In growing adolescents, caution must be taken when inserting the implants in the median suture zone as the maxilla is continuously expanding in the transverse direction during normal growth. This transverse growth results from appositional remodeling of the alveolar processes, leading to the expansion of the dental arches, and growth in the median palatal suture, leading to expansion of the palate. The second contributes more to the development of maxillary width than does the first.[7] An average increase of 2.8 mm in maxillary width through median sutural growth at the level of the molars was seen in radiographs between posterior implants for eight boys aged 10–18 years, with the largest increase between 13 and 15 years.[8] On the basis of morphology, the development of the median suture could be divided into three stages.[9] In the first stage, the suture is short, broad and Y-shaped; in the second stage the course is more sinuous, and in the third stage interdigitation is heavy. During adolescence, the median palatal suture is in the second stage, and bone availability for implant placement might be limited. The degree of obliteration of the median palatal suture increases with age but is still very variable. Since orthodontic treatment is most often started during adolescence, it is important to know if the insertion of palatal implants in the median suture might cause problems either through an influence on normal transverse maxillary development or through insufficient bone to provide the required osseointegration. An experimental study with dogs has shown that transverse maxillary growth was reduced by the presence of implants and suggested that an alternative insertion site should be considered in adolescents.[10,11]

Several studies have demonstrated that the parasagittal region can provide enough bone support to allow for adequate osseointegration of palatal implants. In a more recent study, bone height and bone mineral density were assessed at different potential implantation sites for palatal implants.[12] The thickest part of the palate was detected at (a) 3.0 mm posterior to the incisive foramen and at 6.0 mm distance lateral from the median line of the palatine bone (paramedian); (b) 6.0 mm posterior to the incisive foramen and at 6.0 mm distance paramedian; and (c) 6.0 mm posterior to the incisive foramen and at 9.0 mm distance paramedian. Bone mineral density was greatest exactly on the midline at 6 mm, 9 mm and 12 mm posterior to the incisive foramen. Bone mineral density appeared to correlate negatively with bone height.

The optimal position of a palatal implant will be individual for each patient. Analysis of the lateral cephalometric radiograph should be used to determine the optimal insertion site and the length of the implant to be

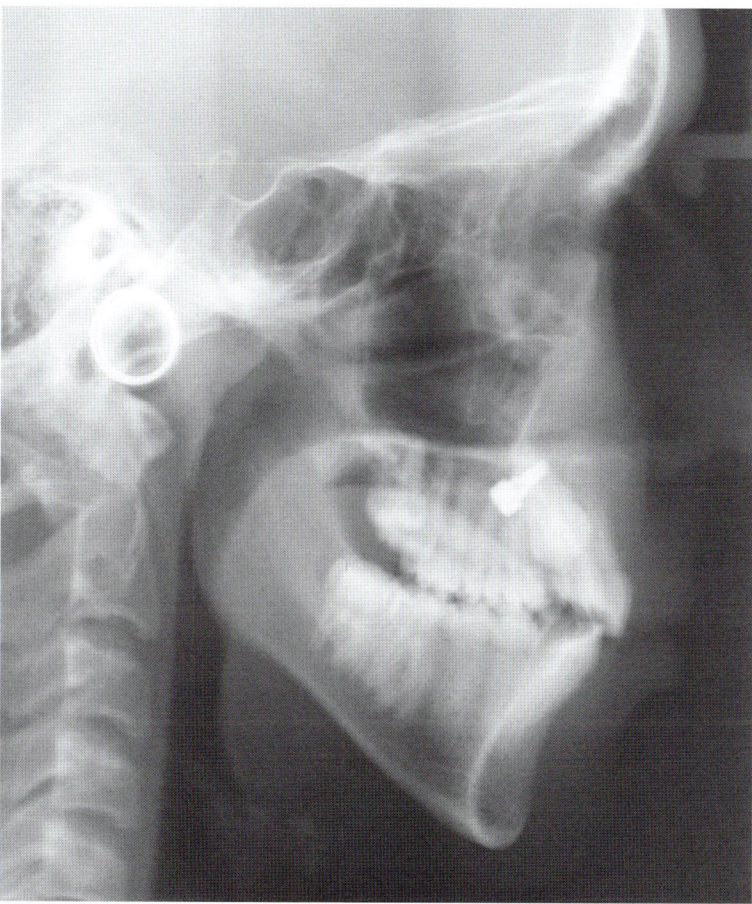

Fig. 7.1 Lateral cephalometric radiograph showing a palatal implant inserted at the level of the first premolars with a direction perpendicular to the palate.

used (Fig. 7.1). As a general rule in adults, the median palatal suture at the level of the first or second premolars is the most stable site for implant insertion. In addition, short implants should be used. In adolescents, the paramedian region (3.0 to 6.0 mm lateral to the midline) at the level of the first premolars is the area of choice.

However, for correction of a Class II, division 2 malocclusion by maxillary molar distalization and torquing of the maxillary anterior teeth, the implant must be inserted even more distally in order to avoid possible root contact with the central incisors when they are torqued.

Several devices have been developed specifically for the palatal region: the BIOS implant system (not commercially available, similar design and dimensions as the ITI-Bonefit Screw Implant [Straumann, Waldenburg, Switzerland] but in biodegradable material),[13] the Straumann Orthosystem (Straumann, Basel, Switzerland),[14] the Frialit-2 Implant System (Friadent, Mannheim, Germany),[15] the Midplant system (HDC, Sarcedo, Italy),[16] the short epithetic implants (Brånemark, Nobel Biocare, Göteborg, Sweden)[17] and the Onplant System (Nobel Biocare).[18]

The Onplant System and the Straumann Orthosystem have been studied most extensively and, therefore, these types will be described in more detail in this chapter. The descriptions and clinical considerations are more or less the same for all implant types that have been developed for palatal insertion.

DENTAL IMPLANTS

While conventional titanium endosseous dental implants have been used as sources of direct anchorage, there are some disadvantages in their use for orthodontic–prosthetic implant anchorage, mainly related to the requirement for an edentulous area with adequate bone support and a fully

grown patient. Another disadvantage is the treatment complexity. Treatment must be coordinated by multiple specialists (including a periodontist or surgeon, a prosthodontist or restorative dentist, and an orthodontist).[2] If the restorative treatment plan involves a dental implant, it may be beneficial to use the implant itself as anchorage for treating concomitant orthodontic problems.[19]

Once the implant has been placed and after an appropriate healing period of 3–4 months, no movement will occur because of osseointegration. Therefore, the exact position of all teeth after treatment must be determined in a pretreatment set-up on casts to aid in the precise placement of implant(s) prior to commencing treatment. This is difficult to do exactly as tooth movements cannot be predicted with 100% precision and bone morphology and bone biology vary between patients.[20]

ONPLANTS

The Onplant System is designed as an implant anchor for insertion in the midpalatal region.[18]

Design

The Onplant is a two-stage subperiosteal implant. The device is a titanium alloy disk (2 mm thick and 10 mm diameter) with a textured side opposing bone that is coated with a 75 μm layer of hydroxyapatite (see Fig. 3.3). The side facing soft tissue is smooth titanium alloy with a threaded hole in the center into which abutments are placed.

Insertion Site and Surgical Procedures

The Onplant is placed subperiosteally on the posterior aspect of the hard palate with a "tunneling" procedure. A full-thickness mucoperiosteal incision is made on the anterior aspect of the hard palate and tunnels are reflected posteriorly. These tunnels allow the Onplant to be placed away from the incision, thus reducing the potential for soft tissue inflammation, which can prevent osseointegration. A healing screw is placed, and 10 to 12 weeks are allowed for osseointegration. After this healing period, the disk is exposed by a punch technique and a ball-shaped abutment is connected to which orthodontic devices can be attached. The abutment is designed to receive a 1.3 mm wire (see Fig. 3.2).

The main problems of this type of implant are that primary stability often cannot be achieved by mechanical retention and that clinical assessment of integration is not easy.

To remove the implant, osteotomes are used; removal of a large portion of soft tissue is needed and might cause postoperative discomfort for the patient.

There is only one study in which the success rates of onplants were evaluated.[21] A group of 29 children (mean age 14.0 years) each had an Onplant inserted. Orthodontic treatment comprised extraction of two maxillary premolars (in most cases, also two mandibular premolars) followed by fixed appliances in both jaws. The Onplant provided additional indirect anchorage on the maxillary first molars. After the healing period, one Onplant was still unstable and was removed. Another two were tilted (although osseointegrated), and so it was not possible to take impressions in order to fabricate the palatal bars. The success rate in this study, defined by the authors as "suitable to provide stationary anchorage," was 89.6%.

ORTHOSYSTEM IMPLANTS

The Orthosystem implants can be placed in areas of decreased bone height and so can be used as palatal anchorage.[14] The implant may replace compliance-dependent extraoral anchoring aids for orthodontics and makes bonding and alignment of the mandibular dental arch for the application of Class II elastics unnecessary.

Design

The fixture is designed for a one-stage application. The endosseous part of the implant is cylindrical, has a self-tapping thread and is made of pure titanium (Fig. 7.2). It has a diameter of 3.3 or 4.0 mm and a length of 4.0 or 6.0 mm. The implant has a sandblasted and acid-etched surface because palatal implants are meant to osseointegrate in bone and the surface treatment provides a larger contact area between the implant and the bone. There is an abutment above the polished transmucosal neck on which the desired suprastructure is soldered or laser welded.

Which size of implant should be used depends on cephalometric data. Usually, the 3.3 mm diameter implant is used, with 4.0 or 6.0 mm in

length. The 4.0 mm diameter implant is a replacement implant that can be used if primary stability does not establish. The benefit of using longer (6.0 mm in length) implants was assessed in a study on human cadavers, which indicated that quality of implantation and bone structure are more important for stability than the length of the implant.[22] When there is any doubt about the available bone height, shorter implants should be used (4.0 mm in length).

Insertion Site and Surgical Procedures

The insertion site can be in the median or paramedian palatal region and provides anchorage in the maxilla.

The insertion procedure (Fig. 7.3) itself is relatively easy and fast when performed by an experienced surgeon.

Under local anesthesia (palatine nerve on both sides and incisive nerve), the palatal mucosa is removed with the aid of the mucosa trephine and an elevator. The implantation site is marked with a round bur (diameter 2.3 mm) and the cortical bone is indented. The implant bed is prepared using the corresponding profile drill. Drilling must be continued until a complete seat is created, maximally to the stop. To prevent excessive heat build-up, the speed of rotation should not exceed 750 rpm. The drills must be sharp and abundant external cooling of the drill with sterile physiological saline or Ringer's solution should be provided. The self-tapping implant is inserted by hand as far as possible and if necessary a ratchet can be used to tighten the implant into its final position. If there is no primary stability of the implant, because of an enlarged implantation bed, the implant bed should be widened with a spiral drill (diameter 3.5 mm) so that a wider implant can be placed (4.0 mm diameter instead of the standard 3.3 mm).

After implant insertion, a healing cap or a healing screw must be placed on top of or in the implant (Fig. 7.3D). Postoperative check-ups are scheduled after 1 day, 1 week, 1 month and 2 months.

The first weeks after insertion, the patient must be instructed not to "play" with the implant with the tongue, as this might destabilize the implant and prevent proper osseointegration. A covering plate can be used for 2 months after implant placement to prevent tongue pressure on it (Fig. 7.3E).

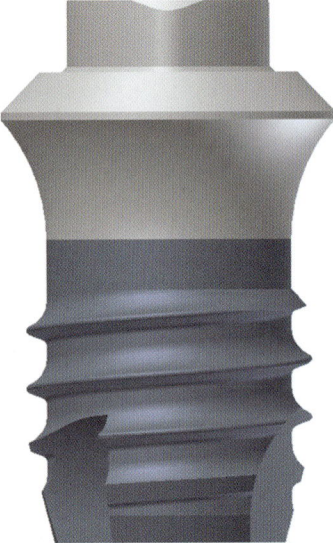

Fig. 7.2 The Straumann Orthosystem implant with a smooth transmucosal neck and a surface-treated endosseous part.

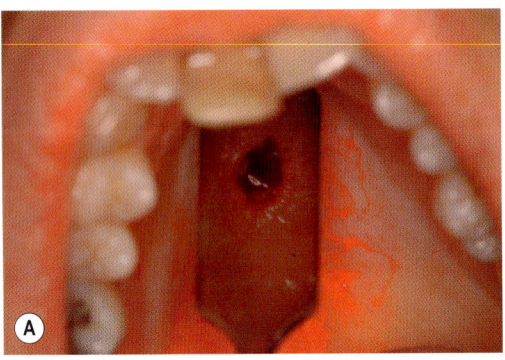

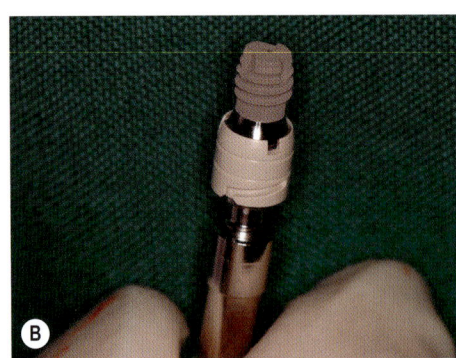

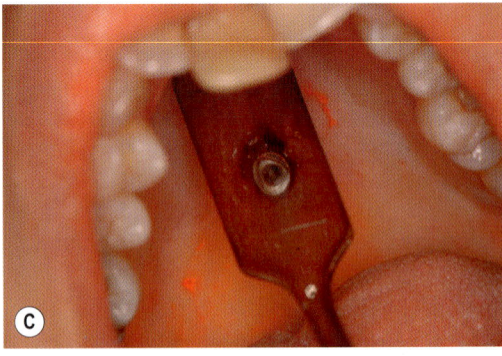

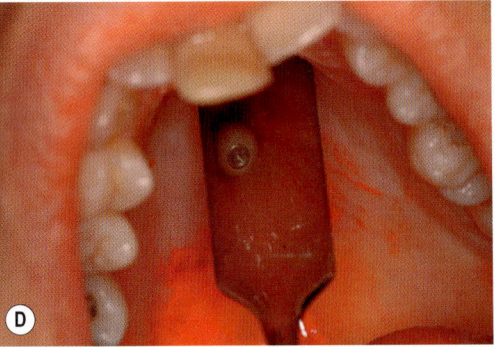

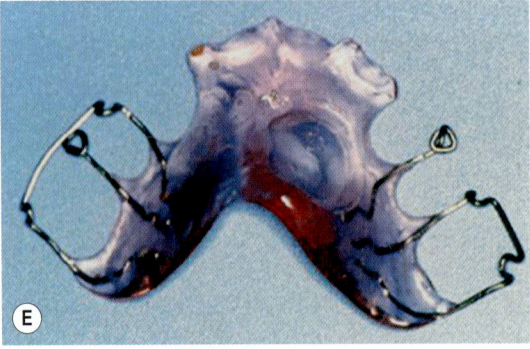

Fig. 7.3 Insertion of a palatal implant. (A) Preparation of implant bed. (B) Insertion of the palatal implant manually. (C) The implant inserted. (D) Healing cap placed on the implant immediately after insertion. (E) A covering acrylic plate, which can be used to prevent tongue pressure on the implant during the healing phase.

Fig. 7.4 Palatal mucosa immediately after implant removal (A) and 3 months later (B).

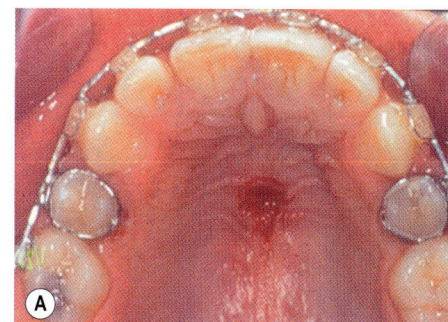
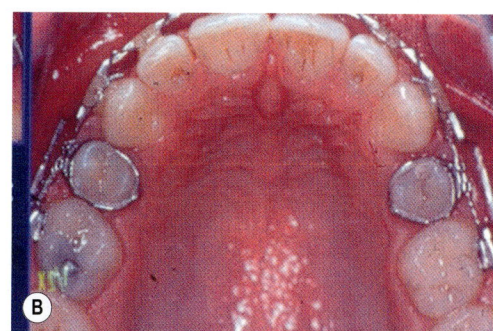

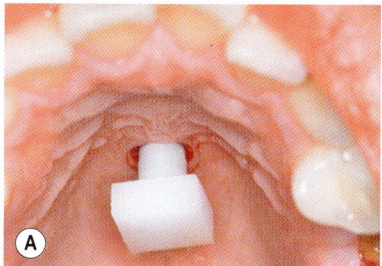
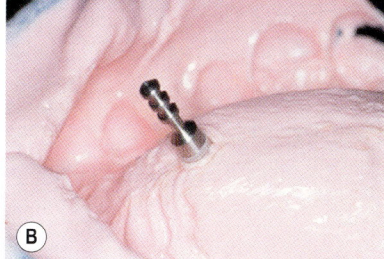
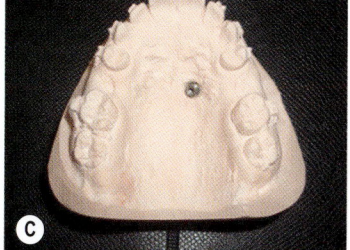
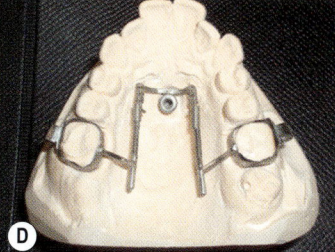

Fig. 7.5 Impression procedure and construction of the suprastructure. (A) Placement of the transfer coping on the implant. (B) Inserting the analogue in the transfer coping. (C) The steel coping placed on the analogue on the dental cast. (D) Fabrication of the suprastructure.

The implant should not be cleaned with a toothbrush up until the seventh postoperative day, but the mouth should be rinsed three times daily with a chlorhexidine digluconate solution. The implant may be cleaned carefully with a toothbrush from the eighth postoperative day, and rinsing with chlorhexidine should be continued until day 14 (twice daily). After this, the implant is cleaned during normal tooth brushing twice to three times daily using a normal toothbrush. In the event of soft tissue inflammation around the implant, the mouth should be rinsed with chlorhexidine according to medical need. A healing period of 10 to 12 weeks is most often advocated before orthodontic loading is started.

Since no findings on "sleeping orthodontic implants" have been published to date, the implant should be retrieved after use. The orthodontic connection is removed and the implant is covered until explantation with a healing cap or a healing screw. Local anesthesia is administered as for the implantation. Since implants osseointegrate, most often the implant is removed together with the surrounding bone. There are two possible options for reaching bone level with the explantation drill. The transmucosal cylinder can be exposed by cutting around it with a scalpel (approximately 1 mm margin) and then removing the sleeve. Otherwise, the mucosa can be removed by the drill, set at approximately 400 rpm. Via the guiding cylinder, drilling is performed down to bone level while soft tissue remnants are rinsed away. Explantation proceeds at 400–700 rpm accompanied by continuous cooling with precooled physiological saline or Ringer's solution. The bone should be trephined down to two-thirds of the implant length. If the implant cannot be removed with extraction forceps and gentle rotation, trephining must be continued to the mark corresponding to the endosseous implant length. The implant is then removed. Simple wound management is indicated after explantation. No flap preparation or suturing is necessary. Healing of the palate after removal is uneventful in most patients. After 1 week, the palatal mucosa is usually closed and the original rugae are restored by 3 months after explantation (Fig. 7.4).

Post-orthodontic evaluation of paramedianly placed fixtures by means of dental scans (General Electric, Milwaukee WI, USA) sometimes reveals a close contact between the well-osseointegrated fixture and the nasal cavity or the adjacent teeth, making removal by trephine drilling potentially harmful.[22] A possible option is to remove the implant with a manual torque device by counterclockwise untightening. This is possible when implants exhibit a stability of more than −5 periotest units (Periotest device; Periotest, Gulden, Germany).[23] Fixtures showing stability values equal to or less than −5 periotest units cannot be removed in this way and removal of the transmucosal part of the implant and sealing of the internal screw hole is proposed in order to allow complete "creeping" mucosal covering of the implant.

Impression Procedure and Construction of Suprastructure

A healing period of 10 to 12 weeks is allowed before an impression is taken. During this time, the implant has sufficient time for osseointegration. Successful implant integration can be concluded if (a) the patient has no subjective symptoms, (b) there is no inflammation with suppuration around the implant, (c) there is a high-pitch sound on percussion and (d) the implant is immobile.

If no healing abutment was placed after implant insertion, mucosa might have grown over the borders of the transmucosal neck, preventing proper placement of an impression cap. In such a situation, a healing cap might be placed several days before the impression. This will remove the mucosa from the borders (Fig. 7.3D).

An impression cap or transfer coping is placed in position on the implant (Fig. 7.5A). Then an impression is made and an analogue is placed in the impression cap (Fig. 7.5B). A master cast is fabricated and the steel coping is placed on the analogue (Fig. 7.5C). The fabricated suprastructure (Fig. 7.5D) is welded or soldered to the steel coping. The steel coping with the suprastructure can be fixed to the implant in the patient's mouth with a small screw.

There are few studies examining success rates with Orthosystem implants, with values ranging from 90% to 95.4%.[24–27] The largest study was a retrospective analysis on prognostic parameters contributing to palatal implant failures in which 11 of 239 Orthosystem implants that were used for orthodontic anchorage purposes failed.[27] The main conclusions of the study were that implant losses occurred mainly early in the healing phase, and that "surgeon's experience" is the cornerstone of palatal implant success.

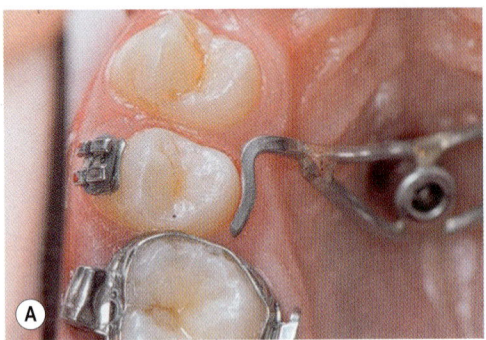
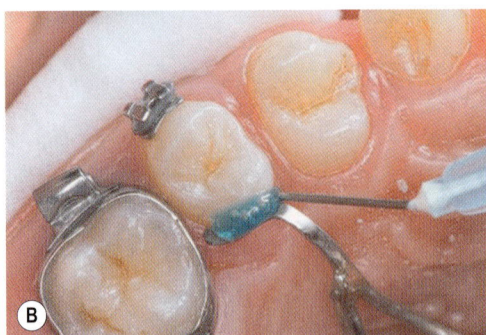
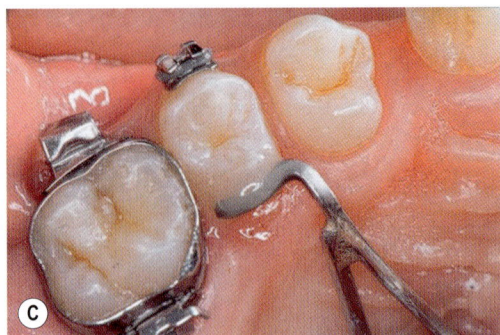

Fig. 7.6 Connection of the transpalatal arch (TPA) to the teeth. (A) Sandblasting of TPA and tooth. (B) Etching of the second premolar with phosphoric acid. (C) TPA bonded to the second premolar.

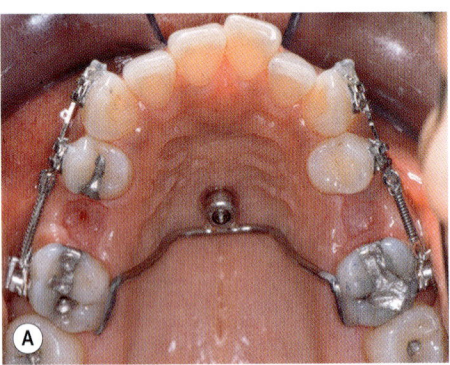
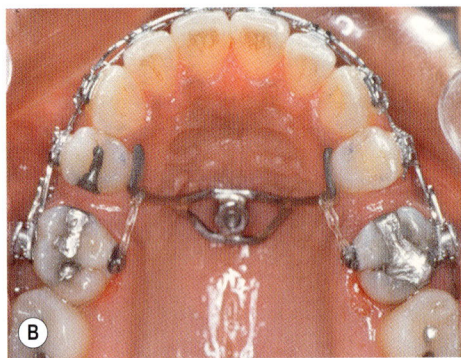
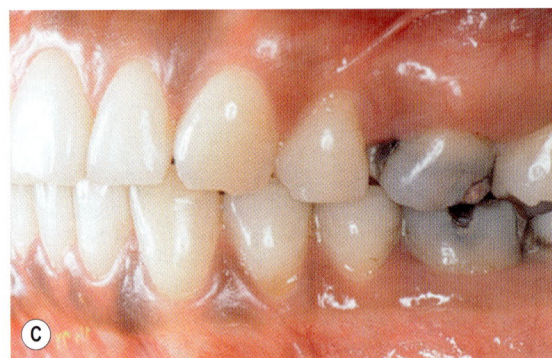

Fig. 7.7 Case presentation after extraction of the maxillary second premolars. (A) The transpalatal arch is connected initially to the first molars to reinforce anchorage for the retraction of the anterior dental segment. (B) After anterior teeth retraction, the arch is connected to the first premolars, to protract the maxillary molars. (C) Lateral view after treatment. (From Asscherickx et al.,[25] with kind permission from Elsevier.)

CLINICAL INDICATIONS FOR PALATAL IMPLANTS IN CLASS II TREATMENT

For the correction of Class II malocclusion, palatal implants can be used to provide either direct or indirect anchorage.

INDIRECT ANCHORAGE

A transpalatal arch can be fixed to the implant and to the teeth (usually the second premolar) to be used as anchorage unit.[24] The arch can be attached to the anchoring teeth by bonding with composite material (Fig. 7.6). Both the transpalatal arch and the tooth are sandblasted. After etching, the tooth is rinsed and dried, and the adhesive is applied and light cured. With a flowable composite, the transpalatal arch is attached to the tooth to give a secure bonding that is both smooth and hygienic.

If the maxillary second premolar is extracted, the transpalatal arch can be connected to the maxillary molars to support retraction of the maxillary anterior segment. Once the anterior segment is retracted into a neutral occlusion, a new transpalatal arch can be connected to the first premolars to start mesialization of the molars (Fig. 7.7). This illustrates the versatility of the system.

If there is no extraction, the implant can be connected with a transpalatal arch to the maxillary second premolars and coils can be used on the buccal side to distalize molars (Fig. 7.8). This type of distalization is indicated particularly when molars present an extreme mesial-in rotation before orthodontic treatment. Once the maxillary molars are distalized into a Class I occlusion, a new transpalatal arch can be connected to the first molars to start distalization of the premolars and anterior teeth retraction.

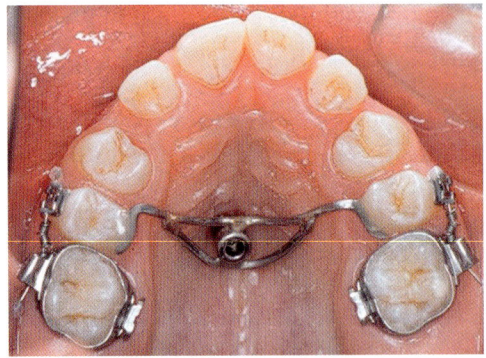

Fig. 7.8 Transpalatal arch connected to upper second premolars to provide stationary anchorage for mesial-out rotation and distalization of the maxillary first molars. (Courtesy of B. Van de Vannet.)

DIRECT ANCHORAGE

Palatal implants can support an implant-anchored distalizer (IAD) in order to distalize maxillary molars (Fig. 7.9). Once the molars have been distalized, the IAD can be made passive to keep the molars secure and stable while retracting the premolars, the canines and the frontal dental segment.

Fig. 7.10 illustrates the use of the IAD for a slight Class II malocclusion with lack of space in the maxillary arch. By using an IAD, treatment can be started in the maxillary arch only, with an almost invisible appliance. Only after distalization of the maxillary posterior teeth fixed appliances are placed on both maxillary and mandibular arches to finish treatment. This substantially reduces treatment time with visible appliances, and buccal tipping of the mandibular anterior teeth by Class II elastics can be avoided.

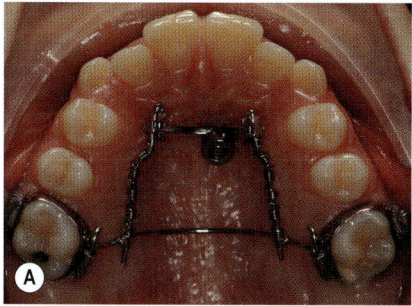 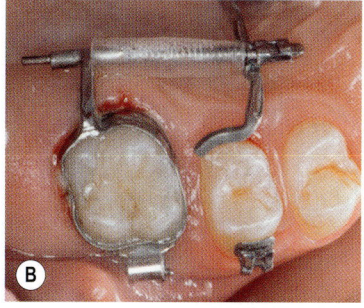 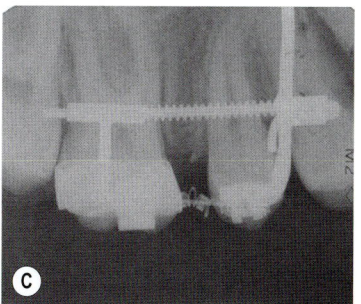 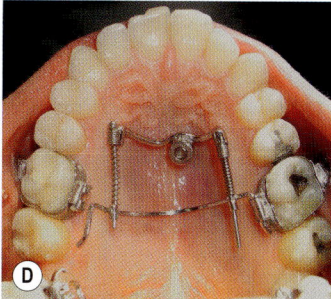

Fig. 7.9 The implant-anchored distalizer. (A,B) Clinical views. (C) Radiography showing the point of force application very near to the center of resistance of the first molar and bodily movement. (D) Activation of the transpalatal arch of the implant-anchored distalizer with antirotation bends to prevent mesiopalatal rotation of the first molars. (Implant-anchored distalizer designed by B. Vande Vannet and J. Aerts.)

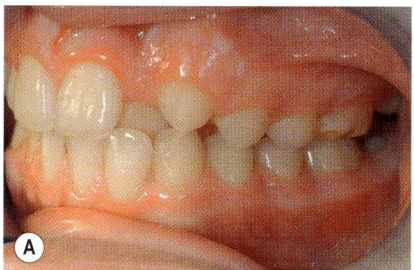 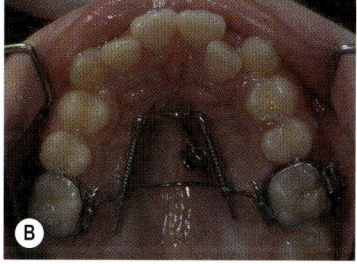 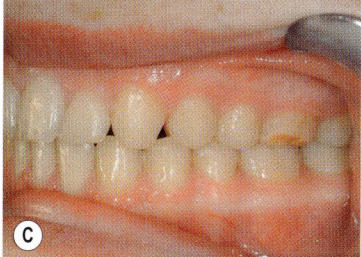 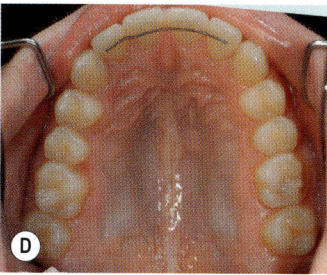

Fig. 7.10 Case presentation for use of the implant-anchored distalizer. (A) Lateral view before treatment. (B) Occlusal view after installation of the implant-anchored distalizer. (C,D) Lateral (C) and occlusal (D) views after treatment. (Courtesy of J. Aerts.)

Important in this type of distalization is to make sure that the force application is at the level of resistance of the maxillary molars to ensure bodily movement during distalization. The point of force application is very near to the center of resistance of the first molar, which is located at the bifurcation of its roots (Fig. 7.9C).

Since the distalization force is applied on the palatal side of the center of resistance of the molars, mesiopalatal rotation can occur. This side effect can be prevented by incorporating antirotation bends in the transpalatal arch (Fig. 7.9D). However, these bends might slow the distal movement of the molars.

CONCLUSIONS

Palatal implants specially designed for orthodontic purposes can be of great benefit in the treatment of Class II malocclusion. Using these implants, stationary anchorage control can be obtained and better oral hygiene can be achieved than with classical conventional anchorage means such as the Nance button.

A prospective randomized controlled clinical trial compared the anchorage capacity of osseointegrated and conventional anchorage systems.[21] Anchorage loss was seen with headgear anchorage and transpalatal bar but both the Onplant and the Orthosystem implant provided stable anchorage. There were more technical problems with the Onplant, resulting in more failures, and the system required additional surgery to place the abutment. The authors concluded that the Orthosystem palatal implant should be the anchorage of choice if maximum anchorage is required but the major disadvantages were the requirement for minor surgery, the need for a healing period and the extra cost.

The need for minor surgery means that implants should be inserted by an experienced surgeon, requiring good communication between the orthodontist and the surgeon.[28] The pain associated with placement of a palatal Orthosystem implant and premolar extraction in adolescent patients was assessed using a visual analogue scale, with the latter having a higher score.[28] A questionnaire assessment of 85 patients whose orthodontic treatment included the use of a palatal implant showed that most patients got used to the implant in about 2 weeks, while 86% of the patients would recommend the treatment to others.[29] This would suggest that the surgical steps should not be a good reason for the orthodontist to exclude palatal implants from a treatment plan.

Another possible disadvantage of the use of osseointegrated implants is that a healing period is required. If carefully planned, this should not be a problem. If extraction is part of treatment and the implant will support a palatal arch to anchor the posterior teeth, leveling of the teeth can be accomplished during the healing phase of the implant and the implant can be loaded when retraction is to be started. With an IAD, the patient has only a small healing abutment in the oral cavity during the 3 months before initiation of treatment. A randomized clinical trial examined immediate loading of palatal implants compared with conventional loading after a healing period of 12 weeks.[25] Immediate loading had equivalent success rates as conventional loading with 4 N after 6 months. However, further follow-up of this group is necessary before a general conclusion can be made that palatal implants can be loaded immediately.

The problem of the higher cost cannot easily be solved. Major advantages of the palatal implants are that only one implant is necessary to provide sufficient anchorage control on both sides of the maxillary arch and that the success rate for palatal implants is relatively high, ranging from 90 to 95.4%. This might compensate partially for the high cost. When MIs are used in the palate to support an intraoral distalization appliance, usually two MIs are recommended and their success rate is not as high as that of palatal implants.

If maximum anchorage is required, anchorage reinforcement by the use of palatal implants seems to be an ideal approach. The minor surgery needed for insertion (and removal) of the implants is well accepted by the patients. The healing period needed before loading of the implants with orthodontic forces may not be needed but further studies are required to support this consideration.

REFERENCES

1. Roberts WE. Bone tissue interface. J Dent Educ 1988;52:804–9.
2. Kokich VG. Managing complex orthodontic problems: the use of implants for anchorage. Semin Orthod 1996;2:153–60.
3. Mah J, Bergstrand F. Temporary anchorage devices: a status report. J Clin Orthod 2005;39:132–6.
4. De Pauw GA, Dermaut L, De Bruyn H, et al. Stability of implants as anchorage for orthopedic traction. Angle Orthod 1999;69:401–7.
5. Thilander B, Ödman J, Gröndahl K, et al. Osseointegrated implants in adolescents: an alternative in replacing missing teeth? Eur J Orthod 1994;16:84–95.
6. Wehrbein H, Merz BR, Diedrich P. Palatal bone support for orthodontic implant anchorage: a clinical and radiological study. Eur J Orthod 1999;21:65–70.
7. Björk A, Skieller V. Growth in width of the maxilla studied by the implant method. Scand J Plast Reconstr Surg 1974;8:26–33.
8. Björk A, Skieller V. Growth of the maxilla in three dimensions as revealed radiographically by the implant method. Br J Orthod 1977;4:53–64.
9. Melsen B. Palatal growth studied on human autopsy material: a histologic microradiographic study. Am J Orthod 1975;68:42–54.
10. Asscherickx K, Hanssens JL, Wehrbein H, et al. Orthodontic anchorage implants inserted in the median palatal suture and normal transverse maxillary growth in growing dogs: a biometric and radiographic study. Angle Orthod 2005;75:826–31.
11. Asscherickx K, Wehrbein H, Sabzevar MM. Palatal implants in adolescents: a histological evaluation in beagle dogs. Clin Oral Implants Res 2008;19:657–64.
12. Lai RF, Zou H, Kong WD, et al. Applied anatomic site study of palatal anchorage implants using cone beam computed tomography. Int J Oral Sci 2010;2:98–104.
13. Glatzmaier J, Wehrbein H, Diedrich P. Die Entwicklung eines resorbierbaren Implantatsystems zur orthodontischen Verankerung. Fortschr Kieferorthop 1995;56:175–81.
14. Wehrbein H, Glatzmaier J, Mundwiller U, Diedrich P. The Orthosystem: a new implant system for orthodontic anchorage in the palate. J Orofac Orthop 1996;57:142–53.
15. Keles A, Erverdi N, Sezen S. Bodily distalization of molars with absolute anchorage. Angle Orthod 2003;73:471–82.
16. Maino BG, Mura P, Gianelly AA. A retrievable palatal implant for absolute anchorage in orthodontics. World J Orthod 2002;3:125–34.
17. Bernhart T, Freudenthaler J, Dortbudak O, et al. Short epithetic implants for orthodontic anchorage in the paramedian region of the palate. A clinical study. Clin Oral Implants Res 2001;12:624–31.
18. Block MS, Hoffman DR. A new device for absolute anchorage for orthodontics. Am J Orthod Dentofacial Orthop 1995;107:251–8.
19. Heymann G, Tulloch C. Implantable devices as orthodontic anchorage: a review of current treatment modalities. J Esthet Restor Dent 2006;18:68–80.
20. Smalley WM. Implants for tooth movement: determining implant location and orientation. J Esthet Dent 1995;7:62–72.
21. Feldmann I, Bondemark L. Anchorage capacity of osseointegrated and conventional anchorage systems: a randomized controlled trial. Am J Orthod Dentofacial Orthop 2008;133:339.
22. Gedrange T, Hietschold V, Mai R, et al. An evaluation of resonance frequency analysis for the determination of primary stability of orthodontic palatal implants: a study in human cadavers. Clin Oral Implants Res 2005;16:425–31.
23. Grognard N, van de Vannet B. Aspects in post-orthodontic removal of Orthosystem implants. Clin Oral Implants Res 2008;19:1290–4.
24. Bantleon HP, Bernhart T, Crismani A, et al. Stable orthodontic anchorage with palatal osseointegrated implants. World J Orthod 2002;3:109–16.
25. Crismani AG, Bernhart T, Schwarz K, et al. Ninety percent success in palatal implants loaded 1 week after placement: a clinical evaluation by resonance frequency analysis. Clin Oral Implants Res 2006;17:445–50.
26. Asscherickx K, van de Vannet B, Bottenberg P, et al. Clinical observations and success rates of palatal implants. Am J Orthod Dentofacial Orthop 2010;137:114–22.
27. Jung BA, Kunkel M, Göllner P, et al. Prognostic parameters contributing to palatal implant failures: a long-term survival analysis of 239 patients. Clin Oral Implants Res 2012;23:746–50.
28. Feldmann I, List T, Feldmann H, et al. Pain intensity and discomfort following surgical placement of orthodontic anchoring units and premolar extraction: a randomized controlled trial. Angle Orthod 2007;77:578–85.
29. Günduz E, Schneider-Del Savio TT, Kucher G, et al. Acceptance rate of palatal implants: a questionnaire study. Am J Orthod Dentofacial Orthop 2004;126:623–6.

Orthodontic anchorage using a locking plate and self-drilling miniscrew implants for the posterior maxilla

Hideharu Hibi, Kiyoshi Sakai, Minoru Ueda and Masaru Sakai

8

INTRODUCTION

Single miniscrew implants are typically used in the alveolus and palate where bone quality and quantity are adequate to support them since they are only mechanically retained. However, in order to avoid complications, the implant must be positioned within the attached mucosa and without any contact with the root surfaces of the underlying teeth. These requirements restrict the location of insertion, inclination and dimensions of the miniscrew implants. In contrast, miniplates are associated with fewer location restrictions, although their insertion requires a more complicated and invasive procedure, as well as higher costs.

The use of miniplates as anchor devices is, therefore, particularly likely for the treatment of Class II malocclusion when there is need for positioning in the posterior maxilla, with only a thin bony wall, in order to retract the anterior teeth and/or for the treatment of open bite in order to intrude the maxillary molars. In this challenging environment, skeletally anchored miniplates using conventional miniscrew systems may become unstable over time,[1] whereas osteosynthetic systems with locking mechanisms between the plates and the miniscrews provide more stability.[2] This chapter examines an effective method of using a locking plate and self-drilling miniscrew implant (Compact lock 2.0, Synthes Maxillofacial, PA, USA) for skeletal anchorage in the posterior maxilla.

INSERTION TECHNIQUE

This system has self-drilling screws of diameter 2.0 mm and L-shaped miniplates that have five threaded holes, three to be used to secure the miniplate with miniscrew implants to the bone and two to be used for application of orthodontic forces. The stabilization miniscrew implants can be locked together with the miniplates via the threaded holes.

Prior to insertion, the L-shaped miniplate is bent into a "crank" form, but it remains straight across its longitudinal portion (Fig. 8.1). Under local anesthesia, two vertical incisions are introduced in the mucogingival junction of the posterior maxilla, each 3 mm long and approximately 1 cm apart (Fig. 8.2A,B). To tunnel these two incisions, the mucosa is supraperiosteally undermined with a mucosal elevator (Fig. 8.2C). The longitudinal portion of the plate is inserted into the tunnel superiorly through the lower incision wound and placed on the periosteum (Fig. 8.2D). Based on the distance between the plate and the underlying bone, a 4 or 6 mm miniscrew is inserted without pilot drilling into the bone through the opened upper incision wound and screwed and tightened through the miniplate threaded hole (Fig. 8.2E). A second miniscrew is placed into the adjacent hole in the same manner, thereby providing complete stability to the plate (Figs 8.3 and 8.4). A bending plier is used to adjust the external portion of the plate for appropriate orthodontic use (Fig. 8.2G). The wounds require no suturing and have almost healed after a week, with minimal postoperative morbidity. The miniplate can be loaded with orthodontic forces immediately after insertion, serving as a temporary orthodontic anchorage device (Fig. 8.2H).

INDICATIONS

Patients undergoing this procedure should generally be healthy and have no intrasinus lesions in the maxilla before placement of the anchorage device. Radiopaque images should not show thickened mucosal lining or retained fluid. In general, the anterior area of the infrazygomatic rim provides and represents the most adequate fixation site because its bony wall is thicker than 1.4 mm, which is regarded as the critical thickness for miniscrew implant stability.[4]

ADVANTAGES

The advantages of using the current locking osteosynthetic system include:

- higher stability, owing to lower incidence of screw loosening[5] and solid frame construction of the miniplate and miniscrews[2]
- faster wound healing and resistance to infection, owing to supraperiosteal placement of the plate
- a wider range of indications for use.

Additional advantages of the self-drilling miniscrews used include:

- less contamination
- shorter operating time
- lower risk because a drill-free procedure is required for their insertion
- less miniplate movement because of the greater contact achieved between the miniscrews and the miniplate.[6]

DISCUSSION

Commercially available skeletal anchored miniplates comprise one part that is specially designed for orthodontic purposes (e.g. hooks or tubes to

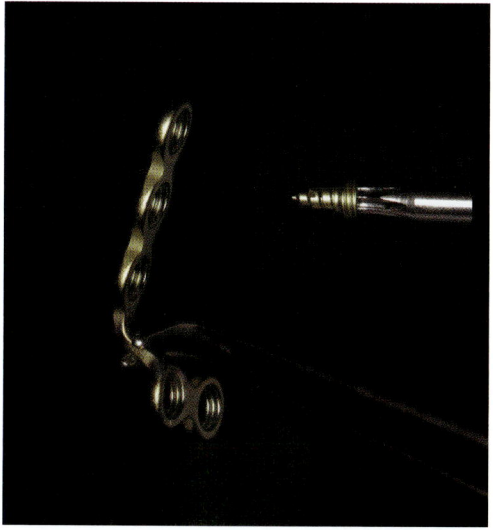

Fig. 8.1 A prebent miniplate and a self-drilling screw. (From Hibi et al. 2006[3] with permission from Elsevier.)

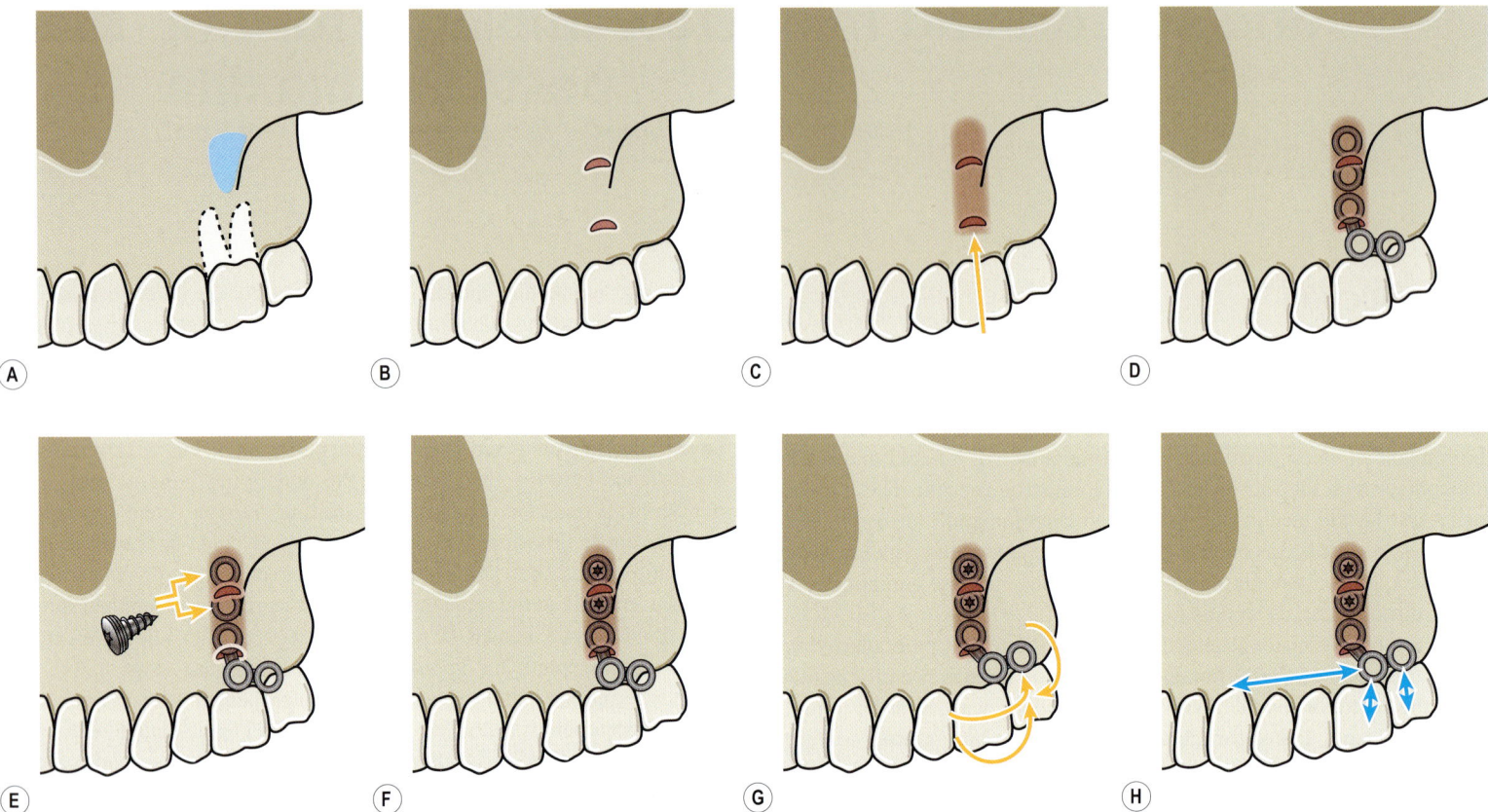

Fig. 8.2 Surgical steps. (A), Anterior area of the infrazygomatic rim adequate for screw fixation (hatch). (B) Two mucosal incisions approximately 3 mm long. (C) Submucosal tunneling. (D) Longitudinal portion of the plate placed on the periosteum in the submucosal tunnel. (E) Self-drilling screws inserted through the upper wound. (F) Plate locked with screws and stabilized. (G) External portion of the plate adjusted for orthodontic use with a bending plier. (H) Plate, ready for use as skeletal anchorage.

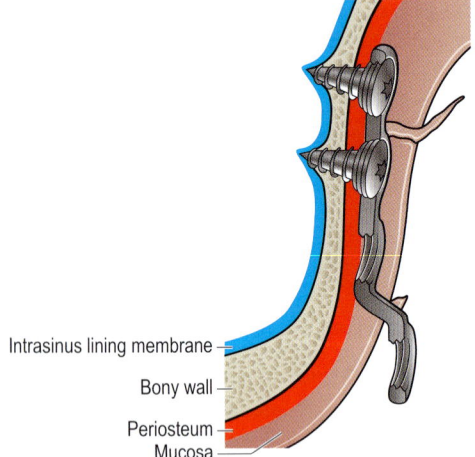

Fig. 8.3 Skeletal anchorage combining a locking plate and self-drilling screw system supraperiosteally applied to the frontal wall of the maxilla. (From Hibi et al. 2006[3] with permission from Elsevier.)

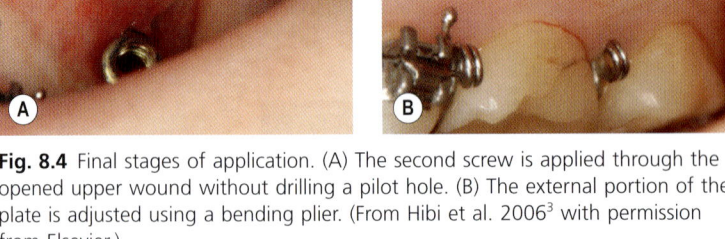

Fig. 8.4 Final stages of application. (A) The second screw is applied through the opened upper wound without drilling a pilot hole. (B) The external portion of the plate is adjusted using a bending plier. (From Hibi et al. 2006[3] with permission from Elsevier.)

allow application of orthodontic forces), and another conventional osteosynthetic part used for fixation on bone. The stability of these systems is affected by compression forces acting on the miniplate by the bone and the miniscrew heads, and thus the underlying bony surface under pressure may resorb over time.[5] This resorption impairs miniplate stability and the resulting unstable osteosynthesis may induce an inflammatory response and promote infection.[7]

In contrast, the locking miniplate and screw systems have a number of positive features in addition to a lower incidence of screw loosening. The threaded holes on the miniplates engage and finally stop the miniscrews in a fully seated position, and hence avoid any stripping of the bony hole.

The screws, miniplate and bone form a solid frame construction, which results in significantly higher stability.[2] This configuration eliminates the need for a plate adaptation procedure for the bony surface and allows supraperiosteal plate placement. Periosteal attachment has less postoperative morbidity and also preserves bone vascularity, which can facilitate wound healing and infection resistance. Moreover, supraperiosteal application of the plate prevents bone apposition over the plate, which is relatively rare but is sometimes observed with traditional plates seated subperiosteally on the bone. This phenomenon can cause complications, such as screw breakage, during removal.[8]

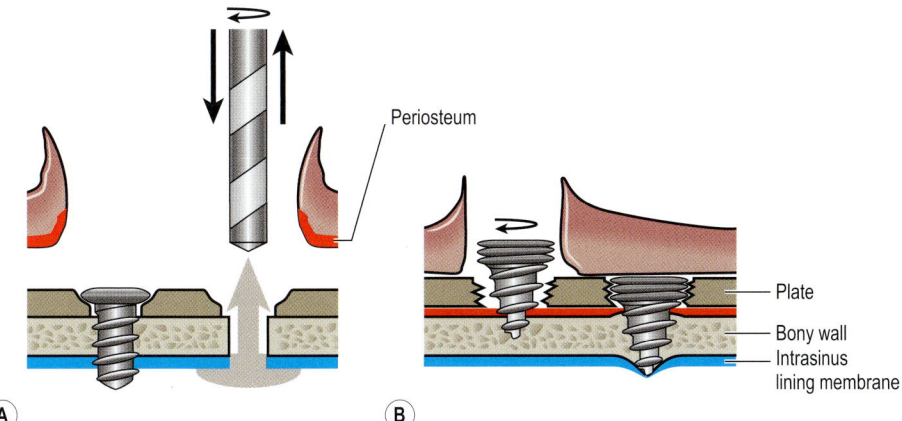

Fig. 8.5 Plate and screw system applied to the maxillary wall. (A) Conventional system. (B) Locking plate and self-drilling screw system. (From Hibi et al. 2006[3] with permission from Elsevier.)

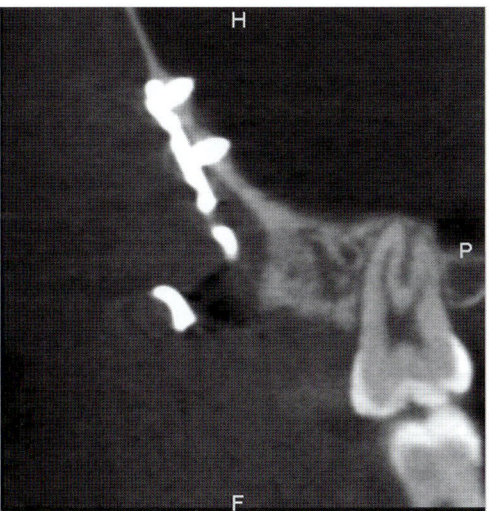

Fig. 8.6 Cone beam CT acquired during follow-up, showing a locking plate and self-drilling screw applied to the frontal maxillary wall for skeletal anchorage. Note that bone thickening resulted from a screw supporting the tent of the lining membrane similar to maxillary sinus elevation. (From Hibi et al. 2006[3] with permission from Elsevier.)

of membrane with or without the inner bony surface in a similar manner to sinus elevation.[9] This can facilitate thickening inward and outward over time (Fig. 8.6).

Although the technique described, with two self-drilling miniscrews and a locking plate for anchorage, achieves higher and longer-lasting stability, the form of the external portion of the miniplate may not be adequate for all possible orthodontic applications. In this sense, specially designed miniplates for orthodontic purposes may be more effective.

REFERENCES

1. Cheng SJ, Tseng IY, Lee JJ, et al. A prospective study of the risk factors associated with failure of mini-implants used for orthodontic anchorage. Int J Oral Maxillofac Implants 2002;19:100–6.
2. Gutwald R, Schön R, Metzger M, et al. Miniplate osteosynthesis with four different systems in sheep. Int J Oral Maxillofac Surg 2011;40:94–102.
3. Hibi H, Ueda M, Sakai M, et al. Orthodontic anchorage system using a locking plate and self-drilling screws. J Oral Maxillofac Surg 2006;64:1173–5.
4. Hibi H, Sakai K, Oda T, et al. Stability of a locking plate and self-drilling screws as orthodontic skeletal anchorage in the maxilla: a retrospective study. J Oral Maxillofac Surg 2010;68:1783–7.
5. Haug RH, Street CC, Goltz M. Does plate adaptation affect stability? A biomechanical comparison of locking and nonlocking plates. J Oral Maxillofac Surg 2002;60:1319–26.
6. Kim JW, Ahn SJ, Chang YI. Histomorphometric and mechanical analyses of the drill-free screw as orthodontic anchorage. Am J Orthod Dentofacial Orthop 2005;128:190–4.
7. Ellis E, Graham J. Use of a 2.0-mm locking plate/screw system for mandibular fracture surgery. J Oral Maxillofac Surg 2002;60:642–5.
8. Cornelis MA, Scheffler NR, Mahy P, et al. Modified miniplates for temporary skeletal anchorage in orthodontics: placement and removal surgeries. J Oral Maxillofac Surg 2008;66:1439–45.
9. Le Gall MG. Localized sinus elevation and osteocompression with single-stage tapered dental implants: Technical note. Int J Oral Maxillofac Implants 2004;19:431–7.

The use of self-drilling miniscrews ensures their primary stability and eliminates various problems accompanying initial predrilling of pilot holes for self-tapping screws, particularly in regions of thin cortical bone (Fig. 8.5). Predrilling increases operating time, can cause thermal or mechanical damage to the bone and results in perforation of the membranous lining of the maxillary sinus. Without prior disinfection of the inner membrane surface, the returning pilot drill can carry microorganisms and contaminate the operating field. In contrast, the use of short self-drilling miniscrews enables the tips to remain under or within the membrane. If the screw tip does penetrate the membrane, the inherent one-step procedure minimizes the risk of contamination. The self-drilling miniscrews may support a tent

9

Miniscrew implants for temporary skeletal anchorage in orthodontic treatment

Moschos A. Papadopoulos and Fadi Tarawneh

INTRODUCTION

Anchorage, resistance to unwanted tooth movement, is a prerequisite for the orthodontic treatment of dental and skeletal malocclusions. Absolute or infinite anchorage is defined as no movement of the anchorage unit (zero anchorage loss) as a consequence of the reaction forces applied to move teeth. Such an anchorage can only be obtained by two means, using ankylosed teeth or using implants, both relying on bone for their anchorage.

Currently, there are several skeletal anchorage devices that are used for orthodontic purposes, for example orthodontic implants, palatal implants or onplants, zygoma ligatures, zygoma anchors or miniplates, as well as miniscrews, microscrews or miniscrew implants (MIs).

Miniscrew implants are small screw-type self-tapping implants, which in contrast to conventional dental or orthodontic implants have smooth, machine-polished surfaces and are designed to be loaded immediately after their insertion and removed easily after treatment (see Fig. 6.1). They carry special heads with or without holes to accommodate auxiliaries or wires for application of orthodontic forces (see Fig. 6.2).

The use of MIs to obtain absolute anchorage has become very popular since they provide a non-compliance approach for reinforcing anchorage, ease of use and low cost.[1]

Currently, there are a large number of commercially available MI systems for orthodontic use in the market (Table 9.1).

TERMINOLOGY

Terms such as mini-implant, miniscrew, microimplant and microscrew all refer to devices with smaller dimensions than conventional dental implants and that are removed following treatment; consequently, their use should not be synonymous with conventional dental or orthodontic implants.

The terms orthodontic implant and mini-implant refer to systems that require osseointegration in order to be retained in the bone, whereas mini-screws to self-tapping devices that do not require osseointegration and are only mechanically retained.[2] Other terms used to describe temporary anchorage devices are intraoral or extradental anchorage systems, but the Moyer's Symposium in 2004 agreed that the term mini-implant should be applied to palatal implants, mini-implants, miniscrews and microscrews.[2] Nevertheless, the term mini-implant should be restricted to small prosthetic implants of diameter larger than 2 mm that are osseointegrated and are used to stabilize removable prostheses.

The prefixes mini- and micro- are currently used in the literature to describe implants or screws of the same dimension without any differentiation. However, we advocate the use of the term miniscrew implant and this term is used throughout this textbook.

HISTORICAL DEVELOPMENT

Skeletal anchorage concepts in orthodontics developed from two areas. The first was from osseointegrated dental implants to give orthodontic implants that were smaller but had similar surfaces and so also osseointe-grated and were difficult to remove after treatment. The second was from surgical miniscrews used to fix osteosynthesis plates and resulted in the development of orthodontic MIs, designed for loading shortly after insertion and easy removal.

The first clinical use of miniscrews for absolute anchorage was the treatment of a patient with a deep overbite using a vitallium bone-screw inserted in the anterior nasal spine.[3] A mini-implant specifically made for orthodontic use was described in 1997[4] and a screw with a bracket-like head in 1998.[5] Since then, several types of MIs have been introduced, each presenting different designs and features.

COMPOSITION OF MINISCREW IMPLANTS

With the exception of the Orthodontic Mini Implant (Leone, Firenze, Italy), which is fabricated from SS, all other systems are manufactured from pure titanium or titanium alloys (medical type IV or type V titanium alloy; see Chapter 5). While both materials are biocompatible, a layer of connective tissue is usually formed around SS implants while direct bone contact and true osteogenesis occurs with pure titanium or titanium alloys.[6,7] The rationale for using SS for MIs is that they are less prone to breakage and have less osseointegration than titanium devices. However, a study comparing three different MIs, two SS and one titanium, concluded that overall material performance of SS MIs was inferior to titanium MIs because of their lower yield or tensile strength.[7]

Removal of MIs is more related to thread design, MI shape and the drill–screw diameter ratio.[7]

Titanium alloys are favored over pure titanium because of their higher strength, excellent corrosion resistance, biocompatibility and favorable mechanical properties.[8,9]

OSSEOINTEGRATION

Osseointegrated implants are largely used for skeletal anchorage purposes as they remain stable under orthodontic loading.[10] However, they do have several disadvantages:[11]

- they cannot be immediately loaded with orthodontic forces since several months are needed for proper osseointegration
- they require an invasive technique for both insertion and removal, which should be done by a surgeon
- there is always need for supraconstruction and laboratory work
- they can only be inserted in edentulous areas (or in the palate) with sufficient bone quantity and quality
- they are expensive.

MIs were introduced in an attempt to avoid some of these problems. Their osseointegration is less than half that of conventional dental implants.[5,12] A histomorphometric examination of titanium MIs retrieved following clinical use in alveolar bone found randomly organized osseointegration islets on the MI surfaces despite the smooth surface and immediate loading pattern of these implants, although it was associated with an extended period of retention (>6 months) (Fig. 9.1).[13]

Table 9.1 Commonly used miniscrew implant systems

Product	Company	Address
Aarhus Anchorage System	American Orthodontics	1714 Cambridge Av, Sheboygan, WI, USA (www.americanortho.com)
AbsoAnchor System	Dentos	258 BunJi, Dong-In Dong, Jung-Gu, Taegu, Korea (www.dentos.co.kr)
Ancotek system	Tekka	ZI de Sacuny, BP 82, 118 Ave Marcel Mérieux, 69530 Brignais, France (www.tekka.eu)
Benefit System	PSM Medical Solutions	Moltkestrasse 41, D-78532 Tuttlingen, Germany (distributed by Mondeal-PSM, North America, PO Box 142, 49950 Jefferson St, Indio, CA 92201, USA) (www.psm.ms)
C-Implant	Dentium	3105 Korea Trade Tower 159 Samsung-dong, Gangnam-gu, 135–729 Seoul, Korea (www.implantium.com)
Cizeta Titanium Miniscrew	Cizeta Surgical	Via Caselle, 76 San Lazzaro di Savena, 40068 Bologna, Italy (www.cizetasurgical.it)
Dual-Top Anchor System	Jeil Medical Corporation	775–3 Daesung B/D, Daelim 3 Dong Youngdeungpoku, Seoul, Korea (www.jeilmed.co.kr); distributed by RMO Inc. PO Box 17085, Denver, CO 80217, USA (www.rmortho.com)
IMTEC Mini Ortho Implant	IMTEC Corporation	2401 N. Commerce, Ardmore, OK 73401, USA (www.imtec.com)
Infinitas Mini Implant System	DB Orthodontics	Ryefield Way, Silsden, BD20 0EF, UK (www.dborthodontics.co.uk)
Lin/Liou Orthodontic Mini Anchorage Screw (LOMAS)	PSM Medical Solutions	Moltkestrasse 41, D-78532 Tuttlingen, Germany (www.psm.ms); distributed by Mondeal-PSM, North America, PO Box 142, 49950 Jefferson St, Indio, CA 92201, USA
Micro Implant Universal Skeletal Anchorage System	Stryker Corporation	Stryker Leibinger Micro Implants, 750 Trade Centre Way, Portage, MI 49002, USA (www.stryker.com)
Miniscrew Anchorage System (MAS)	Micerium S.p.a.	Via Marconi 83, 16030 Avegno, Italy (www.micerium.it)
OMI – Orthodontic Ancor System	OsteoMed	3885 Arapaho Rd Addison, TX 75001, USA (www.osteomed.com)
Orlus	Ortholution	207 Dunchon B/D., 416–1, Seongnae-dong, Gangdong-gu, Seoul 134–844, South Korea (www.ortholution.com)
Ortho Easy system	Forestadent	Westliche Karl-Friedrich-Str. 151, 75172 Pforzheim, Germany (www.forestadent.de)
Orthoanchor K1 System	Dentsply Sankin Corporation	Tokyo, Japan (www.dentsply-sankin.com)
Orthodontic Mini-implant	Ortholution	Joongwon-gu, Seongnam-si, 462–725 Kyunggi-do, Korea (www.ortholution.com)
Orthodontic Mini Implant	Leone S.p.A.	Via P. a Quaracchi 50, 50019 Sesto Fiorentino, Florence, Italy (www.leone.it); distributed by Leone America, 501 W. Van Buren, Avondale, AZ 85323, USA
Orthodontic screw	KLS Martin Group	Ludwigstaler Str. 132, 78532 Tuttlingen, Germany www.klsmartin.com)
Spider Screw Anchorage System	HDC	Via dell'Industria 19, 36030 Sarcedo, Italy (www.hdc-italy.com)
Temporary Mini Orthodontic Anchorage System (TOMAS)	Dentaurum	Turnstrasse 31, D-75228 Ispringen, Germany (www.dentaurum.de)
VectorTAS	Ormco	1717 West Collins Ave, Orange, CA 92867, USA (www.ormco.com)

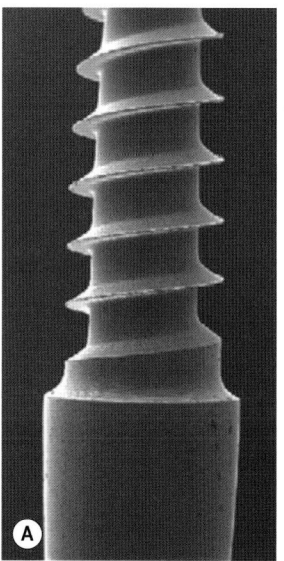 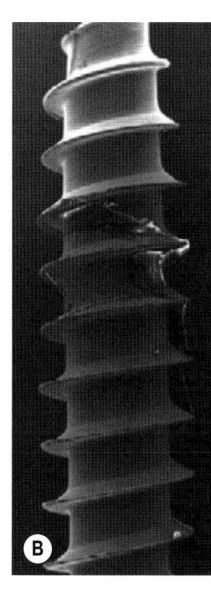 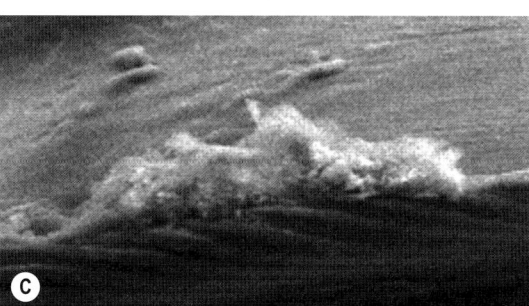

Fig. 9.1 Secondary electron microscopy of miniscrew implants (MIs). (A) Unused MI. (B) Retrieved MI after >6 months inserted in alveolar bone, with integument in the middle third of threaded area. (C) Higher magnification showing organized osseointegration islets on the surface of the retrieved MI. (From Eliades et al., 2009[13] with permission.)

Table 9.2 Available head designs of the miniscrew implants

Head	Indications	Coupling elements	Advantages	Disadvantages
Crossed-slot (bracket)	Translation, space closure, intrusion, extrusion, uprighting	Elastic chains. coil springs, round/square/rectangular wires	Direct/indirect anchorage easily achieved; more than one coupling element can be used; easy orientation	None
Single slot (bracket)	Translation, space closure, intrusion, extrusion, uprighting	Elastic chains. coil springs, round/square/rectangular wires	Square/rectangular wires can be used; direct and indirect anchorage possible	Orientation of slot important but could be compensated by wire bending
Hook	Translation, space closure, intrusion	Elastic chains, coil springs, round wires	Coupling elements can be easily attached	Orientation of hook is crucial; hook can be bent or broken; indirect anchorage difficult
Button	Translation, space closure, intrusion	Elastic chains, coil springs, round wires	Coupling elements can be easily attached; orientation not needed	Indirect anchorage difficult to achieve
Hole	Translation, space closure, intrusion	Elastic chains, coil springs, round wires		Orientation of hole crucial

Since reduced osseointegration is advantageous for removal of MIs after clinical use, most are fabricated with smooth surfaces to achieve good bone–implant contact but not osseointegration.

The quality and quantity of cortical bone is considered one of the most important factors for achieving mechanical stabilization and retention of MIs. Although a dense trabecular bone is desirable, cortical bone is more important for primary stability of MIs and this is directly related to its thickness: the thicker the cortical plate the better the survival rate.[14,15]

MINISCREW IMPLANT DESIGNS

MIs are designed to provide both direct and indirect anchorage as well as to decrease tissue irritation. Chapter 6 discusses the significance of the various components of a MI – head, neck, endosseous body and thread, tip – in detail.

HEAD

The head of the MIs serves two important purposes; to apply torque to the thread during insertion and to act as a point for orthodontic force application. Table 9.2 summarizes the different designs currently available, their indications and coupling methods. The most frequently used shape is the bracket-like design with a single or a double (crossed) slot (e.g. Aarhus Anchorage System, AbsoAnchor System, Ancotek system, Dual-Top Anchor System, Ortho-Easy system, Spider Screw, Temporary Mini Orthodontic Anchorage System) as it can accommodate square and rectangular wires in its slot plus additional auxiliaries such as elastics and ligatures. It can be used for direct and indirect anchorage for uprighting, intrusion, extrusion and mesial and distal translation. The use of rectangular wires also allows for three-dimensional control in contrast to round wires, thus providing an important advantage over other designs.

Other MI head shapes, such as the button-like, sphere, double sphere and hook (Aarhus Anchorage System, AbsoAnchor System, Dual-Top Anchor System, IMTEC Mini Ortho Implant, Lin/Liou Orthodontic Mini Anchorage Screw, Miniscrew Anchorage System, Orthoanchor K1 System, Spider Screw) can be used for mesial and distal translation, space closure and intrusion, but attachment of square or rectangular wires is not possible and indirect anchorage is unattainable or very hard to achieve. Furthermore, correctly orientating the hook-shaped MI during insertion is crucial for its use.

One design has a hole or eyelet through the head (usually 0.6–0.8 mm in diameter), which can accept tension springs, elastic chains and round

wires; this is mostly used for direct anchorage. With this type of head, three-dimensional control is not possible since square and rectangular wires cannot be used. Another disadvantage is the fact that MI heads equipped with holes could be more at risk of fracture during their insertion or removal, since this might make the material around the head less rigid and weaker.

NECK (COLLAR)

The transgingival neck (or collar) connecting the head to the body of the MI is smooth and intended to form a non-irritant seal to protect against inflammation and infection of the surrounding soft tissue (see Fig. 6.6).

Most common collar shapes are conical (tapering towards the body) or cylindrical but there are also polyangular collars.[8,9] Depending on the insertion angle of the MI, pressure areas are formed on the soft tissue in the area of the collar, which appears to be less in conical collars. The diameter of collars is for most MIs identical to the threaded body but having the collar wider than the body, as in the top of a conical collar, is advantageous in terms of providing a good seal between the MI and soft tissue. Ideally, and in order to achieve the best possible seal and hygiene, the diameter of the head should also be smaller or equal to the collar.[8,14] However, most MIs have heads that are larger in width than the collar, which can create areas/undercuts that can be more difficult to clean and easier for plaque to accumulate. Consequently, systems with MI heads smaller in diameter than the collars (e.g. Spider Screw, the Ortho-Easy, Temporary Mini Orthodontic Anchorage System, AbsoAnchor systems) are advantageous. As gingiva width varies between 1 and 4 mm in different locations in the oral cavity,[8,9,16,17] systems that provide a variety of collars in their inventory are useful. Gingival thickness at the site of insertion should be measured before chosing the MI and this can only be done only after local anesthesia, delaying the selection until just before the insertion procedure. This necessitates the orthodontist having a large range of available MIs, which could be impractical in clinical practice. Fortunately, the most popular sites for MI insertion are covered with 1–2 mm gingiva, and MIs with a collar with 2 mm length are usually sufficient apart from for the palatal gingiva, which could reach 3–4 mm and requires a longer collar.[8,9,16,17]

THREAD

The body of the MI is a threaded part that is inserted into the bone (Fig. 9.1A). The body's primary function is the retention of the MI in the bone initially after insertion (primary stability) and afterwards during orthodontic force loading (secondary stability), and its shape and design can influence the stability of the MI as well as the force (torque) needed for insertion and removal. The body can be either conical (e.g. Aarhus Anchorage System, AbsoAnchor System, Miniscrew Anchorage System) or cylindrical (e.g. the Orthodontic Mini Implant) (see Fig. 6.3). The thread design can be a uniform helix rotating either clockwise or counterclockwise with fixed helix angles and pitches or it can be a dual-thread design formed by two different helixes with different angles and pitches in the thread (see Fig. 6.13).[18,19] The thread design can influence the bone–implant contact, the stress load of the bone and the insertion and removal torque.[8,9,18,19] An ideal MI body shape should allow for a high insertion torque that would sustain the MI, but at the same time not damage bone and cause necrosis, and also allow a high enough removal torque to avoid unwanted pullout but at the same time facilitate MI removal without complications.

Conical MI threads have been shown to have an increasing insertion torque compared with cylindrical threads, which require less torque, and a more constant torque, throughout the insertion procedure.[7,18,19–23] This makes cylindrical MIs more desirable for insertion, minimizing the risk of bone necrosis, but their higher removal torque makes them more prone to fracture. Dual-thread MIs also have a high insertion torque but with a gentler increase in comparison with conical MIs.[18]

DIAMETER

The diameter of the MIs is a significant factor that may influence (a) the possibility of injuring the neighboring roots when inserted inter-radicularly, (b) the tendency for breakage, and (c) success/failure rates. Chapter 6 discusses in detail the effect of diameter on these issues. Essentially, smaller-diameter MIs have less risk of root contact but a greater risk of fracture, while it is more difficult to achieve an optimal placement torque for good primary stability with narrower MIs. Based on success rates, 1.2 mm can be considered the minimum diameter required to achieve adequate implantation success.[2,7,24–26] Diameters of 1.5 mm and 1.6 mm represent a satisfactory compromise.

In clinical practice, however, the use of MIs of larger diameter for insertion inter-radicularly can be very difficult to accomplish without the risk of injuring adjacent roots, particularly when the roots are close to each other. In such circumstances, the choice of insertion site should be reconsidered, which may mean adjusting the force application system and applying appropriate orthodontic biomechanics to achieve the required result for the new chosen site of insertion. This is not an issue for palatal insertion, where larger-diameter MIs can be used, eliminating the risk of both MI fracture and root damage. Careful clinical and radiological examination, preparation and measurement to plan the insertion site and the MI diameter before insertion will minimize the risk of breakage failure.

Stress distribution within bone is affected by the diameter of MIs. In cortical bone, the thicker the MI diameter, the more favorable the stress distribution.[9,27] Three-dimensional finite element analysis has shown that a 1.4 mm diameter implant placed in 1.2 mm thick cortical bone can tolerate 150 g of orthodontic forces, while a 1.8 mm diameter implant can tolerate 350 g of orthodontic forces.[9] Therefore, the planned orthodontic forces should also be taken into consideration when selecting the appropriate MI diameter.

LENGTH

Length generally refers to the threaded portion of the MI rather than the entire head-to-tip length but care needs to be taken with catalogues to check that total length is not given. Here lengths refer to the threaded part. In general, it is considered that the longer the MI the higher the success rate.[28,29]

Miniscrew implants are usually provided with lengths ranging from 4.0 to 12.0 mm, although some of them are also available in larger lengths up to 21 mm. The choice of length is determined by the depth and quality of bone, the MI angulation, the soft tissue thickness and the adjacent vital structures.[26] Based on hard and soft tissue depths in 20 patients, MIs of 4–6 mm in length were considered safe in most regions, but individual patient variations dictate individual evaluation of bone depth before surgery.[5] Although MIs of 6–8 mm have been recommended by most authors,[5,8,9,30] MIs shorter than 8 mm are more susceptible to failure[26,31] and longer MIs with small diameter can be more prone to breakage and bending. In this regard, longer MIs should also be thicker in diameter, but anatomical limits restrict the use of very long and thick MIs in clinical practice.

The length of MIs has less effect than diameter on the distribution of stress, and the majority of the load is borne within the cortical bone.[9] The force above which implant length and implant diameter are statistically significant in influencing implant stability was found to be 1 N.[21] At low force (0.5 N), no statistically significant difference in displacement according to implant length and implant diameter was observed. However, at high force (2.5 N), MIs of 9 mm length displaced significantly less than the 7 mm MIs, and the 2 mm wide MIs displaced significantly less than their 1.5 mm wide counterparts.[21] Further, insertion and removal torques seem to be higher in long MIs.[32]

The thickness of soft tissue at the insertion site should also be taken into consideration when choosing the appropriate length of MI. Thick gingival tissue sites demand longer MIs. In general, MI lengths of 6–8 mm are recommended for use in the mandible and of 8–10 mm in the maxilla. Nonetheless, individual patient variations in soft tissue and cortical bone thickness should be considered prior to insertion of any MI.[8,9]

MODE OF INSERTION

All types of MI are self-tapping/self-cutting. The term self-tapping relates to the ability of a screw to create a thread as it advances into the bone. This is sometimes achieved by having a cutting flute, a groove in the thread, that drills away the material to make the hole for the screw.

Some MIs require a pilot drill before their insertion (non-self-drilling MIs), while others have a fine tip that enables their direct insertion into bone (self-drilling MIs). The diameter of a pilot drill is preferably 0.2–0.3 mm thinner than the diameter of the MI thread, otherwise insertion torque values are significantly decreased and MI primary stability is reduced.[8,33,34] Although the length of the pilot drill is determined by the length of the selected MI, deeper holes decrease insertion torque and so it is recommended that drills with depth markings and depth stops should be used.[8,34] Occasionally, a pilot drill is needed even for a self-drilling MI; such as in cases where the cortical bone is thicker than 2 mm, as dense bone would eventually bend the fine tip of the MI.

Self-drilling MI systems include the Aarhus Anchorage System, the AbsoAnchor System, the Dual-Top Anchor System and the Lin/Liou Orthodontic Mini Anchorage Screw, while Spider Screw offers both non-self-drilling and self-drilling MIs.

The advantage of the self-drilling over non-self-drilling MIs is the elimination of the pilot drilling step during insertion, which makes the whole procedure less invasive, less time consuming and more easily accepted by the patient, particularly to young patients and their parents. In addition, since the insertion of the self-drilling MIs is less complicated, they can be easily inserted by orthodontists themselves without requiring referral to a surgeon.

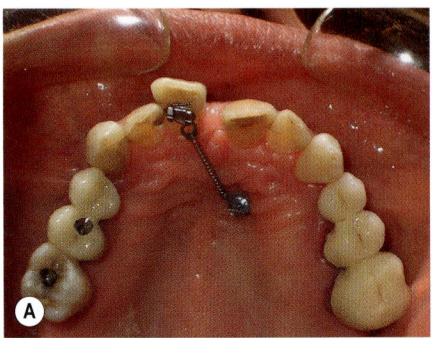

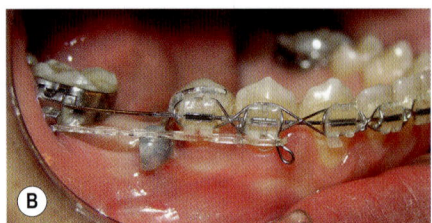

Fig. 9.2 Anchorage. (A) Direct anchorage for the intrusion of a maxillary central incisor. (B) Indirect anchorage for the mesialization of a mandibular second molar after first molar extraction.

Table 9.3 Advantages and disadvantages of direct and indirect anchorage

Type	Advantages	Disadvantages
Direct	Simple mechanics Easy to apply No dental anchorage loss	Load applied directly to implant may cause mobility or loss Should be monitored closely as mechanics used are not fail-safe Placement site for direct anchorage not always achievable or possible
Indirect	Less load applied to implant Fail-safe mechanics Placement site usually easy and preferable	Loss of anchorage in the anchorage teeth group is possible More complicated mechanics and installment

TYPES OF ANCHORAGE

Miniscrew implants can provide two different types of anchorage: direct and indirect. When used for direct anchorage, MIs directly receive the reactive forces used to move the teeth by acting themselves as an anchor unit (Fig. 9.2A). In indirect anchorage, MIs are connected through bars or wires to the teeth of the reactive unit supporting their anchorage (Fig. 9.2B).

Special considerations should be given to the design of the MI head and the placement site for the type of anchorage to be used. Different head designs are more suitable for one type of anchorage over the other, while placement site could play a major role in determining the type of anchorage. Advantages and disadvantages of direct and indirect anchorage are summarized in Table 9.3.

PROPERTIES OF THE MINISCREW IMPLANTS

Currently available MIs vary in their material, diameter and length of threaded portion, design of the head, the existence of a collar and the method of insertion. An ideal MI used for orthodontic anchorage should present some specific properties and characteristics:

- fabricated from a biocompatible material
- provided in different diameter and length sizes
- available in different designs (i.e. button or bracket head)
- self-tapping and self-drilling
- easily and safely inserted in various sites without complicated and invasive approaches
- immediately loaded
- removed without the need for complicated accessory equipment or invasive approaches
- inexpensive (cost beneficial).

LOADING

Some authors have suggested a waiting period of 1 to 2 weeks before loading with orthodontic forces but most agree that, since in contrast to dental implants MIs are mechanically retained in bone sufficiently, they can sustain immediate light orthodontic loading without compromising their clinical stability.[5,35,36] Only a few studies, mostly on animals, have investigated tissue reaction to immediate loading of MIs; all suggest that immediate loading with orthodontic forces can be performed without any complications.[14,37,38]

A finite element analysis found that immediate loading should be limited to 50 cN for a 2 mm diameter MI.[39] One clinical study of 134 titanium MIs concluded that immediate loading is possible if the applied force is less than 200 cN,[14] which is in agreement with a study showing no association between success rates of MIs and the mode of loading.[40] This study concluded that vertical forces seem to be responsible for more failures than horizontal forces.[40]

The ability of MIs to provide absolute anchorage was shown in a study measuring anchorage loss with the use of MIs and conventional molar anchorage for canine retraction.[41] A meta-analysis has shown that the use of MIs significantly decreased or negated loss of anchorage, particularly when compared with other conventional orthodontic means such as headgears, transpalatal arches or other biomechanical force systems.[42]

However, it is questionable if MIs remain stationary throughout their period of loading. In some patients, MIs were shown to move under orthodontic loading,[43] and it is, therefore, advised to allow 2 mm of safety clearance between the MI and dental roots of the adjacent teeth.

COMPLICATIONS

Complications associated with the use of MIs include inflammation, infection and tissue irritation, injuries to adjacent structures, and failure or fracture of the MI during insertion or removal.[44]

INFLAMMATION, INFECTION AND TISSUE IRRITATION

Inflammation and irritation of the tissues around the MI site might occur, although infection is not generally noted (Fig. 9.3). Meticulous oral hygiene maintained around the MI and the use of 0.2% chlorhexidine mouth rinses or dental floss dipped in 2% chlorhexidine can help to avoid inflammation or infection, or control any that might occur.[44] If a patient presents with purulence, palor or inflammation, definitive management with an appropriate antibiotic is indicated.

The risk of tissue inflammation is lessened if the MIs are inserted into keratinized attached gingiva avoiding areas of frenum, muscle tissues and mobile mucosa (non-attached gingiva).[14,26,45] Hypertrophy of mucosa covering an implant may occur as a complication of placing the MI in

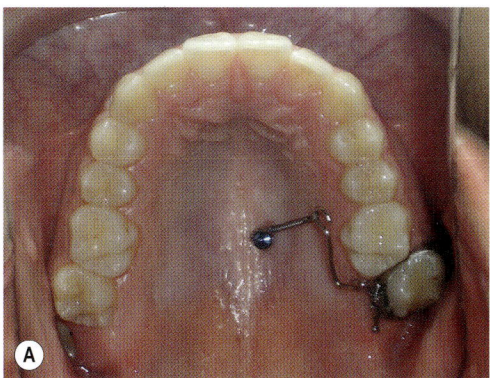 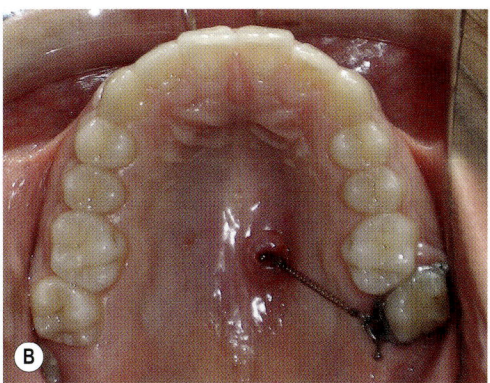 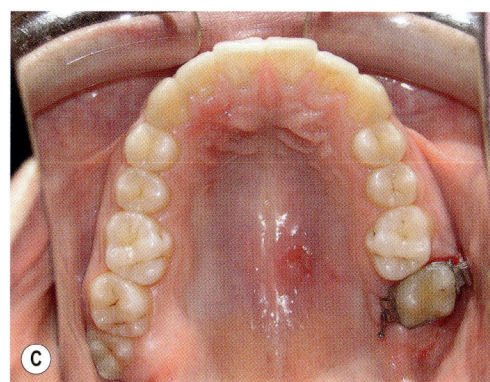

Fig. 9.3 Inflammation around a miniscrew implant inserted in the palate for the correction of the crossbite of the maxillary left second molar. (A) Immediately after insertion. (B) Presence of inflammation. (C) After removal of the implant.

non-keratinized gingiva. With such a placement, a healing cap abutment is recommended at the time of insertion. Alternatively, the mucosa could be allowed to cover the MI head if there is an attached wire or an auxiliary that emerges into the oral cavity passing through the mucosa.[44]

INJURIES TO ADJACENT STRUCTURES

The incidence of root injuries caused by trans-alveolar MIs used for temporary intermaxillary fixation of fractured mandibles is very low[46] and it could be assumed that the incidence of root damage using MIs for orthodontic anchorage would be even lower as they are inserted after careful planning rather than as an emergency situation.

Nonetheless, injuring of the adjacent roots, periodontal ligaments, nerves and blood vessels could occur during MI insertion and is usually indicated by symptoms such as pain on percussion and mastication, or, in cases of root injury, sensitivity to hot and cold.[47,48] Under such circumstances, the MI should be removed immediately.

The prognosis of an injured tooth will depend on whether there has been injury to the pulp. Histological examination of roots of teeth that had been damaged by MI placement demonstrated an almost complete repair of the periodontal structures 12 weeks after removal of the MIs.[49,50] Only in severe injury with displacement of root fragments ankylosis of the lamina dura was noted. External root resorption in response to root injury, as well as evidence of inflammatory infiltrate or necrosis in the pulp tissue or on the injured root surfaces, was not found in any of the injured teeth.[49,50]

FAILURE OF MINISCREW IMPLANTS

Although it is still not clear what precisely affects the success and failure rates of MIs, some factors have been identified:[51]

- patient-related factors, e.g. sex, gender, malocclusion, oral hygiene
- clinician-related factors, e.g. experience, learning curve
- MI-related factors, e.g. length, diameter, thread design
- insertion-related factors, e.g. cortical bone thickness, cortical notching, flap surgery, insertion torque, insertion angle
- treatment-related factors, e.g. loading time, tooth movement
- outcome-related factors, e.g. inflammation, mobility.

A MI can be lost or become loose through various factors such as inflammation (Fig. 9.3), improper placement, inadequate cortical bone at the chosen site or operator inexperience.[47] Based on current evidence, the quality and quantity of the available bone at the insertion site are considered as the most important factors affecting primary stability of MIs. Although most studies have reported success rates of more than 80%,[20,28,41,52] or a failure rate of about 16%,[53] there is no consensus about how to define

clinical success or failure and many authors define failure in a general way as a state where a MI is not clinically usable.

According to Melsen,[52] the insertion angle should be kept stable during insertion, and the threaded part should be inserted totally into bone in order to avoid MI failures.

Orthodontic loading may also affect the success of MIs. The magnitude and direction of force applied to MIs is one of the most important factors associated with MI failure. Loading with orthodontic forces applied perpendicular to the long axis of the MIs is preferable;[54] the strain obtained by loading a MI perpendicular to its long axis with 50 cN was shown to lead to loss of primary stability when the cortex is 0.5 mm or smaller.[55] Further, if a MI is used indirectly with a cantilever to a bracket-like head, the clinician should avoid the application of moments around the MI long axis in a counterclockwise direction since it could unscrew the MI, which can lead to loosening and failure.[54]

Cortical bone thickness is a significant factor in that greater thickness supports better success rates but can have negative effects through greater chance of MI fractures, overheating and necrosis. A clinical cortical bone thickness threshold of 1 mm increased success rate.[20]

A MI diameter below 1.3 mm should be avoided,[14,24,25] and longer lengths tended to give higher success rates (see above).[28]

Patients with high mandibular plane angles may not be suitable candidates for MIs because they often have thin cortical bone, while statistically significant higher success rates have been found in patients with a deep bite.[14,40] Success rates for white patients were found to be higher than for Asian patients[40] but there was no effect of gender apart from a general willingness to cooperate with treatment that was better for girls than boys.[20] Some studies have also correlated age with success rates, as failure rates were reportedly higher in adolescents than in adults.[26,56]

Placement in attached/keratinized gingiva has been associated with higher success rates of MIs,[14,26,40,45] while root proximity has been reported as a major risk factor for MI failure.[57]

A recent meta-analysis has found that MI failure was not associated with patient gender, age and insertion site but was significantly associated with jaw of insertion, insertion torque, cortical bone thickness and root contact.[51] No definitive conclusion could be drawn for the other factors discussed above. However, more MI failures were observed in the posterior region than the anterior in the maxilla and more failures lingually than buccally in the mandible. Orthodontic MIs overall presented a modest small mean failure rate of 13.5%, indicating their usefulness in clinical practice.[51]

FRACTURE OF MINISCREW IMPLANTS

Fracture of MIs may occur during their insertion or their removal if ones of small diameter are employed (<1.2 mm) or if the collar is too narrow (≤1.3 mm) or is equipped with holes.[8,45]

If a MI has to be inserted into high bone density, predrilling should be carried out to minimize the risk of fracture.

If a MI fractures during insertion, the shaft might need to be removed with a trephine and a new site should be selected for insertion of a fresh MI.

CLINICAL APPLICATIONS OF MINISCREW IMPLANTS IN ORTHODONTICS

In general, the various MI systems can be used when dental elements lack quantity or quality, such as periodontally involved teeth and partial edentulism, as well as when there is a necessity to undertake tooth movements and minimizing or completely neutralizing undesired side effects of the reactive forces.[58]

Melsen suggested using MIs as anchorage for tooth movements that could not otherwise be achieved, such as in patients with insufficient number of teeth for the application of conventional anchorage, where the forces on the reactive unit would generate adverse side effects, in patients with a need for asymmetrical tooth movements in all planes of space, and as an alternative to orthognathic surgery.[44]

In general, MIs can be used to support anchorage of anterior or posterior teeth; for mesialization or distalization of teeth; for intrusion, extrusion and uprighting; and for palatal expansion and interarch coordination.[8,9] More specifically, MIs have been used for the correction of deep or open bite, closure of extraction spaces, correction of a canted occlusal plane, alignment of dental midlines, extrusion of impacted canines, extrusion and uprighting of impacted molars, molar intrusion, maxillary molar distalization, distalization of mandibular teeth, en masse retraction of anterior teeth, molar mesialization, maxillary third molar alignment, intermaxillary anchorage for the correction of sagittal discrepancies and for correction of vertical skeletal discrepancies that would otherwise demand orthognathic surgery.[8,9,37,59–61]

CONCLUSIONS

In summary, MIs present several advantages and some disadvantages when used for orthodontic anchorage reinforcement.

The advantages are:

- their insertion and removal does not require any particular surgical procedures, in contrast to other means available, such as orthodontic implants, miniplates and onplants, which require flap surgery
- they can be easily inserted chair-side in one appointment, usually by the orthodontist him or herself
- there is no need for complicated clinical and laboratory procedures (fabrication of acrylic resin splints through taking imprints with additional implant copying systems to accurately transfer the implant position to the cast models) in order to facilitate safe and precise implant insertion
- they can be immediate loaded (there is no need for a waiting period for osseointegration, in contrast to orthodontic implants), which reduces the total treatment time
- they offer a great variety of possible locations for insertion, in contrast to conventional dental implants used for orthodontic anchorage, which require edentulous areas
- they provide absolute anchorage, which eliminates any undesirable effects on the teeth that otherwise would have been normally used as anchorage
- patient cooperation is limited to maintaining an immaculate oral hygiene

- they can be easily removed
- they present reasonable cost relative to other conventional methods used for anchorage, while being much cheaper than orthodontic implants.

The disadvantages are

- if no proper attention is given during insertion, damage of the adjacent tissues or root injuries might occur
- irritation, inflammation of the peri-implant tissues, and consequent failure of the MI is possible, particularly in patients presenting poor oral hygiene
- when an oral surgeon is involved for their insertion (mainly when predrilling is required), there is an additional cost and increased stress to the patient.

REFERENCES

1. Papadopoulos MA, Tarawneh F. The use of miniscrew implants for temporary skeletal anchorage in orthodontics: a comprehensive review. Oral Surg Oral Med Oral Pathol Oral Radiol Endod 2007;103:e6–15.
2. Carano A, Melsen B. Implants in orthodontics. Prog Orthod 2005;6:62–9.
3. Creekmore TD, Eklund MK. The possibility of skeletal anchorage. J Clin Orthod 1983;17:266–9.
4. Kanomi R. Mini-implant for orthodontic anchorage. J Clin Orthod 1997;31:763–7.
5. Costa A, Raffaini M, Melsen B. Miniscrews as orthodontic anchorage: a preliminary report. Int J Adult Orthodon Orthognath Surg 1998;13:201–9.
6. Christensen FB, Dalstra M, Sejling F, et al. Titanium-alloy enhances bone-pedicle screw fixation: mechanical and histomorphometrical results of titanium-alloy versus stainless steel. Eur Spine J 2000;9:97–103.
7. Carano A, Lonardo P, Velo S, et al. Mechanical properties of three different commercially available miniscrews for skeletal anchorage. Prog Orthod 2005;6:82–97.
8. Ludwig B, Baumgaertel S, Bowman J. Mini-implants in orthodontics: Innovative anchorage concepts. Hanover Park, IL: Quintessence; 2008.
9. Lee J, Kim J, Park Y, et al. Applications of orthodontics mini-implants. Hanover Park, IL: Quintessence; 2008.
10. Bantleon HP, Bernhard T, Crismani AG, et al. Stable orthodontic anchorage with palatal osseointegrated implants. World J Orthod 2002;3:109–16.
11. Fritz U, Ehmer A, Diedrich P. Clinical suitability of titanium microscrews for orthodontic anchorage: preliminary experiences. J Orofac Orthop 2004;65:410–18.
12. Vande Vannet B, Sabzevar MM, Wehrbein H, et al. Osseointegration of miniscrews: a histomorphometric evaluation. Eur J Orthod 2007;29:437–42.
13. Eliades T, Zinelis S, Papadopoulos MA, et al. Characterization of retrieved orthodontic miniscrew implants. Am J Orthod Dentofacial Orthop 2009;135:10.
14. Miyawaki S, Koyama I, Inoue M, et al. Factors associated with the stability of titanium screws placed in the posterior region for orthodontic anchorage. Am J Orthod Dentofacial Orthop 2003;124:373–8.
15. Stahl E, Keilig L, Abdelgader I, et al. Numerical analyses of biomechanical behavior of various orthodontic anchorage implants. J Orofac Orthop 2009;70:115–27.
16. Costa A, Pasta G, Bergamaschi G. Intraoral hard and soft tissue depths for temporary anchorage devices. Semin Orthod 2005;11:10–15.
17. Chaimanee P, Suzuki B, Suzuki EY. "Safe zones" for miniscrew implant placement in different dentoskeletal patterns. Angle Orthod 2011;81:397–403.
18. Hong C, Lee H, Webster R, et al. Stability comparison between commercially available mini-implants and a novel design. Angle Orthod 2011;81:692–9.
19. Lim SA, Cha JY, Hwang CJ. Insertion torque of orthodontic miniscrews according to changes in shape, diameter and length. Angle Orthod 2008;78:234–40.
20. Motoyoshi M, Yoshida T, Ono A, et al. Effect of cortical bone thickness and implant placement torque on stability of orthodontic mini-implants. Int J Oral Maxillofac Implants 2007;22:779–84.
21. Chatzigianni A, Keilig L, Reimann S, et al. Effect of mini-implant length and diameter on primary stability under loading with two force levels. Eur J Orthod 2011;33:381–7.
22. Siegele D, Soltesz U. Numerical investigation of the influence of implant shape on stress distribution in the jaw bone. Int J Oral Maxillofac Implants 1989;4:333–40.
23. Kim JW, Baek SH, Kim TW, et al. Comparison of stability between cylindrical and conical type mini-implants: mechanical and histological properties. Angle Orthod 2008;78:692–8.
24. Wilmes B, Ottenstreuer S, Su YY, et al. Impact of implant design on primary stability of orthodontic mini-implants. J Orofac Orthop 2008;69:42–50.
25. Wilmes B, Rademacher C, Olthoff G, et al. Parameters affecting primary stability of orthodontic mini-implants. J Orofac Orthop 2006;67:162–74.
26. Reynders R, Ronchi L, Bipat S. Mini-implants in orthodontics: a systematic review of the literature. Am J Orthod Dentofacial Orthop 2009;135:564.
27. Gallas MM, Abeleira MT, Fernandez JR, et al. Three-dimensional numerical simulation of dental implants as orthodontic anchorage. Eur J Orthod 2005;27:12–16.

28. Chen CH, Chang CS, Hsieh CH, et al. The use of microimplants in orthodontic anchorage. J Oral Maxillofac Surg 2006;64:1209–13.
29. Berens A, Wiechmann D, Dempf R. Mini- and micro-screws for temporary skeletal anchorage in orthodontic therapy. J Orofac Orthop 2006;67:450–8.
30. Poggio P, Incorvati C, Velo S, et al. Safe zones: a guide for miniscrew positioning in the maxillary and mandibular arch. Angle Orthod 2006;76:191–7.
31. Chen Y, Kyung HM, Zhao WT, et al. Critical factors for the success of orthodontic mini-implants: a systematic review. Am J Orthod Dentofacial Orthop 2009;135: 284–91.
32. Kim YK, Kim YJ, Yun PY, et al. Effects of the taper shape, dual-thread, and length on the mechanical properties of mini-implants. Angle Orthod 2009;79:908–14.
33. Uemura M, Motoyoshi M, Yano S, et al. Orthodontic mini-implant stability and the ratio of pilot hole implant diameter. Eur J Orthod 2012;34:52–6.
34. Baumgaertel S. Predrilling of the implant site: Is it necessary for orthodontic mini-implants? Am J Orthod Dentofacial Orthop 2010;137:825–9.
35. Ohashi E, Pecho OE, Moron M, et al. Implant vs. screw loading protocols in orthodontics: a systematic review. Angle Orthod 2006;76:721–7.
36. Buchter A, Wiechmann D, Koerdt S, et al. Load-related implant reaction of mini-implants used for orthodontic anchorage. Clin Oral Implants Res 2005;16:473–9.
37. Ohnishi H, Yagi T, Yasuda Y, et al. A mini-implant for orthodontic anchorage in a deep overbite case. Angle Orthod 2005;75:444–52.
38. Labanauskaite B, Jankauskas G, Vasiliauskas A, et al. Implants for orthodontic anchorage: meta-analysis. Stomatologija 2005;7:128–32.
39. Dalstra M, Cattaneo PM, Melsen B. Load transfer of miniscrews for orthodontic anchorage. Orthodontology 2004;1:53–62.
40. Antoszewska J, Papadopoulos MA, Park HS, et al. Five-year experience with orthodontic miniscrew implants: a retrospective investigation of factors influencing success rates. Am J Orthod Dentofacial Orthop 2009;136:158.
41. Thiruvenkatachari B, Pavithranand A, Rajasigamani K, et al. Comparison and measurement of the amount of anchorage loss of the molars with and without the use of implant anchorage during canine retraction. Am J Orthod Dentofacial Orthop 2006;129:551–4.
42. Papadopoulos MA, Papageorgiou SN, Zogakis IP. Clinical effectiveness of orthodontic miniscrew implants: a meta-analysis. J Dent Res 2011;90:969–76.
43. Liou EJ, Pai BC, Lin JC. Do miniscrews remain stationary under orthodontic forces? Am J Orthod Dentofacial Orthop 2004;126:42–7.
44. Melsen B. Mini-implants: Where are we? J Clin Orthod 2005;39:539–47.
45. Park Y, Lee SY, Kim DH, et al. Intrusion of posterior teeth using miniscrew implants. Am J Orthod Dentofacial Orthop 2003;123:690–4.
46. Fabbroni G, Aabed S, Mizen K, et al. Transalveolar screws and the incidence of dental damage: a prospective study. Int J Oral Maxillofac Surg 2004;33:442–6.
47. Melsen B, Verna C. Miniscrew implants: The Aarhus Anchorage System. Semin Orthod 2005;11:24–31.
48. Maino BG, Mura P, Bednar J. Miniscrew implants: The Spider Screw Anchorage System. Semin Orthod 2005;11:40–6.
49. Renjen R, Maganzini AL, Rohrer MD, et al. Root and pulp response after intentional injury from miniscrew placement. Am J Orthod Dentofacial Orthop 2009;136: 708–14.
50. Asscherickx K, Vannet BV, Wehrbein H, et al. Root repair after injury from miniscrew. Clin Oral Implants Res 2005;16:575–8.
51. Papageorgiou SN, Zogakis IP, Papadopoulos MA. Failure rates and associated risk factors of orthodontic miniscrew implants: a meta-analysis. Am J Orthod Dentofacial Orthop 2012;142:577–95.
52. Schätzle M, Männchen R, Zwahlen M, et al. Survival and failure rates of orthodontic temporary anchorage devices: a systematic review. Clin Oral Implants Res 2009;20:1351–9.
53. Wiechmann D, Meyer U, Buchter A. Success rate of mini- and micro-implants used for orthodontic anchorage: a prospective clinical study. Clin Oral Implants Res 2007; 18:263–7.
54. Melsen B, Graham J, Baccetti T, et al. Factors contributing to the success or failure of skeletal anchorage devices: an informal JCO survey. J Clin Orthod 2010;44: 714–18.
55. Dalstra M, Cattaneo PM, Melsen B. Load transfer of miniscrews for orthodontic anchorage. Orthod 2001;1:53–62.
56. Chen YJ, Chang HH, Huang CY, et al. A retrospective analysis of the failure rate of three different orthodontic skeletal anchorage systems. Clin Oral Implants Res 2007;18:768–75.
57. Kuroda S, Yamada K, Deguchi T, et al. Root proximity is a major factor for screw failure in orthodontic anchorage. Am J Orthod Dentofacial Orthop 2007;131:68–73.
58. Fortini A, Cacciafesta V, Sfondrini MF, et al. Clinical applications and efficacy of miniscrews for extra-dental anchorage. Orthodontology 2004;1:87–98.
59. Papadopoulos MA. Orthodontic treatment of Class II malocclusion with miniscrew implants. Am J Orthod Dentofacial Orthop 2008;134:604.
60. Lee J, Park HS, Kyung H. Micro-implant anchorage for lingual treatment of a skeletal class II malocclusion. J Clin Orthod 2001;35:643–7.
61. Bae S, Park H, Kyung H. Clinical application of micro-implant anchorage. J Clin Orthod 2002;36:298–302.

INTRODUCTION

This chapter will focus on the different types of miniscrew implants (MIs) and the factors that are of significance for their success or failure as identified in different studies: clinical, animal and in vitro. Often, success rates in clinical studies are compared with miniplates rather than among MI types. A further method, finite element analysis (FEA), allows comparative assessment of MI designs using computer simulation to examine the effect of design parameters.

FAILURE RATES

CLINICAL STUDIES

The ideal study, the randomized controlled trial, cannot be used to assess MI success for various reasons. Skeletal anchorage is used clinically as an alternative to conventional treatment and also to perform tooth displacements that cannot be done by another method. So a control group is not possible. Clinical studies attempting to identify MI factors having an impact on failure rate are difficult to analyze as often studies are based on a small number of MIs and confounded by a high number of variables, such as selection of patients, type of malocclusion and insertion procedure.[1] Failure rates may be related more to the type of malocclusion and the type of patient selected than the anchorage unit itself.[2,3] Age may be a factor as younger patients seem to have a higher failure rate than older patients.[2,4,5]

A study of 45 MIs with a diameter of 2 mm reported a success rate of 91.1% and ascribed failures to insertion site.[6] A retrospective analysis of three systems – MIs, microimplants and miniplates – in 129 patients found the lowest failure rate with miniplates but concluded that their related costs and need for surgical intervention supported the use of MIs, as microimplants presented a slightly higher risk because of increased fracture risk.[4] A similar sample size of Taiwanese people showed an acceptable failure rate and recommended the use of thinner MIs in the maxilla (<1.4 mm) and thicker MIs in the mandible (>1.4 mm).[7] A larger study, of 905 temporary anchorage devices in 455 patients, showed the lowest failure rate (6%) for MIs and miniplates, but the "screws," whether mini- or micro-type, exhibited the lowest inflammation rate.[8]

ANIMAL STUDIES

Beagle dogs have been the preferred animals for many studies. These studies rarely identify differences between different MI types, most likely because they have focused on other variables such as failure rate.[9]

Several studies have focused on the tissue reaction associated with the insertion and loading of MIs, using histology and micro-CT to assess bone–implant contact. Insertion of MIs with predrilling in the mandible of beagle dogs indicated that longer MIs (10 mm) had a better survival rate than shorter MIs (6 mm),[10] that early loading did not have a negative impact on the tissue reaction adjacent to the MIs[10] and that time of loading did not influence tissue reaction and osseointegration,[11] although this last study lost 11 out of 20 MIs through lack of primary stability. In contrast, a study in the maxilla of beagle dogs recommended a waiting period of 3

weeks before loading.[12] The different conclusions may reflect differences in bone quality between the maxilla and the mandible, the latter allowing more primary stability. An assessment of bone–implant contact in beagle dogs supported this by finding no influence of loading time when mandible and maxilla results were pooled in a histological and micro-CT study.[13]

A study in mini-pigs used 102 AbsoAnchor (Dentos, Daegu, South Korea) and 98 Dual-Top (Jeil Medical, Seoul, South Korea) MIs in eight animals.[14] A loading of 100–500 cN was applied and maintained for 72 days, while some of the MIs were kept unloaded as controls. Only loading over 900 cN led to failure. These results, however, cannot be extrapolated to the clinical situation in humans since the cortical thickness in mini-pigs exceeds by far that of humans.

IMPLANT DESIGN

IN VITRO STUDIES

The influence of the design of MIs can best be studied by computer simulations or by in vitro studies. In vitro studies allow comparisons of different brands, different types of loading and variations in insertion torque. Failure of temporary anchorage devices mostly occurs during the first weeks after insertion and is, therefore, attributed to insufficient primary stability. The relationship between insertion torque and primary stability has been repeatedly demonstrated and so insertion torque is often the parameter chosen to express primary stability. However, cortical bone thickness and density, and variations in bone quality for animal bone, will have effects and this makes it difficult to draw clear positive correlations from in vitro studies. In addition, in vivo studies often perceive insertion torque values as resistance to loading forces.

A comparison of insertion torque for 12 different MIs used porcine ilium bone since its thickness was considered to be comparable to human maxillary and mandibular bone.[15] Insertion torque was significantly affected by the design of the 12 different MIs tested: the Orlus (Ortholution, Seoul, South Korea) and the Aarhus (Medicon eG, Tuttlingen, Germany) had the highest insertion torques. A follow-up study evaluated the effect of bone quality and implant site preparation.[16] The torque applied to insert the MIs into resin-embedded porcine iliac crest was significantly correlated with the thickness of the compact bone when inserting the Dual-Top MIs. This correlation was much weaker for TOMAS pins (Dentaurum, Ispringen, Germany). The results of this study underlined the importance of the design of the threading.

Five different MIs: FAMI2 (Gebr. Martin, Tuttlingen, Germany), Orlus, TITAN (Bernhard Förster, Pforzheim, Germany), TOMAS pin and VectorTAS (Ormco, Glendora, CA, USA) were inserted into bovine femoral heads in a region where the bone quality was judged to be identical to that of human jaws and both insertion torque and resistance to pullout, axially and at 20 and 40°, were examined.[17] The highest insertion torque after predrilling with a cylindrical bur was found with conical MIs, as expected. Without predrilling, the cylindrical MI required the highest insertion torque, while a high number of TOMAS pins fractured during insertion. At the pullout tests, the highest forces were found with cylindrical MIs. The differences between the MIs were, however, smaller when the pullout direction was 40° with respect to the long axis. A similar study of five

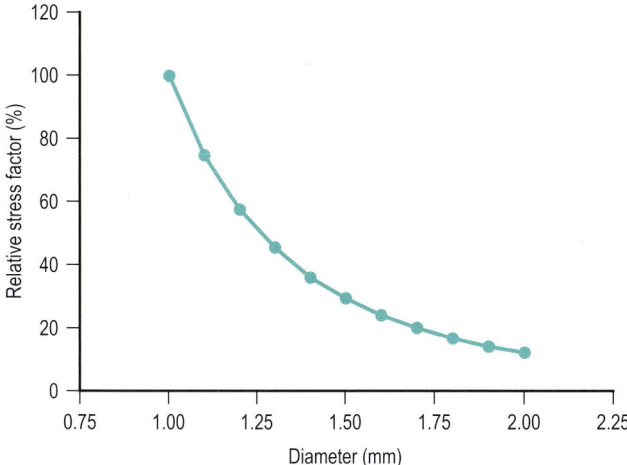

Fig. 10.1 Stress factor for a constant bending moment depending on diameter of the miniscrew implant. An increase in the diameter from 1 to 2 mm reduces the bending stresses by eight-fold.[23]

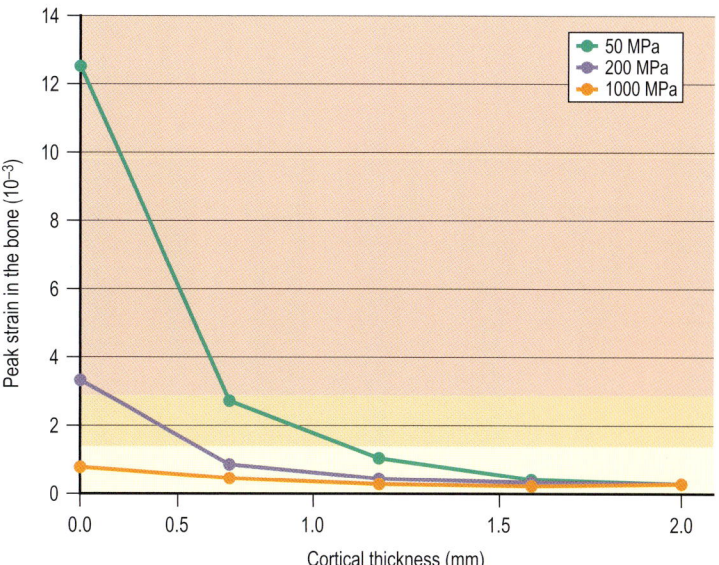

Fig. 10.2 Peak strains in the trabecular bone surrounding a miniscrew implant depend on the stiffness of the bone (50, 200 and 1000 MPa, corresponding to low, medium and high bone density) and the cortical thickness. The colors of the background correspond to Frost's mechanostat windows of physiological use (yellow), mild overuse (orange) and excessive overuse (red).[23]

different MI types inserted into three different bone types found a significant positive correlation between insertion and removal torques, with the insertion torque being significantly higher than the removal torque.[18] Self-drilling MIs with a diameter less than 1.3 mm were not suitable for insertion into bone with a density higher than 641 kg/m^3 (40 lbs/ft^3). This was corroborated by other studies reporting an increased fracture rate for thin MIs (Fig. 10.1).

Resistance to lateral force was assessed for self-tapping MIs requiring predrilling and self-drilling MIs; although the self-tapping MIs could be inserted with less torque, both types had the same resistance to lateral forces.[19] Similarly, mobility of the Aarhus and the LOMAS (MONDEAL Medical Systems, Mühlheiman der Donau, Germany) MIs inserted in bovine bone was the same with a low force, while the Aarhus was more resistant to a high force.[20] The conclusion was that both length and diameter of a MI are of importance.[20]

The stability of two connected MIs in bovine bone was compared when they were linked with a stiff wire or a miniplate; the latter created a larger resistance to pullout.[21] No differences were found between three drill-free MI systems (the Aarhus MI, the Spider Screw (Ortho Technology, Tampa, FL, USA), and the Miniscrew Anchorage System (Micerium, Avegno, Italy) inserted into rabbit femoral condyles when resonance frequency was assessed as an indicator of primary stability.[22]

COMPUTER SIMULATIONS

Influence of MI designs can be studied by computer simulations of the stress distribution and screw-to-bone load transfer. Different designs, virtually positioned in the same piece of surrounding "bone" and loaded in exactly the same way, can be used to neutralize the potential effects of variations in bone structure and quality or insertion procedure.

An examination of the effect of the thickness of the cortical shell and the quality of the underlying cancellous bone following loading of Aarhus MIs provided insights to the way loads are transferred from a MI to the surrounding bone.[23] As load transfer primarily takes place in the cortical shell, its thickness is the prime determinant of a MI's mechanical stability. This stability would be seriously compromised by placing a MI in bone with less than 0.5 mm cortical thickness and low-density (osteoporotic) underlying cancellous bone (Fig. 10.2). A similar model examined the influence of MI length and various interface conditions between MI and bone (simulating no, partial or complete osseointegration) on load transfer with the Miniscrew Anchorage System.[24] The simulation was validated by

inserting the MIs into a photoelastic material, an epoxy resin, and applying various forces to the heads to generate photoelastic fringe patterns in the resin related to the local stresses and visible under polarized light. These patterns showed the closest resemblance to the calculated stresses for the FEA where complete osseointegration was assumed. Varying the MI length from 7 to 14 mm showed that the maximum stress intensity in surrounding bone tended to decrease with an increase in MI length up to 11 mm. A MI length of 14 mm, surprisingly, displayed the highest stress intensity in the surrounding bone, possibly caused by a more pronounced "wiggling" effect of the MI tip because of its longer body length. The authors concluded that a medium length (9–11 mm) yielded the most favorable mechanical conditions.[24] An FEA of 14 different commercially available MIs compared load transfers with variation in cortical thickness and stiffness of the cancellous bone and with variation in the load angle of the force applied to the head of the MI.[25] The TOMAS and AbsoAnchor designs yielded the highest stresses and the Aarhus and Dual-Top the lowest, but no details were given for the other MI designs nor was any attempt made to explain the results from the design characteristics of the MIs.

An FEA of 10 commercially available MIs compared the stresses generated in the surrounding bone for various loading modes.[26] The intraosseous part of the MI was standardized to the length of the Aarhus design and the native extra-osseous parts were replaced by that of the Aarhus MI using computer-aided design software (Fig. 10.3A). This way, any confounding effects from the length itself or the way the external load was applied to the head were excluded, and any differences in the generated stresses would purely originate from the variations of the MI thread design. The loading modes assumed were axial pullout (Fig. 10.3B), transverse flexure and torsional moment. For the pullout mode, the ranking of the designs according to the maximum pullout load based on the lowest stress peaks in the bone was IMTEC (3M IMTEC, Ardmore OK, USA) (100%), Aarhus (84%), AbsoAnchor and MONDEAL (MONDEAL Medical Systems) (80%), OASI (Lancer Orthodontics, Vista, CA, USA) (76%), LOMAS (76%), TOMAS (73%), VectorTAS (62%), Miniscrew Anchorage System (59%) and Ace (ACE Surgical Supply, Brockton, MA, USA) (57%). Similar rankings were found for the other loading modes. The results showed, in addition, that parameters such as thread height, pitch

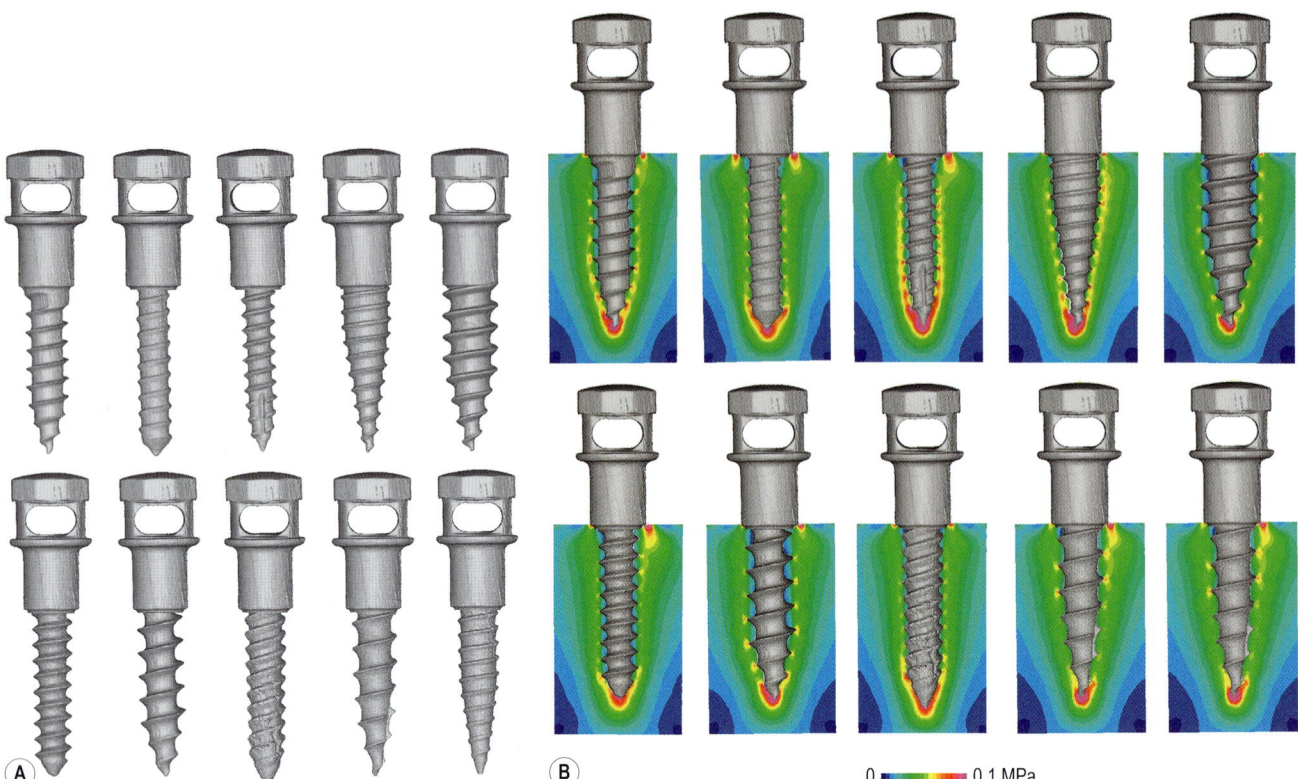

Fig. 10.3 Finite element modeling of 10 designs to examine the influence of miniscrew implant (MI) thread on load transfer on the surrounding bone. (A) In order to exclude confounders such as the length of the intraosseous part and the design of the extra-osseous part, all MI designs were normalized to the Aarhus design, replacing the native head with that of the Aarhus design and keeping the length of the intraosseous part the same as that of the Aarhus design. (B) The distribution of stress intensity (von Mises stresses) in the surrounding bone with a vertical pullout force of 100 cN for the 10 designs. Note that the overall load transfer is similar for all designs and that local differences are limited to the bone at the tip of the MIs, and closely around the threads. Top row (from left to right): Aarhus, AbsoAnchor, Ace, IMTEC and LOMAS; bottom row: Miniscrew Anchorage System, MONDEAL, OASI, TOMAS and VectorTAS.

length and pitch angle had little or no significant correlation with the stress peaks in the surrounding bone. The total volume of the intraosseous part and the inner and outer diameters of the MI were found to have high negative correlations with the stress peaks. This was particularly true for the flexural and torsional loading modes, as those parameters determine the flexural and torsional stiffness of the MIs. A thinner, and thus a more flexible, design (mechanically dictated by the geometry's so-called second moment of inertia) under the same external load would become more deformed, thus enforcing larger deformations on the surrounding bone. In addition, some degree of stress shielding of the bone was observed between two consecutive windings of the thread, resulting in medium to high negative correlations of the thread's valley length. In conclusion, the authors found that any thread variable that makes the design stiffer, though not necessarily thicker, would have a favorable effect on a MI's mechanical stability. It should be noted, however, that potentially higher pre-stresses in the bone inherent to the insertion of a bulkier MI were not taken into consideration.[26]

The influence of the cut of the threading, its angulation and depth, has not been subjected to detailed studies. One study did examine threading of MIs and found that a pitch angle of 7.5° and a flank angle of 12–15° improved the primary stability and minimized the damage, thus leading to a low failure rate.[27] These values correspond closely to the values of the Aarhus MIs (see Fig. 6.10).

USE OF PREDRILLING

Torque values during predrilling were examined in acrylic resin-embedded jaws from mini-pigs, using Dual-Top MIs.[28] The forces applied to insert the MIs were correlated with the root contact assessed on histological sections, with root contact increasing the resistance and resulting in higher torque values. However, one reason for recommending drill-free MIs has been that manual insertion is more susceptible to changes in resistance and, therefore, less risky with respect to root damage.

INSERTION SITE

The insertion procedure and insertion site are important parameters for the primary stability of MIs. Sufficient bone thickness is needed for primary stability and avoidance of root contact is also important for the success of skeletal anchorage. The risk of root contact is minimized with thinner MIs but the risk of fracture and lack of primary stability increases to unacceptable levels with diameters below 1.3 mm.[14,23,29] Ludwig et al.[30] recently published comprehensive anatomical guidelines for insertion of inter-radicular MIs based on cone beam CT in 70 adolescents and adults of white origin. The inter-radicular site is frequently chosen since it results in minimum discomfort, and it is possible to perform a wide range of tooth movements from this site using the MIs either directly or indirectly. Inter-radicular bone width and cortical thickness at different levels were assessed in sections parallel to the occlusal plane and sections passing through the contact points to give graphs indicating safe, less safe and dangerous zones. However, optimal zones were often unacceptable from a comfort point of view.[31] This could be compensated with an anatomically oblique MI insertion. Cortical thickness and insertion torque were positively correlated with primary stability in a clinical study of 76 MIs.[32] The best cortical thickness was found close to the midpalatal suture anteriorly in the palate, which has, therefore, been recommended for palatal insertion of MIs.[33]

The success rate of MIs is also influenced by mucosa levels and failure rates increase if MIs are not surrounded by keratinized gingiva.[34,35]

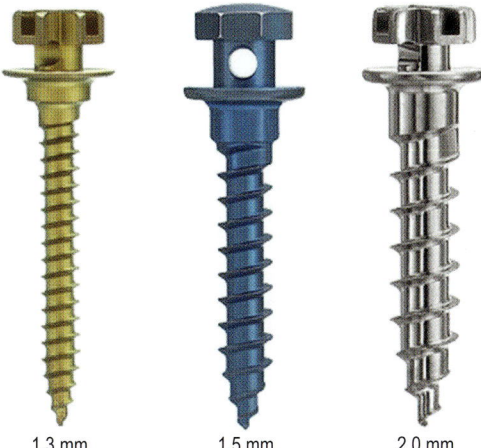

1.3 mm   1.5 mm   2.0 mm

Fig. 10.4 Different versions of the Aarhus MI with increasing thickness.

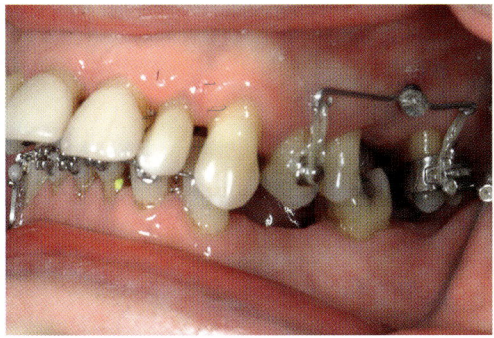

Fig. 10.5 Miniscrew implant with a bracket-like head for the attachment of wires.

DESIGN OF THE EXTRA-OSSEOUS PART

The extra-osseous part of a MI comprises the neck, the collar and the head (see Fig. 6.1). The neck passes through the mucosa and should be smooth in order to minimize infection risk; it also needs a slightly larger diameter than the threaded part so it is possible to feel when the neck reaches the bony surface. Overturning beyond this point can lead to loosening as it can destroy bone adjacent to the threaded part.[36]

To avoid plaque retention, the collar should also be smooth and in addition it should be slightly larger than the head to prevent irritation of the mucosa surrounding the MI through the ligatures tied to the MI's head (Fig. 10.4).

The design of the head depends on the use of the MI (see Fig. 6.2). If only coil springs or elastics are fixed to the MI, a one-point contact is sufficient and a hook or a ball can be chosen as a head. If the point of force application needs to be displaced, a bracket-like head is necessary (Fig. 10.5).

CONCLUSIONS

The type of MI has only a minor impact on failure rates, which seem to be influenced more by factors relating to the patient (bone quality and quantity) and doctor (biomechanics and loading). Nevertheless, when these variables are standardized, there are significant differences in the stress generated with different intraosseous designs. An asymmetrically cut cylindrical MI seems to be preferential. A bracket-like head (e.g. Aarhus MIs) offers the advantage of indirect anchorage, the possibility to vary the point of force application and of having more points of force application for each MI.

REFERENCES

1. Kalha AS. Is anchorage reinforcement with implants effective in orthodontics? Evid Based Dent 2008;9:13–14.
2. Moon CH, Park HK, Nam JS, et al. Relationship between vertical skeletal pattern and success rate of orthodontic mini-implants. Am J Orthod Dentofacial Orthop 2010;138:51–7.
3. Miyawaki S, Koyama I, Inoue M, et al. Factors associated with the stability of titanium screws placed in the posterior region for orthodontic anchorage. Am J Orthod Dentofacial Orthop 2003;124:373–8.
4. Chen YJ, Chang HH, Huang CY, et al. A retrospective analysis of the failure rate of three different orthodontic skeletal anchorage systems. Clin Oral Implants Res 2007;18:768–75.
5. Lee SJ, Ahn SJ, Lee JW, et al. Survival analysis of orthodontic mini-implants. Am J Orthod Dentofacial Orthop 2010;137:194–9.
6. Tseng YC, Hsieh CH, Chen CH, et al. The application of mini-implants for orthodontic anchorage. Int J Oral Maxillofac Surg 2006;35:704–7.
7. Wu TY, Kuang SH, Wu CH. Factors associated with the stability of mini-implants for orthodontic anchorage: a study of 414 samples in Taiwan. J Oral Maxillofac Surg 2009;67:1595–9.
8. Takaki T, Tamura N, Yamamoto M, et al. Clinical study of temporary anchorage devices for orthodontic treatment-stability of micro/mini-screws and mini-plates: Experience with 455 cases. Bull Tokyo Dent Coll 2010;51:151–63.
9. Ohmae M, Saito S, Morohashi T, et al. A clinical and histological evaluation of titanium mini-implants as anchors for orthodontic intrusion in the beagle dog. Am J Orthod Dentofacial Orthop 2001;119:489–97.
10. Freire JN, Silva NR, Gil JN, et al. Histomorphologic and histomorphometric evaluation of immediately and early loaded mini-implants for orthodontic anchorage. Am J Orthod Dentofacial Orthop 2007;131:704–9.
11. van de Vannet B, Sabzevar MM, Wehrbein H, et al. Osseointegration of miniscrews: a histomorphometric evaluation. Eur J Orthod 2007;29:437–42.
12. Zhao L, Xu Z, Yang Z, et al. Orthodontic mini-implant stability in different healing times before loading: a microscopic computerized tomographic and biomechanical analysis. Oral Surg Oral Med Oral Pathol Oral Radiol Endod 2009; 108:196–202.
13. Cha JY, Lim JK, Song JW, et al. Influence of the length of the loading period after placement of orthodontic mini-implants on changes in bone histomorphology: microcomputed tomographic and histologic analysis. Int J Oral Maxillofac Implants 2009;24:842–9.
14. Büchter A, Wiechmann D, Gaertner C, et al. Load-related bone modelling at the interface of orthodontic micro-implants. Clin Oral Implants Res 2006;17: 714–22.
15. Wilmes B, Ottenstreuer S, Su YY, et al. Impact of implant design on primary stability of orthodontic mini-implants. J Orofac Orthop 2008;69:42–50.
16. Wilmes B, Drescher D. Impact of bone quality, implant type, and implantation site preparation on insertion torques of mini-implants used for orthodontic anchorage. Int J Oral Maxillofac Surg 2011;40:697–703.
17. Florvaag B, Kneuertz P, Lazar F, et al. Biomechanical properties of orthodontic miniscrews: an in-vitro study. J Orofac Orthop 2010;71:53–67.
18. Chen Y, Kyung HM, Gao L, et al. Mechanical properties of self-drilling orthodontic micro-implants with different diameters. Angle Orthod 2010;80:821–7.
19. Su YY, Wilmes B, Honscheid R, et al. Comparison of self-tapping and self-drilling orthodontic mini-implants: an animal study of insertion torque and displacement under lateral loading. Int J Oral Maxillofac Implants 2009;24:404–11.
20. Chatzigianni A, Keilig L, Reimann S, et al. Effect of mini-implant length and diameter on primary stability under loading with two force levels. Eur J Orthod 2011;33: 381–7.
21. Leung MT, Rabie AB, Wong RW. Stability of connected mini-implants and miniplates for skeletal anchorage in orthodontics. Eur J Orthod 2008;30:483–9.
22. Veltri M, Balleri B, Goracci C, et al. Soft bone primary stability of 3 different miniscrews for orthodontic anchorage: a resonance frequency investigation. Am J Orthod Dentofacial Orthop 2009;135:642–8.
23. Dalstra M, Cattaneo PM, Melsen B. Load transfer of miniscrews for orthodontic anchorage. Orthodontics 2004;1:53–62.
24. Gracco A, Cirignaco A, Cozzani M, et al. Numerical/experimental analysis of the stress field around miniscrews for orthodontic anchorage. Eur J Orthod 2009;31: 12–20.
25. Stahl E, Keilig L, Abdelgader I, et al. Numerical analyses of biomechanical behavior of various orthodontic anchorage implants. J Orofac Orthop 2009;70:115–27.
26. Stavaras F. The effect of geometrical variations of the thread of orthodontic miniscrews on the load transfer mechanism of the surrounding bone. Master Thesis, Aarhus University, Denmark; 2010.
27. Ungethüm M, Blomer W, Reichle V. [Experimental study of improved threading of bone screws.]. Aktuelle Traumatol 1983;13:128–32.
28. Wilmes B, Su YY, Sadigh L, et al. Pre-drilling force and insertion torques during orthodontic mini-implant insertion in relation to root contact. J Orofac Orthop 2008;69:51–8.
29. Park HS, Jeong SH, Kwon OW. Factors affecting the clinical success of screw implants used as orthodontic anchorage. Am J Orthod Dentofacial Orthop 2006;130: 18–25.

30. Ludwig B, Glasl B, Kinzinger GS, et al. Anatomical guidelines for miniscrew insertion: vestibular interradicular sites. J Clin Orthod 2011;45:165–73.

31. Poggio PM, Incorvati C, Velo S, et al. "Safe zones": a guide for miniscrew positioning in the maxillary and mandibular arch. Angle Orthod 2006;76:191–7.

32. Motoyoshi M, Yoshida T, Ono A, et al. Effect of cortical bone thickness and implant placement torque on stability of orthodontic mini-implants. Int J Oral Maxillofac Implants 2007;22:779–84.

33. Kang S, Lee SJ, Ahn SJ, et al. Bone thickness of the palate for orthodontic mini-implant anchorage in adults. Am J Orthod Dentofacial Orthop 2007;131:S74–81.

34. Cheng SJ, Tseng IY, Lee JJ, et al. A prospective study of the risk factors associated with failure of mini-implants used for orthodontic anchorage. Int J Oral Maxillofac Implants 2004;19:100–6.

35. Chen J, Esterle M, Roberts WE. Mechanical response to functional loading around the threads of retromolar endosseous implants utilized for orthodontic anchorage: coordinated histomorphometric and finite element analysis. Int J Oral Maxillofac Implants 1999;14:282–9.

36. Wawrzinek C, Sommer T, Fischer-Brandies H. Microdamage in cortical bone due to the overtightening of orthodontic microscrews. J Orofac Orthop 2008;69:121–34.

Patient expectations, acceptance and preferences for miniscrew implant treatment

Fraser McDonald and Martin Baxmann

INTRODUCTION

The initial use of dental implants for the replacement of missing teeth has extended into use for the support of orthodontic treatment in many forms, particularly for en masse retraction of teeth, and the development of the miniscrew implant (MI). With the growing acceptance that functional appliances and other orthodontic techniques do not work on all patients, with a failure rate of around 30% (to such a level that intention-to-treat statistical evaluation becomes a necessary part of study analysis), there are more patients who wish to receive orthodontic treatment that is less dependent on their own compliance. Equally, the increasing range of commercial products and numbers of orthodontists chasing a static market can mean that patients are being offered unrealistic treatment approaches. This chapter considers patients' expectations, acceptance of treatment requirements and preferences.

EXPECTATIONS

Expectations relate to all aspects of dental treatment and include:

- convenient timing of treatment
- minimal time spent in the dental surgery
- ideally pain-free treatment
- efficient treatment
- unobtrusive treatment
- the ability to treat all types of malocclusion
- economical/affordable care delivery.

CONVENIENT TIMING OF TREATMENT

Major malocclusions can be treated by "functional" therapy at a stage of a patient's growth and development that will allow some form of modification of soft and hard tissues. The age of peak growth velocity is clearly ideal, but for many reasons patients still request treatment past this age. Often this may lead on to complex orthognathic and orthodontic care, but the provision of implant-supported anchorage offers an interim pathway of care that could facilitate the management of a significant number of patient problems.

MINIMAL TIME SPENT IN THE DENTAL SURGERY

With a growing number of young and mature adults seeking orthodontic care, patients' concerns for job security and time for maintaining daily life, there is a need for limiting the time spent in the dental surgery/office. The problems of long periods of time away from employment (e.g. time spent in hospital or recuperating following surgery) become increasingly significant as does attending surgery during the working day. Consequently, flexible appointment systems with extended opening times for busy patients or treatment of certain professionals either late at night or early in the morning are becoming more common but do have a limited capacity.

IDEALLY PAIN-FREE TREATMENT

Patients often associate dentistry with pain; therefore, any way of reducing discomfort and ensuring patient compliance has to be seen as a benefit. There is clear evidence that the majority who do not attend the dental surgery are cautious about both their own past experiences and reports of others.[1]

EFFICIENT TREATMENT

The current generation of clients expect delivery of results instantly and consistently, have only superficial understanding of how treatment is delivered and the belief that once treated orthodontic alignment is for life. The "downside" of treatment in the form of risks is often neglected and the patients' full engagement in risk–benefit analysis as part of the informed consent process is questionable.

UNOBTRUSIVE TREATMENT

The basis of care delivery has to fit into a patient's acceptable level of social and professional activity. Procedures that are too obvious in adults can impinge on their confidence in many aspects of their lives, for example a decline in reaching work targets or in promotion. Consequently, the search for the invisible brace (ranging from lingual appliances, through tooth-colored fixed apparatus to clear aligners) continues relentlessly and often with commercial interests over-riding patient considerations.[2]

THE ABILITY TO TREAT ALL TYPES OF MALOCCLUSION

Patients anticipate that all malocclusions can be treated regardless of the causation. The concept of the perfect long-lasting smile seems the focus of all despite the knowledge that many images seen in publications of all types have been improved by software. In addition, media focus on obscuring the aging process can lead to aspirations that are unrealistic in many and even to psychiatric syndromes of addiction to corrective surgery.

ECONOMICAL/AFFORDABLE CARE DELIVERY

In addition to the need for minimizing the time spent on care delivery, constraining costs is also important for patients. At present, orthodontics is not associated with convincing evidence of its need in terms of health although many individuals report improvement in self-esteem.

ACCEPTANCE

Acceptance of the need to be compliant with treatment can be implicit in the positive act of arranging follow-up appointments beyond the original consultation, signing appropriate relevant contracts, particularly when financial implications exist, and following instructions offered by a healthcare practitioner. Compliance is an issue. For example, even though fluoride mouthwash is offered free and there is significant positive enforcement, compliance can be as low as 10%.[3] It may be assumed that this is because there is no instantaneous outcome to bolster compliance. By comparison, orthodontic treatment has an immediate feedback, for example with the reduction of an overjet following wear of Class II elastics.

Patient compliance in orthodontics is strongly influenced by issues of pain and discomfort. Pain is linked to both unpleasant sensations of actual or potential tissue damage and emotional responses and can lead to failure to complete treatment.[4–7] A number of procedures in orthodontic treatment can cause pain and discomfort, for example during separations, initial archwire changing and bracket/band removal.[8–10]

Pain is reported to lead 1 in every 10 orthodontic patients to fail to finish treatment.[4] Information about pain caused by MIs is scarce,[11–13] as few studies have addressed the postoperative discomfort caused by MIs. Together with assessing treatment efficacy, it is also necessary to examine to what extent patients can tolerate the intended treatment processes.[12] Assessment of patient discomfort or pain during treatment can be made with various tools and three have been evaluated[14] and proven to be reliable and suitable, although no one solution is deemed to be optimal:

- the visual analogue scale (VAS)
- the numerical rating scale (NRS)
- the verbal rating scale (VRS).

The VRS is mostly used to assess pain quality, while the NRS is applied to measure pain intensity.[6,13,15] Both scales provide a discrete form of categorization. In contrast, the VAS uses a continuous or analogue range of values.[13,16,17] One of the greatest difficulties when applying the VRS is finding a significant clinical rating classification. A recently published study has used the NRS to categorize pain and discomfort into five areas.[6]

Studies have concentrated on comparing pain during MI treatment with other potentially painful dental treatments, for example tooth extraction,[6,12] other dental interventions/pathology[18,19] or discomfort caused by various forms of anchorage equipment.[20,21]

Although the use of self-drilling MIs, which can only be introduced by manual procedures, and the insertion of MIs after predrilling using a dental handpiece are both everyday procedures in orthodontic practice,[22] exactly which method the patient tolerates or prefers has not been well explored. Similarly, little is known regarding the use of a local anesthetic. A prospective study has examined patient expectations, acceptance and preferences for two insertion techniques for MIs and two different anesthesia techniques.[23] The most important result was that it made no difference to the patients whether the orthodontist drilled before MI insertion or whether a self-drilling MI was used. The patients found the noise from the dental handpiece more unpleasant than the pain, and the pressure from the self-drilling MIs more unpleasant than the pain.

PREFERENCES

En masse retraction with the help of MIs has proven to be extremely efficient[19,24] and the orthodontist usually selects the treatment plan based on the clinical situation, whereby ideal occlusion and function are the treatment objectives. In general, patients can only influence the treatment through their compliance and degree of cooperation.

The method of delivering MI-based treatment can have significant implications for the patients' perceptions. MIs can be inserted by either hand-delivered forces or a handpiece method.[22] Many clinicians prefer hand-delivered forces and this mechanism is also least compromising for the patient's experience.

There is ample evidence for successful implementation of both self-cutting MIs requiring predrilling (i.e. non-self-drilling) and self-drilling MIs without a need for predrilling.[25] The difference between these two types in terms of success rate and degree of postoperative discomfort has been briefly investigated[13,24,26] but no study has compared the two methods from the patient's perspective.

There are many dental studies addressing the effectiveness of local anesthetics,[27] but none deals with injection techniques for the placement of MIs. This is particularly surprising because for MI insertion orthodontists utilize anesthetic methods that have an effect only on the superficial soft tissues and periosteum while not anesthetizing either the dental pulp of the neighboring teeth or other important structures close by, such as the inferior mandibular nerve (thus avoiding iatrogenic damage). A prospective study evaluated two injection techniques for local anesthesia in patients requiring skeletal anchorage reinforcement.[23] The most important result was that it made no difference to the patients whether the orthodontist drilled before MI insertion or whether a self-drilling MI was used. In both methods, the patients found the pain less unpleasant than the mechanics of insertion – noise from the dental handpiece or pressure from the self-drilling MI. As both methods are successful, the orthodontist can decide which method to use based on the clinical situation or personal preference.[25] However, patient preferences regarding anesthetic injection method demonstrate how important it is to respect the patient's tolerance levels concerning treatment as this can differ considerably from the opinion of many clinicians. Patients have revealed a significant preference with regard to the anesthetic injection method, preferring injections directly into the area where the MIs were to be inserted. Their reasons for this were the shorter period of numbness after treatment and the potentially quicker therapy. Using this method, MIs can be inserted just seconds after the injection, whereas a wait of 3 minutes is necessary using the standard infiltration technique. Surprisingly, patients found this delay more important than the pain intensity during the injection itself. Pain intensity was higher with the injection directly in the MI insertion area than with the standard technique. Interestingly, a prosthetic replacement meant to cover an implant during the healing phase caused more discomfort than the actual surgical procedure.[12]

Another study focusing on the patient's pain during insertion procedures compared the soft tissue punch as preparation prior to the actual MI insertion (Fig. 11.1) and a "direct" transgingival placement of the implant.[6] Patients described the soft tissue punch as significantly more unpleasant, so this is a questionable approach. Obviously it is also of clinical relevance if this technique has an influence on primary stability, and consequently on the survival rate of the implant. Therefore, a follow-up study is currently being conducted to examine primary stability or survival rate of MIs placed with either a soft tissue punch or transgingivally. Preliminary results show no significant differences.

If extractions are needed, a dental practitioner or oral surgeon can perform the premolar extraction but an experienced and specially trained orthodontist is required to place the MI. It is debatable whether these two steps of the insertion stage would benefit the patient if they took place during one session, even though this requires more complex logistics for the clinicians.

During the removal of MIs, patients reported the same preferences as described in the insertion study, clearly favoring a manual procedure over a mechanical one.[22] The most important finding nevertheless was that pain levels produced by the injection were greater than the pain produced by the removal without anesthesia.

CONCLUSIONS

Although no one of the various rating scales for pain seems to be optimal, the established approach for assessing acute pain involves the analysis of the intensity of discomfort with the VAS, since there are convincing reports

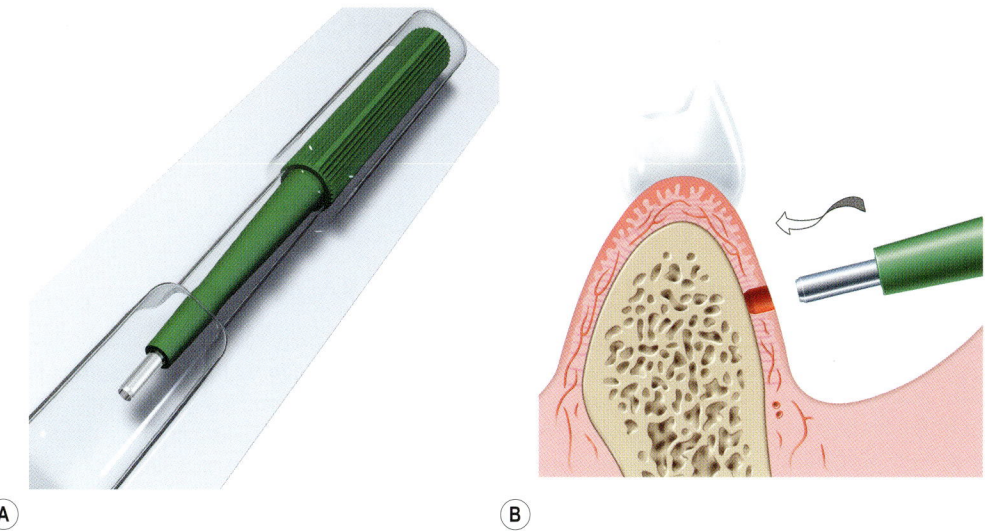

Fig. 11.1 The TOMAS punch. (A) Method of use. (B) A soft tissue punch. (Courtesy of Dentaurum KG, Ispringen, Germany.)

in the scientific literature demonstrating this scale as being quite reliable.[15,16]

A comparison of patient discomfort with regard to manual and mechanical insertion methods as well as with regard to the removal of MIs revealed significant differences. Patients clearly preferred manual techniques. The noise associated with the handpiece during these procedures led to more discomfort than the pain itself. Pain intensity varied from moderate to low. There were no significant differences in the way patients perceived treatment with self-drilling as opposed to non-self-drilling MIs.

There were also significant differences in patients' perceptions concerning the anesthetic injection techniques when inserting the MIs. A low-dose local anesthetic in the immediate MI insertion area was favored over higher doses injected using the standard injection method. During MI removal, the injection itself caused more discomfort than the actual surgery with the result that the patients preferred MI removal without anesthesia. The perceived symptoms were equal to or less intense than expected.

Surgery for MIs seems to be a well-accepted treatment option, with significantly lower pain levels than for tooth extractions. In addition, transgingival placement of MIs was clearly favored by patients, since this does not need soft tissues to be removed before MI insertion. Since the soft tissue punch does not seem to lead to improved primary stability or survival rate, utilization of this technique appears to be of low clinical relevance, particularly as patients did not care for it.

REFERENCES

1. Liddell A, May B. Some characteristics of regular and irregular attenders for dental check-ups. Br J Clin Psychol 1984;23:19–26.
2. Wright N, Modarai F, Cobourne MT, et al. Do you do Damon? What is the current evidence base underlying the philosophy of this appliance system? J Orthod 2011;38:222–30.
3. Alexander SA, Ripa LW. Effects of self-applied topical fluoride preparations in orthodontic patients. Angle Orthod 2000;70:424–30.
4. Patel V. Non-completion of orthodontic treatment: a study of patient and parental factors contributing to discontinuation in the hospital service and specialist practice. Master Thesis, University of Wales, Cardiff; 1989.
5. Sergl HG, Klages U, Zentner A. Pain and discomfort during orthodontic treatment: causative factors and effects on compliance. Am J Orthod Dentofacial Orthop 1998;114:684–91.
6. Baxmann M, McDonald F, Bourauel C, et al. Expectations, acceptance, and preferences regarding microimplant treatment in orthodontic patients: a randomized controlled trial. Am J Orthod Dentofacial Orthop 2010;138:250, discussion 250–1.
7. Bergius M, Kiliaridis S, Berggren U. Pain in orthodontics: a review and discussion of the literature. J Orofac Orthop 2000;61:125–37.
8. Bondemark L, Fredriksson K, Ilros S. Separation effect and perception of pain and discomfort from two types of orthodontic separators. World J Orthod 2004;5:172–6.
9. Erdinc A, Dincer B. Perception of pain during orthodontic treatment with fixed appliances. Eur J Orthod 2004;26:79–85.
10. Giannopoulou C, Dudic A, Kiliaridis S. Pain discomfort and cervicular fluid changes induced by orthodontic elastic separators in children. J Pain 2006;7:367–76.
11. Scheffler NR. Patient and provider perceptions of skeletal anchorage in orthodontics. Am J Orthod Dentofacial Orthop 2006;29:843.
12. Feldmann I, List T, Feldmann H, et al. Pain intensity and discomfort following surgical placement of orthodontic anchoring units and premolar extraction. Angle Orthod 2007;77:578–85.
13. Lee TCK, McGrath CPJ, Wong RWK, et al. Patients' perceptions regarding microimplant as anchorage in orthodontics. Angle Orthod 2008;78:228–32.
14. Williamson A, Hoggart B. Pain: a review of three commonly used pain rating scales. J Clin Nurs 2005;14:798–804.
15. McQuary H, Moore A. An evidence-based resource for pain relief. Oxford: Oxford University Press; 1998. p. 14–18.
16. Seymour RA, Simpson JM, Charlton JE, et al. An evaluation of length and end-phrase of visual analogue scales in dental pain. J Pain 1985;21:177–85.
17. von Bayer CL. Children's self-reports of pain intensity: scale selection, limitations and interpretation. Pain Res Manag 2006;11:157–62.
18. Kvam E, Gjerdet NR, Bondevik O. Traumatic ulcers and pain during orthodontic treatment. Community Dent Oral Epidemiol 1987;15:104–7.
19. Versloot J, Verkamp JSJ, Hoogstraten J, et al. Children's coping with pain during dental care. Community Dent Oral Epidemiol 2004;32:456–61.
20. Cornelis MA, Scheffler NR, Nyssen-Behets C, et al. Patients' and orthodontists' perceptions of miniplates used for temporary skeletal anchorage: a prospective study. Am J Orthod Dentofacial Orthop 2008;133:18–24.
21. Wehrbein H, Göllner P. Skeletal anchorage in orthodontics: basics and clinical application. J Orofac Orthop 2007;68:443–61.
22. Lehnen S, McDonald F, Bourauel C, et al. Expectations, acceptance and preferences of patients in treatment with orthodontic mini-implants. Part II: Implant removal. J Orofac Orthop 2011;72:214–22.
23. Lehnen S, McDonald F, Bourauel C, et al. Patient expectations, acceptance and preferences in treatment with orthodontic mini-implants: a randomly controlled study. Part I: insertion techniques. J Orofac Orthop 2011;72:93–102.
24. Basha A, Shantaraj R, Mogegowda S. Comparative study between conventional en-masse retraction (sliding mechanics) and en-masse retraction using orthodontic micro implant. J Oral Implantology 2010;19:128–36.
25. Chen Y, Kyung HM, Zhao WT, et al. Critical factors for the success of orthodontic mini-implants: a systematic review. Am J Orthod Dentofacial Orthop 2009;135:284–91.
26. Kuroda S, Sugawara Y, Deguchi T, et al. Clinical use of miniscrew implants as orthodontic anchorage: Success rates and postoperative discomfort. Am J Orthod Dentofacial Orthop 2007;131:9–15.
27. Nakai Y, Milgrom P, Mancl L, et al. Effectiveness of local anesthesia in pediatric dental practice. J Am Dent Assoc 2000;131:1699–705.

12 Insertion and removal of orthodontic implants
Thomas Bernhart and Adriano Crismani

INTRODUCTION

Many patients with dental and skeletal anomalies have fully intact dental arches so the alveolar region is not available for implant placement. For the maxilla, the median sagittal and paramedian region of the hard palate are appropriate sites as they have keratinized mucosa and are accessible surgically (see Chapter 7). There are, however, certain restrictions related to implant geometry.

ORTHODONTIC IMPLANTS INSERTED IN THE PALATE

Bone quantity in the vertical dimension of the palate and the presence of the midpalatal suture can create problems, implying a possible need for implants of shorter length (<10 mm) (Fig. 12.1). A recent meta-analysis, however, has indicated that success rate is dependent on implant surface rather than length in the region of the anterior maxilla.[1]

The first implant designed for insertion in the palate had reduced length (down to 4 mm) and a sandblasted and acid-etched surface.[2]

PREOPERATIVE DIAGNOSTICS

Because of the risk of perforation of the inferior nasal cavity and the need for a good assessment of bone quantity, radiography is needed in addition to clinical diagnosis.

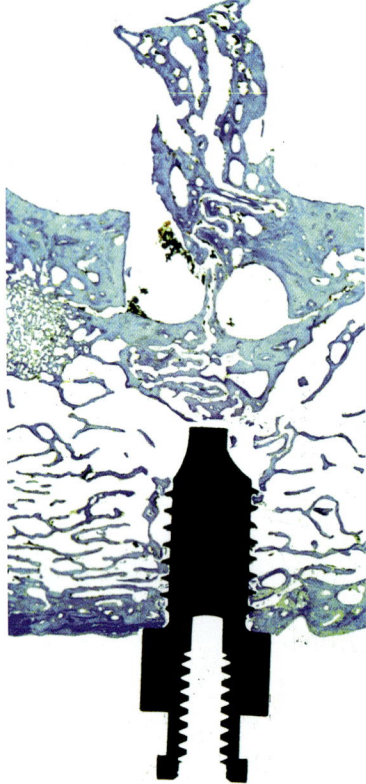

Fig. 12.1 Histological specimen showing a palatal implant.

LATERAL CEPHALOMETRIC RADIOGRAPHY

Lateral cephalometric radiography is the basic radiological diagnostic tool on which all subsequent orthodontic treatment is based and so this is the primary assessment to make. Postoperative lateral cephalometric radiography revealed perforation of the implant into the nose in five patients even though intraoperative probing of the implant bed had not indicated any perforation.[3]

A study in labeled skulls showed that the uppermost bony boundary of the palate in lateral cephalometric radiographs corresponded mainly to the structure of the nasal floor, and not to the nasal septum located in a median–sagittal direction. Therefore, vertical bone in the anterior and median third of the hard palate is at least 2 mm higher than visualized in the lateral cephalometric radiographs, but a safety margin of at least 2 mm to the nasal floor was recommended (Fig. 12.2).[3]

The major problem is the transfer of data measured on the cephalometric radiograph to the intraoperative site. Wehrbein et al.[3] used the incisive foramen as the topmost medial boundary of the palate, as depicted on the cephalometric radiographs. However, these images are often blurred in this area; in addition, use of the radiographic information would necessitate a complete mobilization of the palatal mucosa during surgery. Consequently, use of a ball-marked splint during lateral cephalometric radiography is recommended.

DENTAL COMPUTER TOMOGRAPHY

Since the midpalatal suture may not be fully ossified (closed) even in adults, restricting the utility of the surrounding area for orthodontic implants, the paramedian region is an appropriate alternative site (see Chapter 14).

By using low-dose CT protocols, reduction of radiation dose is achievable without loss of accuracy. For planning orthodontic implants, the usual dental CT protocol is recommended (thickness of layer, 0.5 mm; integrated feeding table, 0.5 mm; fast scan mode, 120 kV, 75 mA, 1 s scan, tilt of cutting plane after the hard palate).

The image data are reformatted in the midsagittal plane on a multiplanar level and a tangential line can be established along the hard palate on the oral side (Fig. 12.3A). Perpendicular to the oral tangential line, paracoronal layers are reconstructed at a distance of 3, 6, 9 and 12 mm (Fig. 12.3B,C). In 95% of patients assessed, there was adequate vertical bone volume for the insertion of a palatal implant of 4 mm in length; 93% had at least 3 mm of vertical bone volume located 4 mm distal to the incisive foramen and 3 mm lateral to the median suture of the palate.[4] The greatest amount of bone in the midsagittal plane was observed 6 mm distally from the incisive foramen. The highest mean value (paramedian) was 7.8 mm and was observed in the median sagittal "plane 3" at a distance of 3 mm from the median.

CONE BEAM COMPUTER TOMOGRAPHY

Use of cone beam CT provides three-dimensional images (3D) (Fig. 12.4). A comparison of the accuracy of cone beam CT and lateral cephalometric radiography in 18 skulls indicated that the former gave higher vertical bone

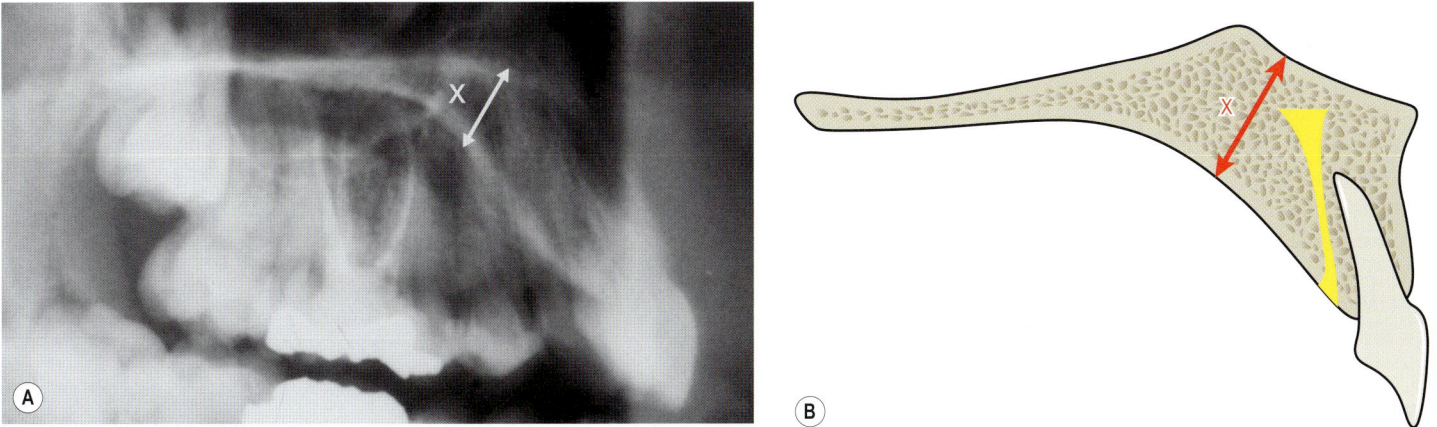

Fig. 12.2 Assessment of bone quantity in the palate. (A) Lateral cephalometric radiograph. (B) Cephalometric tracing of the maxilla. Maximum bone quantity (x) is marked. The maximum length of the implant should be 2 mm less than x.

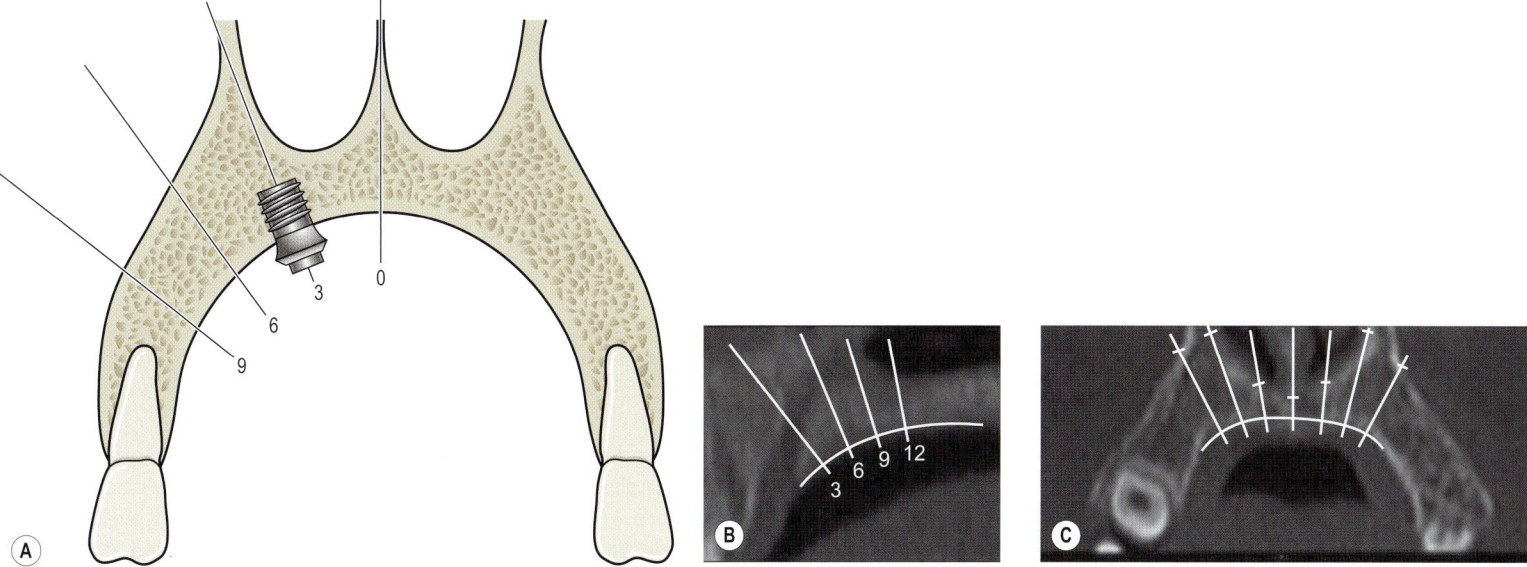

Fig. 12.3 CT of the hard palate. (A) Planes 3, 6 and 9 with planned implant insertion positions every 3 mm on the paramedian side. (B) Multiplanar reformation of the hard palate at the median–sagittal plane. (C) Multiplanar reformation, visualizing the measuring method for distances 0 to 9 mm, 6 mm away from the incisive foramen

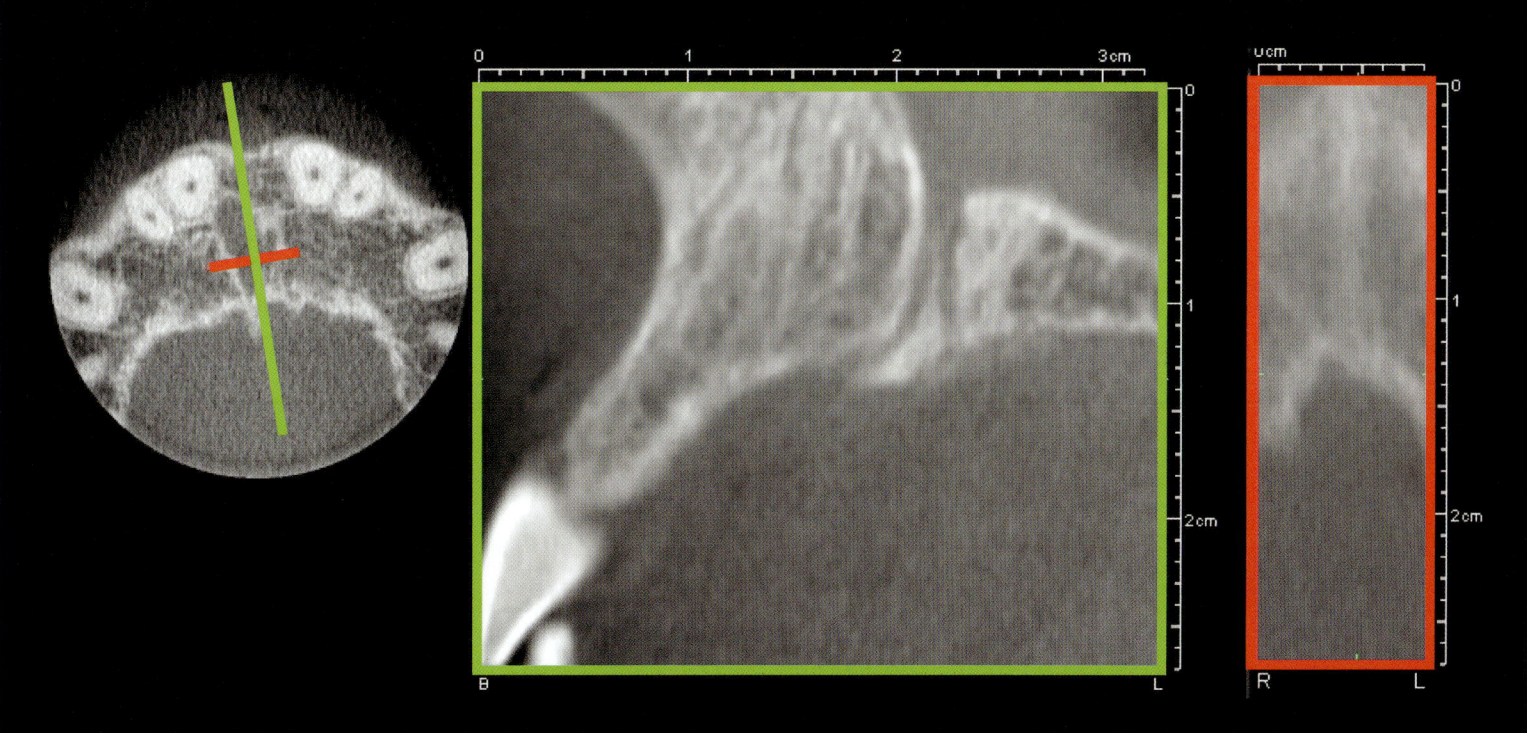

Fig. 12.4 Hard palate reconstruction from cone beam CT (green frame, orthoradial reconstruction in the mid-plane; red frame, panoramic reconstruction of the frontal region).

heights: mean 8.98 ± 3.4 mm compared with 6.6 ± 3.2 mm.[5] In the paramedian region, the two approaches were both within the range of the first premolars in a positive linear relation. It was concluded that lateral cephalometric radiographs show a minimum of vertical bone height paramedian and not the maximum in the median sagittal plane.[5] Therefore, preoperative CT or cone beam CT was recommended if lateral cephalometric evaluation reveals a marginal quantity of bone volume.[5]

A retrospective clinical cohort indicated that 97.8% (89 out of 91) of the patients showed adequate bone volume in lateral cephalometric radiographs. One of the remaining two patients showed inadequate bone volume (<4 mm) in a further cone beam CT evaluation.[6]

SUMMARY

According to these results, the following diagnostic conclusions may be drawn:

- a safety margin of at least 2 mm to the nasal floor should be considered in implant planning when using lateral cephalometric radiographs, thus avoiding possible perforation; a radiological marked splint may be helpful
- CT should only be used if the lateral cephalometric radiograph reveals a bone volume less than 4 mm in the premolar region
- a low-dose protocol is recommended for dental CT.

BONE QUANTITY AND LOCALIZATION

An analysis of bone quality in the hard palate using histomorphometric analysis of autopsy material from 22 adults (18–63 years)[7] indicated three areas for implant placement:

- the anterior part of the medial palate, 7 mm behind the incisive foramen in the area of the first premolars
- the middle part, in the area of the second premolars
- the posterior part, in the area of the first molars.

Age had no influence on bone density. There was adequate bone quality in all areas of the medial palate for primary implant stability plus a mean bone depth–volume ratio that was relatively high (>68%).[7]

Quantity and quality of bone in the posterior palate corresponded to the requirements for palate implant placement.[7]

The paramedian region is of particular interest when treating children, because the midpalatal suture will still be developing. Two studies have examined bone depth in the paramedian region.[4,8] Cone beam CT in 183 adolescents aged 10–19 years showed that 93.2% of the boys and 91.9% of the girls had sufficient vertical bone volume in the paramedian region to host a 3 mm implant with practically no root interference.[8]

SURGICAL INSERTION OF ORTHODONTIC IMPLANTS IN THE PALATE

The requirements for a good palatal implant are that it should be simple to handle surgically, it should produce minimal surgical trauma and it should be simple to connect to orthodontic appliances. The Straumann Palatal Implant (Straumann, Basel, Switzerland), a transmucosally inserted implant, fulfills these needs and is recommended for insertion in the median or paramedian region of the palate. The surgical approach for implant insertion described below is for this type of implant.

The Straumann Palatal Implant is a single unit system made of pure titanium with an endosseous implant part (4.1 and 4.8 mm), a transmucosal smooth neck and a screw-operated abutment (see Fig. 7.2). The endosseous part has a self-cutting thread with a sandblasted and acid-etched surface and a length of 4.2 mm. The transmucosal part has a high-gloss polished neck.

After assessing local bone quantity, adequate local anesthesia is applied to the area of intended implant placement, followed by removal of the palatal mucosa with a mucosal punch (Fig. 12.5A) and a periosteal elevator (Fig. 12.5B).

Palatal compact bone is granulated with a round bur (Figure Fig. 12.5C) and the implant bed is prepared with a twist drill (Fig. 12.5D). The initial preparation with the round bur prevents sliding of the twist drill. Preparation of the implant site should be done under continuous cooling with precooled (5°C [41°F]) physiological saline at a maximum speed of 800 rpm.

The self-cutting implant is then removed from the blister and inserted in the bone without tilting (Fig. 12.5E).

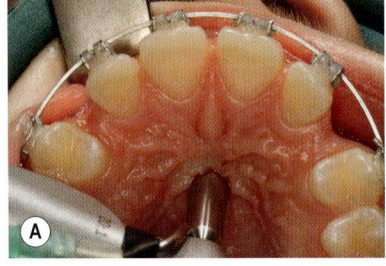 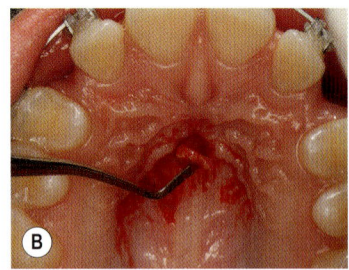 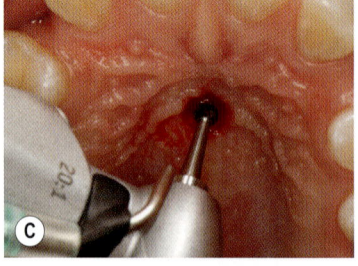 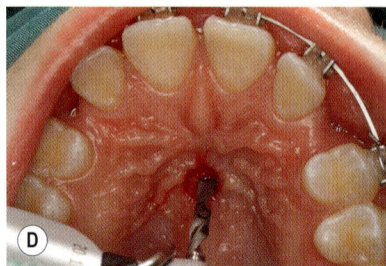
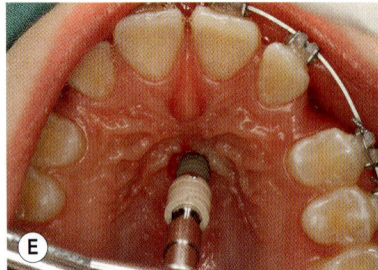 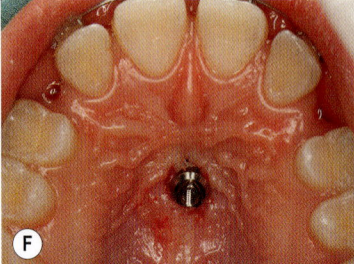 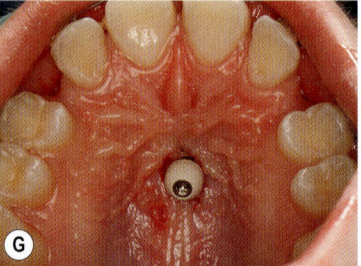 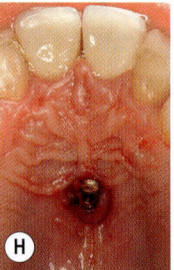

Fig. 12.5 Surgical insertion of an orthodontic implant in the palate. (A) Removal of the palatal mucosa with a special punch. (B) Removal of the mucosa with a periosteal elevator. (C) The round bur as it is marking the implant position. (D) The twist drill preparing the implant bed. (E) Insertion with the special implant insertion device and the manual torque wrench. The implant is driven to its final position at the high-gloss polished shoulder. (F) Immediately after insertion. (G) Postoperative view subsequent to insertion of a healing abutment. (H) Peri-implantitis, caused by inadequate hygiene, observed following removal of the orthodontic device.

Fig. 12.6 Removal of a palatal implant. (A) Using a special guiding cylinder with a trepan bur. (B) Use of extraction forceps.

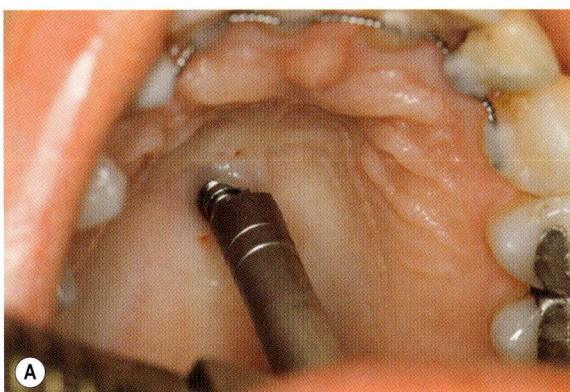
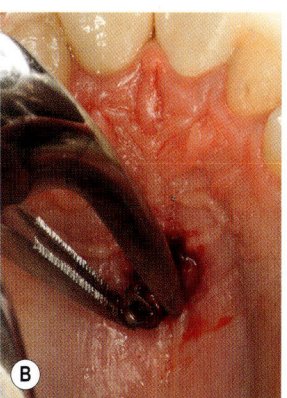

The final positioning of the implant may be achieved using a torque wrench (Fig. 12.5F). Afterwards, the insertion device is removed and a healing cap is attached manually to the implant to protect the inner threads (Fig. 12.5G).

For postoperative care (the first 10 days), it is recommended to rinse several times a day with chlorhexidine digluconate (0.2%), avoiding any mechanical cleaning.

During the orthodontic loading period, thorough cleaning with a toothbrush is essential to avoid infections that could lead to peri-implant complications or implant loss (Fig. 12.5H).[9]

REMOVAL OF ORTHODONTIC IMPLANTS

Once treatment is completed, the implant is removed using a special guiding cylinder with a trepan bur (Fig. 12.6A). The trepan bur has two scales on the outside (6 and 4 mm), for the relative implant length, in line with the deep-seated preparation. Again, sufficient cooling is necessary during surgery. After preparation, the implant is removed with surrounding bone. Extraction forceps and slight rotation may support the explantation (Fig. 12.6B) or controlled rotation without mechanical preparation can be used. A special adapter aids in gripping the implant, and the bone–implant contact can be fractured by a counterclockwise rota-

tion. Up to 40 Ncm of extraction torque is needed, requiring a mechanical torque wrench.

REFERENCES

1. Pommer B, Frantal S, Willer J, et al. Impact of dental implant length on early failure rates: a meta-analysis of observational studies. J Clin Periodontol 2011;38:856–63.
2. Wehrbein H, Merz BR, Diedrich P, et al. The use of palatal implants for orthodontic anchorage: design and clinical application of the Orthosystem. Clin Oral Implants Res 1996;7:410–16.
3. Wehrbein H, Merz BR, Diedrich P. Palatal bone support for orthodontic implant anchorage: a clinical and radiological study. Eur J Orthod 1999;21:65–70.
4. Bernhart T, Vollgruber A, Gahleitner A, et al. Alternative to the median region of the palate for placement of an orthodontic implant. Clin Oral Implants Res 2000;11:595–601.
5. Jung BA, Wehrbein H, Heuser L, et al. Vertical palatal bone dimensions on lateral cephalometry and cone-beam computed tomography: Implications for palatal implant placement. Clin Oral Implants Res 2011;22:664–8.
6. Jung BA, Harzer W, Wehrbein H, et al. Immediate versus conventional loading of palatal implants in humans: a first report of a multicenter RCT. Clin Oral Invest 2011;15:495–502.
7. Wehrbein H. Bone quality in the midpalate for temporary anchorage devices. Clin Oral Implants Res 2009;20:45–9.
8. King KS, Lam EW, Faulkner MG, et al. Vertical bone volume in the paramedian palate of adolescents: a computed tomography study. Am J Orthod Dentofacial Orthop 2007;132:783–8.
9. Männchen R, Schätzle M. Success rate of palatal orthodontic implants: a prospective longitudinal study. Clin Oral Implants Res 2008;19:665–9.

INTRODUCTION

Miniplates offer excellent stability as temporary anchorage devices and have a wide range of applications including distalization of the entire dental arch, maxillary protraction and molar intrusion. Consequently, malocclusions that are challenging to treat with conventional orthodontic mechanics can be managed by the orthodontist with the use of miniplates.

The application and removal of miniplates is more complex and time consuming than that for palatal implants and miniscrew implants, particularly since miniplate surgery requires transmucosal access, bone surface preparation and insertion of two to four screws per plate. The miniplate protocol includes minor surgery for placement and removal by a maxillofacial surgeon. Despite these drawbacks, there are considerable advantages, including maximal anchorage and safer placement away from the roots of adjacent teeth.[1]

Maxillary sites for miniplate fixation are limited to the zygomatic buttress[1,2] and the apertura piriformis (anterior nasal aperture).[3] Maxillary fractures and Le Fort I osteotomies are also stabilized through these areas by miniplates. The zygomatic region has the thickest cortical bone in the maxilla.[2,4]

The mandible has a thicker cortical bone than the maxilla; the outer cortical bone layer of the mandible is strong and thicker at the external oblique line and in the symphyseal region and is ideal for miniplate screw stability.

Primary stability of the miniplates is essential for absolute anchorage as is secondary stability throughout treatment. Orthodontic forces may be applied immediately upon insertion and there is no need to wait for osseointegration. However, a small waiting period is recommended until primary soft tissue healing is achieved.

TYPES OF MINIPLATES

Because patients vary in anatomy, bone quality and quantity and the desired orthodontic movement, a range of miniplate sizes is needed. The distance from the archwire to the anchorage head should be planned before surgery and the miniplates should be selected accordingly.

Standard miniplates, used in maxillofacial surgery, are also used for orthodontic anchorage but the emergence area is not rounded and they have sharp corners (Fig. 13.1A), which can cause delayed wound healing and more soft tissue irritation.

Titanium miniplates designed for specific orthodontic purposes include the Skeletal Anchorage System (SAS),[5] the Ballard miniplate (Surgitec, Brussels, Belgium),[6] the C-tube (0.036" diameter tube formed by curving the end of the miniplate; Martin, Tuttlingen, Germany)[7] and miniplates designed for the zygoma, apertura piriformis and symphysis regions (Tasarım Med, İstanbul, Turkey)[4] (Fig. 13.1B–D).

Miniplates and screws are classified based on the diameters of the fixation miniscrews, such as 1.0, 1.5, 2.0 or 2.3 mm systems. The surface areas of 2.0 mm or 2.3 mm screws are considerably larger than that of the 1.5 mm screw and they have greater mechanical strength; however, the risk of root damage increases as the diameter widens. When the diameter is smaller than 2 mm, mechanical stability of the screw may not be sufficient for orthodontic anchorage. Both self-tapping and self-drilling screws can be used for fixation of miniplates.

The point where the plate arm is exposed or perforates the oral mucosa is called the emergence point of the plate and is one of the most critical aspects that has to be taken into consideration during insertion.

ZYGOMATIC ANCHORAGE

Miniplates used for skeletal orthodontic anchorage are inserted to the zygomatic process, apertura piriformis, mandibular symphysis and mandibular oblique ridge (Fig. 13.2), with the zygomatic process most frequently used.

Anterior, infratemporal and orbital surfaces of the maxilla converge at the zygomatic process. Anteriorly, the process merges into the facial surface of the body of the maxilla. Posteriorly, it is concave and continuous with the infratemporal surface. Superiorly, it is roughly serrated for articulation with the zygomatic bone. Inferiorly, a bony arched ridge, the zygomaticoalveolar ridge of the jugal crest, separates the facial and infratemporal surfaces.

The zygomatic area may be used for molar distalization, posterior en masse distalization, incisor retraction and en masse retraction in Class II malocclusion as well as for molar intrusion in patients with open bite. This area may even be used for the correction of Class III malocclusion by using Class III elastics.

SURGICAL TECHNIQUE

Placement and removal of miniplates is performed under local anesthesia and sedation, although general anesthesia may also be indicated. Following

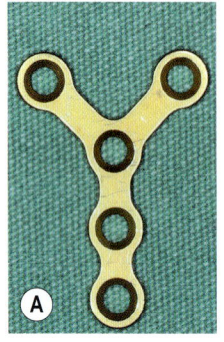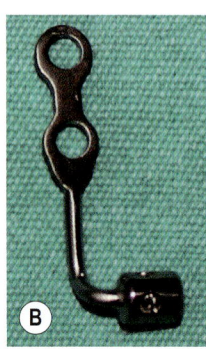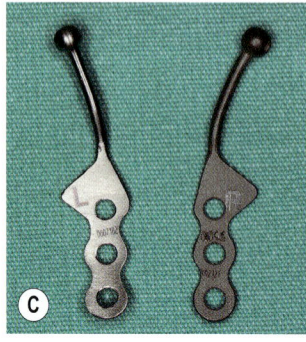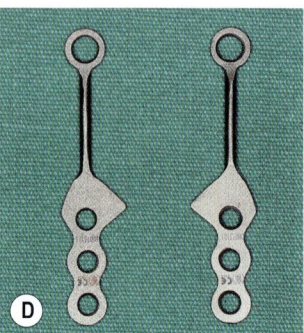

Fig. 13.1 (A) A miniplate used in maxillofacial surgery for fixation of bony segments. (B–D) Different types of miniplates used as skeletal anchorage for orthodontic purposes.

infiltration or posterior superior alveolar block with 4% articaine and 1/100 000 epinephrine (Ultracaine HCl) (Fig. 13.3A), a vertical or horizontal incision (depending on the clinician's preference or anatomy of the buttress) is made at the buccal vestibule adjacent to the first and second molars, 1.5 cm above the coronal gingiva, while maintaining contact with the bone (Fig. 13.3B). Buccal muscle attaches to the buccal alveolus of molar teeth but, mostly, a zygomatic incision does not affect, or only minimally affects, this muscle. If the incision is made too high, there is a higher risk of bleeding. Stenson's duct orifice should be identified as this is the

most important anatomical structure in this area; generally it is away from the incision region but heavy retraction may cause inflammation at the orifice of the duct and thus postoperative pain through inadequate drainage and saliva retention.

A full-thickness mucoperiosteal flap should be raised and stripped with periosteal elevators, exposing the zygomatic process of the maxilla (Fig. 13.3C). A soft tissue retractor is placed as soft tissue tension is very high at this site and specially designed retractors may be helpful to overcome this tension (Fig. 13.3D). Plates should be chosen for each patient based on the anatomy of the buttress area and the emergence point. Plates should be bent and adapted precisely in all planes to achieve a passive bone–plate fixation (Fig. 13.3E). Locking systems (special plates that have treads and hold the screw) may also be used for zygomatic anchorage. The locking screw has a special double-thread design that allows the threaded screw head to engage the corresponding threaded plate holes on the miniplate during insertion.[8]

At least two miniscrews should be inserted to avoid rotation and to resist the orthodontic forces applied but three screws are preferred. The insertion of the miniplate as high as possible accesses a better quality and quantity of bone but retraction of soft tissues and insertion of the upper screws of the miniplate are technically more difficult if the insertion is done under local anesthesia. The first miniscrew should not be completely tightened so that some rotation is available for adjustment of the plate to an ideal position. Following insertion of the first miniscrew, the remaining screws are fixed with a hand driver. Although bone thickness at the zygoma region is better than in other areas of the maxilla, cortical bone quantity may still not be sufficient for screw fixation particularly if the maxillary sinus is highly pneumatized. Zygoma plates are fixed with either 2.0 mm or 2.3 mm diameter screws to increase stability. Surgical closure is performed with 4-0 sutures (Fig. 13.3F). Following surgery, pain killers (acetaminophen 500 mg three times a day), chlorhexidine gluconate (mouthwash

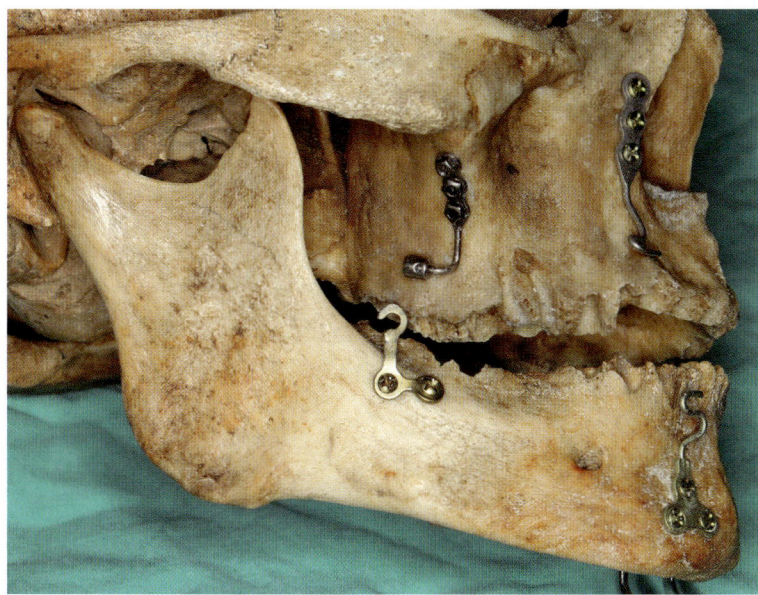

Fig. 13.2 Sites for insertion of miniplates for orthodontic anchorage purposes in the maxilla and the mandible.

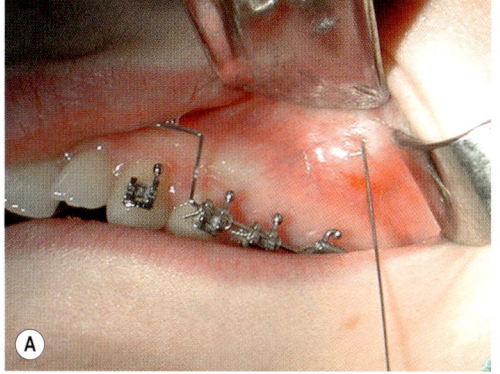
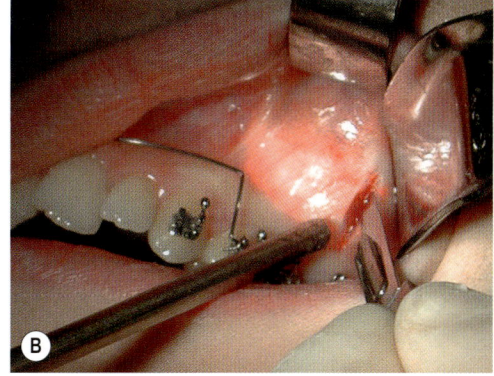
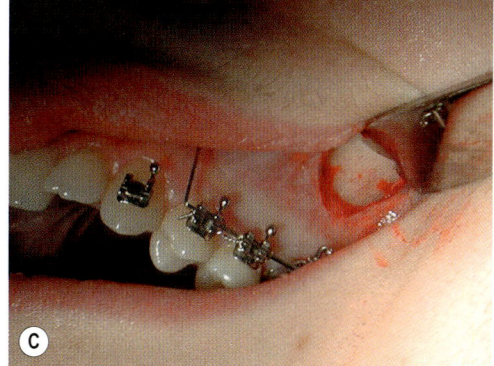
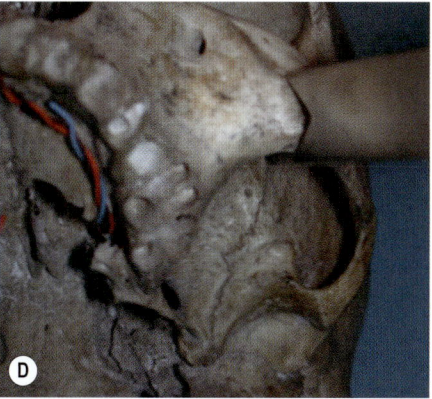
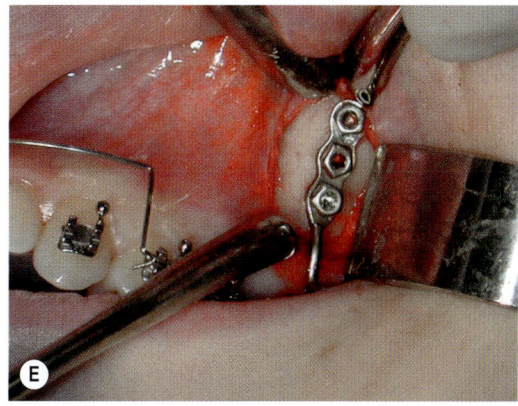
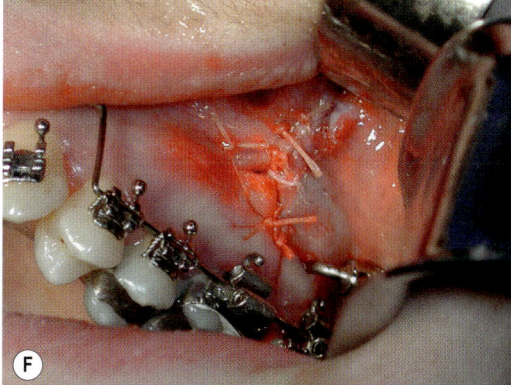

Fig. 13.3 Miniplate attachment for zygomatic anchorage. (A) Application of infiltration anesthesia. (B) Vertical incision at buccal vestibule adjacent to the first and second molars, 1.5 cm above the coronal gingiva. (C) Exposure of the zygomatic buttress of the maxilla following elevation of periosteum. (D) A specially designed retractor for zygomatic region. (E) Adaptation and fixation of the miniplate to the zygomatic buttress with three screws. (F) Closure of the incision with 4-0 sutures.

three times daily) and amoxicillin trihydrate (500 mg three times a day) for 4 days are prescribed.

Some problems may be encountered during surgery. The width of attached gingiva may be too narrow in some patients for the emergence point to be in attached keratinized gingiva or at least at the mucogingival junction. If it is at the mobile (non-attached) gingiva, irritation of the surrounding soft tissues, postoperative inflammation and infection can occur, leading possibly to affect bone and cause loosening of the miniscrews. Cheek or lip irritation may also occur during orthodontic treatment, which can be avoided by precise bending of the exposed loop during surgery. If bending of the loop is attempted postoperatively, the part close to the bone should be held with one set of pliers while bending is performed with another set in order to avoid excessive forces on the bone–screw interface.

Other factors that can lead to loosening of screws are use of rectangular miniplates, non-homogeneous force distribution along the miniplate, insertion technique, duration of the applied orthodontic force and the patient's oral hygiene.

Patients should comply with the instructions regarding maintenance of immaculate oral hygiene. Miniplates should be cleaned daily to prevent inflammation. Moderate postoperative facial swelling generally occurs and may remain a few days after surgery. Applying ice packs every 15 minutes in the early postoperative period may reduce the edema.

There may be moderate levels of discomfort and pain associated with the placement surgery. An evaluation of pain perception in 15 patients who had undergone miniplate insertion indicated that patients were concerned about the surgical procedure before insertion.[9] At 7 days after surgery, their score on a visual analogue scale (VAS) decreased remarkably. Before removal surgery, patients were again anxious as they had experienced pain during the insertion procedure but their VAS score had reduced significantly 24 hours after surgery and 88% stated that they would be prepared to undergo this treatment modality in the future.[9] Effective communication between patients and doctors can help to address the concerns of patients with regard to treatment-related pain.

Patients should be clearly informed of the pain that they might experience during miniplate insertion and removal and of possible complications that might occur.

MINIPLATES ON APERTURA PIRIFORMIS

The anterior part of the medial nasal wall is also the lateral wall of the anterior nasal aperture. This structure is a relatively new site for orthodontic anchorage (Fig. 13.4). In addition to Class II elastics, indications for this site include maxillary protraction using face masks in patients with Class III malocclusion and intrusion of maxillary incisors in patients with deep bite.

The apertura piriformis is close to the maxillary midline and growing areas; therefore, the incision must be made away from the midline and incisions and dissections should not be wide. The most important anatomical landmarks are the lateral nasal branch of the facial artery, branches of the infraorbital and angular arteries and the nasalis muscle. However, all these structures are away from the incision line and the risk of damage is unlikely in apertura incision for miniplate insertion. If the canine has not erupted and is positioned deeply in the maxilla, there is a risk of tooth damage as the plate and screws are inserted directly on the canine region.

SURGICAL TECHNIQUE

A mucoperiosteal incision is made at the labial vestibule between the maxillary lateral incisors and canines and a mucoperiosteal flap is elevated,

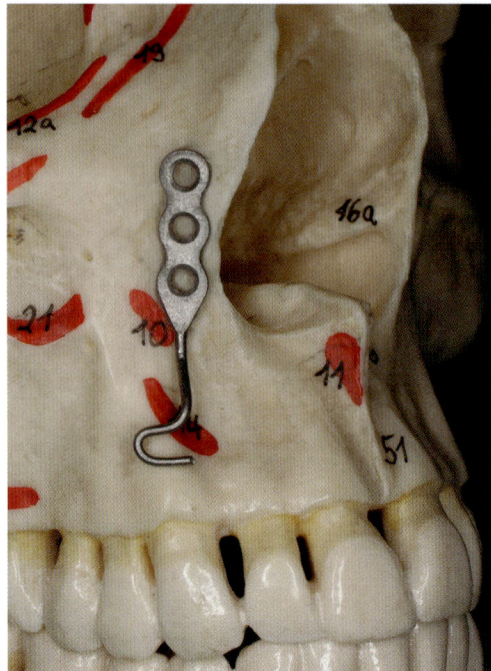

Fig. 13.4 Positioning of a miniplate lateral to the aperture piriformis on an anatomical skull model.

thereby exposing the lateral nasal wall of the maxilla on both sides (Fig. 13.5A). An appropriate cortical bone area is found for the miniplates, with particular care to avoid any damage to the erupting canines. Miniplates are shaped according to the underlying anatomical structure and fixed in position with two monocortical miniscrews (diameter 1.5–2.0 mm, length 7 mm) (Fig. 13.5B). The incisions are sutured with 3-0 vicryl, exposing the third hole of the plate into the oral cavity (Fig. 13.5C). Specially designed plates are used to avoid any soft tissue problems. If the height of the maxilla is sufficient, insertion of three miniscrews may also be possible but insertion and removal of the third screw is usually difficult. Consequently, a third screw is only placed if the stability of the first two screws is insufficient and the bone-plate interface is not rigid enough.

Drilling is performed bicortically at this area to achieve maximum bone contact and stability. As the total thickness of the bone is limited to a few millimeters, drills may cause nasal mucosal perforation and bleeding. To avoid this, a periosteal elevator should be inserted into the gap between the lateral nasal wall and nasal mucosa.

SYMPHYSEAL ANCHORAGE

Miniplates are inserted into the symphysis region to anchor fixed functional appliances in growing patients with skeletal Class II malocclusion, and also for Class III elastics and intrusion of mandibular incisors in patients with deep bite.

The symphysis region is one of the best areas for screw insertion as the cortical bone is relatively thick and the area can be reached easily (Fig. 13.6). Anteriorly, the upper external surface shows an inconstant faint median ridge, which indicates fusion of the halves of the fetal bone at the symphysis menti. Inferiorly, this ridge divides to enclose a triangular mental protuberance; its base is centrally depressed but raised on each side as a mental tubercle. The mental protuberance and mental tubercles constitute the chin. The mental foramen, from which the mental nerve and vessels emerge, lies below either the interval between the premolar teeth or the second premolar tooth.

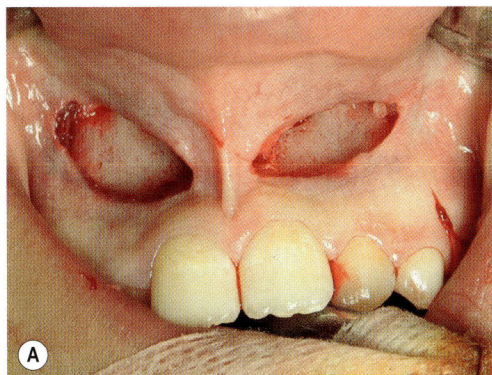 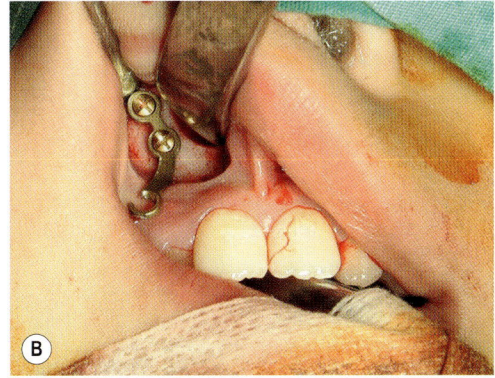 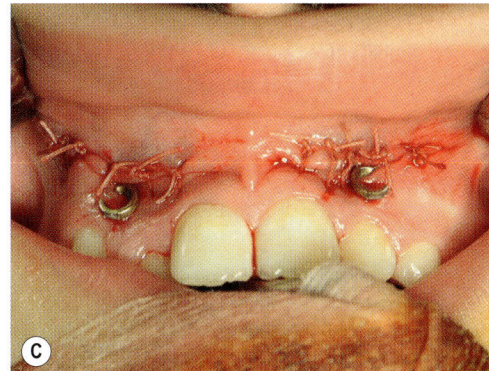

Fig. 13.5 Miniplate attachment to the apertura piriformis. (A) Mucoperiosteal incisions at the labial vestibule of the maxilla on both sides. (B) Adaptation and fixation of miniplates, lateral to the aperture piriformis. (C) Sutures exposing the third hole of the miniplate into the oral cavity.

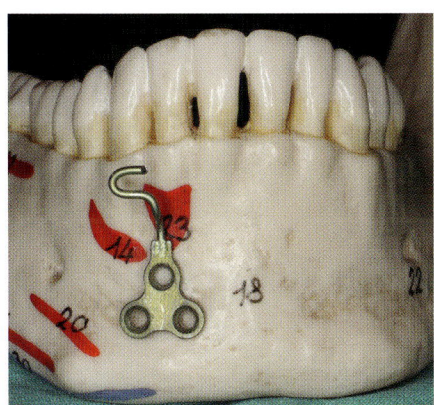

Fig. 13.6 Positioning of a miniplate on the symphyseal region on an anatomical skull model.

SURGICAL TECHNIQUE

Following bilateral injection of articaine or lidocaine with 1/100 000 epinephrine supraperiosteally (infiltrative) to buccal and lingual sites, a 1 cm horizontal incision is made transecting the mental muscle at both sides. Care must be taken not to merge the two incisions; there should be a gingival bridge of at least 1 cm between the incisions. This is extremely important in order to avoid the unpleasant postoperative complication of lip ptosis, caused by partial loss of function of the mental muscle. This complication is intolerable in growing children.

Following dissection through the basis of the anterior mandible (Fig. 13.7A), the plates should be adapted accurately to be passive at the bone surface without interacting with incisor roots, erupting canine or base of the mandible. There are no major anatomical structures in this region; the frenulum of the lower lip and mental nerve, artery and vein are the most apparent. The parasymphyseal incision is anterior to the mental foramen and so vessel and nerves are generally away from the incision line. After bending the plates, the emergence point alignment should be made to perforate the mucosa at the attached gingiva. Otherwise, inflammation and screw loosening during the postoperative period can be seen. The plate should be bent about 90° at the level of mucosal perforation to avoid pressure over the soft tissues after screw tightening.

Screws, usually 2.0 mm diameter, are inserted to fix the plate in position; overtightening should be avoided to decrease stresses on cortical bone (Fig. 13.7B). Stability is double-checked and the wounds are closed by 4-0 vicryl resorbable sutures. The mental muscle is sutured first and then the mucosa; this double-layer closure helps the mental muscle to heal properly and sustains its function.

Following suturing of the mucosa, a final suture that turns around the neck of the plate helps healing of the most critical area by sealing the soft tissues tightly. Medication is prescribed as for zygomatic anchorage. Surface sutures are removed at the sixth postoperative day and orthodontic force is applied at the tenth day.

MINIPLATES ON THE RETROMOLAR (ANGULUS) AREA

The retromolar (angulus) area is another site for miniplate insertion (Fig. 13.8). A faint external oblique line ascends backwards from each mental tubercle and becomes more marked as it continues into the anterior border of the ramus. The lateral surface of the mandibular ramus is relatively featureless and bears the external oblique ridge in its lower part. The anterior border is thicker below where it is continuous with the external oblique line. Near the second and third molar teeth, the external oblique line is superimposed upon the buccal plate. The external surface of the alveolus adjacent to the molar teeth gives attachment to the buccinator. A number of muscles of facial expression are attached to the lateral surface of the mandible.

Miniplates inserted at this area are used for anchorage to obtain skeletal correction in growing patients with Class II malocclusion using Class II elastics and for mandibular molar intrusion in open bite.

This area has even better bone quality than the anterior mandible and is an ideal region biomechanically for initial screw stability. Miniplates are also inserted to this area following angular fractures or sagittal split ramus osteotomies in maxillofacial surgery.[8] The main disadvantages include the requirement for adaptation of the plate and drilling. Since the area is located posteriorly, insertion of miniscrews and drilling are relatively difficult and miniscrew insertion at 90° to the bone surface may not always be possible. However, angled insertion of the screws does not jeopardize the biomechanics as the screw will have a longer length in bone.

SURGICAL TECHNIQUE

Anesthesia is with buccal infiltration of 1 ml of 4% articaine or lidocaine with 1/100 000 epinephrine; alternatively a nerve block of the inferior alveolar nerve and buccal nerve (branches of the mandibular nerve) can be used. Generally, infiltration anesthesia is adequate for painless insertion of the plates in young children. A 1.0–1.5 cm anteroposterior incision is made at the buccal sulcus of the mandibular second molar. The incision should not extend through the ascending ramus as damage to the buccal nerve (sensory branch of the mandibular nerve that innervates the mucoperiosteum of molar area) is possible. Soft tissues including the periosteum are dissected and retracted. Plates are adapted and held at the desired position before fixing with miniscrews (diameter 2.0 mm). As the bone is thick and dense in this region, overtightening is possible and should be avoided

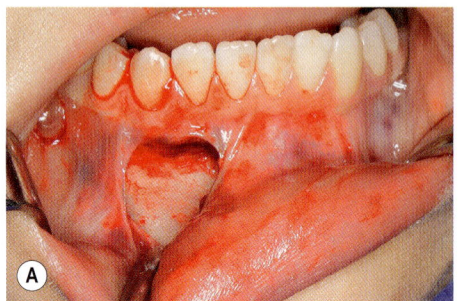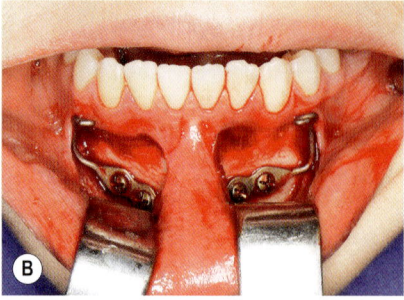

Fig. 13.7 Miniplate attachment to the symphysis region. (A) Exposure of the cortical bone following the dissection of the periosteum at the symphyseal region; (B) Implantation of miniplates with two miniscrews in the symphyseal region of the mandible. It is crucial to keep the frenulum labii inferior and mentalic muscle between two miniplates safe.

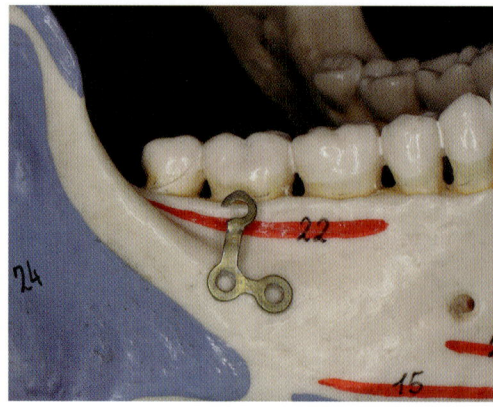

Fig. 13.8 Positioning of a miniplate on the retromolar region of an anatomical skull model.

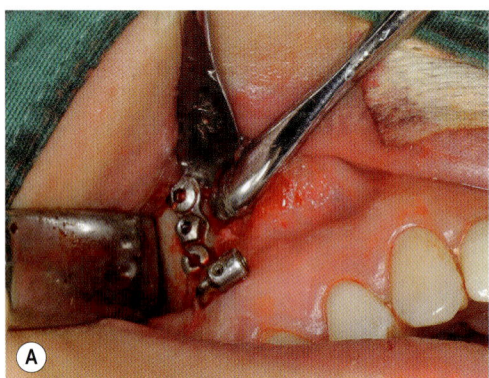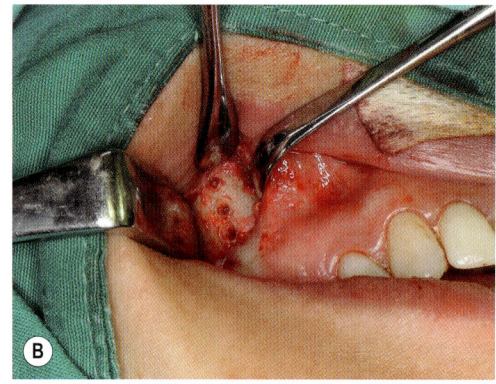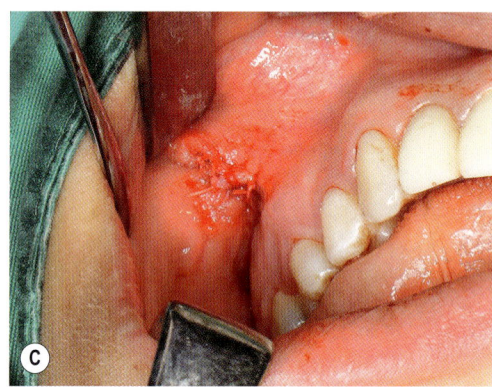

Fig. 13.9 The procedure for removal of a miniplate. (A) The exposed miniplate. (B) A specially designed screwdriver is used to remove the miniscrews. (C) The incision is sutured.

in order not to cause necrosis due to pressure. Soft tissues are closed by 4-0 vicryl sutures. Medication is prescribed as for zygomatic anchorage and the sutures are removed at the sixth postoperative day.

REMOVAL OF THE MINIPLATES

Miniplate removal requires a mucoperiosteal incision under local anesthesia to expose the plate and screws (Fig. 13.9A). Although complete osseointegration of the miniscrews does not occur, there will be some new bone deposition around the plates and the screws and rotational equipment may be necessary to remove the bone over the miniscrew head. In contrast, some screws may be loosened and even a small bony defect may occur. Any granulation tissue should be removed by small bone curettes. Screwdrivers should be inserted very carefully over the riffle of the miniscrew heads to avoid wear to the heads (Fig. 13.9B). Finally the incision is sutured with 4-0 vicryl (Fig. 13.9C) and the patient is instructed to use chlorhexidine mouth rinses for 2–3 days after surgery. The soft tissue repair is inspected and the sutures removed after 6 days. Recovery is mostly smooth and no scar tissue remains following this period.

CONCLUSIONS

New types of miniplate design with more variability in length or prebent to fit specific anatomical sites would be advantageous. In addition, the use of resorbable materials such as poly-L-lactic/polyglycolic acid would avoid the need for removal surgery.

ACKNOWLEDGMENTS

The authors wish to thank the faculty of the Department of Anatomy, School of Medicine, Baskent University, for their valuable contributions.

REFERENCES

1. Chung KR, Kim YS, Linton J, et al. The miniplate with tube for skeletal anchorage. J Clin Orthod 2002;36:407–12.
2. Ding P, Zhou YH, Lin Y, et al. Miniplate implant anchorage for maxillary protraction in Class III malocclusion. Zhonghua Kou Qiang Yi Xue Za Zhi 2007;5:263–7.
3. De Clerck H, Geerinckx V, Siciliano S. The zygoma anchorage system. J Clin Orthod 2002;36:455–9.
4. Erverdi N, Usumez S, Solak A. New generation open-bite treatment with zygomatic anchorage. Angle Orthod 2006;76:519–26.
5. Sugawara J, Kanzaki R, Takahashi I, et al. Distal movement of maxillary molars in nongrowing patients with the skeletal anchorage system. Am J Orthod Dentofacial Orthop 2006;129:723–33.
6. De Clerck HJ, Cornelis MA. Biomechanics of skeletal anchorage. Part 2: class II nonextraction treatment. J Clin Orthod 2006;40:290–8.
7. Chung KR, Kim YS, Lee YJ. The miniplate with tube for skeletal anchorage. J Clin Orthod 2002;36:407–12.
8. Oguz Y, Saglam H, Dolanmaz D, et al. Comparison of stability of 2.0 mm standard and 2.0 mm locking miniplate/screws for the fixation of sagittal split ramus osteotomy on sheep mandibles. Br J Oral Maxillofac Surg 2011;49:135–7.
9. Tseng YC, Chen CM, Wang HC, et al. Pain perception during miniplate-assisted orthodontic therapy. J Med Sci 2010;26:603–8.

14

Insertion and removal of orthodontic miniscrew implants

Fadi Tarawneh and Moschos A. Papadopoulos

INTRODUCTION

In general, insertion of miniscrew implants (MIs) should be as non-invasive as possible, in order to reduce postoperative patient discomfort and to avoid irritation and inflammation of the peri-implant tissues. The insertion procedure for a MI is usually given by the manufacturer; however, certain general issues should be taken into consideration and these are outlined in this chapter

PREPARATIONS BEFORE INSERTION

ANESTHESIA

Soft tissue anesthesia is usually sufficient for the insertion of MIs and can usually be achieved with topical anesthetics, gels or creams; some patients may need a small amount of local anesthetic. Block anesthesia is rarely required and should be avoided as it could mask signs of root contact during insertion, which could lead to root injury.[1]

SOFT TISSUE PREPARATION

Self-drilling MIs can usually be inserted directly through the gingival tissue or the mucosa without any need for soft tissue or bone manipulation. In contrast, non-self-drilling MIs are inserted only after removal of the soft tissue covering the insertion site, either through a gingival flap incision or a soft tissue punch (see Fig. 11.1).[1–3]

Raising a gingival flap has been associated with pain, discomfort and inflammation that might last up to a week after surgery but use of the procedure does not influence success rates.[4] Use of a flap has been advocated in some circumstances, such as for insertion in the mandibular symphysis. When a MI has to be inserted in the frenum area, a frenectomy is suggested to prevent possible mechanical irritation around the implant during function.[2] If possible, these areas should be avoided to simplify the soft tissue issues.

PILOT DRILLING

Self-drilling MIs do not require pilot drilling except when they have to be inserted in sites presenting with thick cortical bone where the high force required can cause excessive bone compression, which might decrease secondary stability of MIs or lead to MI fracture during insertion. In general, buccal cortical bone thickness seems to be greater in the mandible than in the maxilla, and increases gradually in the apical direction.[5,6] Males and adults have thicker cortical bone than females and adolescents.[5,6] A pilot hole is most important for inserting self-drilling MIs in the mandible and in an apical location, more specifically between the first and second mandibular molars.[5]

A pilot drill is always necessary for insertion of non-self-drilling MIs. The procedure is performed in a surgical environment and if possible by an oral surgeon. The soft tissue from the site is either incised or removed using a soft tissue punch (see Fig. 11.1). Then, the pilot hole is drilled, usually using a handpiece (see Fig. 18.6D). A speed of 500–1000 rpm is usually sufficient for cortical bone perforation but should not exceed 1500 rpm.[1,2] Copious irrigation and cooling with sterile saline helps to minimize overheating, which can lead to bone necrosis and implant failure. Cortical bone can be predrilled manually with a sharp drill of high cutting efficiency to minimize heat production. Pilot drilling is an invasive procedure with the potential to introduce microbial contamination and so it is recommended that the drill is not reinserted into the hole once it is made. To avoid fractures and high bone stresses, optimum pre-drilling diameters should be chosen: the pilot drill must be approximately 0.2–0.3 mm thinner than the diameter of the MI to be used. Although drilling a pilot hole makes the procedure more complicated and more time consuming, it provides a fixed path of insertion for the MI, which, in turn, minimizes the risk of injuring adjacent roots or insertions into the sinus.

INSERTION OF MINISCREW IMPLANTS

Insertion of implants can be performed either manually with the use of screwdrivers (Fig. 14.1A) or mechanically with a specially angled handpiece that permits adjustment of torque through altering the speed of the handpiece (see Fig. 16.5C). For implant insertion, a speed up to 30 rpm is usually adequate and should not exceed 60 rpm.[1,2] Ratchets are also available that help to work with MIs in different locations (Fig. 14.1B). Some even provide an adjustable torque control ranging from 5 to 30 Ncm. Once the desired torque is reached, the ratchet bends preventing further force application.[1]

Insertion torque magnitude depends on factors such as bone thickness, bone quality, size and design of the MI, as well as method and velocity of insertion.[1] It is recommended that insertion of MIs should be carried out at a slow and steady rate, with low and continuous forces so that the load

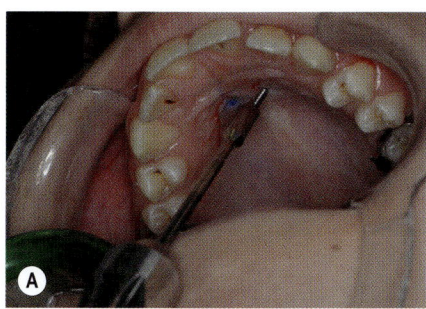

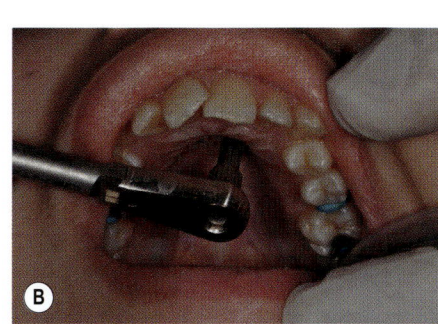

Fig. 14.1 Manual insertion of a MI using a screwdriver (A) and a rachet (B).

on both the MI and bone is kept low. Motoyoshi et al.[7] have recommended an insertion torque of 5–10 Ncm to avoid bone damage.

Controlling torque magnitude, particularly for insertion, seems to be clinically very significant but is not always easy to achieve, particularly when using self-drilling MIs inserted manually.[1] Insertion torque and direction is easier to control with non-self-drilling MIs, which require a pilot hole. The required insertion torque is also lower and so there is less risk of bone compression or MI fracture.[8,9] However, both non-self-drilling and self-drilling MIs show similar resistance to lateral forces.[10] There is still the potential for trauma if the predrilling procedure is not carefully controlled to avoid overheating.

There is more risk of root injury with self-drilling MIs because of the increased difficulty in controlling the insertion path. There is also a greater risk of excessive bone compression because of the higher torque values needed, particularly when the cortical bone is thicker than 1.5 mm, leading to loss of secondary stability.[8,11] Some reports suggest that self-drilling MIs have less mobility and more bone–implant contact than the non-self-drilling types.[1,12]

As a general guideline, self-drilling MIs are favored by most clinicians, particularly when cortical bone is thin, such as in several sites in the maxilla, while non-self-drilling MIs are preferable in sites where the cortical bone is thick, as in the mandible. Placement recommendations according to cortical bone thickness are shown in Table 14.1.

DIRECTION OF MINISCREW IMPLANT INSERTION

Placing MIs perpendicular to the bone surface is not always possible, particularly when teeth are present and root injury is to be avoided.[13] Many authors recommend a more oblique insertion rather than perpendicular if this achieves better implant–cortical bone contact.[14] Inter-radicular space increases in an apical direction but so does movable mucosa. If the available space between two adjacent roots is small, a more oblique direction of insertion seems to be favorable to minimize the risk of root contact.[2]

In the maxilla, it is recommended to insert MIs at an oblique angle in an apical direction with an angulation of 30–45° to the long axes of the

teeth, except in the area of the maxillary sinus, where a more perpendicular angulation is favored in order to avoid any damage to the sinus.[15] In the mandible, the MIs should be inserted as parallel to the roots as possible if teeth are present, or with a 10–20° angulation.[15,16]

POSSIBLE SITES FOR PLACEMENT OF MINISCREW IMPLANTS

Determination of the best site for placement of a MI is made using radiography, casts and clinical examination to assess buccolingual depth and thickness of the cortical bone, soft tissue characteristics, inter-radicular distance, sinus morphology, nerve location, biomechanical considerations and accessibility.[5]

MAXILLA

Possible sites for MI placement in the maxilla include the area below the nasal spine, the palate (on the median or paramedian area), the infrazygomatic crest, the maxillary tuberosities and the alveolar process (both buccally and palatally between the roots of the teeth) (Fig. 14.2).

In the maxilla, the more anterior and the more apical the location, the safer for insertion of a MI.[5,16] The optimal site in the anterior region is between the roots of the central and the lateral incisor, approximately 6 mm from the cementoenamel junction. Buccally, the optimal sites are between the second premolars and the first molars and between the first and second molars (see Fig. 40.1C,D).

Palatally, the best site is between the first and second premolars, since it presents the highest cortical bone thickness. The least amount of bone was found to be in the tuberosity and at the wisdom teeth, which was not considered suitable for MI insertion.

Within the palate, the paramedian region is considered as the safest site for MI placement as it has the greatest amount of ossified tissue in the palate and is away from the roots of neighboring teeth. Alternative to the median region of the palate, the greatest amount of bone support was found 6–9 mm posterior to the incisive foramen and 3–6 mm paramedially;[19] a more recent study showed that orthodontic MIs could be effectively inserted in palatal areas if placed approximately 3 mm posterior to the incisive foramen and 1–5 mm the paramedian.[20]

The midpalatal suture has sufficient bony support for implants with a diameter ranging from 4 to 6 mm (see Fig. 16.5).[19,20] However the suture is sinuous and interdigitized and may not be fully ossified (closed) even in adults;[19,22] consequently, since MIs are provided with a maximum diameter of 2.3 mm, their insertion in the midpalatal suture area should be avoided since there is an increased possibility that a significant part of their endosseous surface would be within the suture and so not in contact with bone.

Table 14.1 Placement recommendations according to cortical bone thickness	
Cortical bone thickness (mm)	**Recommendation**
<0.5	Implant placement not recommended
0.5–1.5	Predrilling not necessary
1.5–2.5	Predrilling of the cortical plate recommended in order to decrease compression and unwanted effects to the bone

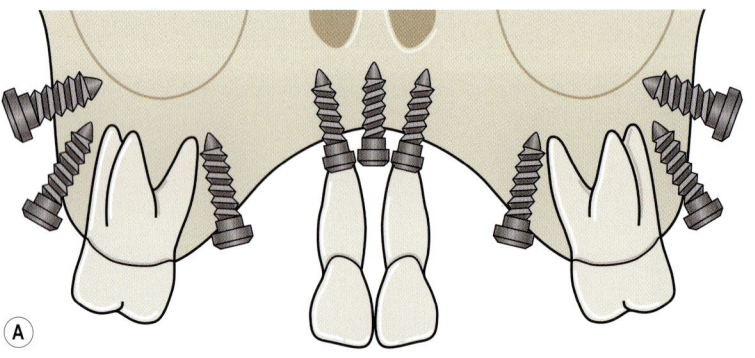
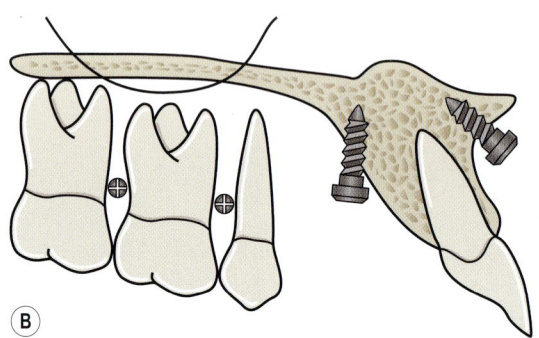

Fig. 14.2 Examples of possible sites for miniscrew implant placement and direction of insertion in the maxilla in frontal (A) and lateral (B) view.

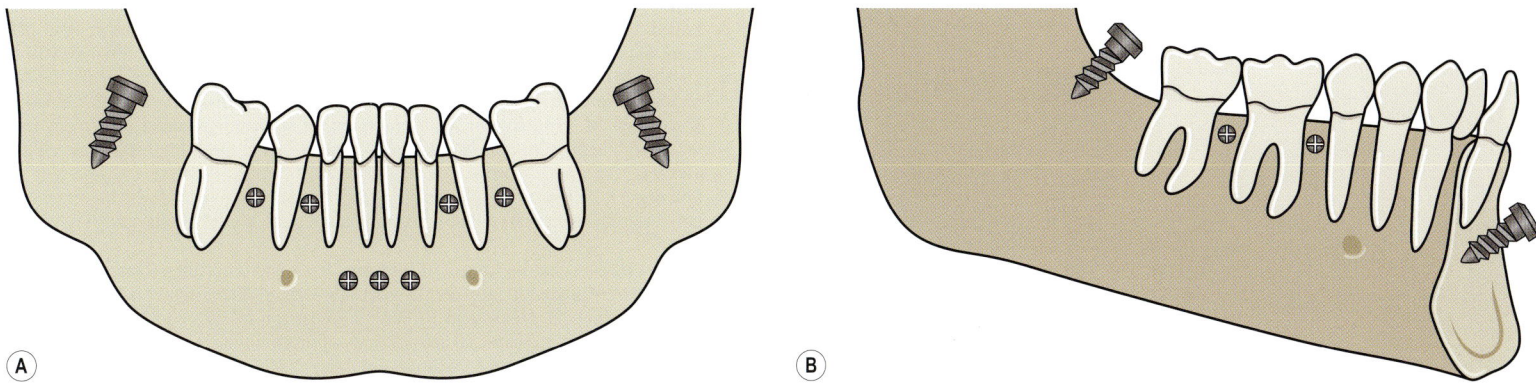

Fig. 14.3 Examples of possible sites for miniscrew implant placement and direction of insertion in the mandible in frontal (A) and lateral (B) view.

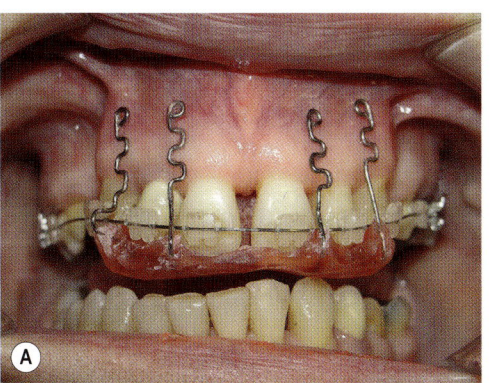
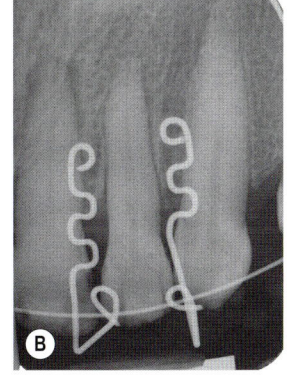
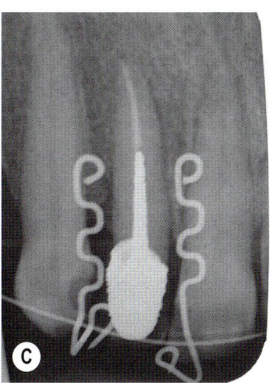

Fig. 14.4 Determination of insertion location for a miniscrew implant using a surgical guide. (A) The surgical guide equipped with several custom-made wire extension arms in the mouth of the patient. (B,C) Periapical radiographs of the anterior teeth of the same patient depicting the position of the wire extensions for the evaluation of the quality of the bone, the dimensions of the inter-radicular spaces and the height of the alveolar bone in the possible insertion areas.

MANDIBLE

Possible sites for the insertion of MIs in the mandible include the symphysis or parasymphysis, the alveolar process (between the roots of the teeth) and the retromolar area (Fig. 14.3).[15]

The safest sites are between the lateral incisor and the canine at 6 mm from the cementoenamel junction, between the first molar and second premolars, and between the first and second molars (see Fig. 40.1C,D).[5,23] However, while adequate bone is located more than halfway down the root length, this area is likely to be covered by movable mucosa and so there is more risk of soft tissue irritation. To overcome this problem, modification of the MI head design or placement technique (such as using an oblique insertion direction) may be necessary.[23]

SOFT TISSUE CONSIDERATIONS FOR MINISCREW IMPLANT INSERTION

Placement within the attached gingiva, where proper soft tissue sealing can occur, has been associated with fewer soft tissue complications and failure risks in comparison with placement in the movable mucosa.[1,7]

INTER-RADICULAR SPACE CONSIDERATIONS FOR MINISCREW IMPLANT INSERTION

It is considered that a minimum of 3 mm space is needed for the safe placement of MIs when they are inserted inter-radicularly.[16,23,24]

Taking an intraoral radiograph with a surgical guide greatly assists in identification and assessment of a specific inter-radicular region for MI insertion site (Fig. 14.4).[15] An adjustable surgical guide, usually fabricated from wires, silicone and acrylic material, or a stent can be used for placement of MIs.[25,26] Chapters 16–18 contain more details of the use of surgical guides.

INFECTION CONTROL AFTER INSERTION

Infection control is vital to avoid peri-implantitis and consequent premature loss and failure of MIs (see Fig. 9.3).[1,27] The risk of infection and inflammation can be reduced by ensuring a sterile environment during MI insertion, placing the implants in attached gingiva and following the advised insertion procedures. After this, the patient must maintain an immaculate oral hygiene, similar to that after tooth extraction, but with specific instructions on attention to the MI during teeth brushing and how to properly clean the area surrounding the MI as well as the head of the MI. Antibiotics are not needed, but mouthwashes and disinfectant rinses help the patient to maintain good oral hygiene. The patient must be instructed to avoid manipulating the MI with fingers, tongue or lips, or with foreign objects such as pens or pencils.

Healing and health of the peri-implant gingival tissues and the status of the patient's oral hygiene must be regularly reviewed by the clinician throughout the time that the MI remains in function.

REMOVAL OF MINISCREW IMPLANTS

Usually, the removal of MIs is uncomplicated and easily accomplished in one appointment using the same screwdriver as for the insertion. Local

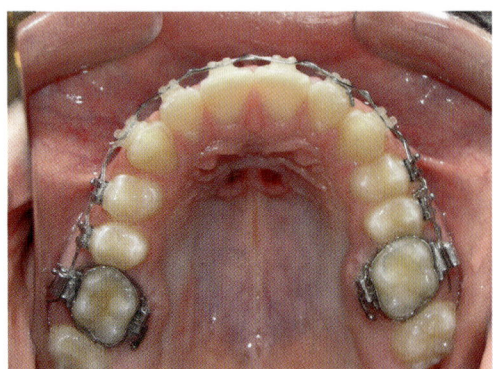

Fig. 14.5 The wound seen immediately after removal of two miniscrew implants that were inserted in the paramedian region of the anterior palate.

anesthetic is not usually needed, although it might be used to avoid patient discomfort or if there is tissue covering the MI. The linking elements of the orthodontic mechanism are first removed and then the MI is simply unscrewed. The resulting small wound requires no special care beyond normal dental hygiene and can be gently swabbed with 0.2% chlorhexidine. The wound left from the removal of a MI is minimal and usually closes within a few days (Fig. 14.5). In most cases, healing continues uneventfully.

If a MI is very tight and cannot be removed at once, it is advised to wait 3 to 7 days before retrying as microfractures or bone remodeling at the peri-implant surfaces following the initial attempt at removal will lead to loosening of the MI. If during removal the MI fractures flush with the bone, the shaft might need to be removed with a trephine. In such cases, referral to an oral surgeon or periodontist might be needed to remove the retained fractured part of the MI.[2]

REFERENCES

1. Ludwig B, Baumgaertel S, Bowman J. Mini-implants in orthodontics: innovative anchorage concepts. Hanover Park, IL: Quintessence; 2008.
2. Lee J, Kim J, Park Y, et al. Applications of orthodontics mini-implants. Hanover Park, IL: Quintessence; 2008.
3. Kuroda S, Sugawara Y, Deguchi T, et al. Clinical use of miniscrew implants as orthodontic anchorage: Success rates and postoperative discomfort. Am J Orthod Dentofacial Orthop 2007;131:9–15.
4. Moon CH, Lee DG, Lee HS, et al. Factors associated with the success rate of orthodontic miniscrews placed in the upper and lower posterior buccal region. Angle Orthod 2008;78:101–6.
5. Fayed MM, Pazera P, Katsaros C. Optimal sites for orthodontic mini-implant placement assessed by cone beam computed tomography. Angle Orthod 2010;80:939–51.
6. Ono A, Motoyoshi M, Shimizu N. Cortical bone thickness in the buccal posterior region for orthodontic mini-implants. Int J Oral Maxillofac Surg 2008;37:334–40.
7. Motoyoshi M, Hirabayashi M, Uemura M, et al. Recommended placement torque when tightening an orthodontic mini-implant. Clin Oral Implants Res 2006;17:109–14.
8. Sowden D, Schmitz JP. AO self-drilling and self-tapping screws in rat calvarial bone: an ultrastructural study of the implant interface. J Oral Maxillofac Surg 2002;60:294–9.
9. Wilmes B, Drescher D. Impact of insertion depth and predrilling diameter on primary stability of orthodontic mini-implants. Angle Orthod 2009;79:609–14.
10. Su YY, Wilmes B, Hönscheid R, et al. Comparison of self-tapping and self-drilling orthodontic mini-implants: an animal study of insertion torque and displacement under lateral loading. Int J Oral Maxillofac Implants 2009;24:404–11.
11. Böhm B, Fuhrmann R. Clinical application and histological examination of the FAMI screw for skeletal anchorage: a pilot study. J Orofac Orthop 2006;67:175–85.
12. Kim JW, Ahn SJ, Chang YL. Histomorphometric and mechanical analyses of the drill-free screw as orthodontic anchorage. Am J Orthod Dentofacial Orthop 2005;128:190–4.
13. Dalstra M, Cattaneo PM, Melsen B. Load transfer of miniscrews for orthodontic anchorage. Orthodontology 2004;1:53–62.
14. Motoyoshi M, Yoshida T, Ono A, et al. Effect of cortical bone thickness and implant placement torque on stability of orthodontic mini-implants. Int J Oral Maxillofac Implants 2007;22:779–84.
15. Carano A, Velo S, Leone P, et al. Clinical applications of the Miniscrew Anchorage System. J Clin Orthod 2005;39:9–24.
16. Poggio P, Incorvati C, Velo S, et al. Safe zones: a guide for miniscrew positioning in the maxillary and mandibular arch. Angle Orthod 2006;76:191–7.
17. Bernhart T, Vollgruber A, Gahleitner A, et al. Alternative to the median region of the palate for placement of an orthodontic implant. Clin Oral Implants Res 2000;11:595–601.
18. Moon SH, Park SH, Lim WH, et al. Palatal bone density in adult subjects: Implications for mini-implant placement. Angle Orthod 2010;80:137–44.
19. Henriksen B, Bavitz B, Kelly B, et al. Evaluation of bone thickness in the anterior hard palate relative to midsagittal orthodontic implants. Int J Oral Maxillofac Implants 2003;18:578–81.
20. Gahleitner A, Podesser B, Schick S, et al. Dental CT and orthodontic implants: Imaging technique and assessment of available bone volume in the hard palate. Eur J Radiol 2004;51:257–62.
21. Melsen B. Palatal growth studied on human autopsy material: A histologic microradiographic study. Am J Orthod 1975;68:42–54.
22. Persson M, Thilander B. Palatal closure in man from 15 to 35 years of age. Am J Orthod 1977;72:42–52.
23. Schnelle MA, Beck FM, Jaynes RM, et al. A radiographic evaluation of the availability of bone for placement of miniscrews. Angle Orthod 2004;74:832–7.
24. Chaimanee P, Suzuki B, Suzuki EY. "Safe Zones" for miniscrew implant placement in different dentoskeletal patterns. Angle Orthod 2011;81:397–403.
25. Kitai N, Yasuda Y, Takada K. A stent fabricated on a selectively colored stereolithographic model for placement of orthodontic mini-implants. Int J Adult Orthodon Orthognath Surg 2002;17:264–6.
26. Suzuki EY, Buranastidporn B. An adjustable surgical guide for miniscrew placement. J Clin Orthod 2005;39:588–90.
27. Park HS, Jeong SH, Kwon OW. Factors affecting the clinical success of screw implants used as orthodontic anchorage. Am J Orthod Dentofacial Orthop 2006;130:18–25.

15

Selecting a suitable site for miniscrew implant insertion

Antonio Gracco and Giuseppe Siciliani

INTRODUCTION

The choice of site for orthodontic miniscrew implants (MIs) is fundamental to success for many reasons, including primary stability, protection of neighboring anatomical structures, biomechanics to apply and patient comfort.

Several anatomical sites for the insertion of MIs have been proposed (Table 15.1). Factors determining suitability include:

- ease of access to the insertion site
- soft tissue characteristics
- bony tissue characteristics
- anatomical characteristics.

These are discussed in this chapter.

EASE OF ACCESS TO THE INSERTION SITE

Two factors influence ease of access: the position of the orthodontist with respect to the patient's head and the use of screwdrivers specific for the site in question.

The orthodontist requires an unimpeded view of the insertion site, either directly or via a mirror, without causing discomfort to either patient or practitioner. As a certain amount of force will be required to counteract the corresponding one generated during MI insertion, the practitioner's hand or indeed the whole body may be needed to supplement the resistance provided by the patient.

Most maxillary and mandibular alveolar areas can be reached with ease using a straight screwdriver of a suitable tip length but some sites, such as the median and paramedian palatal, the maxillary tuberosity and the mandibular retromolar areas, can be more easily reached using a

Table 15.1 Insertion sites for miniscrew implants

Areas	Sites
Alveolar areas	
Maxilla	Buccal alveolus
	Palatal alveolus
	Alveolar crest
	Maxillary tuberosity
Mandible	Buccal alveolus
	Lingual alveolus
	Alveolar crest
	Retromolar area
Non-alveolar areas	
Maxilla	Hard palate (median and paramedian zones)
	Zygomatic crest
Mandible	External oblique line

contra-angle driver. Either could be used for insertion into the zygomatic crest or the external oblique line.

SOFT TISSUE CHARACTERISTICS

TISSUE TYPE

The most suitable site for MI insertion is between the clinically invisible osseous alveolar crest and the clinically evident mucogingival junction (Fig. 15.1).[1] Attached mucosa guarantees greater MI stability and ensures a better seal around the MI neck. If a MI is inserted into unattached gingiva or in the immediate vicinity of a mucosal frenulum, the excessive mobility of the gingiva can lead to soft tissue irritation, compromising MI stability.[1]

Adaptation of the tissues around the MI is considered important for good MI stability. Therefore, in order to prevent capturing of unattached mucosa on the MI thread during insertion, a soft tissue punch or diode laser can be used to remove a portion of the mucosa from the corresponding site (with dimensions approximately equal to the diameter of the MI) prior to MI insertion.

The MI neck is usually smooth to prevent irritation (see Fig. 6.7) but some carry microgrooves to aid connective tissue adhesion and hamper epithelial invagination (see Fig. 6.6). Many MIs also have a platform to compress the gingiva and prevent it riding up and covering the head (see Fig. 6.7). Provisional use of light-cure composite or winding of an elastic around the MI head may also help to prepare the tissues.

MUCOSAL THICKNESS

MI length is chosen to ensure that it will pass through the thickness of the mucosa and have sufficient contact with bone for stability. In the maxilla, the greatest mucosal thickness is generally found on the palatal side of the premaxilla (mean, 3.38 mm) and on the median area of the hard palate (mean, 3.06 mm). In the mandible, the retromolar mucosa tends to be thickest (mean, 3.02 mm) (Fig. 15.2). The thickness of attached gingiva is also influenced by the patient's gender. In males, the following areas feature greater mucosal thickness in both jaws:[2]

- between the central and lateral incisors
- between the lateral incisors and canines
- between the canines and first premolars
- between the first and second premolars.

Soft tissue thickness is evaluated by various methods including the so-called direct methods such as an ultrasonic or a periodontal probe with an endodontic stopper (the latter employed after local anesthesia).[3] Ultrasound shows greater mucosal thickness at the anterior and premolar areas of the labial side of the maxilla than the corresponding areas of the mandible, with the mandibular labial area thicker at the molar region. In contrast, on the palatal side of the maxilla, the greatest thicknesses are

Fig. 15.1 Reference points for MI insertion. (A) Intraoral points. (B) Radiographic points. Black dots, points of interproximal contact; white dashed line, crestal bone; red dashed line, mucogingival border (in A) and lower wall of maxillary sinus (in B).

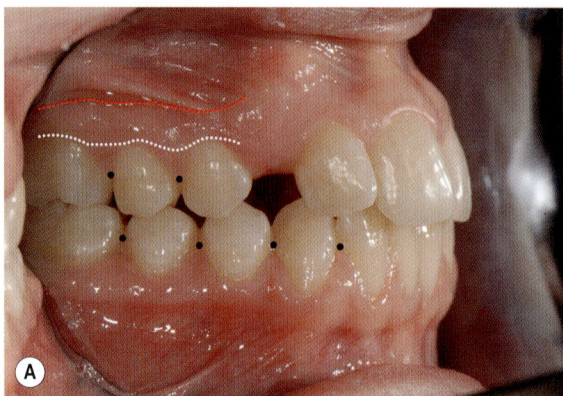 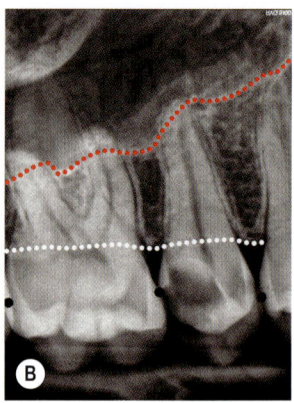

Fig. 15.2 Miniscrew implant inserted into the retromolar triangle in order to upright an impacted second molar. Note the length of the threaded portion of the core that penetrates the bone and the quantity of soft tissue covering the miniscrew implant head.

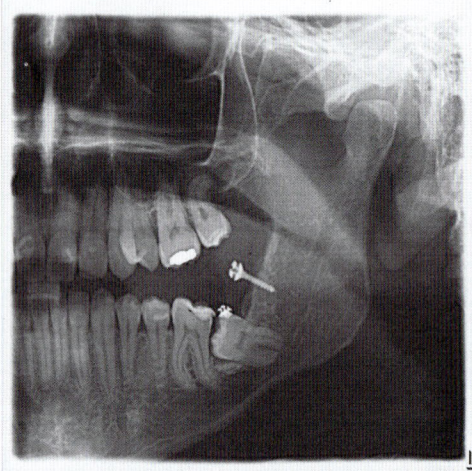

found between the first premolars and the adjacent canines and second premolars.

BONY TISSUE CHARACTERISTICS

TISSUE QUALITY, QUANTITY AND AGE-RELATED DIFFERENCES

The quality of bone refers to its density and thickness, both of which vary with age.

The alveolar process is the part of the maxilla and mandible that forms and supports the dental alveoli. The alveolar walls are lined with compact bone, while spongy bone is found in the areas between the cortical walls. The dimensions of these areas are mainly determined by genetics, but they can be influenced also by the functional forces of the dentition. The greater part of the interdental septa is filled with spongy bone, but the majority of the bone at the labial and palatal surfaces is compact (Fig. 15.3).

The compact bone covering the root surfaces is considerably thicker on the palatal side than the labial side of the maxilla, whereas in the mandible the compact bone at the buccal surface of the incisors and premolars is far thinner than that at the lingual side. This contrasts with the molar region of the mandible, where greater compact bone thickness is present at the labial rather than the lingual surface.[7]

Bone quality is also affected by conditions such as edentulism. After tooth loss, the quality of bone in the surrounding area diminishes with time. Bone quality is also affected by the presence of muscle insertions, pre- or postedentulous parafunctions, hormone and systemic conditions.

The maxilla and mandible are characterized by anatomical regions of varying degrees of mineralization and cortical thickness; based on the ratio of cortical to medullary bone, four types of bone quality can be identified, in order of descending compactness:[4]

- type I: compact bone consisting predominantly of cortical bone
- type II: bone featuring thick, compact cortex and a dense internal network of trabeculae
- type III: bone featuring thinner cortex and less dense spongiosa
- type IV: bone featuring thin cortex and sparsely distributed trabeculae.

A modified version of this classification, based not only on the ratio of cortical to medullary bone but also on the macroscopic characteristics of the bony tissue, was proposed in 1987 by Misch, who identified five different bone densities (D1–D5) (Fig. 15.4).[5] The bone densities pertaining to Misch's classification can be expressed in Hounsfield units (quantitative scale for describing radiodensity) (Table 15.2).

Bone quality can be accurately determined by CT; however, expert surgeons can distinguish D1 and D4 by touch alone.

It seems that bone quality and quantity at the insertion site is linked to mechanical retention rather than to osteointegration.[6] Hence, relative thickness of the cortex becomes an important factor in ensuring primary stability, with a thickness of at least 1 mm being required. It is considered that at least 71.2% of the screw length should penetrate alveolar bone, particularly in the maxilla, where this percentage may need to be even higher.[7] The MI core should penetrate bone to a depth of at least 5 mm in the mandible and 6 mm in the maxilla in order to guarantee stability over the whole period necessary for dental movements.

Even with adequate bone, secondary stability can be compromised by the excessive application of forces during MI insertion, which increases friction and potentially causes bone trauma. Hence, preparation of the insertion site by soft tissue punch (see Fig. 11.1) or by flap elevation and predrilling is recommended for thick cortical bone.

Another means of improving stability is inserting the MI through two layers of cortical bone, thereby considerably reducing the load on the trabecular layer between them (Fig. 15.5).[8]

MAXILLARY INSERTION SITES

Based on these considerations, possible insertion sites in the maxilla include:[9]

- the buccal sides
- the posterior palatal sides
- the median and paramedian palatal areas
- the anterior nasal spine and anterior alveolar bone
- the infrazygomatic crest.

When contemplating insertion into the buccal side of the maxilla, it is worth bearing in mind that the greatest buccopalatal bone width is found

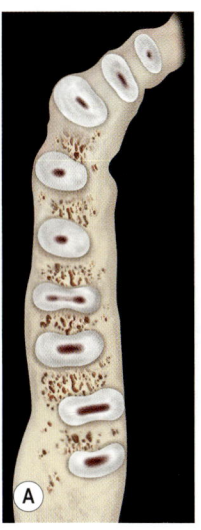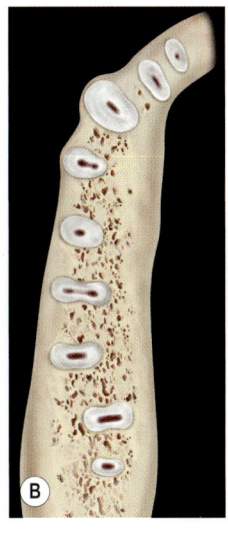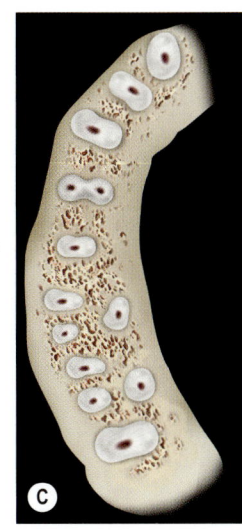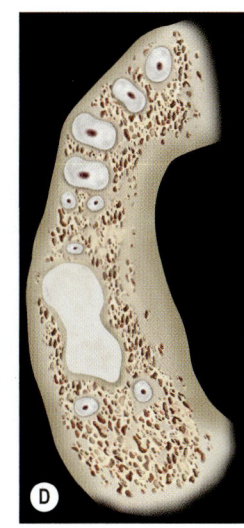

Fig. 15.3 Axial sections of the maxilla to show bone thickness and inter-radicular distances. (A,B) Variation in labial and lingual thickness of cortical bone and in inter-radicular distances between anterior and posterior teeth in a section at the cementoenamel junction (A) and halfway up the root length (B). (C) Section at the central third of the roots showing the greater inter-radicular distances on the palatal than the labial side. (D) Section at the apical third of the roots. Note the appearance of the maxillary sinus, which invaginates between the roots of the posterior teeth.

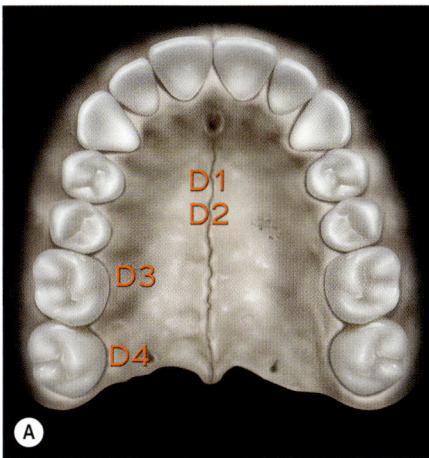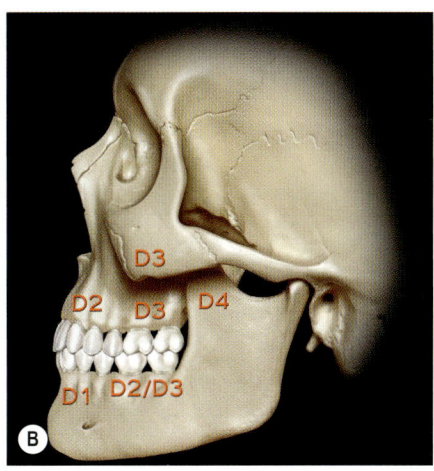

Fig. 15.4 Areas with different bone densities according to Misch's classification on the palatal side of the maxilla (A) and in lateral view of the craniofacial complex (B).

Table 15.2 Misch's classification of bone densities

Type		Bone density	Anatomical site
D1		Compact cortical bone featuring little medulla (>1250 HU)	Mandible: symphyseal and parasymphyseal regions
D2		Bone featuring thick cortex and dense internal trabecular structure (850–1250 HU)	Maxilla: anterior region Mandible: anterior and posterior regions
D3		Thin cortex and wide, cavernous internal trabecular structure (350–850 HU)	Maxilla: anterior and posterior regions Mandible: posterior region
D4		Mainly spongy bone with very little cortex (150–350 HU)	Maxilla: posterior region
D5		Immature bone (<150 HU)	Immature bone

HU, Hounsfield unit.
Source: from Misch, 1990.[5]

between the first and second molars, 5 mm from the alveolar crest (Fig. 15.6B).[9] In contrast, the greatest thickness of cortical bone is located in the inter-radicular space between the first and second premolars.[10]

With regard to posterior palatal insertion, the smallest quantity of bone (0.2 mm) on both the buccopalatal and mesiodistal planes is at the maxillary tuberosity.[9]

One of the most favorable insertion sites is the area around the median and paramedian sutures. This area is characterized by type D1 bone. The width of the palatal cortex decreases incrementally from the anterior to the posterior section. There is a similar trend in total bone depth in the median area, which decreases proportionally to the distance from the midsagittal plane.[11] Consequently, the most favorable palatal sites for MI insertion are located between 6 and 9 mm posterior to the incisal foramen, and in the paramedian area between 3 and 6 mm from the midpalatal suture.

The suitability of a paramedian insertion site will need to be based on the patient's age as the palatal suture in growing patients is unlikely to be completely ossified; consequently, two MIs in the paramedian zone might be preferable to ensure good primary stability.

Patient age is significant for other reasons: areas with unerupted permanent teeth should be avoided and bone density is decreased in growing patients. Therefore, in adolescents, insertion areas with more compact bone are preferred, such as the palate, bearing in mind the necessity to avoid excessive loading of forces (<100–150 g) because of poor bone quality. It does appear that MI failures are far more common in adolescents than in adults.[6]

Fig. 15.5 Finite element modeling of a miniscrew implant inserted into bone. (A) Monocortical anchorage showing the distribution of stresses in the external cortex at the screw–bone interface. (B) The effect of bicortical anchorage.

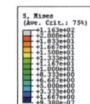
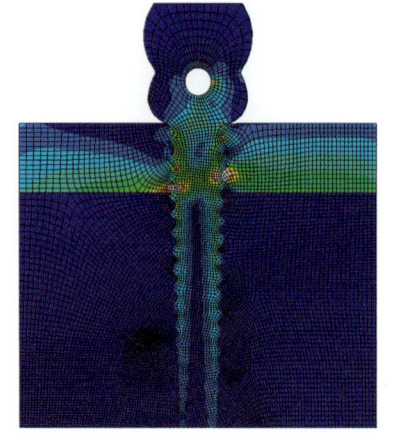
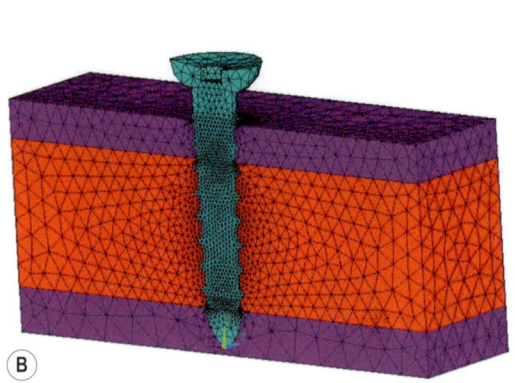

Fig. 15.6 Palatal sites for miniscrew implant (MI) insertion. (A) Tomographic image of a paramedian sagittal section, showing a MI inserted into the palate. Note the tip of the implant penetrates the upper layer of cortical bone, thereby providing bicortical anchorage. (B) Three-dimensional construction from cone beam CT showing a MI inserted into the palate between the first and second maxillary molars.

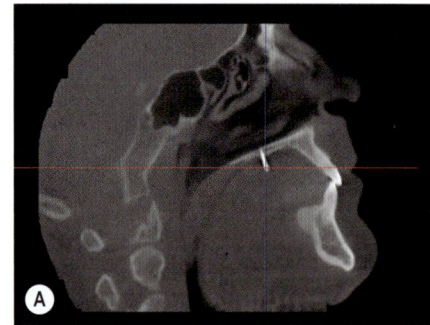
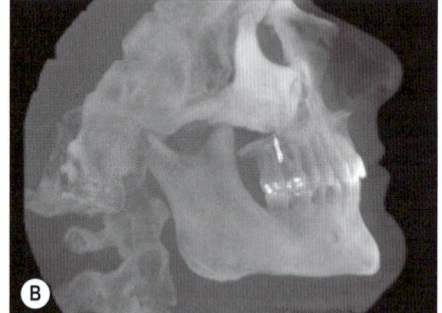

Cortical bone is significantly thicker in adults in all areas except the infrazygomatic crest, between the first and second molars on the buccal side of the mandible and on the posterior paramedian area of the palate.[6,10]

The area around the anterior nasal spine and the anterior alveolar bone has bone of D2 type.[12] The greatest buccolingual thickness in this area is found between the central and lateral incisors, 6 mm from the cemento-enamel junction. The greatest mesiodistal thickness is located between the two central incisors, 6 mm from the cementoenamel junction.[10]

Bone thickness of the infrazygomatic crest at the maxillary first molar is generally between 5.2 and 8.8 mm, allowing a MI insertion angle of 40 to 75° with respect to the upper occlusal plane. Since 6 mm is considered as the minimum thickness of the infrazygomatic crest required to effectively support a MI, the insertion should be performed 14–16 mm above the maxillary occlusal plane at an angle of 55–70° with respect to this plane in order to avoid damage to the mesiolabial root of the first molar (Table 15.3).[13]

MANDIBULAR INSERTION SITES

The bone of the mandible is more compact than that of the maxilla. Although there are no statistically significant differences between maxilla and mandible regarding the total labiolingual bone thickness in the anterior section, differences have been documented in the posterior section. Indeed, in the maxilla, the cortical bone mesial and distal to the inter-radicular sites of the canines is relatively thin, whereas the thickness in the mandible increases gradually moving away from these sites in both anterior and posterior directions.[15]

From all the insertion areas investigated, the greatest thickness of cortical bone appears to be at the buccal side of the mandible.[6] Cortical bone thickness in this area depends on both the inter-radicular site considered for MI insertion and its distance from the alveolar crest.

The greatest thickness of buccal mandibular cortex is found between the first and second molars,[9,10] while the smallest bone quantity is between

the canine and first premolar.[9,14] It is also suggested that MIs should be inserted 4–6 mm away from the alveolar crest since the cortical bone is significantly thicker in this area (Table 15.3).[10,15] Based on bone thickness evaluation, the safest sites for MI insertion in the mandible are the following, in order of decreasing stability:[9]

- between the first and second molars (all depths)
- between the first and second premolars (all depths)
- between the second premolars and first molars, 11 mm from the alveolar crest
- between the canines and first premolars, 11 mm from the alveolar crest.

ANATOMICAL CHARACTERISTICS

SUFFICIENT SPACE

Consideration of inter-radicular distances when inserting MIs is important in order to avoid damage to teeth roots (Fig. 15.7). The minimum inter-radicular space required for safe insertion of a temporary anchorage device appears to be 3.3 mm, which corresponds to a 1.3 mm diameter MI leaving approximately 1 mm on either side as space from the roots of the adjacent teeth.[7]

In general, the inter-radicular distance increases from the cervical to the apical areas of each tooth in both jaws, and the space between the roots is generally greater in the molar than in the incisor areas (Fig. 15.8A). Consequently, the anterior alveolar area, despite its excellent biomechanics and ideal location for intruding the anterior teeth, is a relatively unsuitable insertion site because of its smaller inter-radicular space as well as the continual irritation provoked by the labial muscles (Fig. 15.8B).[7]

In contrast, adequate inter-radicular distances can be found in the posterior sections of both the maxilla and mandible. In particular, the widest spaces in the mandible are found between the first and second

Table 15.3 Bone thickness in the maxilla and mandible

Maxilla	Mandible	Source reference
Palatal bone at paramedian site is thicker in anterior than posterior sites	Greater cortical bone thickness in posterior than anterior sites	6
Greatest cortical thickness at infrazygomatic crest	Greatest cortical thickness at buccal sides	
Small differences in thickness between upper buccal site, maxillary palate and palatal regions		
Greater buccolingual thickness between M1 and M2	Greatest buccolingual and buccal cortical thicknesses between M1 and M2	10
Greatest mesiodistal and buccopalatal distances between P2 and M1	Greatest mesiodistal buccal distance between P2 and M1	
Greatest palatal cortical thickness between central and lateral incisors	Greatest mesiodistal lingual distance between P1 and P2	
	Thickest lingual cortex between canine and P1	
No problems with MI insertion	Greatest mesiodistal bone thickness between M1 and M2 on the labial and lingual sides	14
	Smallest amount of bone in the mesiodistal plane on the labial side between incisors	
	Greatest labiolingual bone thickness between M1 and M2	
	Smallest labiolingual bone thickness between central and lateral incisors	
Greatest buccopalatal bone width between M1 and M2, 5 mm away from the alveolar crest; 0.2 mm bone quantity at tuberosity, 11 mm away from the alveolar crest	Safest sites in the mandible are, in decreasing order: (a) between M1 and M2 (all depths) (b) between P1 and P2 (all depths) (c) between P2 and M1, 11 mm from the alveolar crest (d) between canines and P1, 11 mm from the alveolar crest	9
Thickness of infrazygomatic crest at M1 is 5.2–8.8 mm		13
Buccal cortical thickness increases in the anterior maxillary sector	Greater buccal cortex thickness in the mandible, which increases with increasing distance from the alveolar crest	11
	Significant increase in cortical bone thickness beyond 4–6 mm from the alveolar crest	15

MI, Miniscrew implant; M1, first molar; M2, second molar; P1, first premolar; P2, second premolar.

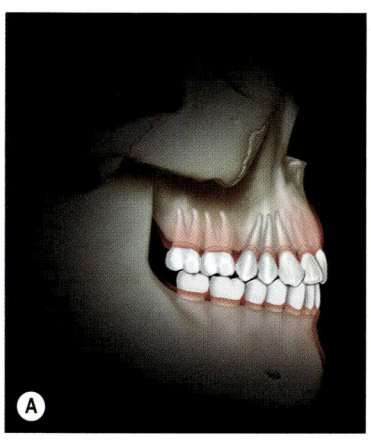 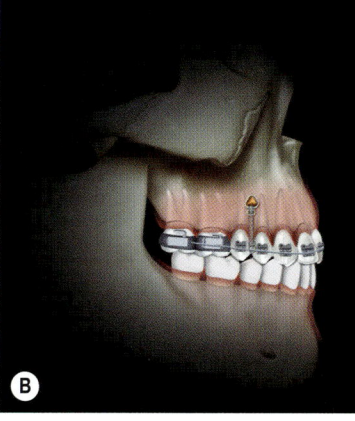

Fig. 15.7 Inter-radicular distances in the maxilla. (A) Root crowding at the canine and both premolars. Root alignment should be instituted as a precautionary measure before miniscrew implant insertion between the two premolars. (B) Miniscrew implant inserted between the premolar roots after orthodontic root alignment.

molars.[8,16–18] However, because of the abundance of blood vessels on the lingual side of the posterior mandible and the possibility of tongue irritation, it is safer to avoid insertion in this area. Both labial and lingual areas are suitable insertion sites in the maxilla, with the greatest inter-radicular space being found between the second premolar and the first molar on both sides.[9]

Interestingly, the width of the inter-radicular space appears to be influenced by the skeletal relationships of the patient. In fact, wider spaces have been reported in the maxilla of skeletal Class II individuals, whereas in Class III patients inter-radicular spaces are greater in the mandible (Table 15.4).[19]

DISTANCE FROM CRITICAL ANATOMICAL STRUCTURES

When choosing a site for MI insertion, it is also important to consider the position of neighboring anatomical structures. In the maxilla, the structures at risk of insertion damage include the maxillary sinus and the palatine neurovascular bundle. In the mandible, structures of importance are the inferior alveolar nerve, the mental foramen and the frenula.

Regarding the maxillary sinus, a perforation of the Schneider membrane of less than 2 mm in diameter is unlikely to become inflamed and will heal completely over a short period of time upon MI removal. Consequently, MIs with diameters of not more than 2 mm should be used in the palatal area of the maxilla.

The palatine neurovascular bundle (including the palatine artery and anterior palatine nerve) exits from the greater palatine foramen, which can vary widely in position, size and shape but is generally found lateral to the third molar or between the second and third molar.[20] The bundle then runs in an anterior direction, between 5 and 15 mm from the gingival margin, towards the incisal foramen. Hence, MIs should be placed medial to the nerve and thus mesial to the second molar.[12]

In the mandible, the inferior alveolar nerve could be damaged in MI insertion.[12] and so panoramic radiography is always advisable before any intervention, although the risk of a lesion is considerably reduced if the appropriate MI insertion angle is chosen to avoid the root apices.[7] MIs should never be positioned in the lingual portion of the mandible because of the rich vascularization of this area and significant tongue interference.

Fig. 15.8 Inter-radicular distances in the mandible. (A) Intraoral radiography of the posterior section showing the greater inter-radicular space between the molars than between the second premolar and first molar. (B) Axial cone beam CT slice taken at the central third of the mandibular tooth roots. Note the lack of space between the roots of the lower incisors.

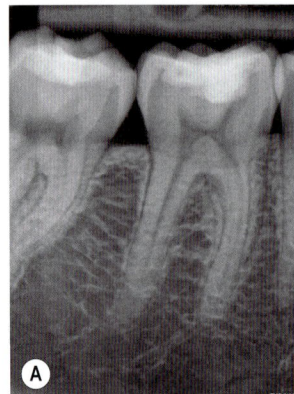

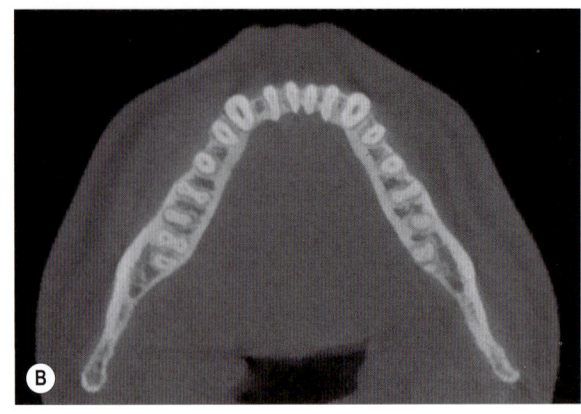

Table 15.4 Inter-radicular widths in the maxilla and mandible

Maxilla	Mandible	Source (sample)
ID in descending order: between M1 and M2, between the P2 and M1 and between the P1 and P2 Care needed to avoid the mental foramen for MI insertions between PMs; a distance of 9 mm from the bony crest is suggested Insufficient space for implantation between incisors		18 (sample size 15; CT)
Anterior area: greater ID between lateral incisors and canines Posterior area: greater ID on buccal side between P2 and M1; on lingual side between P1 and P2	Anterior region: greater ID between central incisors Posterior region: greater ID, palatal and labial, between P2 and M1	10 (sample size 34 maxilla, 66 mandible; CBCT)
Sites with ID >3.1 mm (in descending order): (a) between M1 and M2 (b) between P1 and P2 (c) between P2 and M1, 11 mm from the alveolar crest (d) between canines and P1, 11 mm from the alveolar crest	Sites with ID >3.1 mm (in descending order): (a) palatal between M1 and P2, 2–8 mm from crest and between M1 and M2, 2–5 mm from crest (b) buccal or palatal between P1 and P2 and between canines and P1, both at 5 and 11 mm from crest (c) buccal between P2 and M1, at 5 and 8 mm from crest Greater ID on both labial and palatal areas encompassing P2 and M1	9 (sample size 25; CBCT)
ID >3 mm found between PMs, between the Ms and between P2 and M1, at a distance of 4 mm from the CEJ	ID >3 mm found in anterior region 8 mm from the CEJ and in the posterior region between PMs and between P2 and M1, 4 mm from the CEJ	16 (sample size 30; CT)
ID >3 mm found 11 mm from alveolar crest in all inter-radicular spaces and 8 mm from the alveolar crest in all inter-radicular spaces, except 33–34 and 35–36	ID >3 mm found between P2 and M1 11 mm from alveolar crest	7 (sample size 25; CT)
Greater ID in area between M1 and M2 at least 5 mm from cervical line	Greater ID found in area encompassing P2 and M1, 6–8 mm from cervical line	17 (sample size 20; CBCT)

CBCT, cone beam computed tomography; ID, inter-radicular distance; CEJ, cementoenamel junction; M1, first molar; M2, second molar; P1, first premolar; P2, second premolar.

The mental foramen usually opens on both sides of the mandible in the space between the first and second premolars, at a relatively deep position in the fornix. The mucosa in this region is evidently very mobile and could compromise MI stability, and such a deep position for a MI would be biomechanically unfavorable.

The frenula are also possible impediments to the mechanical stability of MIs and are particularly prone to implantation-related inflammation of the soft tissues.

PRESURGICAL DIAGNOSIS

Thorough radiographic evaluation of each patient should be carried out before initiation of treatment to ensure choice of a good site for MI insertion. Panoramic radiography provides very general information about the implantation site in two dimensions and is subject to varying levels of distortion in different sections of the stomatognathic system. Periapical radiographs provide more precise images, but while they are a useful source of information regarding the mesiodistal bone width, they too have the inherent limitations of two-dimensional imaging. Good three-dimensional images of high diagnostic value are provided by CT, although the radiation dose precludes frequent use. Cone beam CT provides an ideal balance between three-dimensional image quality and radiation dose. It allows precise evaluation of the quantity of bone between roots, of mesiodistal and labiolingual thickness of bone and also of the thickness of the cortex.[9]

In addition to their preparatory use, radiographic techniques using radiopaque pins can simulate implantation and with effective computer-aided design/manufacturing software can support decision making.[21,22]

ACKNOWLEDGMENTS

The authors would like to thank Drs. Claudia Carmen Lombardi, Serena Montefrancesco, Antonio D'Ercole and Maria Larosa for their valued contributions.

REFERENCES

1. Ludwig B, Glasl B, Kinzinger GSM, et al. Anatomical guidelines for miniscrew insertion: Vestibular interradicular sites. J Clin Orthod 2011;45:165–73.
2. Cha BK, Lee YH, Lee NK, et al. Soft tissue thickness for placement of an orthodontic miniscrew using an ultrasonic device. Angle Orthod 2008;78:403–8.
3. Costa A, Pasta G, Bergamaschi G. Intraoral hard and soft tissue depths for temporary anchorage devices. Semin Orthod 2005;11:10–15.
4. Lekholm U, Zarb G. Patient selection and preparation. In: Branemark PI, Zarb GA, Albrektsson T, editors. Tissue integrated prostheses. Berlin: Quintessence; 1985. p. 199–210.
5. Misch CE. Density of bone: effect on treatment plans, surgical approach, healing and progressive bone loading. Int J Oral Implantol 1990;6:23–31.
6. Farnsworth D, Rossouw PE, Ceen RF, et al. Cortical bone thickness at common miniscrew implant placement sites. Am J Orthod Dentofacial Orthop 2011;139:495–503.
7. Biavati AS, Tecco S, Migliorati M, et al. Three-dimensional tomographic mapping related to primary stability and structural miniscrew characteristics. Orthod Craniofac Res 2011;14:88–99.
8. Lombardo L, Gracco A, Zampini F, et al. Optimal palatal configuration for miniscrew applications. Angle Orthod 2010;80:145–52.
9. Poggio PM, Incorvati C, Velo S, et al. "Safe zones": a guide for miniscrew positioning in the maxillary and mandibular arch. Angle Orthod 2006;76:191–7.
10. Fayed MM, Pazera P, Katsaros C. Optimal sites for orthodontic mini-implant placement assessed by cone beam computed tomography. Angle Orthod 2010;80:939–51.
11. Baumgaertel S, Hans MG. Buccal cortical bone thickness for mini-implant placement. Am J Orthod Dentofacial Orthop 2009;136:230–5.
12. Kravitz ND, Kusnotob B. Risks and complications of orthodontic miniscrews. Am J Orthod Dentofacial Orthop 2007;131(Suppl.):43–51.
13. Liou EJ, Chen PH, Wang YC, et al. A computed tomographic image study on the thickness of the infrazygomatic crest of the maxilla and its clinical implications for miniscrew insertion. Am J Orthod Dentofacial Orthop 2007;131:352–6.
14. Hernández LC, Montoto G, Puente RM, et al. "Bone map" for a safe placement of miniscrews generated by computed tomography. Clin Oral Implants Res 2008;19:576–81.
15. Lim JE, Lee SJ, Kim YJ, et al. Comparison of cortical bone thickness and root proximity at maxillary and mandibular interradicular sites for orthodontic mini-implant placement. Orthod Craniofac Res 2009;12:299–304.
16. Lee KJ, Joo E, Kim KD, et al. Computed tomographic analysis of tooth-bearing alveolar bone for orthodontic miniscrew placement. Am J Orthod Dentofacial Orthop 2009;135:486–94.
17. Hu KS, Kang MK, Kim TW, et al. Relationships between dental roots and surrounding tissues for orthodontic miniscrew installation. Angle Orthod 2009;79:37–45.
18. Monnerat C, Restle L, Mucha JN. Tomographic mapping of mandibular interradicular spaces for placement of orthodontic mini-implants. Am J Orthod Dentofacial Orthop 2009;135:428, discussion 428–9.
19. Chaimanee P, Suzuki B, Suzuki EY. "Safe zones" for miniscrew implant placement in different dentoskeletal patterns. Angle Orthod 2011;81:397–403.
20. Jaffar AA, Hamadah HJ. An analysis of the position of the greater palatine foramen. J Basic Med Sci 2003;3:24–32.
21. Ludwig B, Glasl B, Lietz T, et al. Radiological location monitoring in skeletal anchorage: Introduction of a positioning guide. J Orofac Orthop 2008;69:59–65.
22. Liu H, Liu DX, Wang G, et al. Accuracy of surgical positioning of orthodontic miniscrews with a computer-aided design and manufacturing template. Am J Orthod Dentofacial Orthop 2010;137:728, discussion 728–9.

INTRODUCTION

During preoperative assessment of miniscrew implant (MI) insertion, radiological and/or positioning devices are frequently used. These devices improve planning and placement via assessment of the available bone, the root position of adjacent teeth and the suitable MI dimensions. Positioning guides are intended to transfer information from the implant site, accurately and reproducibly, to the patient's mouth during MI insertion.

POSITIONING GUIDES

Early devices were often fabricated in the laboratory and required additional time for production and clinical positioning. Some complex systems involved the positioning device being attached to a fixed orthodontic appliances or coupled to an intraoral radiographic plate holder.[1] Other techniques involved guiding splints, fabricated on replica models, which were based on reconstructed three-dimensional CT images.[2,3]

The metric approach used a mock up of the MI insertion point and a tooth surface point, determined beforehand on a model.[4] The distance between the two was measured using a periodontal probe and this measurement was transferred intraorally.

CONVENTIONAL POSITIONING GUIDES

Conventional positioning guides have wire elements that are temporarily fixed to the teeth (with composite resin or a rim of silicone-impression material) and adjusted above the planned point of insertion. The basic shape is a (repeatedly) bent wire, with a circular wire end that tapers off above the target area[5–7] or tapers off to a point[8] (Fig. 16.1A). This frame is adapted to the contours of the alveolar process and the dental arch but can be fabricated in the laboratory in order to optimize its positional stability during radiography. The adapted wire elements are set in an acrylic resin splint, which covers several adjacent teeth, thus maximizing stability and retention. After evaluation of the diagnostic radiograph (Fig. 16.1B), the insertion point is marked with an explorer probe, creating a bleeding spot.[6–8]

NEWER POSITIONING GUIDES

The X-ray Pin

A common problem with most positioning devices is that the device itself, or the technique, is complex and not entirely suitable for routine orthodontic practice. The X-ray pin is a radiographic auxiliary with a probing function that marks the gingiva at the desired MI insertion point, thus eliminating the need for laboratory procedures and devices with wires that require adjustment (Fig. 16.2). It is easy to use for inexperienced practitioners.

The X-ray pin is a very small auxiliary, fabricated from a SS alloy. It has a thickened ball-shaped head and a tapered conical shaft, ending in a point, for puncturing the gingiva (Fig. 16.2A). The pin is held with a Weingart plier for positioning in both the maxilla and mandible and is particularly useful in sites between the roots of the adjacent teeth (Fig. 16.2C).

Each pin has a total length of 3.5 mm, which is sufficient for safe retention in the gingiva.[9] The head of the pin has a diameter of 1.6 mm and is therefore compatible with the diameter of most MIs (Fig. 16.2A,B). Because of their conical shape, the pins can easily be inserted into the gingiva in many places (Fig. 16.2C). The pin is designed to perforate the gingiva with direct pressure in a single movement. The X-ray pin is reliable, stable and enables an accurate assessment of the insertion area for

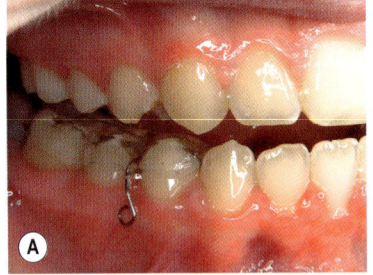 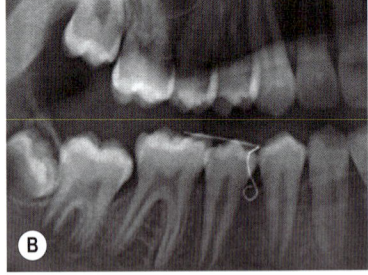

Fig. 16.1 A laboratory-fabricated positioning device with a commercially available wire element (TOMAS-locator, Dentaurum, Ispringen, Germany), incorporating a marking hole that corresponds to the MI insertion site. (A) Intraoral photograph after insertion of the device. Note that the acrylic guide is extended to cover several teeth. (B) Diagnostic panoramic radiograph.

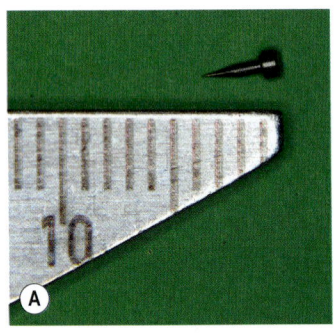 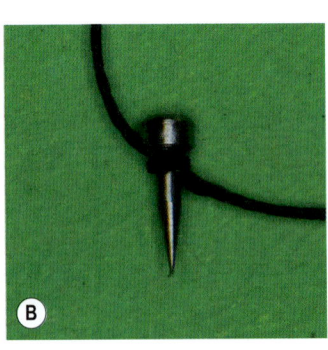 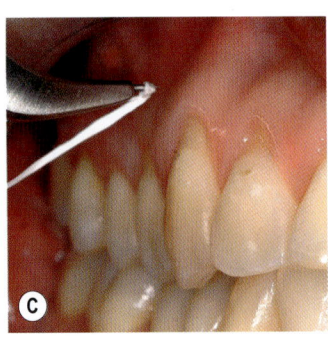

Fig. 16.2 The X-ray pin. (A) The pin includes a puncture point, a conical shaft and a ball head (total length 3.5 mm; working length 2.5 mm, largest diameter 0.75 mm). (B) Securing of pin with dental floss. (C) Intraoral application of the pin at the predetermined point with Weingart plier.

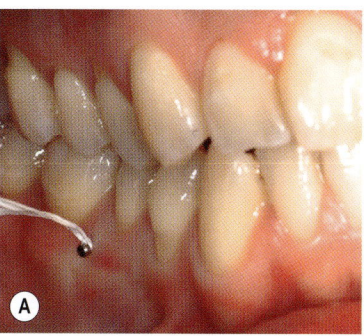
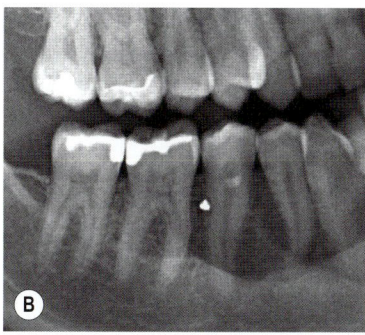
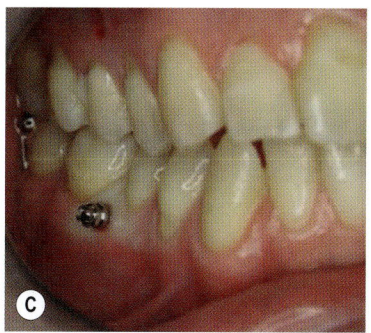
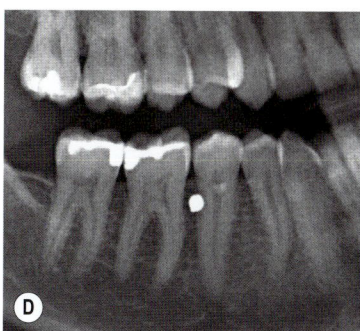

Fig. 16.3 The use of X-ray pins for inter-radicular insertion of microscrew implants in the mandible. (A) Intraoral photograph showing the positioning of the pin. (B) Diagnostic panoramic radiograph showing the pin position and the bone availability of the insertion area. (C) Inserted MI. (D) Panoramic radiograph following MI insertion.

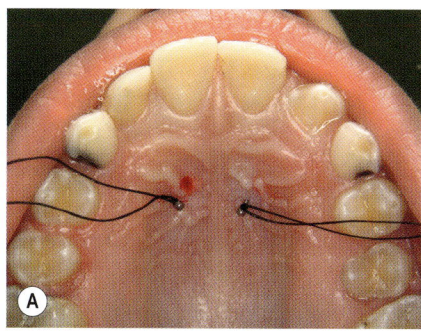
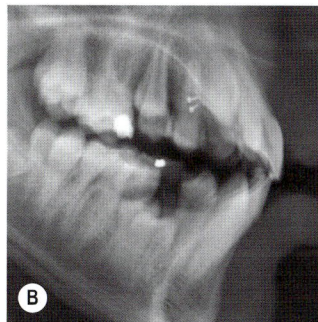
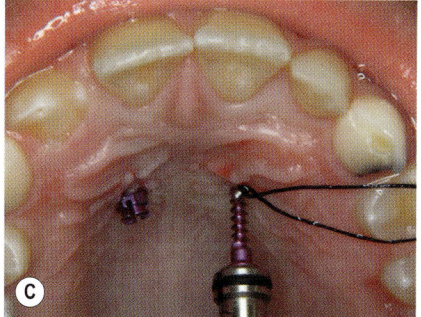
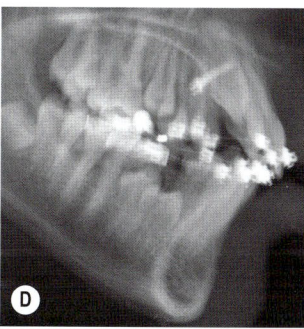

Fig. 16.4 The use of X-ray pins for palatal insertion of miniscrew implants (MI). (A) Intraoral photograph showing the positioning of the X-ray pins. (B) Diagnostic lateral cephalometric radiograph. (C) Intraoral photograph showing MI insertion next to the X-ray pin. (D) Lateral cephalometric radiograph following MI insertion.

safe positioning of MIs. However, this approach does not eliminate the problems of radiographic image distortion or of choosing the angulation during insertion of MIs.

The use of X-ray pins is a minimally invasive procedure, however, from an infection control standpoint, each device is for single use only.

The Individual Vacuum-formed Splint

In some situations, direct positioning of an X-ray pin can be difficult. The use of a vacuum-formed splint, with an incorporated radiopaque tube, is an alternative way to assess the MI insertion site radiographically and to provide a precise guide to control the drilling direction for the MI during its insertion.

CLINICAL APPLICATION OF X-RAY PINS

Prior to use, X-ray pins have to be disinfected and sterilized. Attaching them to dental floss (Fig. 16.2B) and securing them extraorally with an adhesive tape, is recommended for patient safety.

After determining the MI insertion point, the tissue around the area is anesthetized using local infiltration anesthesia, which will also facilitate the insertion of the MI. Initially the area can only be superficially anesthetized and additional local anesthesia will be needed for the insertion of the MI. Figure 16.3 shows the insertion of the pin and the subsequent diagnostic radiograph and MI insertion position. The X-ray pin is stable when positioned and because of its small size and screw-like design, it provides a valuable marker for the MI insertion site. After diagnostic evaluation of the radiographic image, the pin is removed with a slight pull, marking the insertion site for the MI with a bleeding spot.

If the site chosen is shown to be close to, or in contact with, the roots of adjacent teeth, an alternative location can be chosen using the bleeding spot and the position of the X-ray pin on the radiograph as references.

Since the safety of the above procedure is confirmed radiographically, the MI can be inserted securely in the corresponding inter-radicular sites. Finally, a follow-up radiograph shows the correct insertion of the MI (Fig. 16.3D).

PALATAL USE OF X-RAY PINS

Vestibular inter-radicular insertion of MIs has some limitations because of the underlying hard and soft tissues (see Chapter 15). The procedure for X-ray pins can be easily adapted to the palate if additional diagnostic information is required prior to MI placement (Fig. 16.4).

CLINICAL APPLICATION OF THE VACUUM-FORMED SPLINT

A dental impression is taken with alginate or polyvinylsiloxane and a cast is fabricated. A 2 mm vacuum splint (Track E, Forestadent, Pforzheim, Germany) is fabricated in the laboratory and a 2 mm SS tube is heated and inserted into the composite of the splint at the planned MI insertion point. The splint is transferred to the mouth of the patient (Fig. 16.5A) and a radiograph is taken to evaluate the position of the tube and thus the insertion position and angulation of the MI (Fig. 16.5B). Following radiographic assessment, the splint is used as a drilling guide during MI insertion (Fig. 16.5C). After MI insertion, a final radiograph can be taken to ensure proper orientation and position of the MI (Fig. 16.5D).

CONCLUSIONS

Positioning devices can be useful tools for MI insertion. Those made of wire elements require an additional impression appointment, cast construction

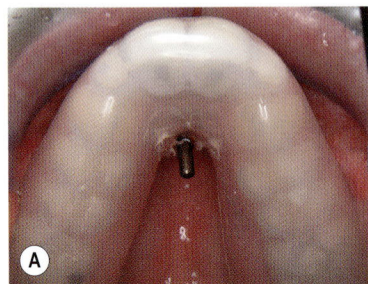 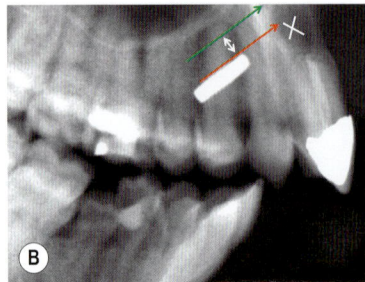 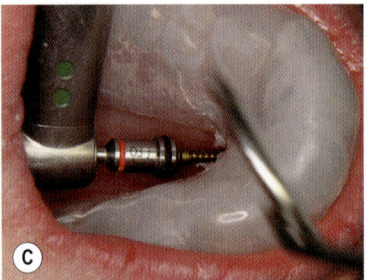 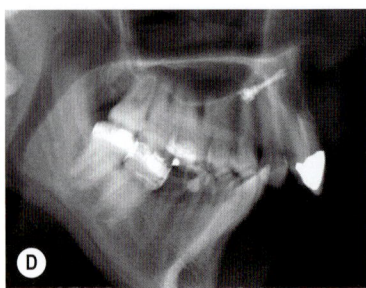

Fig. 16.5 The use of vacuum-formed splints for palatal insertion of microscrew implants. (A) Intraoral photograph showing the fabricated vacuum-formed splint along with the guiding insertion tube applied on the maxillary arch. (B) Diagnostic lateral cephalometric radiograph taken with the splint, showing the radiopaque diagnostic auxiliary tube indicating the position and the suitable direction for the implant insertion. (C) Intraoral photograph showing the use of the now modified splint as a drilling guide during implant insertion. (D) Lateral cephalometric radiograph following insertion.

and may cause gingival irritation due to extensive bends and fixing measures. In addition, manipulation of the film holder can inadvertently move the positioning device during periapical radiography. In general, it is difficult to accurately apply the preoperative diagnostic findings using radiological guides to the designated MI insertion site. A deviation of only 8° from the ideal insertion angle can lead to a deviation of more than 1 mm at the tip of the MI thread.[1] Therefore, some clinicians have suggested leaving the guiding pins used in place for the subsequent predrilling stage.[1,2,9] Most conventional diagnostic positioning devices provide accurate assessment of the vertical dimension but are less than perfect in assessing the ideal insertion angle.

The X-ray pin is a chair-side auxiliary that is diagnostically valuable, clinically efficient and cost effective.[10] It avoids all the complexities of wires and fixing associated with conventional guides and allows a precise determination of the insertion point, bone quality and vertical bone height. Repeated diagnostic radiography is rarely necessary. The vacuum-formed splint is a useful alternative when direct positioning of an X-ray pin is difficult.

There are some limitations with X-ray pins and vacuum-formed splints, such as radiographic image distortion and choosing the angulation for MI insertion; therefore, their role in facilitating MI insertion should not be overestimated.

REFERENCES

1. Estelita Cavalcante Barros S, Janson G, Chiqueto K, et al. A three-dimensional radiographic-surgical guide for mini-implant placement. J Clin Orthod 2006;40: 548–54.
2. Kim SH, Choi YS, Hwang EH, et al. Surgical positioning of orthodontic mini-implants with guides fabricated on models replicated with cone-beam computed tomography. Am J Orthod Dentofacial Orthop 2007;131:S82–9.
3. Kitai N, Yasuda S, Takada K. A stent fabricated on a selectively colored stereolithographic model for placement of orthodontic mini-implants. Int J Adult Orthod Orthognath Surg 2002;17:264–6.
4. McGuire MK, Scheyer ET, Gallerano RL. Temporary anchorage devices for tooth movement: a review and case reports. J Periodontol 2006;77:1613–24.
5. Lietz T. Minischrauben – Aspekte zur Bewertung und Auswahl der verschiedenen Systeme. In: Ludwig B, editor. Mini-Implantate in der Kieferorthopädie: Innovative Verankerungskonzepte. Berlin: Quintessence; 2007. p. 11–71.
6. Bumann A, Wiemer K, Mah J. Tomas – eine praxisgerechte Lösung zur temporären kieferorthopädischen Verankerung. Kieferorthopädie 2006;20:223–32.
7. Morea C, Dominguez GC, Wuo A, et al. Surgical guide for optimal positioning of mini-implants. J Clin Orthod 2005;39:317–21.
8. Maino BG, Bednar J, Pagin P, et al. The Spider Screw for skeletal anchorage. J Clin Orthod 2003;37:90–7.
9. Suzuki EY, Buranastidporn B. An adjustable surgical guide for miniscrew placement. J Clin Orthod 2005;39:588–90.
10. Ludwig B, Glasl B, Lietz T, et al. Radiological location monitoring in skeletal anchorage: introduction of a positioning guide. J Orofac Orthop 2008;69:59–65.

Precise miniscrew implant insertion technique between the roots of maxillary second premolar and first molar (Kim's stent)

17

Tae-Woo Kim and Hyewon Kim

INTRODUCTION

The space between the roots of the maxillary second premolars and first molars is the preferred site for miniscrew implant (MI) insertion because it is wider than other inter-radicular spaces, particularly after leveling with Roth prescription brackets.[1] However, even though this is the widest inter-radicular space, insertion of MIs here may not always be safe. The most common errors when inserting MIs inter-radicularly are encroachment into the periodontal ligament, contact with root surfaces or proximity to the alveolar crest.

There are a number of devices introduced to help in finding a safe MI insertion site, all with some disadvantages (see Chapter 16). Kim's stent, introduced in this chapter, is a guide that can facilitate accurate placement of MIs between roots, it is easy to fabricate in the clinic, and it increases the success rates of MIs by decreasing the chances of root damage.

COMPONENTS OF KIM'S STENT

Kim's stent comprises a positioning gauge and a direction guide (Fig. 17.1).

POSITIONING GAUGE

The positioning gauge is ligated on to the first molar bracket; it has a vertical and a horizontal arm and helps to set the mesiodistal position of the MI. The vertical arm is the vertical portion of the positioning gauge, while the horizontal arm has five to eight pieces of wire acting as a gauge and welded at 1 mm intervals (Fig. 17.1A).

DIRECTION GUIDE

The direction guide is ligated on to the second premolar bracket and indicates the direction of the MI insertion (Fig. 17.1B). The wire lying on the occlusal surface is called the occlusal arm and is placed at the midpoint between the second premolar and the first molar. It passes the contact point of the two adjacent teeth in close contact and approximates the proximal surface. The horizontal angulation of the X-ray beam lies parallel to this occlusal arm. The MI is also inserted parallel to this occlusal arm.

PREPARATION OF THE PATIENT

It is recommended that the posterior teeth are leveled up to 0.019×0.025 inch Ni-Ti (Fig. 17.2) or SS archwire (in 0.022 inch bracket slots). This is a prerequisite because if there is crowding, the roots may make contact with the MIs during further leveling or de-crowding procedures. In addition, after leveling, the regular pattern of root arrangement and inter-radicular distance will provide some consistency in placing the MIs and will also facilitate in avoiding root contact.

FABRICATION OF KIM'S STENT

MATERIAL AND INSTRUMENTS

The following material and instruments are needed for the fabrication of the Kim's stent (Figs. 17.3-17.5).

- *Periapical radiograph.* Adjacent teeth must not overlap (Fig. 17.3A). A panoramic radiograph is not accurate enough and the

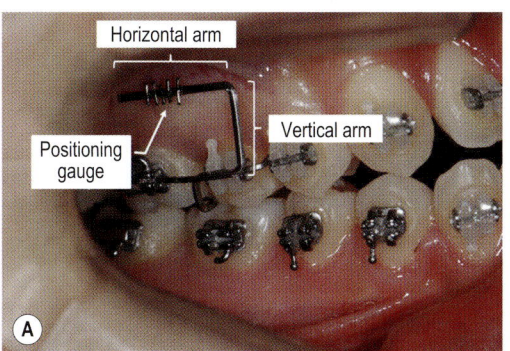

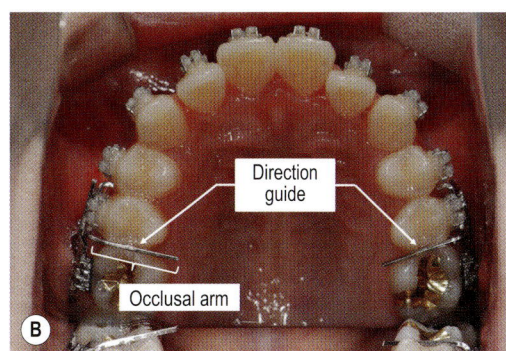

Fig. 17.1 Components of Kim's stent. (A) The positioning gauge, which is ligated into the first molar bracket. (B) The direction guide, which is ligated into the second premolar bracket.

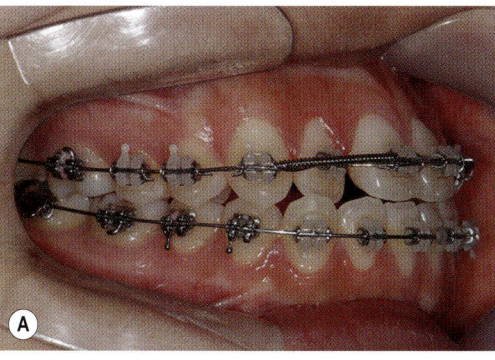

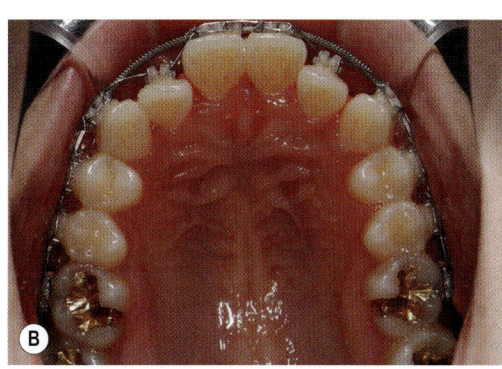

Fig. 17.2 Preparation of a patient before inserting a miniscrew implant (MI) at the maxillary posterior region. After leveling the posterior teeth with an archwire, the MI is placed between the roots of the maxillary second premolar and first molar. This specific patient shows a wide area of attached gingiva, and so the MI can be placed in a higher location.

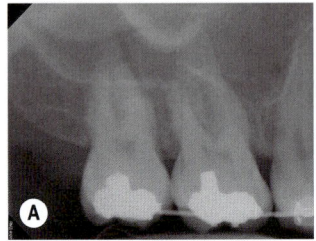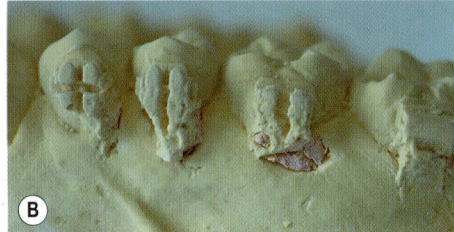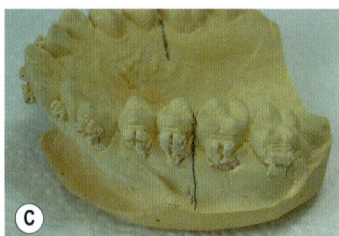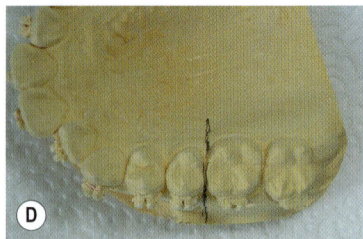

Fig. 17.3 Fabrication of Kim's stent. (A) Periapical radiograph taken before miniscrew implant insertion making sure that the maxillary right second premolar and first molar contact points do not overlap. (B) A good-quality model including the vestibular area with the impression taken after removing the archwire. (C,D) Marking on the study model based on the periapical radiograph. A line is drawn on the model to mark the center of the inter-radicular space (C) and is extended to the occlusal and palatal surfaces (D) in order to choose the direction of MI insertion.

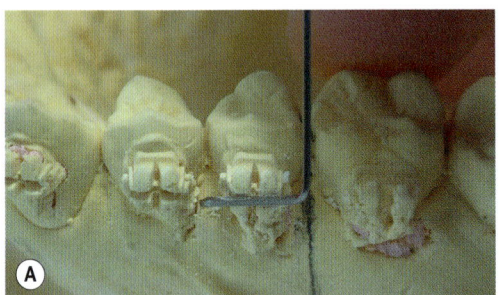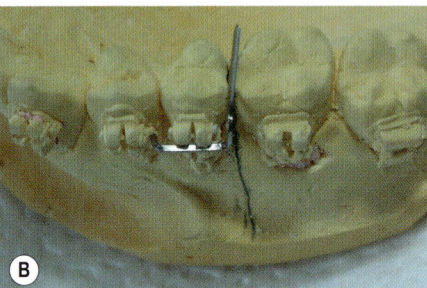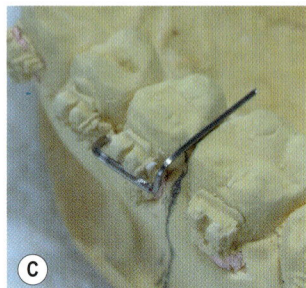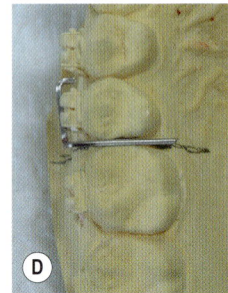

Fig. 17.4 Fabrication of the direction guide. (A) Wire (SS wire 0.022 × 0.028 inch) is inserted into the second premolar bracket, then bent in the occlusal direction at the pencil mark between the second premolar and first molar. (B) The occlusal arm is bent to contact the proximal area while passing through the center of the contact point of the two adjacent teeth. The excessive portion is cut to avoid contact with the tongue or the X-ray sensor (or film) and the direction is adjusted, here a little distally to correspond to the direction of miniscrew implant insertion. (C) The final form of the direction guide. (D) The occlusal arm is bent to follow the direction of the pencil line, which corresponds to the direction of miniscrew implant insertion and the long axis of the X-ray beam.

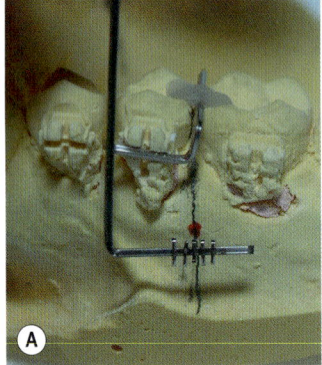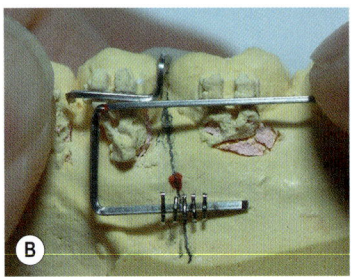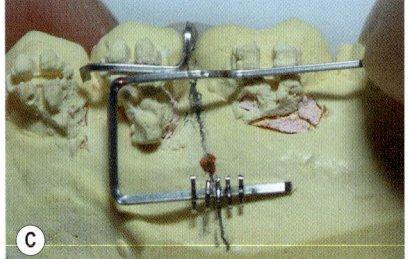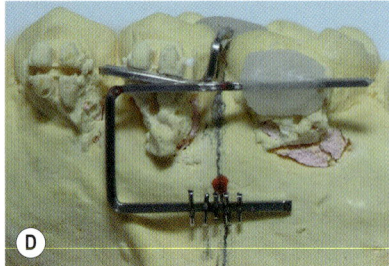

Fig. 17.5 Fabrication of the positioning gauge. (A) Five to eight pieces of the green Elgiloy wire are welded on to the horizontal arm of the positioning gauge at 1 mm intervals and the pins are positioned so that the center pin matches the estimated insertion position of the miniscrew implant (red dot); this will be adjusted after taking a periapical radiograph using the Kim's stent. The vertical arm is bent to have a position near the contact point of the first premolar and second premolars. (B) The wire is bent at 90° at the height of the first molar bracket. (C) A bayonet bend is formed at the mesial end of the first molar tube or bracket to act as a stop, providing also space for the second premolar bracket and the direction guide. (D) Finally, the excessive end is cut and the positioning gauge is ready to be used.

inter-radicular distance is difficult to determine; CT has lower resolution, higher radiation and higher cost.

- *Study model.* An impression is taken with the archwire removed (Fig. 17.3B). Clear views of the buccal vestibule are required. If the archwire is not removed and the buccal vestibule is not duplicated well, it is difficult to precisely manufacture Kim's stent.
- *Brackets.* With 0.022 inch slot.
- *Wires.* SS wire 0.0125 × 0.028 inch (Jinsung Industrial, Seoul, Korea) and 0.014 inch green Elgiloy wire (Rocky Mountain Orthodontics, Denver, CO, USA), which is easily welded on to the 0.022 × 0.028 inch SS wire.
- *Welder device.*
- *Tools.* Tweed loop and helix-forming pliers (043-CK, Orthopli, Philadelphia, PA, USA), cutter and marker.

The cast and periapical radiograph are used for a provisional decision on the position and direction of the MI. With a lead pencil, the corresponding line is drawn on the cast (Fig. 17.3C,D).

FABRICATION OF THE DIRECTION GUIDE

The direction guide is ligated to the bracket of the tooth mesial to the point of insertion (i.e. the second premolar; Fig. 17.1B). Figure 17.4 shows the steps to fabricate the direction guide.

FABRICATION OF THE POSITIONING GAUGE

Five to eight pieces (pins) of the green Elgiloy wire of approximate length 2–3 mm are welded on to the SS wire (0.0215 × 0.028 inch) at 1 mm intervals. Figure 17.5 shows the steps taken to complete the guide.

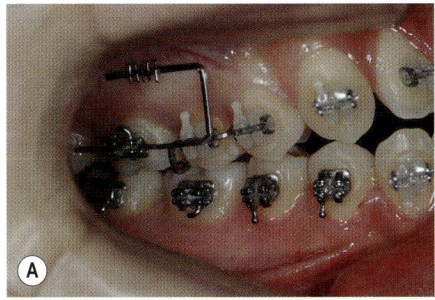 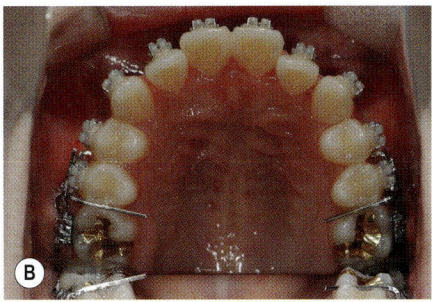

Fig. 17.6 Fixation of Kim's stent. (A) The direction guide ligated into the second premolar bracket before fixing the positioning gauge in place. (B) Occlusal view of the maxillary arch with two Kim's stents fixed bilaterally. The direction guides are positioned as planned on the model.

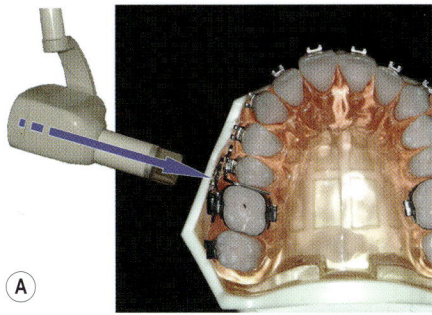 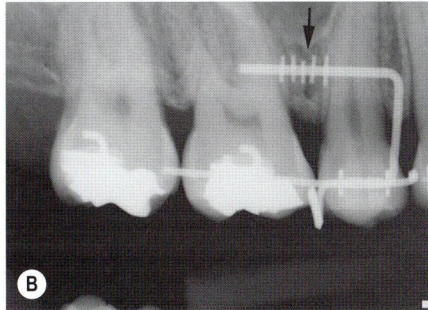

Fig. 17.7 Periapical radiography. (A) The occlusal arm of the direction guide and the long axis of the X-ray beam should be parallel. (B) In this patient, the middle of the second and the third pins from the vertical arm (arrow) indicates the miniscrew implant insertion point.

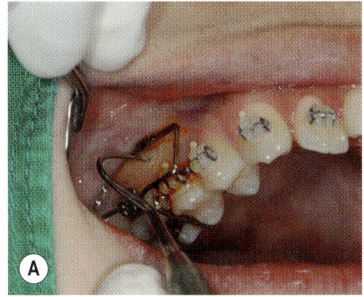 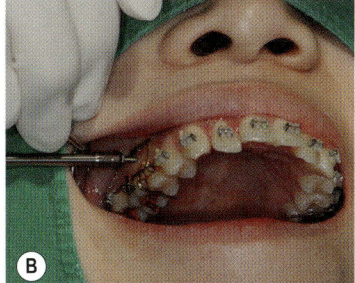 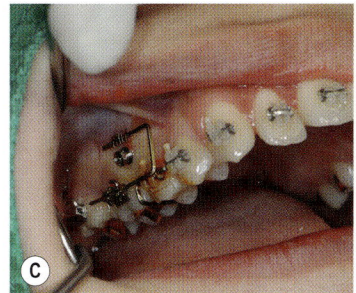 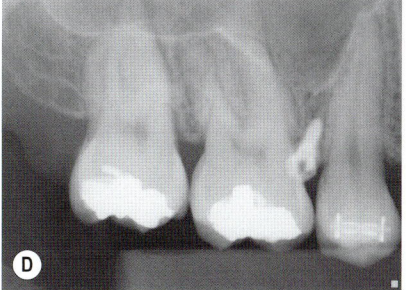

Fig. 17.8 Miniscrew implant (MI) insertion. (A) Using an explorer, the position of MI insertion is marked, the mucosal thickness is measured and the quality of the cortical bone is evaluated. (B) After rotating the screwdriver two or three times, the tip of the MI perforates the cortical bone. With a large mirror, the direction of the MI is checked and adjusted, and the long axis of the screwdriver is positioned parallel to the occlusal arm of the direction guide. (C) A well-inserted MI between the maxillary right second premolar and the first molar. The MI is placed as high as possible on the attached gingiva. (D) Periapical radiograph showing a well-inserted MI.

MINISCREW IMPLANT INSERTION USING KIM'S STENT

ANESTHESIA

After disinfection of the oral cavity and insertion region, local anesthesia (lidocaine plus epinephrine) is injected, ensuring that only buccal mucosa is anesthetized.

FIXATION OF KIM'S STENT

The direction guide is ligated on to the second premolar. If required, the occlusal arm is adjusted at this point. Then the positioning gauge is ligated after appropriate adjustment. Care should be taken that the gauge of the horizontal arm does not interfere with the insertion location of the MI. The gauge should be placed approximately 2 mm above the border of the attached gingiva (Fig. 17.6), while the horizontal arm should be well positioned, almost touching but not impinging on the mucosa.

RADIOGRAPHIC EVALUATION

After fixing the stent on the maxillary arch, a periapical radiograph is performed taking care that the occlusal arm of the direction guide and the horizontal angle of the X-ray beam are parallel (Fig. 17.7A). In an ideal periapical radiograph, the contact point of the second premolar and first molar is clearly visible, while the crowns do not overlap (Fig. 17.7B). The insertion position should be at the center of the inter-radicular space between the second premolar and first molar.

MINISCREW IMPLANT INSERTION

After disinfection of the oral cavity, the soft tissue is marked with an explorer, and at the same time the soft tissue thickness and quality of the cortical bone are determined (Fig. 17.8A).

Using a specially designed screwdriver, the MI is inserted in the highest point of the attached gingiva, perpendicular to the gingival surface (Fig. 17.8B,C). If there is need to insert the MI in an oblique direction, after the MI has pierced the cortical bone the direction of insertion can be altered, having an angle of approximately 15–30° in relation to the soft tissue surface. If there is need for a more oblique direction, the use of predrilling is necessary prior to MI insertion. When viewed from the occlusal surface, the long axis of the screwdriver and the occlusal arm of the direction guide should be parallel. Using a large dental mirror from the occlusal surface may be helpful to determine this direction. Finally, during MI insertion, the long axis of the screwdriver should be kept stable without any jiggling.

EVALUATION OF MINISCREW IMPLANT INSERTION

Immediately after insertion, a further periapical radiograph should be taken to check if the MI is placed in the correct site as initially planned (Fig. 17.8D). If the position is incorrect, the MI should be removed immediately and reinserted in a new position.

REFERENCE

1. Kim T-W, Kim H. Clinical application of orthodontic mini-implant. Seoul, Korea: Myung Mun; 2008. p. 44.

INTRODUCTION

The biggest challenge for insertion of orthodontic miniscrew implants (MIs) inter-radicularly in the buccal or palatal area of the alveolar ridge is to avoid the roots of the neighboring teeth. Availability of adequate bone in the interdental septum is one of the key factors for a successful insertion and this is improved by initial leveling and aligning of the teeth (see Chapter 17). In some individuals, such as those with small clinical crowns, there is still not sufficient space for insertion. In these cases, space can be opened with an open coil spring or an alternative location can be chosen.

In all cases where there is a possible risk of root contact or root perforation, the precise insertion of MIs using surgical guides (conventional or stereolithographic) is suggested to minimize the risks.

CONVENTIONAL SURGICAL GUIDES

The principle for constructing a conventional surgical guide[1,2] is similar to that used for dental implants, but because the placement of the MI must be precise, only non-self-drilling MIs should be used. The aim of the surgical guide is to control the bur used for pilot drilling in all three dimensions so that the MI can be inserted precisely into the planned position. This is achieved using a metallic sleeve in the body of the surgical guide.

Initially, a plaster cast of the dental arch is used to identify the ideal insertion point based on the mechanics that are going to be used. As described in other chapters, ideally an insertion site in the attached gingiva as close as possible to the mucogingival line is chosen but if needed insertion in the alveolar mucosa can be considered. However, in the latter situation, a miniflap should be elevated before drilling to avoid any tissue being trapped during pilot drilling (see Chapter 14).

Sometimes a vertical depression is visible on the attached gingiva between the two neighboring teeth where the clinician is planning to insert the MI. This depression follows the middle of the septum and can be used as a guide (Fig. 18.1A). When the ideal insertion is selected, it is marked with a pencil on the plaster cast (Fig. 18.1B).

The sleeve is fixed to the plaster cast with a sleeve positioner (Fig. 18.2), which is a patented mechanical aid comprising:

- a body incorporating a horizontal blade; the insertion pin is located on the upper part of the body for the paralleling device
- a scrolling identifier moving in apical–coronal direction to allow adjustment in an apical–coronal inclination

- a sleeve holder, which is inserted in one of the two possible holes of the apical–coronal angle keeper and retained firmly by a screw.

The mesiodistal position of the sleeve is determined by the line bisecting the two marginal crests, while the coronal–apical direction of the sleeve can be predetermined on the sleeve positioner and can be varied depending on the anatomical situation of the insertion point. The line is drawn on the cast starting from the middle of the marginal crest towards the contact point of two neighboring teeth. If this line is extended in an apical direction parallel to the long axis of the teeth, it remains between the roots of the neighboring teeth, avoiding any root contact (Fig. 18.2C). On this imaginary line, the appropriate fixation point of the sleeve (i.e. the insertion point of the MI) can be chosen (Fig. 18.2D).

The sleeve positioner is then inserted into the vertical arm of the paralleling device (Fig. 18.2E). The sleeve holder should be parallel to the blade and attached to the body of the sleeve positioner in such a way that, when it is inserted in the paralleling device, if a vertical line is traced through the blade, it hits the center of the sleeve positioner. This allows the scrolling identifier to be moved vertically, thus enabling the sleeve holder to pass through the predefined MI insertion point. The plaster cast is then placed on the table of a paralleling device so that the MI insertion point on the septum midline is located parallel to the vertical arm of the device and perpendicular to the ground (Fig. 18.2F). The inclination of the sleeve holder is also adjusted in order to indicate precisely not only the mesiodistal (Fig. 18.2G) but also the apical–coronal (Fig. 18.2H) angulation of the insertion direction of the MI.

Once the plaster cast has been oriented towards the sleeve positioner device, the coronal–apical indicator is scrolled downwards until the tip of the sleeve holder hits the insertion point marked on the plaster model. At this point, the blade of the body of the sleeve positioner should bisect the marginal line. All of the screws of the adjustable parts should be firmly tightened.

After loosening the retention screw and gently retracting the sleeve holder, a metallic sleeve can then be inserted on the tip of the sleeve holder. After repositioning the tip of the sleeve holder to the surface of the plaster cast in contact with the insertion point, the retention screw of the sleeve holder is tightened again. The position and direction of the sleeve now corresponds to the position and direction of MI insertion. The sleeve is then fixed to the plaster cast using sticky wax placed around its base and the plaster cast is removed from the positioning device.

The extent of the area of teeth and soft tissues that is covered by the surgical guide is determined by placing utility wax around the area to ensure the relief of the retentive areas and area for use of orthodontic appliances such as brackets and tubes (Fig. 18.3).

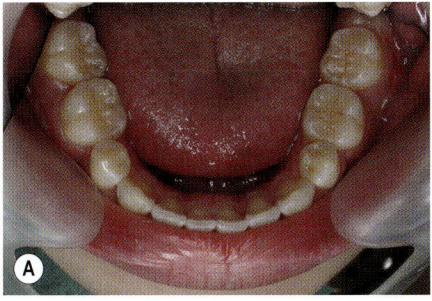
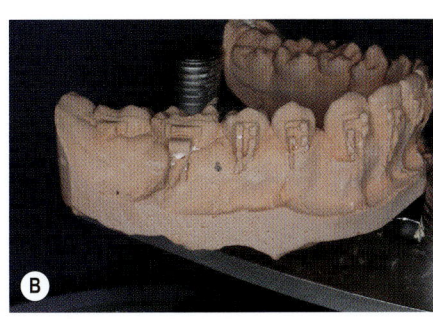

Fig. 18.1 The interdental septum. (A) A gingival depression indicates the middle of the interdental septum between the first and second lower molar. (B) A plaster model on the table of a paralleling device with the insertion point marked. The septum midline needs to be oriented perpendicular to the ground.

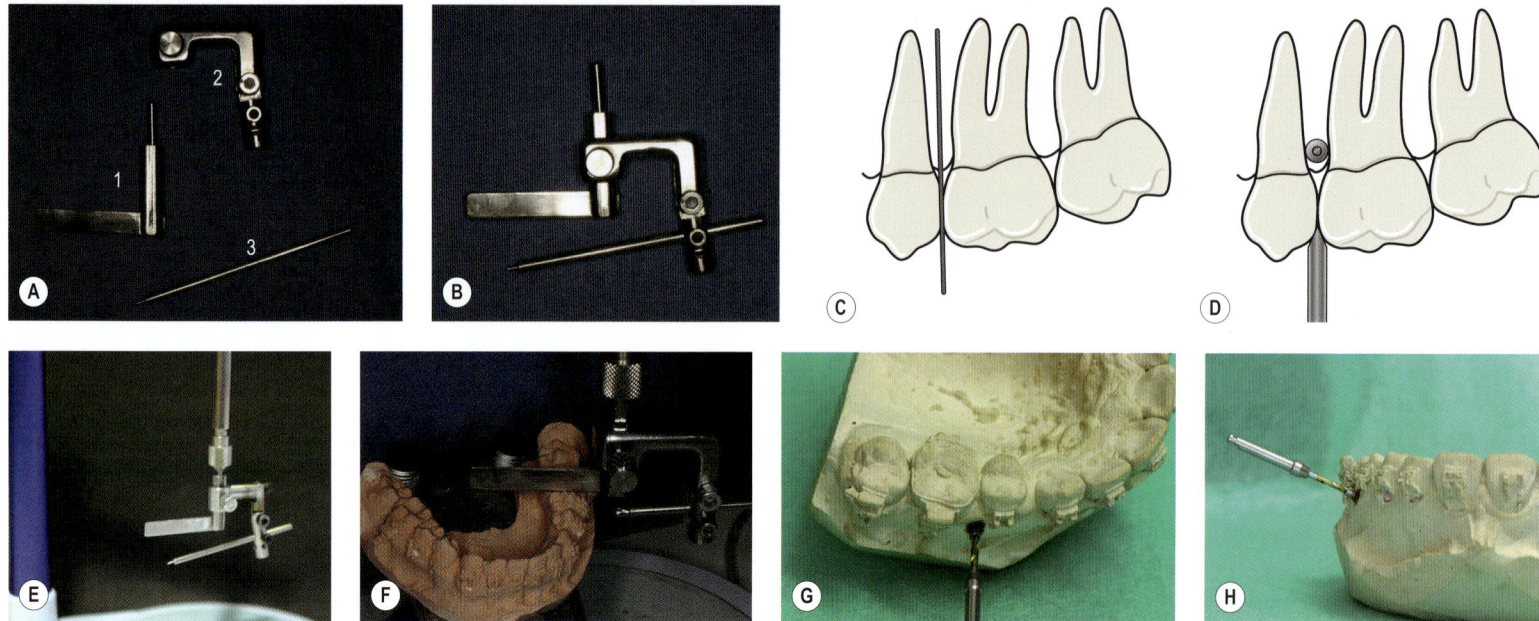

Fig. 18.2 The sleeve positioner. (A) The components are the body with the blade and the insertion pin for the paralleling device (1), the scrolling apical–coronal level identifier (2) and the sleeve holder (3). (B) The assembled sleeve positioner ready to be inserted into the paralleling device. (C) The fixation point of the sleeve is set using a vertical line drawn from the middle of the marginal crest towards the contact point of two neighboring teeth and prolonged in an apical direction parallel to the long axis of the teeth. (D) The blade and the sleeve holder are constructed to be located on the same vertical line. (E) The sleeve positioner inserted into the vertical arm of the paralleling device. (F) Positioning of the plaster cast on the paralleling device and adjustment of the sleeve holder in order to correspond to the insertion position of the miniscrew implant. (G,H) Bur equipped with a sleeve indicating the mesiodistal (G) and the apical–coronal (H) inclination of the insertion direction of the pilot drill.

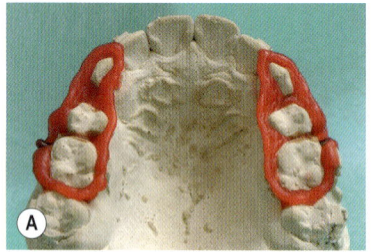
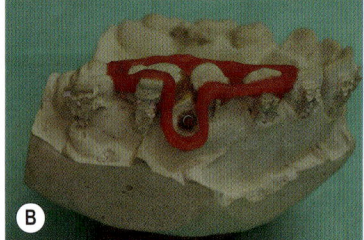

Fig. 18.3 Delimitation of the surgical guide's area with wax in occlusal (A) and lateral (B) view.

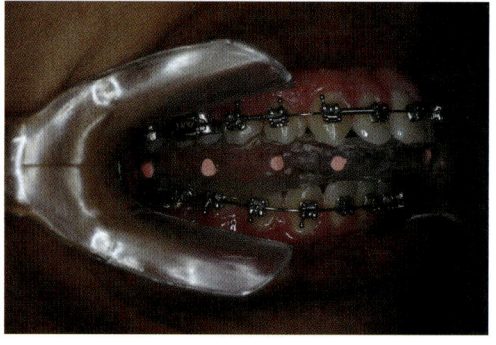

Fig. 18.5 Acrylic splint with 2 mm perforations filled with gutta-percha marks used to capture the cone beam CT images.

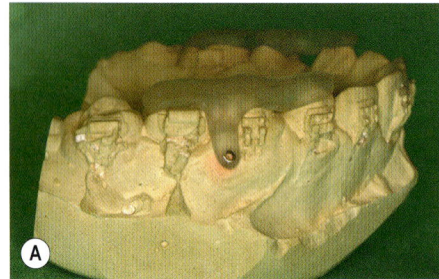
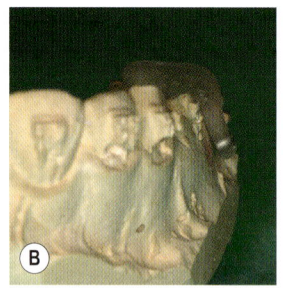
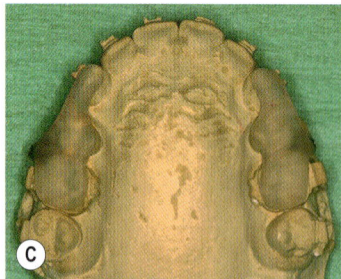
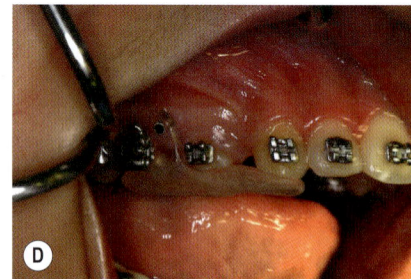

Fig. 18.4 Surgical guide fitting. (A–C) Checking the guide on the plaster model. (D) Checking the guide in the patient's mouth prior to surgery.

After delimitation of the surgical guide's area, the plaster is hydrated in water for 5 minutes and subsequently isolated with Vaseline. Acrylic resin is deposited into the waxed area and polymerized under pressure. Finally, the acrylic resin is trimmed and polished and its fitting is checked on the plaster cast (Fig. 18.4A–C).

If the surgical guide fits correctly, it is cleaned in ultrasound detergent and kept in chlorhexidine solution (1%) until its intraoral use. Prior to surgery, the fitting of the surgical guide, as well as the insertion point and angulation of the sleeve, must be checked again on the patient's teeth (Fig. 18.4D).

STEREOLITHOGRAPHIC SURGICAL GUIDES

There are situations where surgical guides as described above are not feasible, for example where rotated teeth or pneumatization of the maxillary sinus narrows the insertion path or where multiple MIs are needed. In this case, cone beam CT can be used to create a stereolithographic surgical guide.[2–4]

Initially, plaster models of both arches are obtained and the bite is recorded with wax. Using these models, a 5 mm thick occlusal splint is fabricated in the laboratory with acrylic resin. Six perforations, each

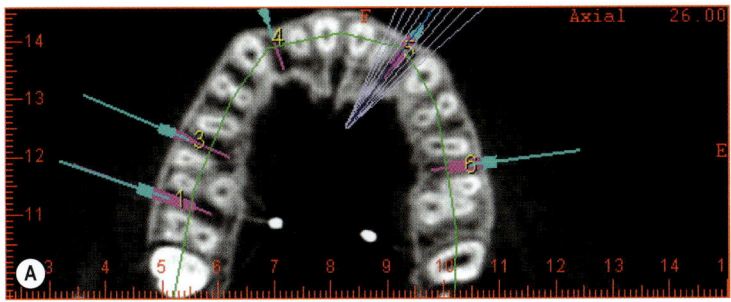
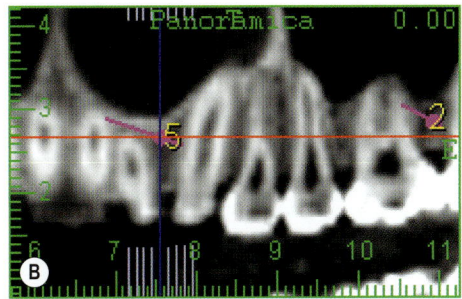
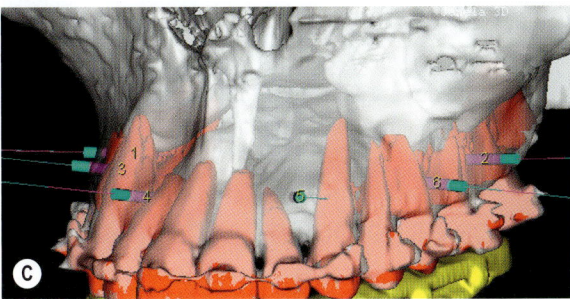
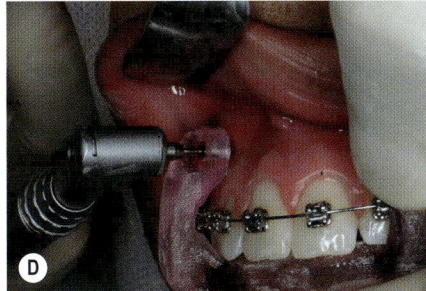

Fig. 18.6 Surgery planning with the stereolithographic approach. (A–C) Simulated surgery for miniscrew implant insertion in transversal (A), panoramic (B) and three-dimensional (C) views. (D) The prototyped surgical guide used to drill a pilot perforation.

of 2 mm diameter, are created in the splint and filled with gutta-percha (Fig. 18.5). Then, the splint is carefully checked in the patient's mouth to ensure a firm fit with no movement.

Cone beam CT is used to take an average of 217 thin slices. The protocol of acquisition is the same for the maxilla and the mandible (6 cm, 40 segments, 0.25 high-resolution voxel). If both arches have to be recorded at the same time, a slightly different protocol should be used for data acquisition (8 cm, 40 segments, 0.25 high-resolution voxel). Two scans are necessary, one of the patient's maxilla and/or mandible and one of the splint itself. The first scan is performed with the patient wearing the fabricated occlusal splint. The patient needs to be positioned with the occlusal plane parallel to the horizontal plane, and the head has to be stabilized to avoid any movements during data capture. In addition, the patient must not swallow until completion of the scan. The second scan is taken using the same acquisition protocol but capturing the splint alone. In order to avoid any density interferences, the splint is positioned on top of a small empty paper box.

The resulting data are exported in DICOM 3 (digital imaging and communications in medicine; Multi-File) format for segmentation using software that generates multiple displays (sagittal, transversal, panoramic and three-dimensional). Then, specific software for image analysis and implant surgery is used with these images for treatment planning: to simulate the insertion location and angulation for the MIs (Fig. 18.6A–C). Using different simulations, the surgeon can check the position of the MIs in all three dimensions.

After planning and defining the MIs' insertion points and angulation, the file is sent back to a laboratory for fabrication of the corresponding prototyped surgical guide. The surgical guide is designed virtually with computer-aided design software to accurately reproduce the positions and angulations of the MIs as they were defined by the surgeon. The design process includes also selection of the type of MI and the surgical kit to be used during surgery.

The surgical guide is manufactured with a rapid prototyping machine using a stereolithographic approach, and the SS sleeves are inserted and fitted perfectly to obtain the planned pilot holes (Fig. 18.6D).

Surgical guides manufactured following this approach are useful for the insertion of conventional MIs.[5] For the insertion of multiple orthodontic MIs, two-component MIs (such as the C-implant, where there is a screw and a separate abutment), other approaches already described in the literature can be used.[3,4]

CONCLUSIONS

Each MI system is unique in terms of design, mechanical resistance and the corresponding surgical kit needed for insertion. Each one of these parameters needs to be taken into consideration before treatment planning. Prototyped surgical guides may be of significant value in ensuring precise MI insertion in the desired position, thus improving success rates.

REFERENCES

1. Morea C, Dominguez GC, Wuo Ado V, et al. Surgical guide for optimal positioning of mini-implants. J Clin Orthod 2005;39:317–21.
2. Suzuki EY, Suzuki B. Accuracy of miniscrew implant placement with a 3-dimensional surgical guide. J Oral Maxillofac Surg 2008;66:1245–52.
3. Kim SH, Choi YS, Hwang EH, et al. Surgical positioning of orthodontic mini-implants with guides fabricated on models replicated with conebeam computed tomography. Am J Orthod Dentofacial Orthop 2007;131:S82–9.
4. Kim SH, Kang JM, Choi B, et al. Clinical application of a stereolithographic surgical guide for simple positioning of orthodontic mini-implants. World J Orthod 2008;9: 371–82.
5. Morea C, Hayek JE, Oleskovicz C, et al. Chilvarquer I. Precise insertion of orthodontic mini-screws with a stereolithographic surgical guide based on cone beam computed tomography data: a pilot study. Int J Oral Maxillofac Implants 2011;26:860–5.

19 Overview of orthodontic implants for the correction of Class II malocclusion

Gero Kinzinger, Heiner Wehrbein, Friedrich K. Byloff and Moschos A. Papadopoulos

INTRODUCTION

Maxillary molar distalization is intended to gain or restore space for the teeth in the arch. This can be achieved by molar distalization, dental arch expansion or extraction of teeth. Among others, the following criteria should be considered when assessing available treatment options:

- the size of the maxillary apical base
- the functional tongue space
- third molar formation
- potential tooth agenesis
- patient's growth pattern
- patient's soft tissue profile
- patient's oral hygiene and their susceptibility to caries
- patient's compliance
- patient's perception of esthetics.

Intraoral non-compliance distalization appliances allow correction of Class II malocclusion with a variety of active components delivering the distalization force (see Chapter 2). Depending on the location of the incorporated force module, they can be classified as appliances with vestibular or palatal force application:

- vestibular force application:
  - magnetic modules
  - loaded coil spring systems: Wilson Distalizing Arch, Ni-Ti springs, Jones Jig, Lokar Distalizing appliance
- palatal force application
  - pendulum appliances
  - loaded coil spring systems: Distal Jet, Keles Slider, First Class Appliance.

These appliances are anchored on the maxillary anterior teeth, usually by means of bands or occlusal wire rests on the premolars, as well as on the anterior palate by means of modified acrylic resin Nance buttons. However, this type of anchorage is not always adequate to withstand the reciprocal forces, and anchorage loss of the anterior teeth, in terms of mesial movement of the premolars and canines and proclination of the incisors are almost always observed after non-compliance maxillary molar distalization. In addition, the temporary partial coverage of the palate causes oral hygiene problems. To avoid these problems, anchorage can be provided for example by osseointegrated implants inserted in the palate. This chapter will discuss anchorage designs using orthodontic implants and maxillary molar distalization appliances or approaches.

IMPLANTS FOR ORTHODONTIC ANCHORAGE

Orthodontic implants of reduced diameter or length inserted in the palate can serve as absolute or auxiliary types of anchorage modalities, providing either direct or indirect anchorage (see Chapter 3):

- *direct anchorage*: the active component is fitted by support elements or special constructions to the implant and applies force directly on the tooth or group of teeth to be moved during treatment
- *indirect anchorage*: the teeth that act as reactive units are indirectly stabilized by the skeletal device via a transpalatal bar connected to the implant
- *absolute anchorage*: only the orthodontic implant resists the reciprocal forces of the distalization systems
- *auxiliary anchorage*: a number of teeth, or more often other anchorage modalities (e.g. a modified acrylic resin Nance button), form part of the anchoring system.

DIMENSIONS OF ORTHODONTIC IMPLANTS

Conventional dental implants have large dimensions and may only be suitable for orthodontic anchorage in patients who have spaces after extraction of teeth, where they may provide viable options not only for the prosthetic rehabilitation of the missing teeth but also to act as absolute anchorage for various orthodontic movements including distalization of molars prior to the prosthetic restoration (Fig. 19.1).

Further, endosseous titanium implants of reduced length inserted in the palate can provide adequate stationary anchorage (see Chapter 7).

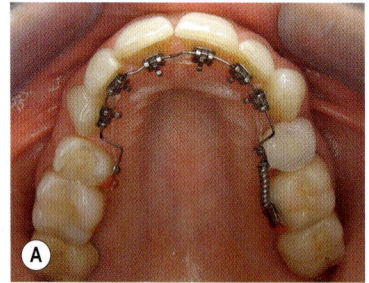 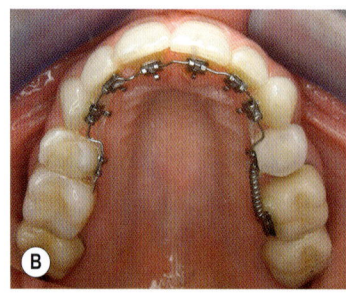 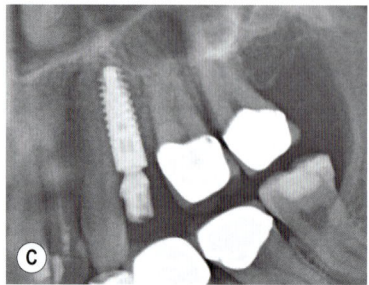 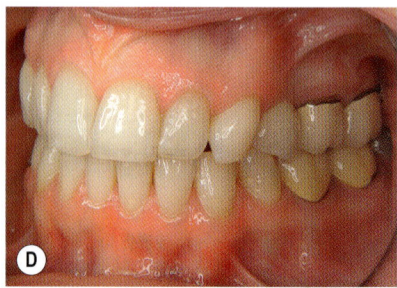

Fig. 19.1 A dental implant used to support maxillary molar distalization and asymmetrical anterior teeth retraction prior to the final prosthetic restoration. (A) Occlusal view immediately after insertion of a dental implant with provisional crown for the second premolar to provide orthodontic anchorage control. Push–pull biomechanics were used (coil spring and elastic chain, respectively) to distalize the molars and move the midline towards the implant simultaneously. (B) In progress occlusal view of the maxillary arch close to the final result. The space mesial to the second premolar is closed and a distal space has opened. (C) Post-treatment radiograph after molar distalization. The left canine was retracted as much as possible, almost touching the implant. (D) Post-treatment lateral view following the final restoration of the left second premolar with the molars in Class I occlusion.

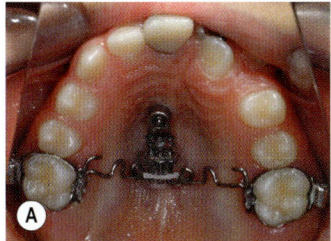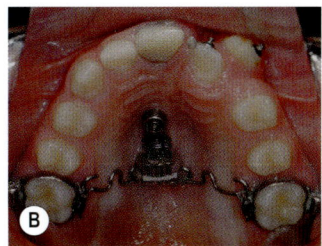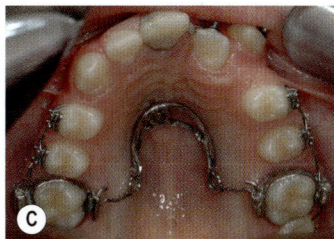

Fig. 19.2 The Mainz Implant Pendulum (MIP). (A) Occlusal view of the maxillary arch after paramedian insertion of an endosseous palatal implant of reduced length (Orthosystem) and placement of the MIP for non-compliance maxillary molar distalization. (B) Occlusal view after distalization of the first molars and drifting of the premolars. (C) Occlusal view following replacement of the MIP with a modified transpalatal bar attached to the molar bands and the palatal implant, providing further stationary anchorage for the anterior teeth retraction. (From Kinzinger et al., 2005,[10] with permission of Springer.)

INSERTION LOCATION

In many patients requiring maxillary molar distalization, the most suitable area for implant insertion is the palate and the issues of palatal insertion are discussed in detail in Chapters 7 and 12. The degree of obliteration of the median palatal suture increases with age but is still very variable and this must be taken into consideration when considering implant position in adolescents.

APPLIANCES FOR NON-COMPLIANCE MAXILLARY MOLAR DISTALIZATION AND IMPLANT-SUPPORTED ANCHORAGE

The two types of appliances used most frequently for non-compliance maxillary molar distalization are pendulum appliances and palatal coil spring systems (e.g. the Distal Jet), which rely basically on two different biomechanical concepts. Pendulum appliances attempt to achieve maxillary molar distalization by distalizing the maxillary molars along a pendulum arc. To counteract this pendulum type of movement, certain modifications of the appliance as well as specific preactivations of the pendulum springs are essential.[1-4] Uprighting activation at the horizontal arm of the pendulum springs is vital to exert an intrusive force and an uprighting moment on the molars while at the same time it applies a reciprocal moment in the opposite direction and an extrusive force on the anchoring unit.[1,4] The anchorage unit should be firm enough to resist this reciprocal distalization force, which can best be achieved using endosseous palatal implants of reduced length[5] or subperiosteal osteosynthetic plates fixed with miniscrews and supported by push-on palatal buttons.[6]

In contrast, in palatal coil spring systems the line of force application determined by the active components runs almost through the center of resistance of the first molars; since the maxillary molars are forced to move on a line parallel to the occlusal plane of the maxillary arch, and no vertical forces and moments are exerted on the anchoring unit, uprighting activations are not needed.

The most commonly used non-compliance distalization approaches in combination with stationary anchorage provided by orthodontic implants are presented below.

THE MAINZ IMPLANT PENDULUM

The Mainz Implant Pendulum (Fig. 19.2) is a skeletonized K-Pendulum appliance with a distal screw that is firmly anchored by means of an endosseously positioned palatal implant of reduced length (Orthosystem, Institut Straumann, Waldenburg, Switzerland).[1,3,5,7] As this is stationary anchorage, there is no need for occlusal wire rests for additional dental anchorage or for an acrylic resin palatal button, which facilitates maintenance of good oral hygiene of the palatal area, particularly around the implant. The

anterior part of the distal screw is attached directly to the soldered or welded cap of the implant by laser welding. The distal part of the screw in which the retentive elements of the pendulum springs are located is coated with plastic.

Before insertion of the appliance in the mouth, the arms of the pendulum springs have to be bent to avoid unwanted effects: (1) uprighting activation of the springs results in an uprighting of the molar roots and counteracts the tendency for distal molar crown tipping, which could occur because the distalization force is applied more occlusally in relation to the center of resistance of the molars; and (2) a toe-in of the pendulum springs avoids undesirable distobuccal rotation of the molars. Regular adjustment of the distal screw allows a larger amount of bodily maxillary molar distalization.[1,2,4,8,9] Since an orthodontic implant is used as anchorage, the reactive forces are absorbed exclusively by bone and there are no effects on the anterior dentition in terms of mesial movement and proclination. In addition, since no occlusal wire rests are used to anchor the appliance on the teeth, spontaneous distal drifting of the premolars and canines takes place. Thus, the severity of the initial malocclusion is reduced and the total time needed for the retraction of the anterior teeth is less. Following distalization, the appliance is removed and the molars are connected by a new fabricated transpalatal bar to the palatal implant, providing for further stationary anchorage for the retraction of the anterior teeth (Fig. 19.2C). Thus, anchorage loss of the molars during this stage of treatment is avoided.

THE AACHEN IMPLANT PENDULUM

The Aachen Implant Pendulum (Fig. 19.3) consists of a Quad Pendulum anchored solely to an endosseously placed palatal orthodontic implant of reduced length (Orthosystem).[5] This implant-supported Pendulum appliance is an interesting option, particularly for the treatment of adults where the preservation of anchorage is usually very challenging owing to significant periodontal involvement.

The four pendulum springs allow a sequential distalization of the first and second molars, distalizing initially the second molars by applying a rather low force. The first molars are not incorporated in the anchoring system at this stage so that they can drift freely distally under the pull of the transeptal fibers. When the second molars are sufficiently distalized, their pendulum springs are deactivated. This way the second molars are kept in place, reinforcing the anchorage unit for the subsequent distalization of the first molars.

The pendulum springs of the Quad Pendulum are removable components, while lingual sheaths originally designed for molar bands are incorporated into the acrylic resin button to ensure a firm hold when they are activated and prevent any slippage out of the acrylic resin. By replacing these springs with longer ones, it is possible to displace the horizontal and sagittal centers of rotation of molars. Prior to the insertion of the appliance, uprighting activation and a toe-in have to be performed at the ends of the pendulum springs, as described above.

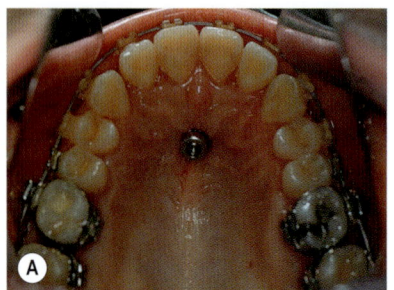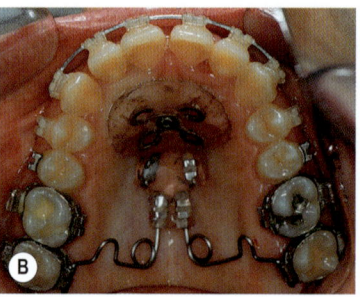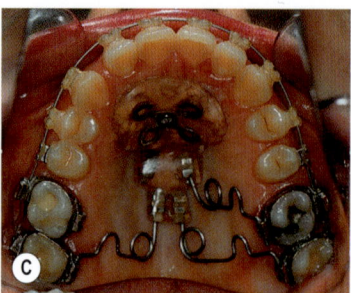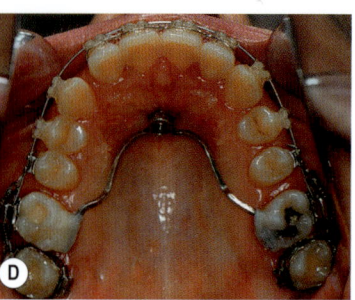

Fig. 19.3 The Aachen Implant Pendulum (AIP). (A) Occlusal view of the maxillary arch after median insertion of an endosseous palatal implant of reduced length (Orthosystem). (B) Occlusal view of the maxillary arch after insertion of the palatal implant and placement of the AIP, initially with two pendulum springs for second molar distalization. (C) Occlusal view of the maxillary arch after distalization of the second molars. Stabilization of the second molars with "active anchorage" and placement of one further pendulum spring to distalize the left first molar. (D) Occlusal view of the maxillary arch after removal of the AIP and placement of a transpalatal bar connected to the first molars to support retraction of the lateral and the anterior teeth.

The modified acrylic resin Nance button serves for the incorporation of the sheaths that hold the pendulum springs and is firmly attached to the neck of the implant through a clamping cap with an octagonal design to resist rotation. Although the acrylic resin has surface contact with the palatal mucosa, it does not provide any additional anchoring capacity to the system. Consequently it can be very thin and slim to decrease discomfort for the patient.

Occlusal wire rests on the premolars and canines are not needed. Following completion of distalization, supporting the distalized molars with a transpalatal bar prevents loss of posterior anchorage (in terms of mesial movement of the molars) during the subsequent stage of Class II treatment involving the retraction of the anterior teeth (Fig. 19.3D).

Compatibility of the Aachen Implant Pendulum with other Pendulum appliances is possible in general. All these exclusively implant-supported appliances are fitted with only one screw, and, therefore, they can be easily removed during treatment by the clinician for reactivations or for ultrasound cleaning.

THE IMPLANT-SUPPORTED DISTAL JET

Although some applications of the Distal Jet appliance in conjunction with palatal implants have been described,[11] most uses of the Distal Jet are associated with miniscrew implants. These applications are presented in detail in Chapters 31 and 32.

THE IMPLANT-SUPPORTED KELES SLIDER

The implant-supported Keles Slider consists of a modified Keles Slider appliance (see Fig. 2.9) attached to a stepped screw titanium palatal implant (diameter, 4.5 mm; length, 8 mm; Frialit-2 Implant System, Friadent, Mannheim, Germany), which is positioned either on the midpalatal suture or in the paramedian area. This modification eliminates the need to use palatal soft tissues, first premolars or anterior teeth to support anchorage, thus avoiding the side effects of maxillary molar distalization using the conventional Keles Slider with a Nance button.

To construct the appliance, the maxillary first molars are banded, and tubes (diameter, 0.045 inch; Leone, Firenze, Italy) are soldered on the palatal side of the first molar bands. A SS wire (diameter, 0.040 inch) is then attached to the palatal implant, positioned approximately 5 mm apical to the gingival margin of the first molars, passing through the tube and oriented parallel to the occlusal plane. A Ni-Ti open coil spring (length, 2 cm; diameter, 0.045 inch; thickness, 0.010 inch; Leone) is placed between the lock on the wire and the tube in full compression in order to exercise the appropriate force for molar distalization. The amount of force generated following full activation of the coil springs is approximately 200 g per side. After appliance insertion, there is a 3-month healing period to allow completion of osseointegration before the palatal implant is loaded with orthodontic forces. The patient is seen at 1-month intervals for regular checks as well as to activate the appliance by compressing the coil springs using the Gurin locks (3M Unitek, Orthodontic Products, Monrovia, CA, USA), which are attached to the SS wire.

This system allows the application of a consistent force close to the center of resistance of the first molars, resulting in an almost bodily distal movement of the molars. In addition, because stationary anchorage is used, no anchorage loss of the anterior segment with maxillary incisor proclination or increase of the overjet is observed after molar distalization. Furthermore, since no occlusal rests are used, first and second premolars drift distally during maxillary molar distalization.

When molar distalization is completed, the coil springs are removed and the Gurin locks are tightened and fixed to the mesial side of the molar tubes, converting the appliance into a passive anchorage device that can be used to reinforce posterior anchorage during the subsequent stage of anterior teeth retraction with fixed orthodontic appliances.

Either some months before the end of the total orthodontic treatment or during the removal of the fixed orthodontic appliances, the palatal implant is easily removed by loosening it with a hollow drill. The implant site heals rapidly, usually within 5 days.

The implant-supported Keles Slider is effective in correcting Class II malocclusion and in resolving maxillary crowding. Maxillary molars are distalized almost bodily without or with minimal crown tipping and without loss of anchorage of the anterior teeth. No patient cooperation is required beyond maintenance of a good oral hygiene.

IMPLANT-SUPPORTED TRANSPALATAL BAR AND COIL SPRINGS

An efficient indirect orthodontic implant anchorage for molar distalization can be constructed relatively simply in terms of appliance design and without extensive laboratory work. A combined tooth–implant anchoring system can be constructed with a transpalatal bar anchored on a palatal implant and connected to the first or second premolars. When the Orthosystem implant (length, 4.0 mm; diameter, 3.3 mm) is used, the individually manufactured transpalatal bar is attached to the implant by means of a clamping cap featuring an eccentric slot and a fastening screw. Alternatively, the cap and the bar may also be soldered or laser welded. In either case, the transpalatal bar is anchored three dimensionally on the palatal implant and bonded on the palatal surfaces of the first or second premolars bilaterally, incorporating these teeth in the anchorage unit. The distalization force is provided by open coil springs, which are attached on sectional or full archwires positioned vestibularly (Fig. 19.4) or palatally (Fig. 19.5).

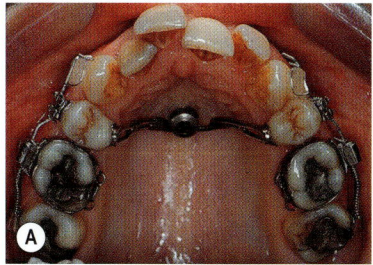 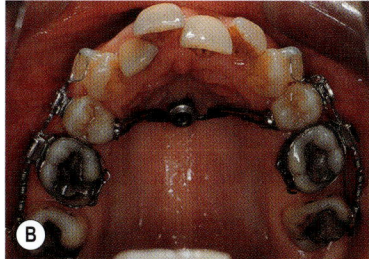 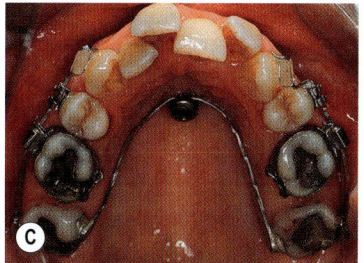 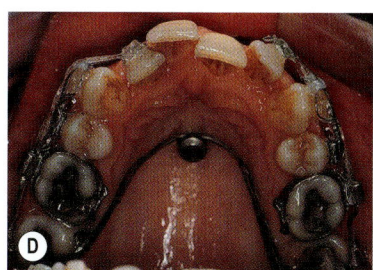

Fig. 19.4 Combination of implant-supported transpalatal bar with vestibular mechanics. (A) Occlusal view of the maxillary arch after median insertion of an endosseous palatal implant of reduced length (Orthosystem). (B) Distalization of the second molars by Nitinol coil springs supported by indirect stationary anchorage. (C) Stabilization of the distalized second molars with a new transpalatal bar attached to the implant and the second molars, and retraction of the first molars with elastomeric chains. (D) Distalization of the first premolars and canines. (Parts B,D from Kinzinger et al., 2005,[10] with permission of Springer.)

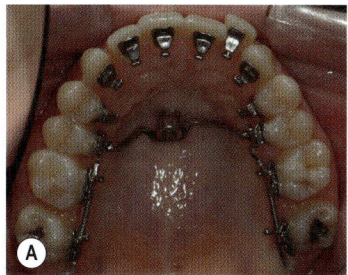 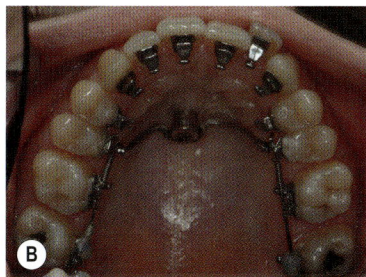 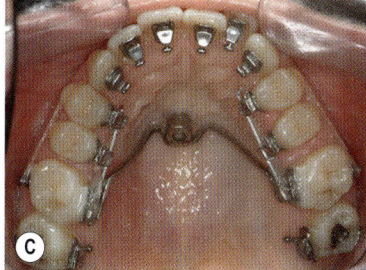 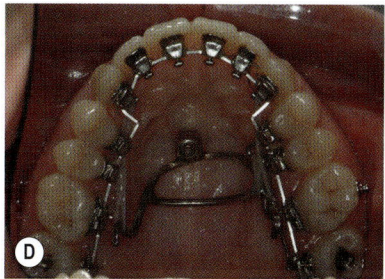

Fig. 19.5 Combination of implant-supported transpalatal bar with palatal mechanics. (A) Occlusal view after median insertion of an endosseous palatal implant of reduced length (Orthosystem). Distalization of the second molars by means of Nitinol coil springs attached to palatal archwires using indirect anchorage. (B) Stabilization of the distalized second molars with composite interlocking. Distalization of the first molars by open coil springs attached between the second molars and first molars. (C) Occlusal view of the maxillary arch after placement of a transpalatal bar with the new one connected to the first molars to support retraction of the lateral teeth. (D) Occlusal view of the maxillary arch during retraction of the anterior teeth. (Parts C,D from Kinzinger et al., 2005,[10] with permission of Springer.)

Table 19.1 Appliance designs for non-compliance maxillary molar distalization featuring orthodontic implants, with their specific characteristics

Appliance	Design and features	Main indications
Mainz Implant Pendulum	Stationary anchorage; skeletonized K-Pendulum appliance and endosseous palatal implant of reduced length Paramedian/median insertion No occlusal rests needed Compatible with various Pendulum appliances Pendulum appliance can be replaced with a TPA after molar distalization	All ages
Aachen Implant Pendulum	Stationary anchorage; Quad Pendulum with an endosseous palatal orthodontic implant of reduced length, supported by a reduced palatal acrylic button Median insertion No occlusal rests needed Compatible with various Pendulum appliances Pendulum appliance can be replaced with a TPA after molar distalization	Adults
Implant-supported Keles Slider	Stationary anchorage; modified Keles Slider with endosseous palatal orthodontic implant Median/paramedian insertion No occlusal rests needed Can be converted into a passive anchorage device after molar distalization	All ages
Implant-supported transpalatal bar with coil springs	Indirect anchorage; endosseous palatal implant connected to the bar Median insertion Transpalatal bar attached (palatally) to first or second premolars bilaterally Compatible with various loaded spring systems Original transpalatal bar can be replaced with a new one after molar distalization	Adults

When the maxillary second molars are erupted, sequential distalization is recommended. Initially, the second molars are distalized while the reciprocally acting forces are absorbed by the anchorage unit incorporating the anchoring teeth and the palatal implant. Following distalization of the second molars, their position is stabilized with a new transpalatal bar connected again with the palatal implant to reinforce posterior anchorage during the subsequent phase of the retraction of the anterior teeth. The initial transpalatal bar is removed and the new one is constructed and attached to the implant and bonded to the distalized second molars. Alternatively, the second molars may be stabilized by composite interlocking, which has the advantage that no transpalatal bar replacement is needed. Finally, the first molars and afterwards the teeth anterior to them can be moved distally along the archwires by means of elastomeric chains or closed coil springs.

CONCLUSIONS

Table 19.1 summarizes the appliances designed for use with orthodontic palatal implants for maxillary molar distalization. Endosseous implants of reduced length inserted into the anterior region of the hard palate provide anchorage that does not result in unwanted mesial proclination of the anterior teeth, which is evident when conventional non-compliance distalization appliances are used. In particular, the combination of palatal implants with Pendulum appliances can be considered as an alternative anchorage design that presents several advantages:

- treatment outcome is not dependent on patient's cooperation
- treatment is possible even with a reduced number of teeth (i.e. with limited dental anchoring capacity of the supporting zone)
- there is no anchorage loss of the anterior dental unit since the anterior teeth are not incorporated in the anchorage unit
- spontaneous distal drifting of the premolars and canines takes place during molar distalization, as well as afterwards, under the pull of the transeptal fibers, since there are no occlusal rests on these teeth
- following molar distalization, the construction of an "active anchorage" of the posterior teeth to support anterior teeth retraction is possible, but usually the appliances connected to the palatal implants are replaced with newly fabricated transpalatal bars connected to molars in order to reinforce posterior anchorage during that stage of treatment.

The disadvantages are that insertion and removal of palatal implants are associated with more complicated and invasive surgical procedures and a higher cost is incurred.

In conclusion, the use of orthodontic implants in conjunction with intraoral non-compliance maxillary molar distalization approaches is a feasible and efficient treatment option that can be applied not only in children and adolescents but also in adults. For this purpose, the use of anchorage designs with orthodontic implants of reduced length seems to be very advantageous compared with use of conventional dental implants.

REFERENCES

1. Kinzinger G, Fuhrmann R, Gross U, et al. Modified pendulum appliance including distal screw and uprighting activation for non-compliance therapy of Class II malocclusion in children and adolescents. J Orofac Orthop 2000;61:175–90.
2. Kinzinger GSM, Wehrbein H, Diedrich PR. Molar distalization with a modified pendulum appliance: in vitro analysis of the force systems and in vivo study in children and adolescents. Angle Orthod 2005;75:484–93.
3. Kinzinger GSM, Diedrich PR. Biomechanics of a modified pendulum appliance: theoretical considerations and in vitro analysis of the force systems. Eur J Orthod 2007;29: 1–7.
4. Kinzinger G, Syree C, Fritz U, et al. Molar distalization with different pendulum appliances: in vitro registration of orthodontic forces and moments in the initial phase. J Orofac Orthop 2004;65:389–409.
5. Kinzinger G, Wehrbein H, Diedrich P. Pendulum appliances with different anchorage modalities for non-compliance molar distal movement in adults. Kieferorthopädie 2004;18:11–24.
6. Byloff FK, Kärcher H, Clar E, et al. An implant to eliminate anchorage loss during molar distalization: a case report involving the Graz implant-supported pendulum. Int J Adult Orthod Orthognath Surg 2000;15:129–37.
7. Brender D, Thole M, Wehrbein H. Skelettale Verankerung in der Kieferorthopädie. Freie Zahnarzt 2004;48:22–8.
8. Kinzinger GSM, Fritz UB, Sander FG, et al. Efficiency of a pendulum appliance for molar distalization related to second and third molar eruption stage. Am J Orthod Dentofacial Orthop 2004;125:8–23.
9. Kinzinger GSM, Gross U, Fritz UB, et al. Anchorage quality of deciduous molars versus premolars for molar distalization with a pendulum appliance. Am J Orthod Dentofacial Orthop 2005;127:314–23.
10. Kinzinger G, Wehrbein H, Byloff FK, et al. Innovative anchorage alternatives for molar distalization: an overview. J Orofac Orthop 2005;66:397–413.
11. Jung BA, Harzer W, Wehrbein H, et al. Immediate versus conventional loading of palatal implants in humans: a first report of a multicenter RCT. Clin Oral Invest 2011;15:495–502.

20

The use of the Straumann Orthosystem as palatal implant in the correction of Class II malocclusion

Adriano Crismani and Michael Bertl

INTRODUCTION

This chapter describes the use of a palatal implant, the Straumann Orthosystem (Institut Straumann, Basel, Switzerland), for treatment of Class II malocclusion.[1]

The implant is a transmucosally placed endosseous titanium screw-type implant with a sandblasted, large-grit, acid-etched surface (see Fig. 7.2). The surface treatment increases implant–bone contact and thus compensates for the implant's reduced length. The implant comprises an endosseous part (length, 4.2 mm; diameter 4.1 or 4.8 mm), a transmucosal neck (length, 1.8 mm; diameter, 4.8 mm) and a threaded orthodontic abutment (length, 3.5 or 5.5 mm; diameter, 4.8 mm).

PALATAL IMPLANTS

Männchen and Schätzle[2] proposed a wide range of indications for the utilization of palatal implants based on the favorable combination of mechanical (cortical) and biochemical (osseointegration) stability (see Chapter 7).

Various factors influence the process of osseointegration, including biocompatibility, design and surface properties of the implant; the volume, structural properties and regenerative capabilities of the surrounding bone; the surgical techniques of preparing the implant bed and insertion; and the timing of functional loading. The process of osseointegration is described in detail in Chapter 4.

The conventional protocol for loading palatal implants suggests a healing period of 3 months before applying any orthodontic load for the maxilla and 6 months for the mandible.[3] However, early loading, defined as the insertion of the restoration (in or out of occlusion) immediately or a few days after implant placement, has been used successfully by a number of clinicians.[4–7] Chapter 4 discusses the evidence for primary and secondary stability of implants with time of loading.

While recent evidence favors early loading protocols for palatal implants, thus shortening overall treatment time, lighter loads or indirect loading may be advisable until the onset of secondary stability and osseointegration.

CONNECTION TO THE PALATAL IMPLANT

Depending on the clinical situation and the orthodontic treatment plan, palatal implants may be loaded directly or indirectly in order to achieve maximum anchorage (see Chapters 7 and 19). Connecting procedures for palatal implants have evolved from prosthodontics-derived transfer impressions involving considerable laboratory input to intraorally bonded adhesive procedures.

The *standard procedure* for connecting the teeth to be stabilized with a palatal implant uses an alginate impression to fabricate a study cast. From this, a custom tray with an occlusal window at the site of the implant (Fig. 20.1) is made at the laboratory and used to create a master cast. The impression coping is screwed on to the implant through this window, a silicon impression is taken (Fig. 20.1B) and the master cast with an implant replica is made at the laboratory. The transpalatal arch (TPA)–palatal implant connector is fabricated by adapting a 1.2 mm SS wire of spring hardness to the palate and soldering it to the implant cap (Fig. 20.1C). Finally, the cap is attached to the implant with a screw and the TPA is bonded to the teeth to be stabilized. Although standard and well established, this procedure needs considerable laboratory input and is considered quite cost and material intensive.[8,9]

A *simpler chair-side procedure* with little laboratory input connects the TPA with the palatal implant using small connectors that are initially soldered to the implant cap and bonded to the TPA. The TPA and connectors are then removed from the mouth and placed in a plaster support for removal of the composite and soldering the connections.[8]

Another *innovative adhesive procedure* avoids the requirement to solder the small connectors to the TPA, thus replacing the time-consuming steps of the approach with a simple bonding technique.[9] Initially, the palatal tubes on the molar bands are opened on the occlusal surfaces with a diamond-studded drill (Fig. 20.2A). A small connector of 0.9 mm SS wire is soldered to the implant cap, which is then placed on the implant and attached with a screw. The wire ends of the small connector should cross the TPA below and are bent from the distal to the mesial above it, thus clasping the TPA (Fig. 20.2B). The area where the small connector crosses the TPA is sandblasted. The TPA is attached to the tubes with 0.010 inch SS ligatures and secured with orthodontic luting composite in order to

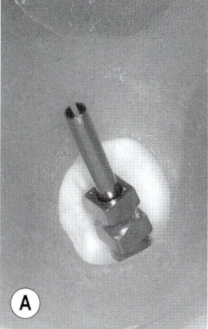
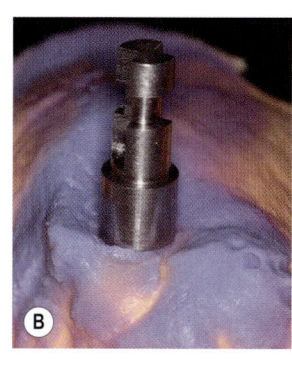
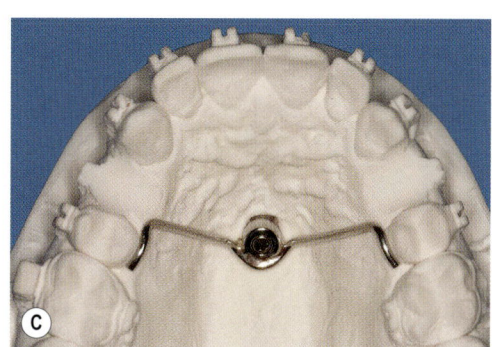

Fig. 20.1 Standard procedure with laboratory and chair-side stages for attaching to an implant. (A) Custom tray with occlusal window and impression coping. (B) Silicon impression with an implant replica. (C) Master cast with the TPA–palatal implant connector soldered to the implant cap.

Fig. 20.2 Adhesive procedure for attaching to an implant. (A) The palatal tubes of the molar bands are opened on the occlusal surfaces. (B) The small connectors bent around the TPA. (C) Bonding of the connectors with the TPA.

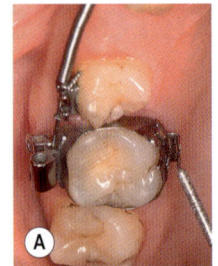
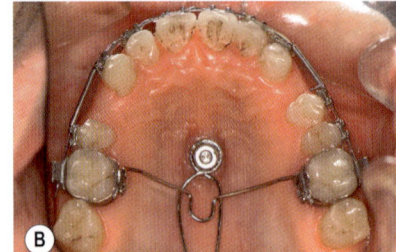
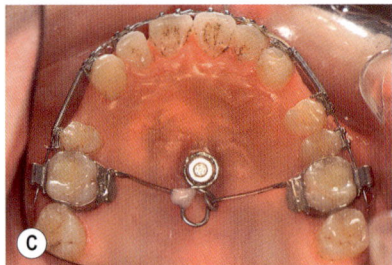

Fig. 20.3 Case 1: unilateral distalization. (A) Pretreatment occlusal intraoral view with the palatal implant providing indirect anchorage for the distalization of the right maxillary molars. (B) After space opening, the right first molar is stabilized with a new TPA and the second premolar is retracted with an elastic chain. (C) Retraction of the right first premolar. (D) Final result.

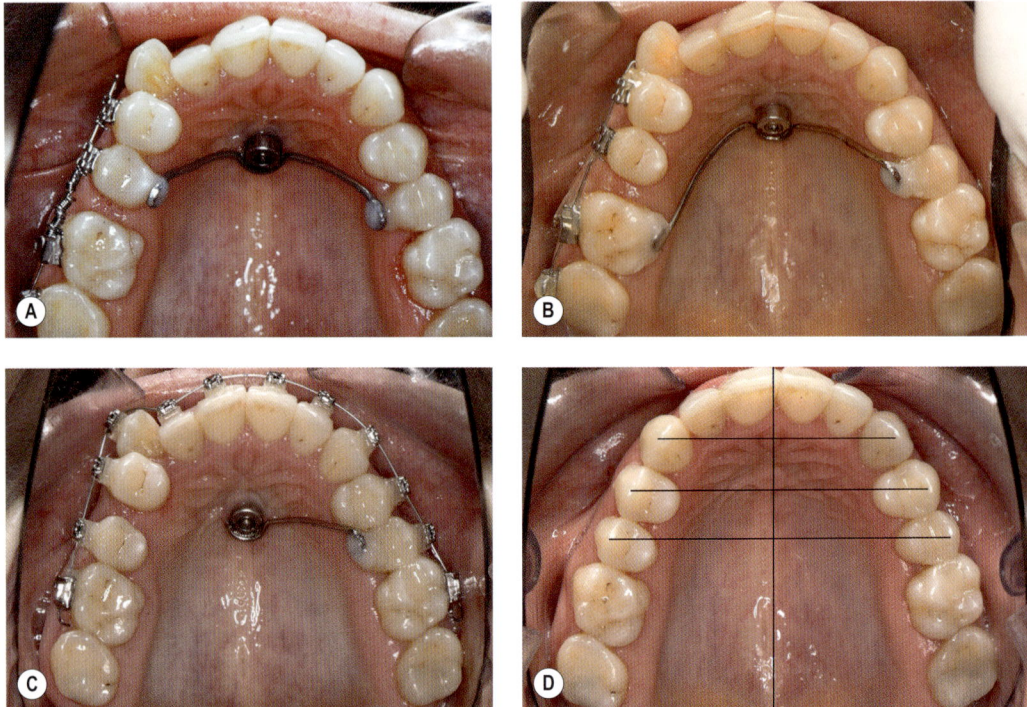

immobilize it for the next step. Metal primer, sealer and composite are applied to the connections and fixed by light curing (Fig. 20.2C). The composite-connected component parts resist breakage up to a mean force of 3323.2 cN and provide absolute stability of the TPA–palatal implant connection in terms of maximum anchorage at forces up to 408.1 cN.[9] These force levels are well within those typically used in orthodontic treatment. In addition, high precision and exact fit are ensured because all the work is carried out intraorally.

While all three methods are comparable in terms of effectiveness and patient comfort, they differ markedly in chair-time and costs. A decision should be made on the basis of local availability of laboratory facilities and ease of integration with patient workflow.

CORRECTION OF CLASS II MALOCCLUSION

Skeletal anchorage techniques have facilitated the decision to opt for a non-extraction treatment, particularly for Class II malocclusion where a Class I relationship of the canines and molars has to be achieved. Distalization of the maxillary teeth is achieved by using palatal implant and a strong connecting wire for a rigid osseous anchorage.

CASE 1: UNILATERAL DISTALIZATION

In this patient, the teeth on the right side of the maxilla were located more mesially than the contralaterals. Because of local crowding, the right

canine was buccally blocked out. Initially, the anterior teeth, including the canines and the teeth in the left quadrant, were left out of treatment. Only four teeth in the right quadrant were bonded (0.018 inch slot system) and a rectangular (0.016 × 0.022 inch) SS wire was engaged. On the palatal side, skeletal anchorage was established using the new adhesive technique with a round SS wire of 1.1 mm, which stabilized the second premolars to the palatal implant. Indirect loading of the implant was carried out with an open coil spring (Sentalloy yellow) positioned between the second premolar and first molar for distalizing the maxillary right first and second molars, delivering a force of 150 cN (Fig. 20.3A).

After successful distalization of the maxillary right first and second molars and subsequent space opening between the second premolar and first molar, anchorage was adapted and a new TPA of 1.1 mm SS was fabricated. By connecting the palatal implant to the right first molar and the left second premolar, the right first molar was anchored in the correct position and the right second premolar was distalized with an elastic chain (Fig. 20.3B).

Following distalization of the right second premolar, a block consisting of the right first molar and second premolar was established, the remaining maxillary teeth were bonded and anchorage was minimized. Again, the distalizing force acting on the right first premolar was introduced by including the blocked-out right canine into the leveling archwire (0.016 inch Sentalloy blue, 100 cN; GAC) (Fig. 20.3C).[9]

After 22 months, the fixed appliances and the palatal implant were removed. At this point the maxillary arch was properly aligned, the right canine was properly incorporated into the arch and symmetry was reinstated (Fig. 20.3D).

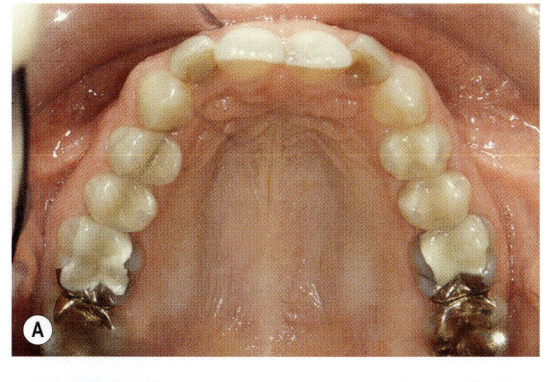
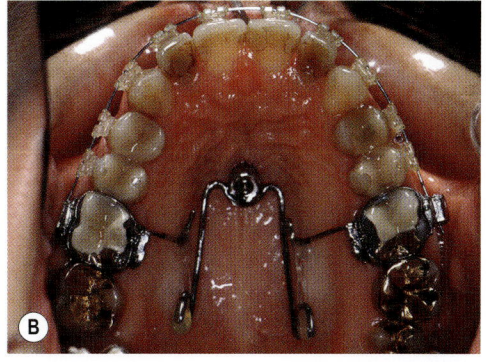
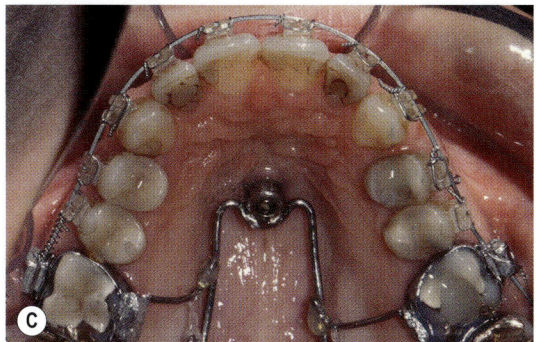
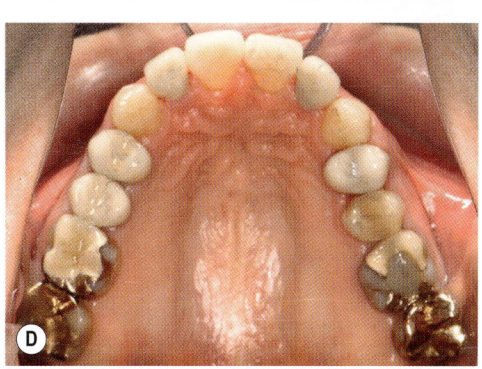

Fig. 20.4 Case 2: bilateral distalization. (A) Pretreatment occlusal view of the maxilla of a patient with Class II division 2 malocclusion, Class II molar relationships and midline deviation. (B) Maxillary molar distalization using a palatal implant and cantilever arms to move the point of force application towards the center of resistance of the molars. (C) Occlusal view after distalization. (D) Post-treatment occlusal view of the maxilla.

CASE 2: BILATERAL DISTALIZATION

This patient had a bilateral Class II molar relationship, an increased overbite, retroclined maxillary incisors, a mandibular midline deviation of 2 mm to the left and mild crowding in both arches (Fig. 20.4A).

The maxillary teeth were bonded (0.018 inch slot system) and the arch leveled. In order to achieve a Class I dentition in this patient, the palatal implant was directly loaded. This means that the distalization force was directly applied between the palatal implant and the first molars, using cantilever arms.[10] Bodily tooth movement was achieved by applying elastic chains (300 cN) between palatal extensions from the implant and cantilever arms attached to the molars' bands, their endings passing close to the centers of resistance (Fig. 20.4B).

By reactivating the force system at each check-up, using new elastic chains (150 cN per tooth), the molars were steadily distalized. Success is evident in Fig. 20.4C, which shows the increased distance between the molar cantilever arms and the palatal implant.

At the end of treatment, a Class I molar relationship was achieved, the overbite was reduced, the crowding resolved and the midlines were corrected (Fig. 20.4D).

CONCLUSIONS

The palatal implant is a valuable and reliable tool to support correction of Class II malocclusions. The introduction of the innovative adhesive technique for connecting the palatal implant with the teeth has simplified the handling of this skeletal anchorage device. From the biomechanical point of view, direct and indirect loading types enable controlled tooth movements in different clinical situations.

REFERENCES

1. Wehrbein H; Merz BR, Diedrich P, et al. The use of palatal implants for orthodontic anchorage. Design and clinical application of the Orthosystem. Clin Oral Implants Res 1996;7:410–16.
2. Männchen R, Schätzle M. Treatment possibilities of different skeletal anchorage systems in view of failures and risk factors. Inf Orthod Kieferorthop 2011;43:111–22.
3. Ganeles J, Wismeijer D. Early and immediately restored and loaded dental implants for single-tooth and partial-arch applications. Int J Oral Maxillofac Implants 2004;19:92–102.
4. Crismani AG, Bernhart T, Schwarz K, et al. Ninety percent success in palatal implants loaded 1 week after placement: a clinical evaluation by resonance frequency analysis. Clin Oral Implants Res 2006;17:445–50.
5. Borsos G, Rudzki-Janson I, Stockmann P, et al. Immediate loading of palatal implants in still-growing patients: a prospective, comparative, clinical pilot study. J Orofac Orthop 2008;69:297–308.
6. Jackson A, Lemke R, Hatch J, et al. A comparison of stability between delayed versus immediately loaded orthodontic palatal implants. J Esthet Restor Dent 2008;20:174–84.
7. Gollner P, Jung BA, Kunkel M, et al. Immediate vs. conventional loading of palatal implants in humans. Clin Oral Implants Res 2009;20:833–7.
8. Crismani AG, Bernhart T, Baier C, et al. Chair-side procedure for connecting transpalatal arches with palatal implants. Eur J Orthod 2002;24:337–42.
9. Crismani AG, Bernhart T, Bantleon HP, et al. An innovative adhesive procedure for connecting transpalatal arches with palatal implants. Eur J Orthod 2005;27:226–30.
10. Sachdeva RCL, Bantleon HP. Cantilever based orthodontics: biomechanical and clinical considerations. In: Sachdeva RCL, Bantleon HP, editors. Orthodontics for the next millennium. Glendora, CA: Ormco; 1997. p. 269–88.

21

Overview of miniplates and zygomatic anchorage for treatment of Class II malocclusion

Ayça Arman Özçırpıcı, Burçak Kaya and Çağla Şar

INTRODUCTION

Miniplates are widely used in maxillofacial surgery as osteosynthesis devices for facial fracture repair and for fixation osteotomies. Miniplates used in the orthodontic practice are modified devices with a connection bar passing through the attached gingiva. They overcome the disadvantages of miniscrew implants (MIs), such as difficulty in finding a suitable site, and can serve as more reliable and long-standing skeletal anchorage units that provide excellent stability. The fixation screws of miniplates can be placed at various regions of the maxilla and mandible (zygomatic buttress or aperture piriformis of the maxilla, posterior cortical bone and symphyseal regions of the mandible; see Chapter 13). Miniplates present however some disadvantages: they are more expensive than MIs, they must be placed by a maxillofacial surgeon in an operating room and both placement and removal may cause swelling and discomfort for the patient.[1]

Minplates have been used for skeletal anchorage for intrusion or distalization of molars, in en masse distalization of the entire dental arch, for buccal segment distalization, for severe skeletal Class III as an alternative to orthognathic surgery or where anchorage teeth are lacking, and to apply orthopedic forces for treatment in both Class II and Class III cases.

A prospective clinical study evaluated maxillary protraction with miniplates in comparison with conventional face-mask therapy and an untreated group.[2] Treatment with miniplate anchorage was more effective in a shorter period of time, eliminating or reducing the undesired effects of conventional face-mask therapy. Miniplates applied laterally to the apertura piriformis region could withstand orthopedic forces of 400–500 g, showing a 93% success rate. Only 2 out of 30 miniplates had to be replaced by an additional surgery. This success is important as the face-mask elastics apply a force vector that can pull miniplate screws out of bone.

Class II malocclusion results from combinations of skeletal and dental components: facial structure, maxillary and mandibular growth patterns and dentoalveolar development. The etiology may include maxillary prognathism, maxillary dental protrusion, mandibular retrognathism, mandibular dental retrusion or any combination of these (see Chapter 1). Accompanying vertical and transversal problems involving the undereruption or overeruption of the anterior or posterior teeth, maxillomandibular rotation and maxillary transverse deficiency can also contribute to the severity of the problem. Differential diagnosis is critical for preparing a problem-based treatment plan.[3] Miniplates can be valuable tools in Class II treatment as they have the advantages of stability and durability even under high orthopedic forces as well as ease of placement at different anatomic locations.

This chapter summarizes the use of miniplate anchorage for the treatment of Class II malocclusion.

TREATMENT OPTIONS

Treatment of Class II malocclusion resulting from maxillary dental protrusion is based on retraction of the maxillary dentition either by buccal segment distalization without extractions or by retraction of the maxillary anterior dentition following maxillary premolar extractions. In maxillary prognathism, the treatment protocol is based on inhibiting the sagittal and downward growth of the maxilla by using extraoral traction during the growth period. Both require adequate extraoral or intraoral anchorage mechanics.[3] Chapters 1 and 2 cover in detail the various methods available for treatment of Class II malocclusion including the various types of intraoral molar distalization devices, their mode of action and the indications for their use.

The move to use implant-supported intraoral molar distalization systems attempted to avoid issues such as mesialization of maxillary premolars, protrusion of maxillary incisors and increase in overjet, which all occur when teeth provide the anchorage. No matter which biomechanical appliance configuration is used, all implant-supported molar distalization appliances obtain anchorage from palatal implants, thus allowing molars to be distalized without anchorage loss of the premolars and incisors. Nevertheless, preventing reciprocal teeth movements is not enough to correct Class II buccal relationship. The maxillary premolars and canines can only be minimally distalized parallel to molar distalization when using palatal implant-supported molar distalization systems, which results in a need for a significant amount of premolar distalization in the subsequent phase of treatment.[4–7]

The use of dentoalveolar MIs with sliding mechanics allowed the segmental distalization of all posterior teeth on rigid archwires: known as buccal segment distalization. Despite the ability to distalize all maxillary posterior teeth together, the distalization obtained using alveolar MIs is limited since the MIs are inserted between the roots of the maxillary posterior teeth on the buccal or palatal side. This type of MI, which has to be of small diameter and have a relatively small surface in contact with the alveolar bone, is relatively fragile and can only withstand low forces: a maximum of 200 g for a MI of diameter 1.2 mm and length 8 mm.[8]

MINIPLATE ZYGOMA ANCHORAGE

Zygoma anchors are miniplates placed on the zygomatico-maxillary buttress and fixed to the bone with two or more miniscrews. Different designs have been introduced by manufacturers, each with its own clinical advantages. Some miniplates are fabricated in I-, T- or Y-shapes for the zygoma anchor to increase stability, while others have modified head sections, which are exposed to the oral cavity, for better control of orthodontic forces.[9–17] The zygoma anchors offer several advantages, particularly in the treatment of patients having severe maxillary protrusion with accompanying vertical problems, either open bite or deep bite.

Zygoma plates are positioned at a safe distance from the roots of the maxillary molars and do not limit the amount of distalization of maxillary posterior teeth as is the case with alveolar MIs.

BUCCAL SEGMENT DISTALIZATION

The use of zygoma anchors for maxillary buccal segment distalization in non-growing patients by Sugawara et al.[11] achieved an average of 3.78 mm crown and 3.20 mm root distalization of the molars, which can be considered as an almost bodily translation. Elastic chains were attached from the maxillary first premolar brackets to the hooks of the zygoma anchors, and

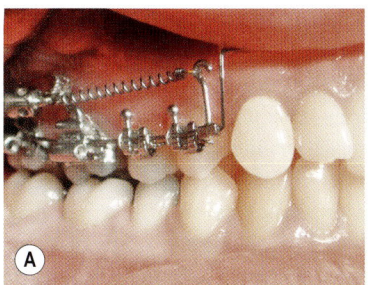 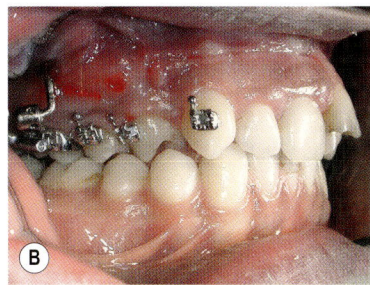

Fig. 21.1 Application of the zygoma anchorage system for buccal segment distalization. (A) During distalization. (B) After distalization.

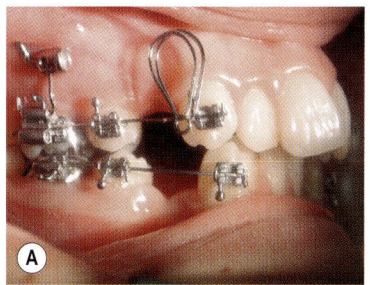 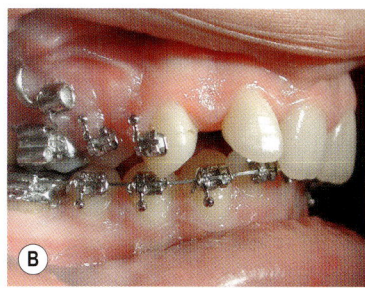

Fig. 21.2 Indirect anchorage reinforcement with zygoma anchors. (A) During canine distalization with a Paul Gjessing spring. (B) After upper maxillary premolar extraction and canine distalization.

the maxillary buccal segments were distalized using sliding mechanics on continuous archwires. The authors noted that when a two-stage procedure is used, with the maxillary first molars initially distalized with an intraoral molar distalization appliance, it is difficult to maintain the distalized position of the molars during the second stage. Therefore, they considered that the distalization obtained with zygoma anchors should be evaluated as true molar distalization since there is no second stage involving retraction of maxillary premolars and anterior teeth that could result in a mesial movement of the maxillary first molars.

In our prospective clinical study sliding mechanics on SS continuous archwires (0.016 × 0.022 inch) were used with anterior bends to achieve maxillary buccal segment distalization (Fig. 21.1A).[9] An average of 4.5–5 mm distalization of all maxillary premolars and molars (maximum 7.5 mm distal movement) was obtained (Fig. 21.1B). This was greater than seen in other implant-supported distalization systems,[4–8,11] which could be attributed to the dental characteristics of the subjects in our study, as most started treatment with a full unit Class II buccal relationship and needed substantial distalization. One of the biggest advantages of the zygoma plates in our experience is that they can be used in the treatment of full step or even more severe Class II relationship as they allow distalization of all posterior teeth.[9]

The force applied on the zygoma plates in our study[9] was approximately twice that achieved with the alveolar MIs in a similar buccal segment distalization method (450 g and 200 g, respectively).[8] This increased distalization force can be achieved because each zygoma anchor is fixed to the dense bone structure of the zygomatico-maxillary buttress with three miniscrews of 2.3 mm diameter and 7 mm in length.[9] Being able to apply high distalization forces, similar to those achieved with cervical headgear,[11] is an important advantage of zygoma anchors. It gives the option of treating patients with severe maxillary skeletal or dentoalveolar protrusion without maxillary premolar extraction or possibly orthognathic surgery.

CANINE DISTALIZATION IN EXTRACTION TREATMENT

Zygoma anchors can be used for reinforcing posterior anchorage in extraction treatment of Class II where maximum anchorage is required. A zygoma anchorage system was used for orthodontic treatment in maxillary first premolar extraction requiring unilateral or bilateral maximum anchorage.[10] The zygoma anchor consisted of an I-shaped miniplate with three screw holes continuing with a round bar and a cylindrical fixation unit at the end. The specially designed cylindrical fixation unit had a vertical slot to place an auxiliary wire (0.032 × 0.032 inch maximum size) and a small locking screw inside the cylinder to fix the wire. A unique power arm fitted in the vertical slot of the maxillary canine bracket with a hook at the end of the arm situated at the canine's center of resistance. Maxillary canines were distalized on continuous archwires using sliding mechanics with Ni-Ti closed coil springs attached between the power arms on the canine bracket and the zygoma anchors. The distalization force applied was

50–100 g and the canines moved distally at an average of 1.14 mm per month.[10]

Zygoma anchorage has been used for orthodontic treatment in maxillary first premolar extraction demanding bilateral maximum anchorage.[18] A passive SS wire (0.017 × 0.025 inch) was placed starting at the vertical slot of the fixation unit of the anchor plate and ending at the auxiliary tube of the maxillary first molar band. This connected the maxillary molars to the zygoma anchors for reinforced anchorage. The maxillary canines were distalized on sectional SS archwires (0.016 × 0.022 inch) with Paul Gjessing (PG) springs between the maxillary canines and second premolars (Fig. 21.2A). A distalization force of 100–150 g was applied with each activation of the PG spring, which was reactivated every 4 weeks. An average of 5.5 mm canine distalization was obtained with only 0.6 mm anchorage loss at the molars, the canines moving distally at an average of 1.20 mm per month (Fig. 21.2B).[18] The advantage of the system described here is that the zygoma anchors were used as indirect anchorage, which is reported to be more stable and less likely to fail.

ANTERIOR SEGMENT OR EN MASSE RETRACTION

Zygoma anchors can also be used as anchorage for the retraction of maxillary anterior teeth in both extraction and non-extraction treatment of Class II malocclusion. Retraction can be performed smoothly with either a two-stage or en masse mechanics using the zygoma anchors as an absolute anchorage unit. As all of the maxillary teeth can be retracted together, the treatment time can be significantly decreased, which is a major advantage.

Maxillary incisors were retruded, overjet was decreased and canine relationship was corrected to Class I using a zygoma anchorage system after a maxillary first premolar extraction.[19] After canine distalization, the patient was instructed to attach intraoral elastics between the zygoma anchor hooks and crimpable hooks placed mesial to lateral brackets.

Zygoma anchorage has been used for en masse retraction of the maxillary anterior segment to correct excessive overjet and increased lip strain during closure.[12] Following extraction of the maxillary first premolars, zygoma anchors were placed and the maxillary six anterior teeth were bonded. An archwire with vertical steps distal to the canine brackets, followed by loops, was bent. The archwire passed through the buccal vestibule and entered the head of the zygoma anchors. A retraction force of 150 g was applied bilaterally with coil springs attached from the loops to the zygoma anchors.

A similar correction of excessive overjet and increased lip strain during closure used zygoma anchors for secondary treatment of an adult who had already had the maxillary first premolars extracted, so first premolar extraction was not a treatment option to gain the appropriate space for anterior teeth retraction.[15] The maxillary second molars were distalized on posterior segmental wires by an open coil spring placed between the first and second molars. Afterwards, a continuous archwire was placed to retract all maxillary teeth with sliding mechanics. The authors emphasized that the use of zygoma anchors provided absolute anchorage and enabled different treatment options that avoided a need for space creation through extraction or the use of extraoral anchorage devices such as headgear.[15] The only treatment alternative would have been orthognathic surgery, which the patient did not want. In our opinion, retraction of the entire maxillary arch using zygoma anchors was the best, and possibly the only, treatment option for this patient.[15]

In our study comparing zygoma anchorage with cervical headgear in buccal segment distalization, maxillary buccal segment distalization was obtained with the zygoma anchorage system.[9] Maxillary premolars and molars were leveled at the beginning and then distalized segmentally on continuous SS archwires (0.016 × 0.022 inch) with a vertical step-up bend at the anterior region. Distalization force was applied on each side with Ni-Ti closed coil springs from the zygoma anchors to the crimpable hooks placed mesial to the first premolar brackets. During this buccal segment distalization stage, no orthodontic force was applied to the canines and incisors. However, at the end of this stage, the maxillary canines, which were initially in Class II relationship or in high vestibule position, moved to Class I relationship. In addition, maxillary incisors were retroclined and retruded with an average of 2.7 mm, under the pull of the transeptal gingival fibers, and overjet was decreased as a result.[9] In the second stage, maxillary anterior teeth did not require any retraction and were only leveled, while the distalized posterior teeth were retained in place with ligature wires tied between the zygoma anchors and maxillary first molars.

Based on evidence presented in the literature and our clinical experience, we consider that zygoma anchor plates have proven to be stable and reliable anchorage units for maxillary anterior retraction. In addition, the option of en masse maxillary retraction via zygoma anchorage has the advantage of shortening treatment time significantly.

CONTROLLING THE VERTICAL COMPONENT OF THE FORCE VECTOR WITH ZYGOMA ANCHORS

With zygoma anchors it is possible to control the vertical component of the distalization or retraction force vector. Vertical position of the posterior and anterior teeth can be altered by changing the direction and application point of force vectors. The vertical component of the retrusion force vector applied from the zygoma anchors to the maxillary teeth can be modified easily by using crimpable power hooks of different lengths (Fig. 21.3).

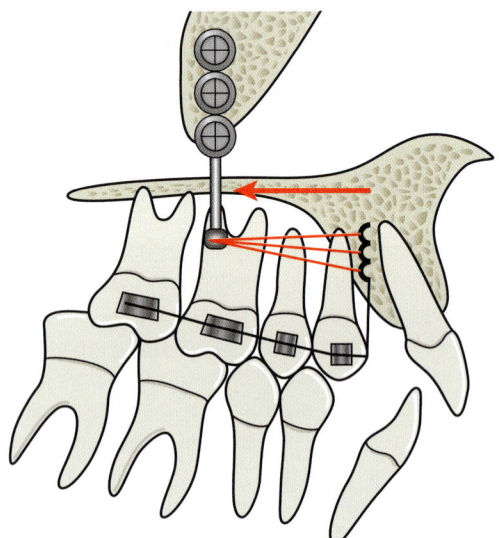

Fig. 21.3 The vertical component of the distalization or retraction force vectors applied from the zygoma anchors can be controlled by using crimpable hooks with different lengths.

The ideal position for exposing zygoma anchors to the oral cavity is the keratinized gingiva or mucogingival junction, which is clearly higher than the maxillary teeth crowns and brackets,[20] and so a retrusion force vector applied away from the brackets with a long hook will pass above the center of resistance of the teeth and result in mesial or anterior rotation. This kind of force vector can be an advantage when treating patients with gummy smile or deep bite, in which extrusion or retroclination of the maxillary anterior teeth is contraindicated. In contrast, applying the retrusion force vector at the same level as the zygoma anchors with a long hook will cause the force vector to approach the center of resistance of the teeth, resulting in an almost bodily parallel movement with translation. This parallel force vector can be preferred in the treatment of patients who do not require vertical tooth movements at the maxillary anterior segment. This was the case in our study described above,[9] where the neck of the zygoma anchor and the crimpable hook were at the same level. No vertical movement or tipping was observed at the premolars where the force was applied and only a minor distal tipping of 5° with no significant vertical movement was perceived at the molars. This was more advantageous than the movement seen with the other implant-supported molar distalization systems.[4–7] The counterclockwise moment force applied to the buccal segment by the closed coil springs was thought to be the reason for the unchanged inclination or minor mesial tipping observed at the premolars.[9]

Because of variations in the thickness of the attached gingiva and morphology of the infrazygomatic crest, it is not always possible to expose the zygoma anchors through the ideal region.[20] The position of the miniplates on the zygomatic buttress can be changed under these circumstances but potential complications that must be considered include contact between the head of the zygoma anchor and brackets, damage to the buccal fat pad, hypertrophy of the buccal mucosa from irritation and injury to adjacent teeth roots. In addition, modifying the position of the zygoma anchor may alter the direction and magnitude of the orthodontic force. The availability of zygoma plates in variable lengths may help to overcome these problems.[20]

One design of zygoma anchor was developed to facilitate application and control of orthodontic force vectors.[11] The subperiosteal body portion is a V-shaped titanium miniplate with three miniscrew holes. The transmucosal arm portion has three possible lengths (short, 6.5 mm; medium, 9.5 mm; long, 12.5 mm) to compensate for individual morphological differences. The head portion has three continuous hooks to adjust the direction and application point of orthodontic force vectors. The anchor plate characteristics can be altered to fit the distance between the implantation site and the dentition, thus allowing retrusion force vectors with individual vertical components based on the patient's needs.[11]

Zygoma anchors can also be used to control the anteroposterior rotation of occlusal and mandibular planes (Fig. 21.4).[13] A zygoma anchor with a special appliance was designed to impact the maxillary posterior teeth. The appliance consisted of bilateral acrylic resin bite blocks connected by palatal arches and buccal wire attachments. Coil springs were attached to the buccal wire attachments and extended to the zygoma anchors, creating an intrusive force of 400 g. Because of the impaction of the maxillary molars, the mandibular plane showed counterclockwise autorotation and overjet decreased as a result.[13] This system has also been used in individuals presenting skeletal Class II relationship with increased overjet, anterior open bite and vertical growth pattern with increased lower anterior facial height. A 3.6 mm intrusion of the maxillary first molars led to changes in the cephalometric angles: an increase of 1.8° in SNB, plus a decrease in ANB of 1.5° and SN-GoGn of 3°. There was a decrease of 2.9 mm in the lower anterior facial height.[14]

A patient with a convex profile, increased overjet and open bite was treated with osteotomy-assisted maxillary posterior impaction with zygoma anchorage.[16] The vertical osteotomy cuts were performed mesial to the first

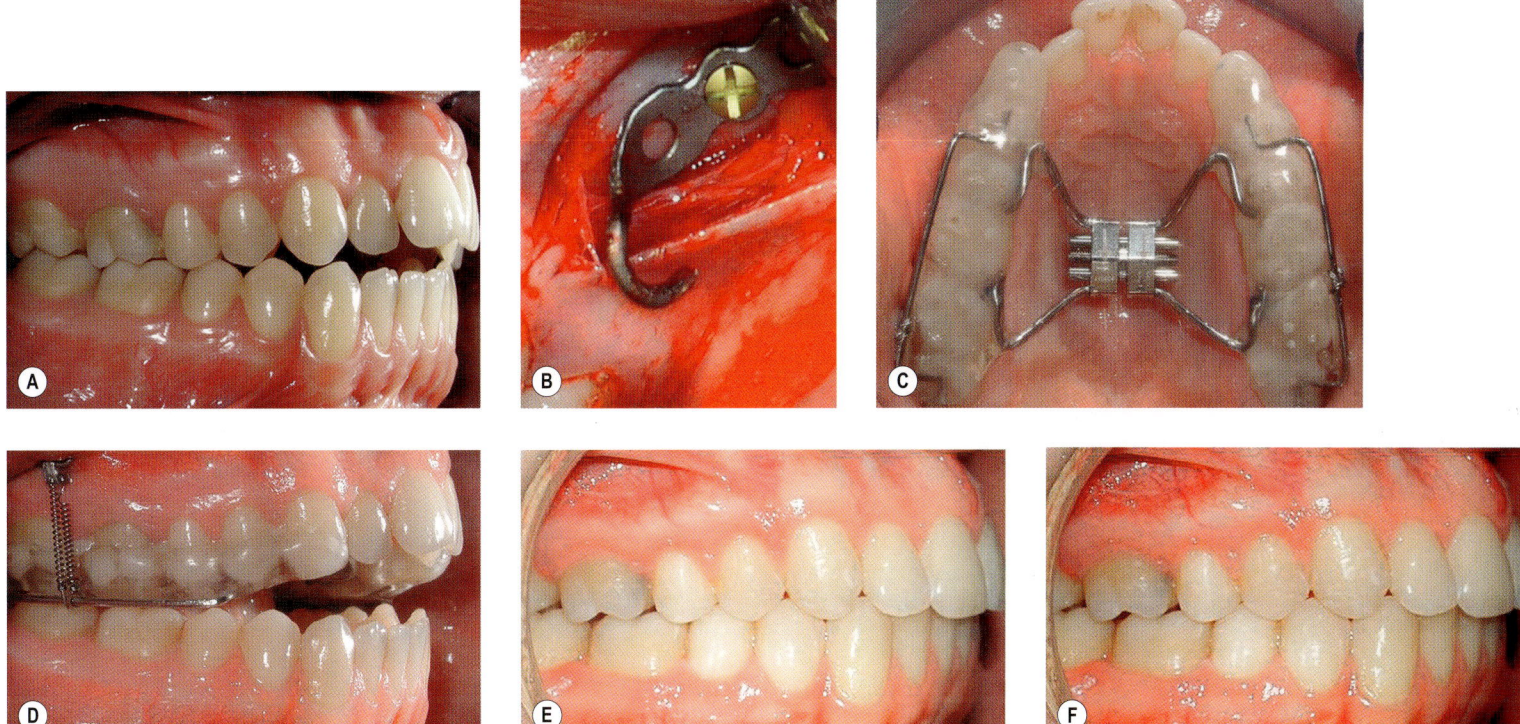

Fig. 21.4 A 22-year-old patient with skeletal Class II malocclusion with open bite. (A) Pre-retreatment. (B) The miniplate bent and prepared for zygomatic anchorage after surgical insertion. (C) Acrylic appliance used for maxillary posterior intrusion with zygoma anchors. (D) An intrusive force of 400 g applied with Ni-Ti closed coil springs extending from the zygoma anchors to the buccal wire attachments of the appliance. (E) Lateral intraoral view after 16 months of treatment. (F) Lateral intraoral view 5 years later. Advancement genioplasty surgery was also performed after the treatment. (Courtesy of Professor Nejat Erverdi, Department of Orthodontics, Faculty of Dentistry, Marmara University, Istanbul, Turkey.)

molars and distal to the second molars while the horizontal osteotomy cut was performed above the apices of the molars on the buccal and palatal alveolar bone. An intrusive force of 250 g was applied by coil springs from the zygoma anchors to the maxillary first and second molar buccal tubes. At the end of the orthodontic treatment, a 4 mm intrusion of the maxillary first and second molars had been achieved. This created a 2° increase in the SNB angle, a 1° decrease in the ANB angle, a 3° decrease in the SN-MP angle, and 3 mm decrease in the lower anterior facial height.[16]

Although MIs can be used as anchorage for en masse retraction, there is a significant correlation between MI failure rate and increased mandibular plane angle;[21] consequently, miniplates may offer a better approach in patients with a high mandibular plane angle. Moreover, the stability and durability of MIs under multidirectional forces is less clear at present. By comparison, zygoma anchors can be used efficiently for both the intrusion of maxillary molars and the en masse retraction of the maxillary anterior segment simultaneously in patients with Class II high mandibular plane angle. A proper occlusion and correction of a convex profile can easily be achieved with retraction of the maxillary dentition and anterosuperior rotation of the mandible at the same time. The system can also be used for the preprosthetic orthodontic rehabilitation in adults presenting sagittal and vertical dentofacial discrepancies (Fig. 21.5).

The vertical control mechanism to intrude posterior teeth with miniplates can be applied at both maxillary and mandibular molar regions.[22] Consequently, miniplate anchorage can be used successfully in patients with Class II high-angle vertical growth pattern plus increased mandibular plane angles to obtain anterosuperior rotation in the mandible as well as to eliminate disto-occlusion with the accompanying convex profile. Hence, the effectively applied multidirectional retraction and intrusion biomechanics can be used in severe cases as an alternative to orthognathic surgery.

ORTHOPEDIC AND SOFT TISSUE CORRECTION WITH ZYGOMA ANCHORS

Palatal implant-supported systems can be used for the dental correction of Class II malocclusions; however, no skeletal or soft tissue improvements are achieved.[4–7] In contrast, maxillary buccal segment distalization with zygoma anchorage systems does also allow significant skeletal and soft tissue correction as the skeletal and soft tissue structures naturally follow the dentoalveolar structures, for example a 0.8 mm distal movement of point A (position of deepest concavity on anterior profile of maxilla), a 1.3° decrease of SNA angle and 0.86 mm upper lip retrusion.[9]

The skeletal and soft tissue improvements obtained with zygoma anchorage are only matched by those achieved with use of cervical or occipital headgear.

FUNCTIONAL TREATMENT OF MANDIBULAR RETROGNATHISM WITH MINIPLATE ANCHORAGE

Mandibular skeletal retrusion seems to be the major contributing factor in Class II malocclusions and the ideal correction is to alter the amount and/or direction of growth of the mandible. The main treatment for this purpose is functional appliance therapy in growing patients. The hallmark of Class II functional appliances is the construction bite, which provokes an anterior displacement of the mandible, inducing muscle stretching with the aim of stimulating condylar growth for supplementary lengthening of the mandible.[23] Functional appliances, including a range of removable (activator, bionator, Twin Block) and fixed (Herbst, Jasper Jumper, Forsus) appliances, are used to alter the position of the mandible

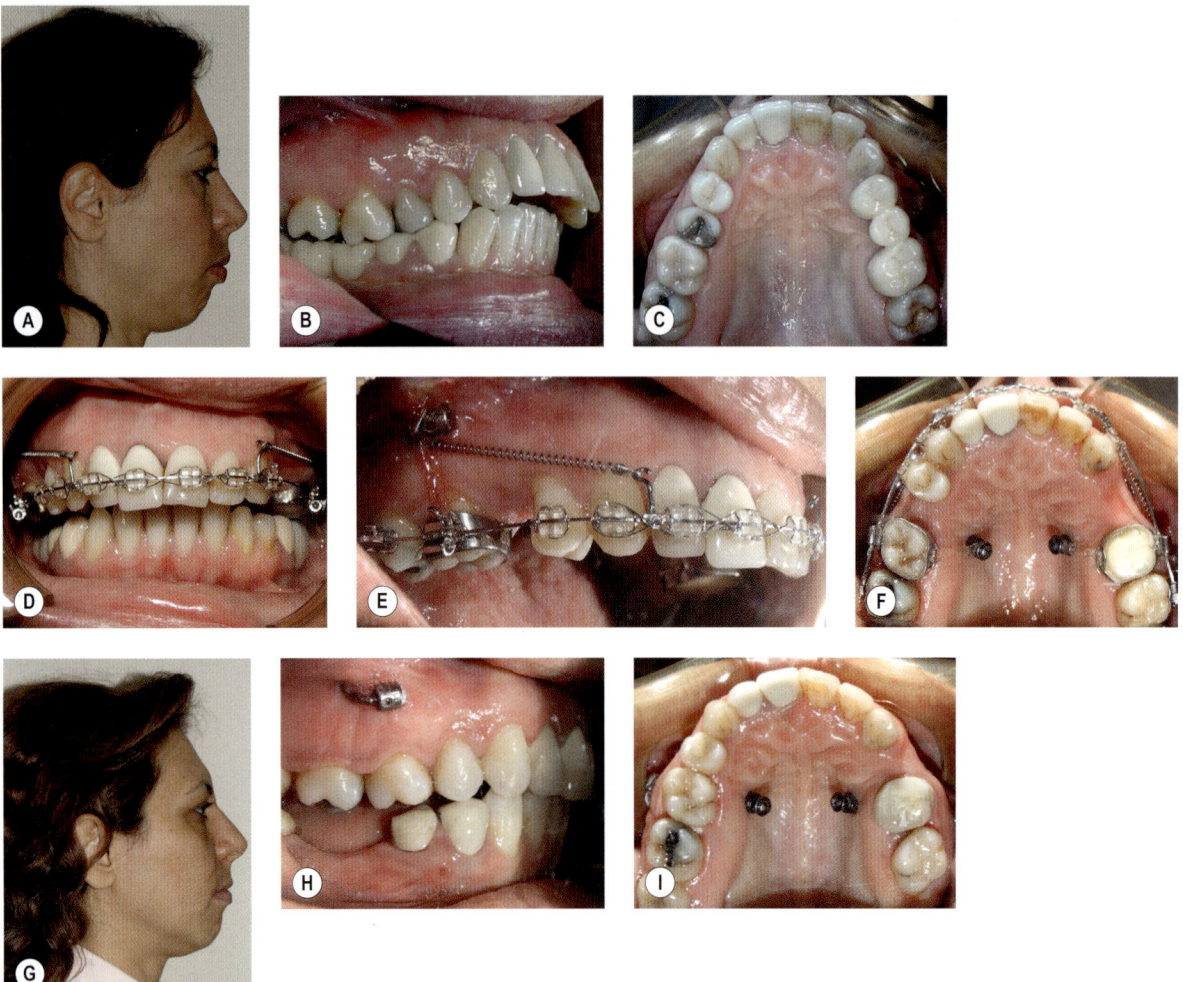

Fig. 21.5 A woman with Class II high mandibular plane angle whose main complaint was that she was unable to close her mouth properly and wrinkles appeared on her chin when she tried to close her lips. Maxillary molars were extruded before the prosthetic rehabilitation of the previously lower edentulous posterior regions. (A–C) Pretreatment extraoral (A), intraoral lateral (B) and occlusal (C) views. Note the severe extrusion of the upper right posterior region causing a deviated occlusal plane and asymmetric smile, plus an inappropriate prosthodontic restoration at the mandibular right region. (D–F) After extraction of upper maxillary right second premolar and upper maxillary left first premolar, and alignment of the teeth, zygoma anchors and palatal miniscrew implants (MIs) were inserted. Elastic chains from both miniplates and the palatal MIs were used to obtain posterior intrusion, while Ni-Ti closed coil springs were used for en masse retraction of the anterior segment simultaneously. (G–I) Extraoral (G), intraoral lateral (H) and occlusal (I) views after 23 months of fixed appliance treatment, which achieved 4 mm maxillary molar intrusion, 7 mm en masse retraction of the maxillary anterior teeth and 9 mm decrease in overjet. Intrusion of the maxillary molars led to a significant autorotation of the mandible causing a 4 mm decrease of the lower facial height and a 2° decrease of the ANB angle. Appropriate vertical spaces for the fixed prosthodontic restorations were also obtained. Afterwards, the patient received advancement genioplasty surgery and prosthodontic restoration for her complete dental rehabilitation.

in both sagittal and vertical planes. Although functional appliances are still considered the best option for treatment of mandibular retrognathism, it is less clear from the literature as to their efficacy.[24,25] A systematic review found the Herbst to be the most effective functional appliance, with a monthly mandibular length increase of 0.28 mm, followed by the Twin Block (0.23 mm), bionator (0.17 mm), activator (0.12 mm) and Frankel (0.09 mm).[26] It has been claimed that most of the correction with functional appliances is from dentoalveolar changes, with only a small amount from skeletal effects.[27,28]

Skeletal anchorage with MIs might provide a solution to overcome the undesired dentoalveolar effects of functional appliances and to increase the amount of mandibular advancement. However, functional fixed appliances exert a heavy force vector and moment that could force MIs out of bone. Miniplates applied to the posterior region of the mandible might serve as more stable anchorage sources. Alternatively, four miniplates (two at the angulus area and two at the apertura piriformis region) could be used.

One study has examined the skeletal and dental effects of the Jasper Jumper applied between maxillary molar tubes and miniplates inserted in the symphyseal region in seven patients (mean age, 13.75 years) and compared the results with those for eight patients who received conventional Jasper Jumper treatment.[29] The miniplates were successful throughout the study period without causing any discomfort or complications, but the combination of Jasper Jumper and miniplates did not produce the expected skeletal results and had no significant effect on growth of the mandible in the sagittal direction. It was suggested that a more rigid fixed functional appliance such as the Herbst appliance or the Forsus Fatigue Resistant Device symphyseal miniplate anchorage might be more effective (Fig. 21.6).

CONCLUSIONS

Miniplates can be used effectively for the treatment of Class II malocclusion resulting from different maxillomandibular skeletal and dentoalveolar components. Ideal treatments for different types of discrepancy can be applied effectively by changing the place, shape and size of the miniplates as well as the force application protocol. With their stability and durability,

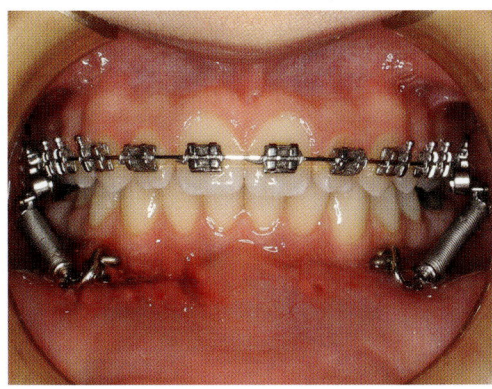

Fig. 21.6 Application of the Forsus Fatigue Resistant Device with symphyseal miniplate anchorage.

miniplates provide an effective treatment alternative to orthognathic surgery and for severe malocclusion.

ACKNOWLEDGMENTS

The authors wish to thank to Drs. Zahire Sahinoglu, Ipek Coskun, Alev Yılmaz, Omur Polat-Ozsoy, Bulem Yuzugullu and Neslihan Arhun for their valuable contributions.

REFERENCES

1. Cornelis MA, Scheffler NR, Nyssen-Behets C, et al. Patients' and orthodontists' perceptions of miniplates used for temporary skeletal anchorage: a prospective study. Am J Orthod Dentofacial Orthop 2008;133:18–24.
2. Şar C, Arman-Ozcirpici A, Uckan S, et al. Comparative evaluation of maxillary protraction with or without skeletal anchorage. Am J Orthod Dentofacial Orthop 2011;139:636–49.
3. Kulbersh R, Pangrazio-Kulbersh V. Treatment of Class II malocclusions. In: English JD, Peltomaki T, Pham-Litschel K, editors. Mosby's orthodontic review. St. Louis, MO: Mosby-Elsevier; 2009. p. 152–77.
4. Mannchen R. A new supra-construction for palatal orthodontic implants. J Clin Orthod 1999;33:373–82.
5. Byloff FK, Karcher H, Clar E, et al. An implant to eliminate anchorage loss during molar distalization: a case report involving the Graz implant-supported pendulum. Int J Adult Orthod Orthognath Surg 2000;15:129–37.
6. Karaman AI, Basciftci FA, Polat O. Unilateral distal molar movement with an implant-supported distal jet appliance. Angle Orthod 2002;72:167–74.
7. Keles A, Erverdi N, Sezen S. Bodily distalization of molars with absolute anchorage. Angle Orthod 2003;73:471–82.
8. Park H, Lee S, Kwon O. Group distal movement of teeth using microscrew implant anchorage. Angle Orthod 2005;75:510–17.
9. Kaya B, Arman A, Uckan S, et al. The comparison of zygoma anchorage system with cervical headgear in buccal segment distalization. Eur J Orthod 2009;31:417–24.
10. De Clerck H, Geerinckx V, Siciliano S. The zygoma anchorage system. J Clin Orthod 2002;36:455–9.
11. Sugawara J, Kanzaki R, Takahashi I, et al. Distal movement of maxillary molars in non-growing patients with the skeletal anchorage system. Am J Orthod Dentofacial Orthop 2006;129:723–33.
12. Erverdi N, Acar A. Zygomatic anchorage for en masse retraction in the treatment of severe Class II division 1. Angle Orthod 2005;75:483–90.
13. Erverdi N, Usumez S, Solak A. New generation open-bite treatment with zygomatic anchorage. Angle Orthod 2006;76:519–26.
14. Erverdi N, Usumez S, Solak A, et al. Noncompliance open-bite treatment with zygomatic anchorage. Angle Orthod 2007;77:86–90.
15. Tanaka E, Nishi-Sasaki A, Hasegawa T, et al. Skeletal anchorage for orthodontic correction of severe maxillary protrusion after previous orthodontic treatment. Angle Orthod 2008;78:181–8.
16. Tuncer C, Ataç MS, Tuncer BB, et al. Osteotomy assisted maxillary posterior impaction with miniplate anchorage. Angle Orthod 2008;78:737–44.
17. Veziroglu F, Uckan S, Ozden UA, et al. Stability of zygomatic plate-screw orthodontic anchorage system: a finite element analysis. Angle Orthod 2008;78:902–7.
18. Cetinsahin A, Dincer M, Arman-Ozcirpici A, et al. Effects of zygoma anchorage system on canine retraction. Eur J Orthod 2010;32:505–13.
19. Bengi AO, Karacay S, Akin E, et al. Use of zygomatic anchors during rapid canine distalization: a preliminary case report. Angle Orthod 2006;76:137–47.
20. Eroglu T, Kaya B, Cetinsahin A, et al. Success of zygomatic plate-screw anchorage system. J Oral Maxillofac Surg 2010;68:602–5.
21. Miyawaki S, Koyama I, Inoue M, et al. Factors associated with the stability of titanium screws placed in the posterior region for orthodontic anchorage. Am J Orthod Dentofacial Orthop 2003;124:373–8.
22. Sugawara J, Baik UB, Umemori M, et al. Treatment and posttreatment dentoalveolar changes following intrusion of mandibular molars with application of a skeletal anchorage system (SAS) for openbite correction. Int J Adult Orthod Orthognath Surg 2002;17:243–53.
23. Moore RN, Igel KA, Boice PA. Vertical and horizontal components of functional appliance therapy. Am J Orthod Dentofacial Orthop 1989;96:433–43.
24. Toth LR, McNamara JA Jr. Treatment effects produced by the twin-block appliance and the Fr-2 appliance of Frankel compared with an untreated Class II sample. Am J Orthod Dentofacial Orthop 1999;116:597–609.
25. Ruf S, Baltromejus S, Pancherz H. Effective condylar growth and chin position in activator treatment: a cephalometric roentgenographic study. Angle Orthod 2001;71:4–11.
26. Cozza P, Baccetti T, Franchi L, et al. Mandibular changes produced by functional appliances in Class II malocclusion: a systematic review. Am J Orthod Dentofacial Orthop 2006;129:599.
27. Janson GR, Toruno JL, Martins DR, et al. Class II treatment effects of the Frankel appliance. Eur J Orthod 2003;25:301–9.
28. Konik M, Panherz H, Hansen K. The mechanism of Class II correction in late Herbst treatment. Am J Orthod Dentofacial Orthop 1997;112:87–91.
29. Gazivekili C. The cephalometric evaluation of Jasper Jumper appliance in conjunction with skeletal bone anchorage in skeletal Class II cases with mandibular retrognathism. PhD Thesis. Istanbul: Marmara University; 1995.

22

Distalization of the maxillary arch with miniplate anchorage

Hugo De Clerck and Hilde Timmerman

INTRODUCTION

Class II malocclusions may reflect maxilla–mandible skeletal disharmony with underdevelopment of mandibular growth and/or maxillary excess, leading to a convex soft tissue profile. Ideally, treatment of Class II malocclusions should focus first on improving the skeletal discrepancy using functional appliances while the individual is still growing.[1] However, dentoalveolar compensations, reducing overjet and the severity of the Class II malocclusion, are still the major effect of functional appliances.[2,3] In adults, repositioning of the maxilla and mandible can be achieved with orthognathic surgery, adjusting the position of both in relation to the cranial base in the three dimensions and improving overall facial esthetics.

Part of the Class II malocclusion can be treated by dentoalveolar compensation alone and a variety of methods have been advocated, as described in other chapters of this book. This chapter concentrates on the use of miniplate anchorage,[4] which makes it possible to insert the anchor close to the infrazygomatic crest and above the apex of the maxillary first molar. The miniplate can be extended to transfer the point of force application close to the fixed appliances (Fig. 22.1). If this extension is an osteosynthesis plate, oral hygiene at the perforation of the soft tissues can be difficult and local infections sometimes occur. An extension with a round section facilitates oral hygiene. Major advantages of miniplate anchorage include the reduced risk of damage to the roots of a tooth during surgery or by orthodontic movement of neighboring teeth, better quality of the anchorage and better biomechanics.

MINIPLATE SURGERY

Bollard miniplates have three holes and an extension round bar with a fixation hook at its end (Fig. 22.1A). The miniplate is fixed on to the infrazygomatic crest by three monocortical osteosynthesis screws with a diameter of 2.3 mm; a screw of 7 mm length is inserted through the upper hole and ones of 5 mm through the middle and lower holes. Alternatively, self-tapping or self-drilling miniscrew implants (MIs) can be used.

Initially, an L-shaped incision is made with anterior convexity (Fig. 22.2A) and a posterior-based mucoperiosteal flap is raised for bone exposure (Fig. 22.2B). The miniplate is slightly bent to obtain good contact with cortical bone (Fig. 22.2C). The bending should be limited to the region between the holes of the miniplate, it should not exceed 10° and can only be performed once to avoid any risk of fracture during or after surgery. The angulation between the miniplate and the neck should not be modified in order to ensure good contact between the lower part of the neck and the alveolar bone. The round bar should also not be bent as that could lead to its later fracture.

The device is positioned so that the round connecting bar of the neck penetrates the soft tissues exactly at the angle of the L-shaped incision, 2 mm below the mucogingival border. The center of the holes of the miniplate should be as close as possible to the top of the infrazygomatic crest oriented parallel to the alveolar bone, with the opening of the hook oriented to the distal. A pilot hole, diameter 1.65 mm, is drilled in the bone through the middle hole of the miniplate using a standard hard steel 1.65 mm twisted drill (Fig. 22.2D). The fixation screws are seated with a standard screwdriver. The first screw is not completely fixed to allow some rotation of the miniplate. The lower hole is drilled and the screw is inserted, followed by the upper one and all are then fixed for a strong and stable retention (Fig. 22.2E).

After rinsing with saline solution, closure is obtained in one plane with 4-0 resorbable sutures. The mucoperiosteal flap is positioned by the first suture just anterior from the neck of the bone anchor. Additional sutures are placed until good closure is obtained (Fig. 22.2F).

PATIENT INSTRUCTIONS

Immediately after surgery the fixation units are covered with wax. The patient replaces the wax after brushing. This protects the cheeks, which may be irritated by the intraoral extension of the miniplate, particularly initially when there will be some tissue swelling. Cooling of the area for 48 hours after surgery is advised and sports should be avoided for 3 days. Patients should rinse twice a day with chlorhexidine for 12 days and several times a day with sparkling water. In addition, patients must be instructed not to touch the extension of the miniplate repeatedly with their tongues or fingers as this is the main reason for some early loss of stability of the anchor. Patients should be clearly warned of the risk of loosening the miniplates and even needing further surgery. Continual clinical checks for any small mobility of the miniplate can minimize any adverse effects. About 10 days after surgery, the patient is given specific instructions on how to clean the soft tissues surrounding the round bar, using a soft

Fig. 22.1 Bollard miniplates. (A) Left and right upper miniplates. (B) Intraoral view 3 weeks after surgery.

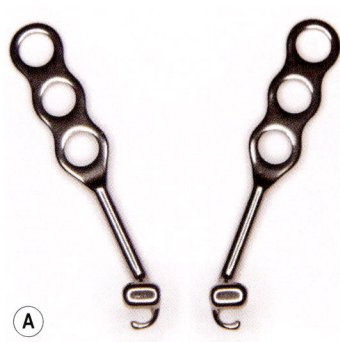

(A)

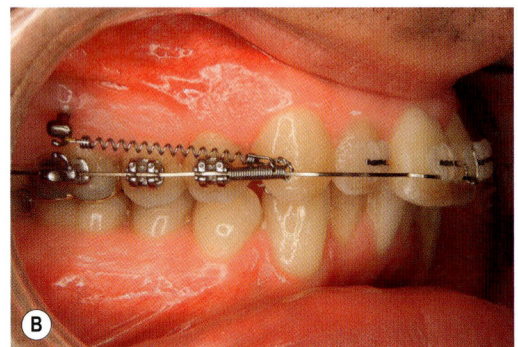

(B)

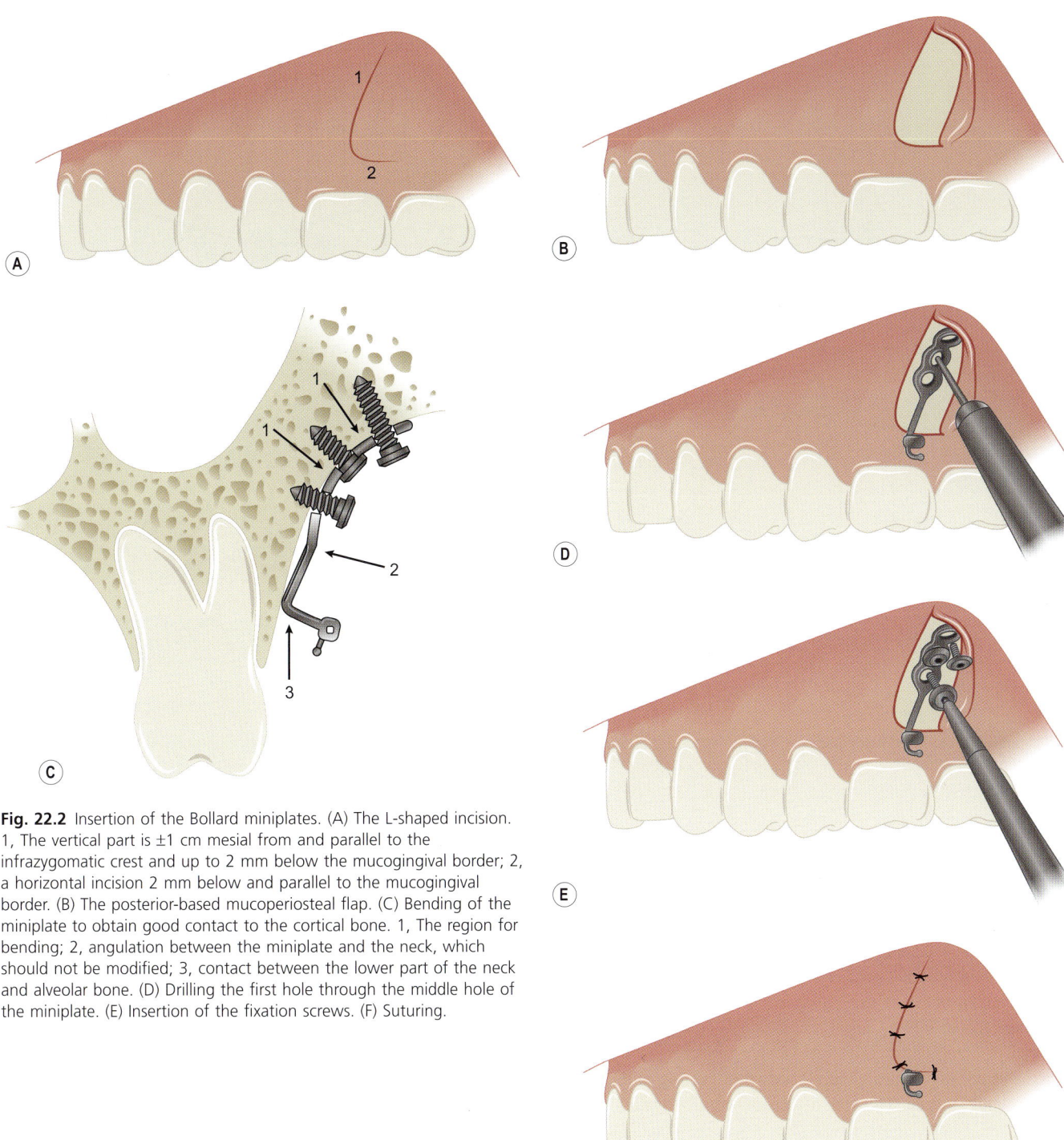

Fig. 22.2 Insertion of the Bollard miniplates. (A) The L-shaped incision. 1, The vertical part is ±1 cm mesial from and parallel to the infrazygomatic crest and up to 2 mm below the mucogingival border; 2, a horizontal incision 2 mm below and parallel to the mucogingival border. (B) The posterior-based mucoperiosteal flap. (C) Bending of the miniplate to obtain good contact to the cortical bone. 1, The region for bending; 2, angulation between the miniplate and the neck, which should not be modified; 3, contact between the lower part of the neck and alveolar bone. (D) Drilling the first hole through the middle hole of the miniplate. (E) Insertion of the fixation screws. (F) Suturing.

conventional toothbrush rather than an electrical one. Orthodontic loading should be started no later than 2 to 3 weeks after surgery, with initial loading no higher than 100–150 g. Loading can increase progressively over the first 3 months but should never exceed 250 g; such high forces are not needed for optimal tooth movement.

MOLAR DISTALIZATION BIOMECHANICS

Because of the oblique inclination of the infrazygomatic crest, the fixation unit is usually located in front of the second premolar. An elastic or a closed Ni-Ti coil spring can be placed from the hook directly to the maxillary canine bracket. The line of force is located below the center of resistance of the canine and so will initially result in distal crown tipping. Binding of the archwire at the mesial and distal border of the bracket generates forces that will upright the root of the canine (Fig. 22.3A).

Consecutive crown tipping and root uprighting finally results in sliding of the canine bracket along the archwire. Because of the repetitive binding between the bracket slot and the archwire, friction is generated, which pulls the archwire posteriorly. The posterior traction on the archwire is further amplified by similar friction generated by binding in the brackets of the premolars and in the molar tubes. All these small distalizing forces are transmitted to the anterior segment and pull the incisors back (Fig. 22.3B).

Where distalization is only needed on one side, a midline deviation results. During canine crown tipping, the archwire in front of the bracket

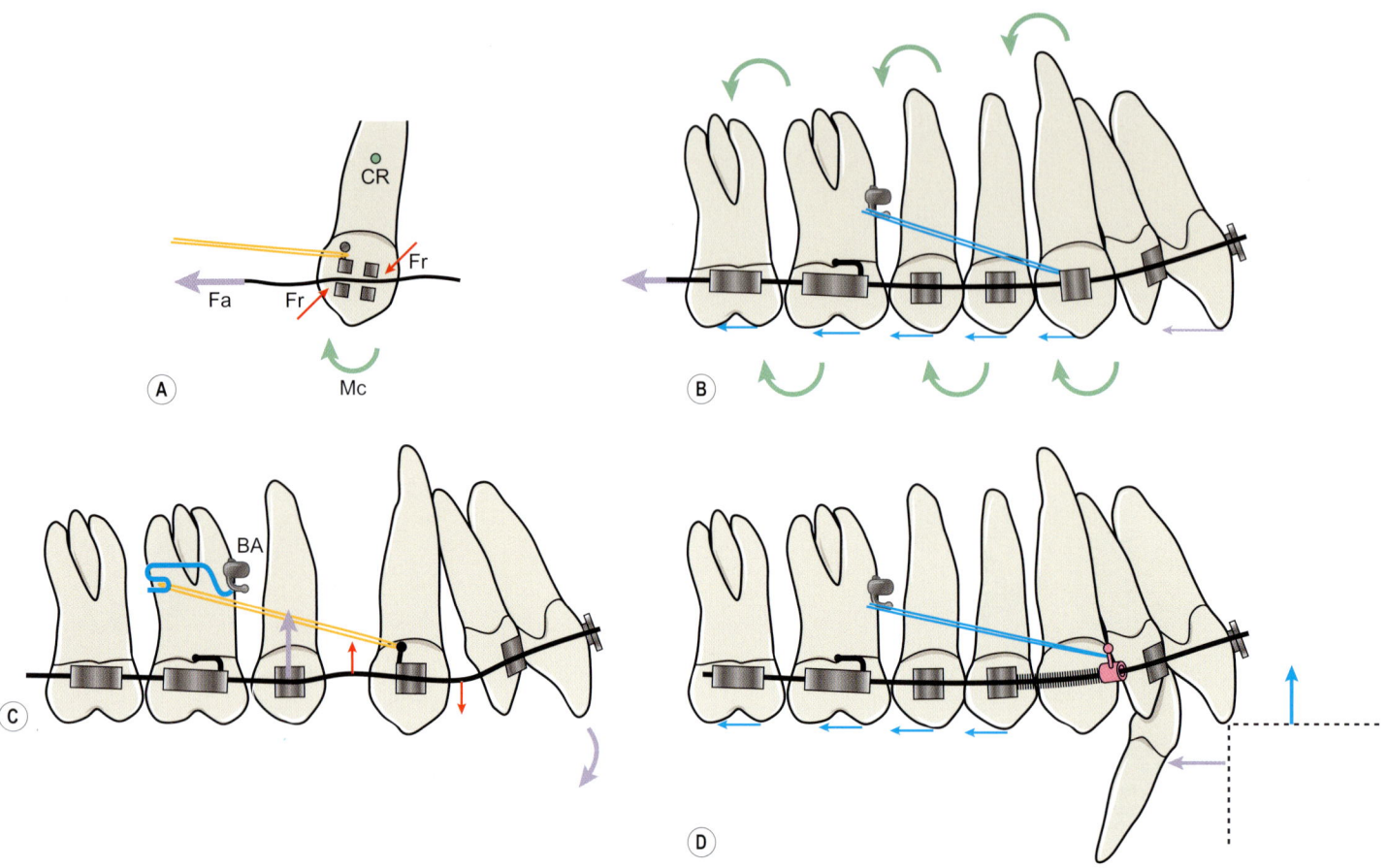

Fig. 22.3 Distalizing forces. (A) Initial crown tipping during canine distalization. The line of force is located below the center of resistance (CR) of the canine. (B) Distalizing forces generated in the lateral segment resulting in a posterior traction on the incisors. (C) Crown tipping of the canine tends to extrude the incisors. (D) A closed coil spring is pushed against the mesial side of the first premolar bracket to act as a rigid sliding jig for posterior movement of the lateral segments.

is pulled down and the archwire behind the bracket is pulled upwards. This results in some extrusion of the incisors and intrusion of the first premolar (Fig. 22.3C).

In increased overbite, the maxillary incisors are blocked by the mandibular incisors and cannot move posteriorly together with the canines and so space will be created between the canine and the lateral incisor. After distalization of the canines into a Class I relationship, the four incisors can only be distalized in combination with bite-opening mechanics such as a T-loop arch in the maxillary dentition combined with leveling of the curve of Spee in the mandibular arch. The lack of vertical control of the incisors during sliding of the lateral segment will slow down the distalization of the whole dental arch. This is a consequence of the two-phase biomechanics: distalization of the lateral segments first followed by retraction of the incisors in combination with elimination of the deep bite.

A better approach is to use a single phase where lateral and anterior segments are moved simultaneously. No bracket is bonded on the maxillary canines at the start of treatment but the second molars are always to be bonded. Crowding in the anterior segment is not corrected during initial leveling to avoid "round tripping" of the incisors. Overlapping or rotation of the incisors is maintained and not corrected by the Ni-Ti archwires. However good alignment of all the premolars and first and second molars is required before initiation of distalization. After alignment of the lateral segments, a round Australian wire is inserted (0.016 inch for a 0.018 × 0.025 inch bracket slot and and 0.020 inch for a 0.022 × 0.028 inch slot). Posterior movement of the lateral segments is started by inserting an SS closed coil spring mesial of the bracket of the first premolar to act as a rigid sliding jig; this has no active inherent force such as that with a compressed open coil spring (Fig. 22.3D).

Distalization starts only after fixation of a stretched Ni-Ti closed coil spring between the hook on the miniplate and the anterior limit of the closed coil spring, which will be pushed against the bracket of the first premolar. The line of force applied to the mesial border of this bracket is located below the center of resistance of the premolar but parallel to the archwire. To avoid rotation of the premolars during distalization, a 0.010 inch SS ligature should be firmly tied around the distal wings of the bracket. This provides better control of rotation and reduces friction. A round archwire generates less friction than a rectangular wire. The main advantage of using a sliding SS coil spring in front of the maxillary canine is the vertical component of force: a lever is created that generates an intrusive force close to the lateral incisors (Fig. 22.4A,B). This vertical force alone, applied to the bracket of the incisors at a distance from their center of resistance, would result in incisor proclination. However, binding at the bracket–archwire interface in the lateral segments will add a continuous distalizing force to the incisors. Clinically, this horizontal force is be big enough to avoid proclination of the incisors and to maintain contact with the antagonists. This is very important in order to avoid a spontaneous overeruption of the mandibular incisors during bite opening.

Although some extrusion may also occur in the posterior segment, this bite opening in the anterior segment will be more restricted when there is extreme retroclination of the maxillary incisors at the start of treatment. Simultaneous displacement of the lateral and frontal segments results in less increase of arch length, and thus fewer archwire replacements are needed. In fact, at the monthly visits it should be checked if there is still sufficient archwire extending behind the second molar tube.

When molars are distalized without retraction of the incisors, the total arch length increases and the amount of archwire distal to the second molar tube can become so short that the sliding movement of the last molar will be blocked. Blocking will, of course, also result in blocking of the distalization of the complete posterior segment. In order to extend the archwire distal to the second molar tube without irritating the cheeks, a horizontal bend parallel to the occlusal plane is advised; the bended extremity should not be too short. Further irritation may also be caused by sliding of the archwire to one side. This can be avoided by bending two stops in the archwire mesial to the brackets of both central incisors (Fig. 22.4C,D). Sometimes, a ligature or chain elastomeric connecting the four incisors is needed to avoid creation of a medial diastema.

The maxillary canines partially follow the movement of the first premolars under the pull of the transeptal fibers, but this only happens when there is no interference with the mandibular canine or by its bracket. Therefore, the lower fixed appliances are only bonded after a nearly Class I occlusion in the canine region is reached.

From an occlusal view, the maxillary arch can be divided into three segments, with the canine (middle segment), the only tooth without a bracket. The lateral segments are pushed back by the sliding closed coil in the rail formed by the labial and palatal cortical plates. This is a movement along a straight line, guided by the walls of the alveolar process but with some possibility of labial or palatal crown tipping. The retromolar region has a high potential for remodeling and so the germs of unerupted third molars are not as a rule removed prior to distalization. Because round archwires are used, the front segment is moved posteriorly mainly by retroclination. This tipping movement is easily obtained because there is little binding friction. The light distalizing force generated by sliding of the lateral segments will be sufficient to maintain contact with the mandibular incisors during bite opening. The amount of movement of the incisors and the reduction of the overjet will depend on the amount of bite opening. Excessive retroclination of the incisors will only be corrected by using rectangular archwires in a later stage of treatment after a Class I occlusion is reached.

The most complex movement is made by the canines, which are guided between the curved plates of the alveolar process. During this spontaneous drift, the canine follows the trajectory with the least resistance, without hitting the outer or inner cortical bone plates, and along the labial surface of the mandibular canine. If a bracket is bonded to the maxillary canine, the movement will be determined by the shape of the archwire. At each monthly appointment, some expansion should be added to the archwire in the canine region. If too much expansion is given, drifting of the canine will be restricted by contact with the outer cortical plate. If not enough, the canine will be stopped by occlusal interference with the mandibular canine. Movement will also be restrained by friction at the bracket–archwire interface. The advantage of not bonding the canine is not only a better vertical control of the maxillary incisors but also a smoother distal drift of the canine and a limited amount of rotation.

Rotation always results when a distalizing force is applied to the hook on the canine bracket; this can be avoided by tying the distal wing of the bracket with an SS ligature to the archwire. However, this will increase friction. When the first premolar is distalized and no bracket is bonded to the canine, the canine will move distally under the pull of the transeptal fibers. Some of these fibers are located at the level of the center of resistance and will not generate rotation but fibers labial from the center of resistance will cause a rotation opposite to the rotation generated by the elastic fibers on the palatal side, thus resulting in distalization with hardly any rotation.

From a labial view, the force of the fibers is applied far below the center of resistance of the canine and so distal crown tipping is commonly observed and root uprighting is needed after a Class I occlusion in the molar region has been reached. To upright the root of the canine, a bracket is bonded and a Ni-Ti archwire inserted. The resistance against root uprighting will be higher than the resistance against mesial crown tipping. A laceback from the canine bracket to the miniplate may restrict mesial crown tipping and help to maintain the Class I relation with the mandibular canine (Fig. 22.5A). This laceback should be passive. To avoid rotation of the canine during root uprighting, the distal wing of the bracket should be firmly tied to the archwire (Fig. 22.5B,C).

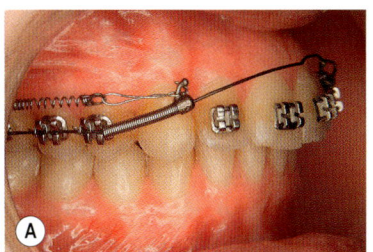 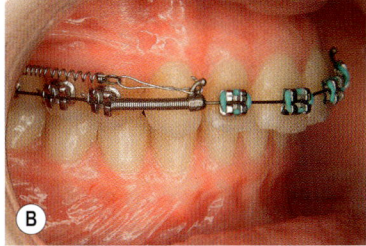 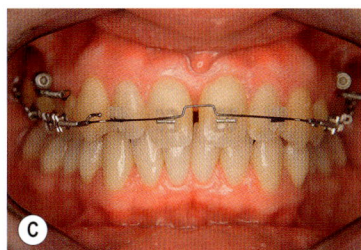 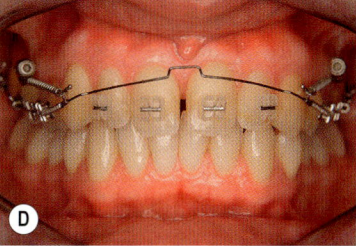

Fig. 22.4 A continuous light intrusive force results in some bite opening during distalization of the lateral segments. (A,B) Lateral view (A) and after (B) insertion of the arch wire Sliding of the archwire to one side is avoided by bending two steps between the brackets of the central incisors: without (C) and with fixation (D) of the open coil spring to the closed coil spring on the archwire.

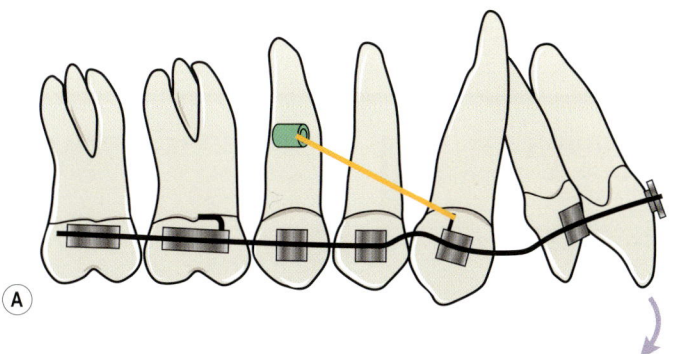 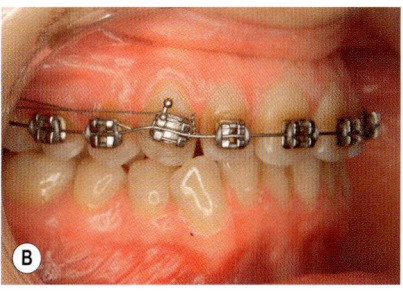 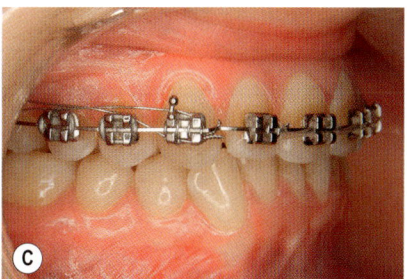

Fig. 22.5 Restriction of mesial crown tipping of the maxillary canine. (A) Laceback from the canine bracket to the miniplate. (B,C) Canine uprighting before (B) and after (C) application of a passive laceback.

Crowding of the maxillary incisors is not corrected at the start of fixed appliance therapy. This usually results in proclination of the incisors and an increased overjet. When there is lack of space and overlapping of the anterior teeth, all the teeth are bonded but the initial leveling wires are only partially inserted into the brackets' slots. In extreme crowding, as in some Class II, division 2, the archwires are fixed below the lower border of the incisor brackets (Fig. 22.6).

To obtain contact with each bracket, some first- and second-order bends have to be made in the main archwire so that the intrusion force generated by the lever arm of the closed coil spring and the retracting force from binding in the lateral segments are transferred to the four crowded incisors. Distal drift of the canines results in an increased intercanine distance and a spontaneous unraveling of the crowded incisors. Only after sufficient space is available should a light Ni-Ti wire be inserted for the first time in the brackets' slots, aligning the anterior teeth with minimal proclination.

When a sliding coil is used to distalize the maxillary premolars without bonding the canines, a dual occlusal plane is often created through intrusion of the incisors and some extrusion of the premolars (Fig. 22.7).

After bonding the maxillary canines and insertion of a straight wire, the archwire will be flattened again by some intrusion of the premolars, but mainly by extrusion of the incisors. During root uprighting of the maxillary canines, additional extrusive forces will be applied to the incisors and, before leveling the maxillary arch, a choice has to be made as to whether incisor extrusion is wanted or not, depending on incisor exposure and smile esthetics. Without precautions, part of the intrusion obtained in the first part of distalizing mechanics will be spontaneously lost. As long as contact with the mandibular incisors is maintained, and once the lower fixed appliance is bonded, the deepening of the bite will be limited and will not affect the Class I occlusion previously obtained. Furthermore, simultaneous leveling of the curve of Spee in the mandibular arch will help to control the overbite. Extrusion of the incisors during uprighting of

the canines can be reduced by adding an intrusion auxiliary arch when there is vertical excess in the front segment. Intrusion auxiliary arches are usually inserted in an additional molar tube. However, the reaction forces will extrude the molars and tip their crowns to the distal. This can be avoided by inserting the intrusion arch in the tube of the Bollard miniplate. Instead of a continuous arch, segmented intrusion arches are easier to adjust. A SS segmented wire (0.018 × 0.018 inch) is inserted into the tube of the miniplate. The wire is cut between the lateral incisor and the canine and a small circle is bent (Fig. 22.8A,B). The anterior part of the wire is pulled down and fixed distal from the lateral incisor to the archwire by means of an SS ligature (Fig. 22.8C). The amount of force is modified by altering the curvature of the segmented wire and different forces may be used on the left and right where there is a canted occlusal plane. The small piece of wire extending behind the tube of the miniplate rarely disturbs the patient but can be bent or covered by a drop of a flowable composite (Fig. 22.8C). It does facilitate removal if necessary during future controls.

The transverse dimension of the maxillary arch will be affected by the sliding mechanics, and the widths between premolars and between molars will become larger. This can be explained by the direction of traction from the sliding hook to the elastic hook on the miniplate (Fig. 22.9). In addition to the sagittal component, there is also a lateral component of force, resulting in some expansion of the premolars.

The increase in intercanine width occurs spontaneously without brackets and without forces from the fixed appliance. The distal drift of the canines, guided by both cortical plates of the alveolar process, positions them more posteriorly in the arch, with an increased distance between left and right center of the alveolar process. This also explains part of the increase in widths between premolars and between molars.

DISCUSSION

The use of miniplates for direct anchorage as described in this chapter can support all the treatment required for distalization of the complete maxillary dental arch with little need for patient compliance during treatment apart from maintenance of oral hygiene. The intraoral tube with a hook, positioned between the maxillary molar and the second premolar, offers unique options for adding intrusion or extrusion auxiliaries.

Sliding mechanics have the advantage that all premolars and molars are moved as one unit and that the canine partly follows the movement of the premolars, thus creating space for the incisors. The light intrusive and retraction forces acting continuously on the incisors during distalization of the lateral segments result in a reduction of the overjet without increase

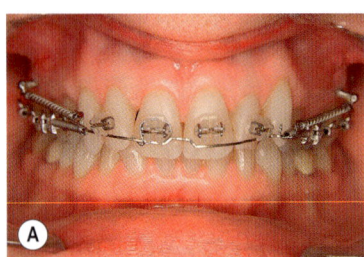
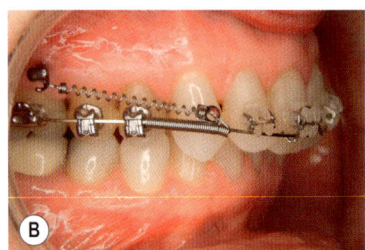

Fig. 22.6 Frontal (A) and lateral (B) intraoral views showing that the archwire is not inserted in the bracket slot in order to avoid excessive proclination during initial alignment.

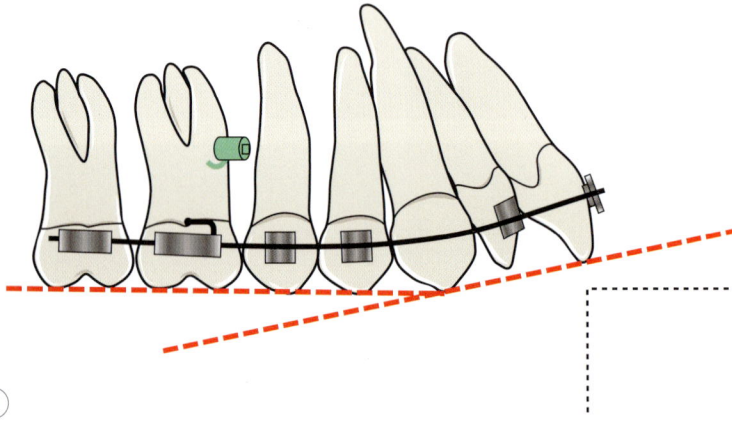
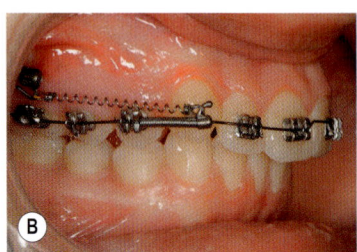
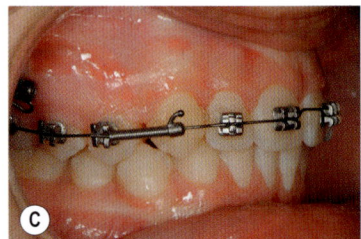

Fig. 22.7 (A) The dual occlusal plane. (B,C) The occlusal plane before (B) and after (C) distalization.

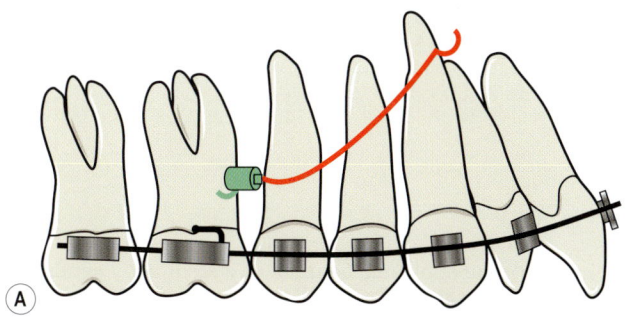

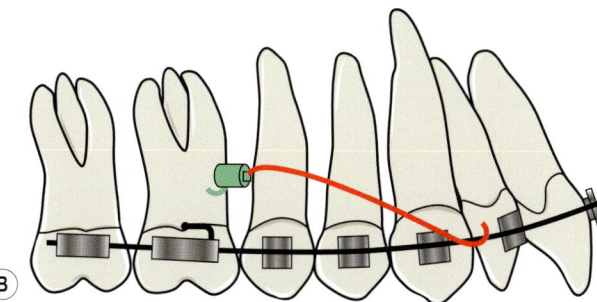

Fig. 22.8 Segmented intrusion arch. (A,B) Before (A) and after (B) activation. (C) The intrusion arch fixed to the archwire between the lateral incisor and canine.

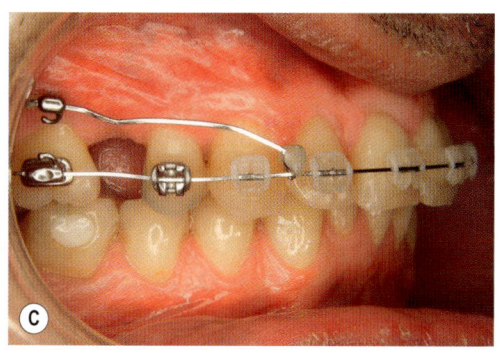

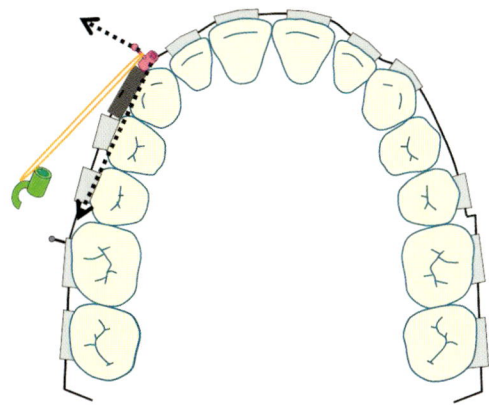

Fig. 22.9 The lateral component of force generated by the open coil spring.

The combination of anteroposterior corrections in the lateral segments with vertical control in the anterior segment results in an efficient posterior displacement of the whole maxillary dental arch in one stage. Where no retraction of the incisors is wanted, the molars, premolars and canines can be distalized to create extra space for the alignment of crowded incisors without proclining them. Obtaining a normal sagittal and vertical overbite of the incisors and a nearly Class I occlusion of the molars within the first year of treatment leaves more time for finishing and detailing of the occlusion and may improve the final outcome of the orthodontic treatment. However, more research is needed to find out how the incisor exposure might change after completion of the fixed appliance therapy and what tendency there is for relapse.

of the vertical overbite, and sometimes with a slight bite opening in the frontal segment.

Very few adaptations have to be made to the archwires during the procedure, which reduces chair-time at the monthly check-ups. As with all other orthodontic treatment approaches, facial esthetics, incisor exposure and smile esthetics should always be taken into consideration. In order to avoid over-retraction of the maxillary teeth, some proclination of the mandibular incisors can be used to compensate any mild skeletal disharmony. This proclination is usually obtained during leveling of the curve of Spee and elimination of some initial crowding of the incisors. Class II elastics should be avoided in order to avoid overproclining the incisors.

REFERENCES

1. O'Brien K, Macfarlane T, Wright J, et al. Early treatment for Class II malocclusion and perceived improvements in facial profile. Am J Orthod Dentofacial Orthop 2009;135:580–5.
2. AAO. Council on Scientific Affairs (COSA). Functional appliances and long-term effects on mandibular growth. Am J Orthod Dentofacial Orthop 2005;128:271–2.
3. Martin J, Pancherz H. Mandibular incisor position changes in relation to amount of bite jumping during Herbst/multibracket appliance treatment: a radiographic-cephalometric study. Am J Orthod Dentofacial Orthop 2009;136:44–51.
4. De Clerck H, Geerinckx V, Siciliano S. The Zygoma Anchorage System. J Clin Orthod 2002;36:455–9.

23

Maxillary molar distalization with the Graz Implant-Supported Pendulum appliance

Friedrich K. Byloff and Hans Kärcher

INTRODUCTION

The Graz Implant-Supported Pendulum (GISP) is a Pendulum appliance with two parts that was developed to distalize maxillary molars in adults.[1,2] A significant characteristic of this device is that the pendulum auxiliary is not integrated and is easily removed for reactivation and control of movement in all planes of space.

DESIGN OF THE GRAZ IMPLANT-SUPPORTED PENDULUM

The GISP has an anchorage part consisting of a surgical miniplate with four miniscrew holes and two cylinders welded at right angles to the center of the miniplate, all made of titanium. This part is directly fixed to the palatal bone via four 5 mm long titanium miniscrew implants (MIs) (Fig. 23.1A). The cylinders perforate the palatal mucosa (Fig. 23.1B), which is folded back to form a mucoperiosteal flap to expose the bone; alternatively, they can be tunneled by an incision. In adults, existing maxillary third molars are removed during the same surgical session to reduce resistance to distalization. In this case a general anesthetic is used; otherwise local anesthesia is sufficient. When there are no maxillary third molars present, the procedure requires "weakening" of the alveolar bone from the occlusal with a bur distal to the second molars in order to facilitate distal movement. Removal of the anchorage attachment during fixed appliance treatment is completed with two longitudinal tunneling incisions in the mucosa under local anesthesia.

The removable part of the appliance consists of a resin body similar to an acrylic resin Nance button. Two cylindrical slots of the acrylic resin button are telescoped over the two cylinders of the anchorage miniplate to avoid compression of the mucosa (Fig. 23.1C). After the surgical procedure, a healing period of 2 weeks allows any swelling to subside. An impression of the maxillary arch and the palate with the two protruding cylinders is then taken. The existing maxillary molar bands are also shown in the impression, so that the distalizing TMA springs (0.032 inch) can be adapted to the lingual sheaths of the bands. After fabricating the acrylic resin Nance button on the cast, the distalizing springs are activated to generate a force of approximately 250 g per side. Intraorally, this removable pendulum is fitted on the two cylinders (Fig. 23.1C). The two springs, which are curved at their ends for better three-dimensional molar control, are fitted into the sheaths. The sheaths have a built-in 8° offset for easier intraoral insertion.

During insertion of the preactivated appliance, the maxillary second molars are bonded and a sectional (leveling) archwire is engaged. This way both molars can be simultaneously distalized (Fig. 23.1D), which has been shown to be the most efficient approach.

IMPROVED DESIGN

To avoid invasive surgery, a new design has the miniplate placed directly on to the palatal mucosa and fixed with four 10 mm long locking MIs (TriLock; Medartis, Basel, Switzerland) (Fig. 23.2A,B). The MIs' heads are sunk into the cavities in the palatal miniplate so that the mucosa is not compressed by pressure from the acrylic resin Nance button when the

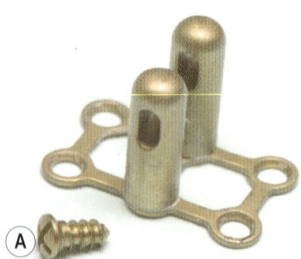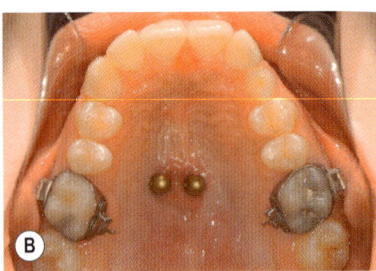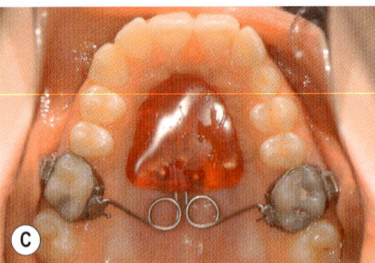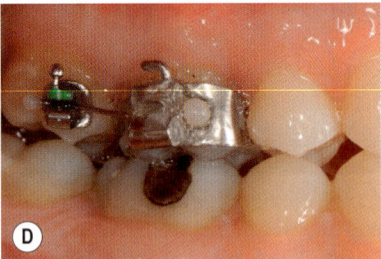

Fig. 23.1 Original design of the Graz Implant-Supported Pendulum appliance. (A) The surgical miniplate and the miniscrew implants. (B) Cylinders perforating the mucosa. (C) Intraoral occlusal view of the appliance; the removable acrylic button with distalizing springs telescoped over the two cylinders of the miniplate. (D) Sectional archwire in place during simultaneous distalization of the first and second molars.

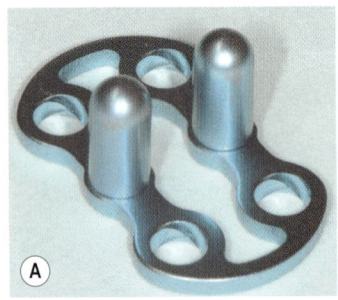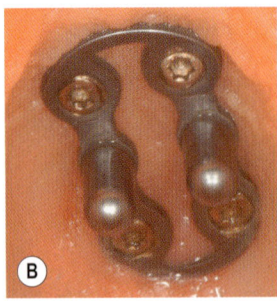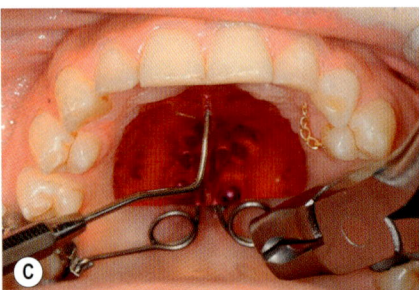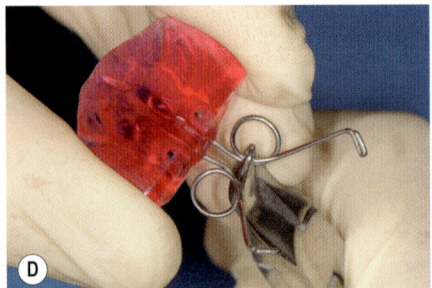

Fig. 23.2 Improved design of the Graz Implant-Supported Pendulum appliance. (A) The new anchorage miniplate. (B) The miniplate fixed on the palatal mucosa. (C) Removal of the acrylic button with Weingart pliers and a probe. The probe is inserted into a tunnel at 45° to the occlusal plane and both instruments are pulled gently down simultaneously. (D) Extraoral reactivation of the distalizing spring.

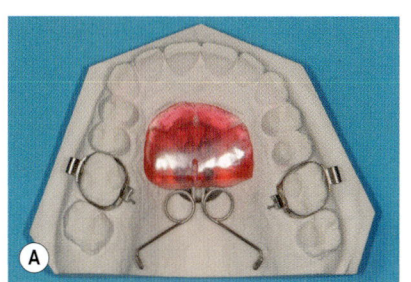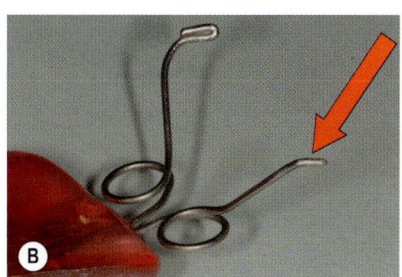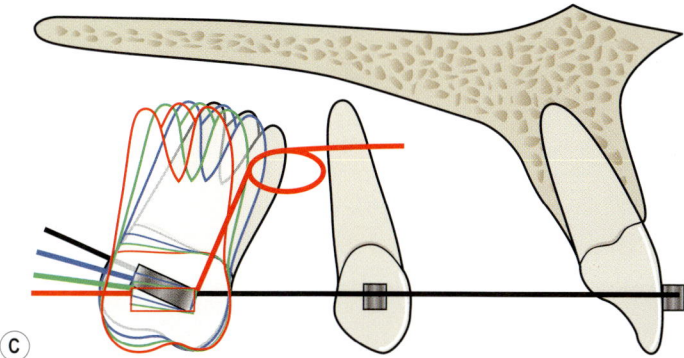

Fig. 23.3 (A) Laboratory-fabricated Graz Implant-Supported Pendulum with pre-reactivated distalizing springs. (B) A specially modified end for the distalizing spring, which allows molar distal root tipping by the leveling wire. (C) Schematic view of root uprighting using a leveling wire with a modified spring end.

springs are activated. With this system, the hole in the miniplate accommodates the MI head in such a way that it is perfectly stabilized. Holes in the bone are predrilled under local anesthesia and the MIs inserted using a manual screwdriver. The cylinders in this modified design are smaller: 7.5 mm in length and 3.6 mm in diameter (Fig. 23.2A). These design improvements enable the alginate impression for construction of the button and embedded springs to be made on the insertion day, immediately following surgery.

A small tunnel at about 45° to the occlusal plane is drilled into the anterior part of the button to allow it to be removed periodically (Fig. 23.2C,D). If desired, the removable acrylic resin button can be miniaturized. This solution offers improved hygiene and gives the tongue more space in the palatal vault.

As with the original GISP, bands are fitted to the maxillary first molars prior to surgery, removed and set aside for use when taking the impression for the construction of the Nance button. The modified Nance button is similar to a Pendulum appliance but without wires bonded to the premolars. One week should be allowed for healing after which an impression is made and the maxillary molar bands are left in the alginate. A simulated internal miniplate with cylinders is inserted into the impression and a plaster cast is fabricated in the laboratory. Once the appliance is made, the springs are fitted passively to the molar palatal sheaths and then activated to exert a force of approximately 250 g per side (Fig. 23.3A). The appliance is inserted into the mouth after the bands have been bonded to the molars; the second molars are bonded and a sectional leveling arch is engaged (Fig. 23.1D). The wire enhances mobilization of the second molars and we also consider that it improves distal movement of both molars simultaneously. Patients are seen every 6 to 8 weeks. If necessary, the removable button is pulled off and the springs are reactivated (Fig. 23.2D). The curved ends of the springs allow the clinician to control vertical and rotational movement, as well as tipping throughout treatment.[3]

INDICATIONS

The GISP is mainly indicated when significant distalization of maxillary molars is required, either unilaterally or bilaterally. Clinical goals achievable include correction of a dental Class II malocclusion without extraction of the maxillary premolars, first or second molars. Mandibular advancement surgery can also be avoided where camouflage treatment is considered possible. In general, a final occlusion with a molar and canine Class I relationship, as provided by nature, is the most harmonious solution that can be achieved through the use of the GISP.

Simplified placement has allowed use of the GISP to be extended from adults to adolescents with permanent dentition. Adolescents and their

parents are now able to decide between the classic Pendulum appliance or the implant-anchored GISP. The advantages of the GISP include:

- it acts as a counterbalance to mesial movement of premolars
- the canines and maxillary incisors are not impinged
- spontaneous distal movement of the premolars takes place during molar distalization
- treatment time is shorter.

In adults, the individual situation will determine the treatment plan. Where there is a third molar in perfect condition and the first or second molar has a root canal treatment, a deep filling or crown, the orthodontic decision might be to keep the third molar and extract the affected molar. There would then be no need for molar implant-supported distalization and conventional dental anchorage might be possible. If premolars or molars are to be extracted, reinforcement of anchorage for molar distalization becomes necessary. If both maxillary molars are to be moved distally, existing maxillary third molars are removed. Decisions to extract third molars, particularly when they are impacted, are generally accepted since they are often not considered to be valuable teeth.

ORTHODONTIC PROCEDURE

Distalization of first and second molars can sometimes take more than 3 months before space mesial to the first molar becomes visible. Distal movement of the premolars under the pull of the transeptal fibers can camouflage space opening for some time, particularly when there is crowding at the start of treatment. Initially with the GISP, the first and second molars are distalized individually with an undersized square SS archwire and a Ni-Ti push-coil spring. The push-coil spring distalizes the second molars, while the distalizing spring on the first molars is also activated. Once the second molars are sufficiently distalized, the force of the push-coil is reduced until it is barely active. As a result, the TMA spring on the first molars becomes dominant and the first molars are moved toward the second molars, eventually closing the space between them, while the coil spring holds the second molars in their distal position.[1] This method was used to treat a patient who did not return for checks for almost 12 months and we found that the first and second molars distalized simultaneously with the single activation at the start of treatment (see Case 1). Based on this, we changed to simultaneous distalization as this required the same time with much less effort and clinical time.

Patients are seen every 6 weeks for an appliance check and, if needed, spring reactivation; the patient also rinses without the removable button in the mouth. The time required to distalize maxillary molars depends on the distance to be covered and on the individual biological response.[4]

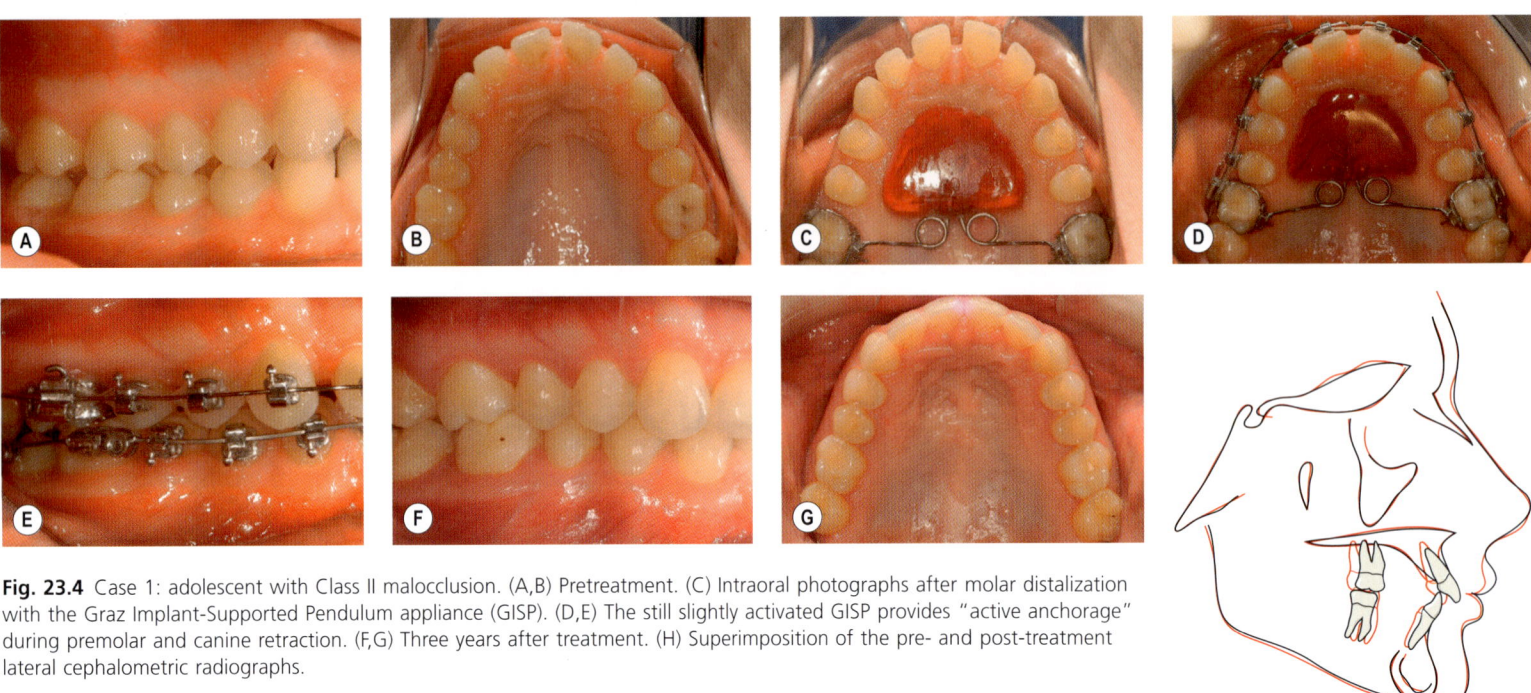

Fig. 23.4 Case 1: adolescent with Class II malocclusion. (A,B) Pretreatment. (C) Intraoral photographs after molar distalization with the Graz Implant-Supported Pendulum appliance (GISP). (D,E) The still slightly activated GISP provides "active anchorage" during premolar and canine retraction. (F,G) Three years after treatment. (H) Superimposition of the pre- and post-treatment lateral cephalometric radiographs.

Generally, 8–12 months is likely for correcting a cusp-to-cusp relationship to a complete molar Class I relationship. During this time, the patient has no other fixed appliances. Fixed appliances are bonded once the molars are sufficiently distalized, ideally to a slightly overcorrected Class I relationship. During the leveling and alignment phase with fixed appliances, the GISP stays in place and the springs are lightly activated to avoid mesialization of the molars. The force of activation is slightly increased during distalization of the premolars and canines to counteract any mesially directed reaction forces ("active anchorage").[1] We consider this to be an advantage over other systems that have only passive anchorage (i.e. rigidly holding the molars in their distalized position).

At the end of distalization, the molars should have no distal tip. If the first molar has to be uprighted, the sectional archwire between the first and second molars is removed toward the end of distalization. If fixed appliance therapy begins and there is a molar that is not sufficiently upright, but the mesial cusp is in a good Class I relationship, one component of the curved end of the spring should be cut off (Fig. 23.3B). This way, there will be enough play in the lingual sheath to allow the leveling wire to upright the root without permitting mesialization of the crown (Fig. 23.3C). Once premolars and canines are positioned in Class I relationship, the acrylic resin Nance button is removed to retract the maxillary anterior teeth. The internal miniplate is removed under local anesthesia. If necessary, Class II elastics are used as anchorage from the maxillary canines to the mandibular second molars. Since patients sometimes postpone the surgical removal of the miniplate for months, it can be concluded that it does not represent a major discomfort.

CLINICAL PRESENTATIONS

CASE 1: ADOLESCENT WITH CLASS II MALOCCLUSION

A 16-year-old boy sought treatment to correct his apparent Class II occlusion, dental deep bite and multiple spaces in both arches (Fig. 23.4A,B). The decision was made to distalize the maxillary molars into Class I relationship and to close all spaces. The third molars were removed during the

insertion of the internal part of the original GISP. After distalization, the molars were in an overcorrected Class I relationship (Fig. 23.4C). The first and second molars were distalized as a unit. During retraction of the premolars and canines with elastic power chains, the GISP provided further "active anchorage" (Fig. 23.4D,E). A clearly visible distalization of the maxillary molars was evident.

At the end of treatment, the occlusion was corrected to Class I, which remained stable, as shown 3 years after treatment (Fig. 23.4F,G). On the superimposition of the pre- and post-treatment radiographs, a 5 mm distal movement of the maxillary molars can be seen (Fig. 23.4H). Due to a Bolton tooth size discrepancy, the crowns of the maxillary lateral incisors were reconstructed with composite.

CASE 2: ADULT WITH CLASS II MALOCCLUSION

A 25-year-old man sought orthodontic treatment to correct his apparent Class II occlusion and protruded maxillary anterior teeth (Fig. 23.5A–C). As he refused to have combined surgical/orthodontic treatment, it was decided to try camouflage treatment by distalizing the maxillary arch with the original GISP. The mandibular left molar had been extracted a long time previously (Fig. 23.5B).

Substantial distalization of the maxillary teeth during treatment, particularly on the left side, could be seen 5 years after treatment (Fig. 23.5D–F). Substantial distal molar movement and uprighting of the maxillary incisors was achieved, as seen in the superimposition of the radiographs before and after treatment (Fig. 22.25G). The final profile met the patient expectations perfectly and was also esthetically acceptable.

DISCUSSION

When palatal anchorage is used, maxillary molars are distalized before the fixed appliances are bonded to the teeth. This shortens the time for wearing the fixed appliances significantly, which is a serious consideration for patients.

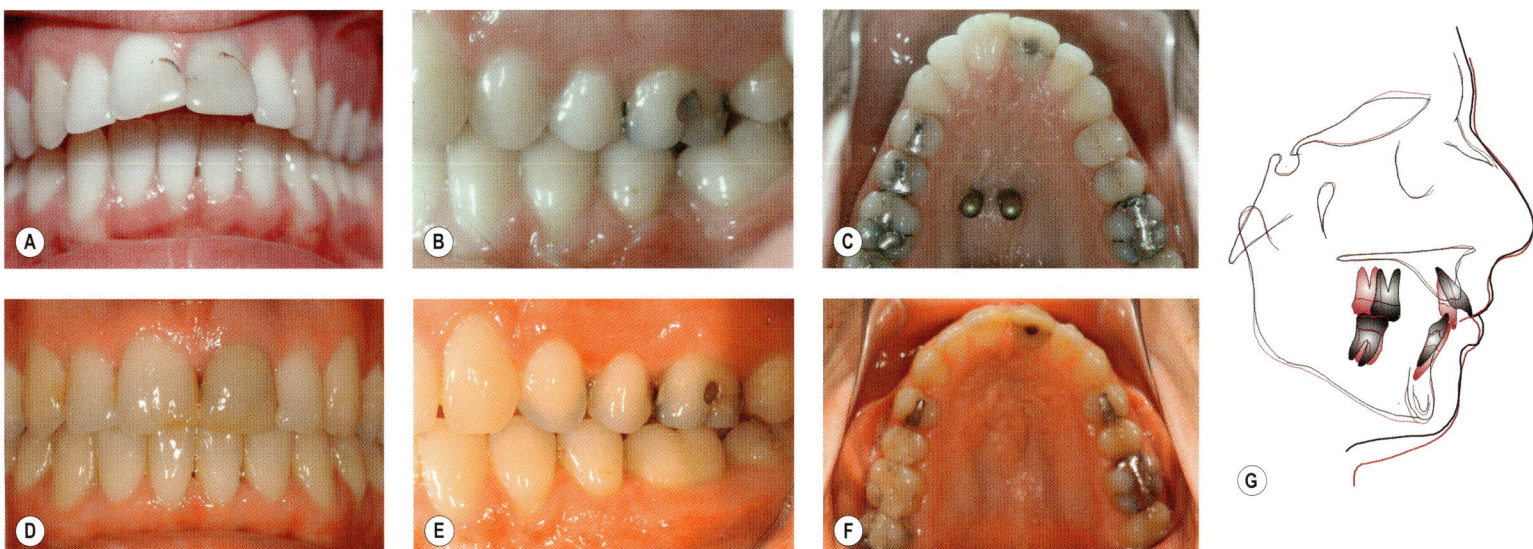

Fig. 23.5 Case 2: adult with Class II malocclusion. (A–C) Pretreatment. (D–F) Five years after treatment. (G) Superimposition of the pre- and post-treatment lateral cephalometric radiographs.

With solid palatal anchorage, the first and second premolars can be spontaneously distalized along with the molars under the pull of the transeptal fibers. If a transpalatal arch is supported by intraosseous MIs, there is some reactive mesial movement of the premolars during molar distalization.[5–7] Simultaneous premolar distalization with molar movement has been reported with a palatal implant used as anchorage.[8] However, placement of palatal implants, unlike a miniplate, is dependent on adequate bone thickness and so radiological examination is required before implant placement. In addition, palatal implants need at least 3 months of healing and osseointegration. By comparison, the GISP can be used immediately after surgical insertion, although 1 week is allowed for mucosal healing. The area where the internal miniplate of the GISP is placed has been demonstrated to be safe,[9,10] thus eliminating the need for pretreatment radiographic examinations. Further, nasal floor perforations of less than 2 mm tend to heal spontaneously.[11] The GISP has no wires attached to the premolars, thus allowing them to migrate distally during molar distalization (Fig. 23.4C).

Insertion of the latest version of GISP requires only minor surgery, as the miniplate is placed directly onto the mucosa and anchored with four MIs, which provides absolute stability and loosening or loss has never occurred. By comparison, failure rates as high as 10–30% have been reported with other MI anchorage systems.[12–15] Surgical protocol, clinician experience, the type of MI and location all play an important role in the failure rates of MIs. Their high failure rate is a clear disadvantage compared with systems with miniplate anchorage.

Other designs using metallic plates fixed by MIs to the palatal mucosa have recently been introduced.[16–18] These systems, like the GISP, have a solidly fixed miniplate that cannot easily become loose. The GISP has the further advantages that the springs can be manipulated to create movements in all directions (i.e. not only distalization, but also intrusion, rotation or expansion) and the button with distalizing springs is easily removed so that activation of the distalizing springs can be made extraorally rather than intraorally, as is the case with most other systems. A device with removable pendulum springs on a Straumann Palatal Implant can be adjusted extraorally but it seems to be more complicated in handling and risks less precise control of the molars due to a looser fit of the springs in their slots.[19]

The GISP allows the clinician to maintain good vertical control of distal molar movement, which is an advantage compared with the Distal Jet appliance and its variations, including the Beneslider.[20] The distally directed push coils used on the Beneslider do not allow any adjustments except for reactivation of the coils.[6–8] Despite the volume of the acrylic resin button of the GISP, patients acclimatize to it within about a week, which is similar to the period needed to get used to a retention plate.

CONCLUSIONS

The GISP seems to be an absolutely stable palatal anchorage system that can be activated without waiting for osseointegration. The removable portion is easy to remove and reinsert, which facilitates and simplifies reactivations. During the retraction phase, springs provide further "active anchorage," a function that a rigid anchoring system without springs cannot provide. Finally, molars can be moved in all directions of space.

REFERENCES

1. Byloff FK, Kärcher H, Clar E, et al. An implant to eliminate anchorage loss during molar distalization: a case report involving the Graz implant-supported pendulum. Int J Adult Orthod Orthognath Surg 2000;15:129–37.
2. Kärcher H, Byloff FK, Clar E. The Graz implant supported pendulum: a technical note. J Craniomaxillofac Surg 2002;30:87–90.
3. Byloff FK, Darendeliler MA, Clar E, et al. Distal molar movement using the pendulum appliance. Part 2: the effects of maxillary molar root uprighting bends. Angle Orthod 1997;67:261–70.
4. Iwasaki L, Haack J, Nickel J, et al. Human tooth movement in response to continuous stress of low magnitude. Am J Orthod Dentofacial Orthop 2000;117:175–83.
5. Gelgor I, Buyukyilmaz T, Karaman A, et al. Intraosseous mini-screw-supported upper molar distalization. Angle Orthod 2004;74:838–50.
6. Kinzinger G, Gülden N, Yildizhan F, et al. Efficiency of a skeletonized distal jet appliance supported by mini-screw anchorage for noncompliance maxillary molar distalization. Am J Orthod Dentofacial Orthop 2009;136:578–86.
7. Kinzinger G, Gülden N, Yildizhan F, et al. Anchorage efficacy of palatally-inserted mini-screws in molar distalization with a periodontally/mini-screw-anchored Distal Jet. J Orofac Orthop 2008;69:110–20.
8. Keles A, Erverdi N, Sezen S. Bodily distalization of molars with absolute anchorage. Angle Orthod 2003;73:471–82.
9. Schlegel K, Kinner F, Schlegel K. The anatomic basis for palatal implants in orthodontics. Int J Adult Orthod Orthognath Surg 2002;17:133–9.
10. Gracco A, Luca L, Siciliani G. Molar distalisation with skeletal anchorage. Aust Orthod J 2007;23:147–52.
11. Ardekian L, Oved-Peleg E, Mactei E, et al. The clinical significance of sinus membrane perforation during augmentation of the maxillary sinus. J Oral Maxillofac Surg 2006;64:77–82.

12. Miyawaki S, Koyama I, Inoue M, et al. Factors associated with the stability of titanium mini-screws placed in the posterior region for orthodontic anchorage. Am J Orthod Dentofacial Orthop 2003;124:373–8.

13. Cheng S, Tseng I, Lee J, et al. A prospective study of the risk factors associated with failure of mini-implants used for orthodontic anchorage. Int J Oral Maxillofac Implants 2004;19:100–6.

14. Fritz U, Ehmer A, Diedrich P. Clinical suitability of titanium microscrews for orthodontic anchorage: preliminary experiences. J Orofac Orthop 2004;65:410–18.

15. Berens A, Wiechmann D, Dempf R. Mini-and micro-mini-screws for temporary skeletal anchorage in orthodontic therapy. J Orofac Orthop 2006;67:450–8.

16. Cozzani M, Zallio F, Lombardo L, et al. Efficiency of the distal mini-screw in the distal movement of maxillary molars. World J Orthod 2010;11:341–5.

17. Itsuki Y, Imamura E. A new palatal implant with inter-changeable upper units. J Clin Orthod 2009;43:318–23.

18. Wilmes B, Drescher D, Nienkemper M. A miniplate system for improved stability of skeletal anchorage. J Clin Orthod 2009;43:494–501.

19. Giancotti A, Muzzi F, Greco M, et al. Palatal implant-supported distalizing devices: clinical application of the Straumann Orthosystem. World J Orthod 2002;3:135–9.

20. Wilmes B, Drescher D. Application and effectiveness of the Beneslider: a device to move molars distally. World J Orthod 2010;11:331–40.

INTRODUCTION

The term functional appliance refers to a variety of appliances designed to transmit forces to the dentition and the basal bone in order to alter the function and position of the mandible. Typically this new sagittal and vertical muscular position results in orthodontic and orthopedic changes. In spite of differences in design, all functional appliances rely on keeping the mandible in a forward position. The fixed functional appliances all act in the same way and their clinical consequences are similar.

Approximately 30% of the Class II correction achieved using fixed functional appliances is attributed to skeletal response, with 70% to dentoalveolar response.[1] Dentoalveolar response is characterized by uncontrolled and unwanted tipping of the mandibular incisors.[2] True treatment of the skeletal malocclusion requires correction of the morphogenetic pattern. Consequently, condylar adaptation and mandibular skeletal growth have to be the main goal in functional treatment. Some investigators claim that rapid labial tipping of the mandibular incisors, which takes place in almost 6 months using functional appliances, limits the time needed to obtain more skeletal response. It can be assumed that direct protrusive force application through the mandibular skeletal bone can prevent labial tipping of the mandibular incisors and, therefore, pure skeletal response of the functional treatment can be observed.

This chapter describes the use of fixed functional appliances with symphyseal bone anchorage and discusses clinical results with three different designs.

PREPARATION OF THE MAXILLARY DENTITION

Before inserting the symphyseal bone-anchored devices, fixed appliances are placed on the maxillary dentition to align and level the teeth. After leveling, a rectangular (0.017×0.025 inch) archwire including a palatal root torque and a transpalatal arch of 0.9 mm SS wire are applied to the maxillary teeth.

THE MINIPLATE FOR CHIN FIXATION

Special titanium alloy (Titanium Alloy Certificate 1210021571000020 01) miniplates to attach to the chin were designed and developed using three-dimensional modeling software (Tasarimmed, Istanbul, Turkey) (see Fig. 13.1C).

The miniplates are constructed to fit either the left or the right side. The retentive plate has three holes (diameter, 2.3 mm) suitable for all surgical miniscrews. An antirotation wedge is constructed in order to balance rotation forces. A round bar extension with a slight mesial curve is designed to carry the point of force application to the level of the canine crown. This round bar can be bent to get the ball ends to the desired position. The ball ends house round tubes that are parallel to the dental arches and are used to fix functional appliances.

POSITIONING THE BALL ENDS

To position the ball ends, an imaginary line is drawn beginning from the cusp tip of the canine and continuing along the root axis; this line represents the *y*-axis. Another line connecting the mesial and distal corners of the canine crown is drawn to represent the *x*-axis. The intersection point of the axes is the central point. The ball ends are placed 4–5 mm buccally and centrally in relation to the central point for hygienic purposes. The round bar extensions with the ball ends exposed to the oral cavity must pass through attached gingiva; peri-implantitis may develop if they pass through mobile gingiva.

SURGICAL INSERTION OF THE MINIPLATES

Under local anesthesia, an incision is made between the premolars along a line passing through the mucogingival junction. The mucoperiosteum is then released along the incision to the level of the bony chin prominence. The miniplates are adjusted for symphyseal topography to ensure that the ball ends arise through the incision lines in the attached gingiva in the correct position. The plates are fixed with three 7 mm titanium miniscrews (2 mm diameter), and the flaps are closed with interrupted 3-0 absorbable polyglycan sutures without any tension (Fig. 24.1). Amoxicillin/clavulanate 1000 mg twice daily is taken for 5 days postoperatively and the sutures are removed at 7 days.

APPLICATION OF FIXED FUNCTIONAL APPLIANCES

JASPER JUMPER

After 7 to 10 days to allow for soft tissue healing, standardized lateral cephalometric radiographs are taken and the Jasper Jumper is applied between the maxillary molar bands to the ball-pins. The correct length for the Jasper is determined by adding 12 mm to the distance between the mesial end of the molar tube and the distal ball ending. The activation protocol is the same as for the conventional method (see Chapter 2). If the size of the appliance is insufficient for activation, it can be applied between the mesial (instead of the distal) end of the molar tube and the ball ends.

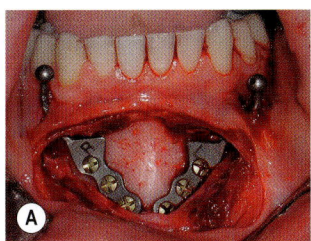
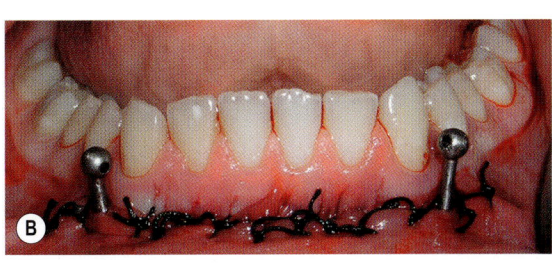

Fig. 24.1 Surgical application. (A) Miniplates fitted to the chin. (B) Ball ends of the miniplates rising up through the mucogingival junction.

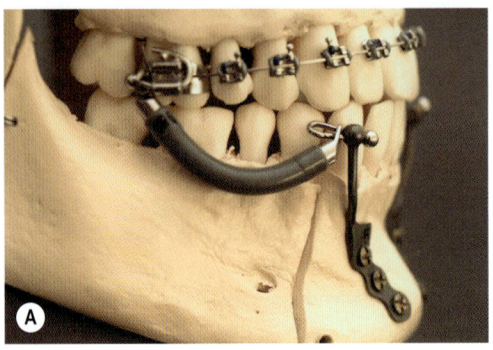
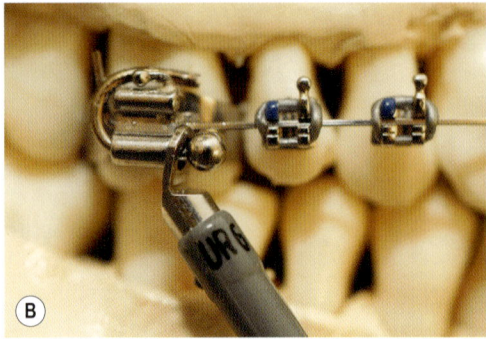
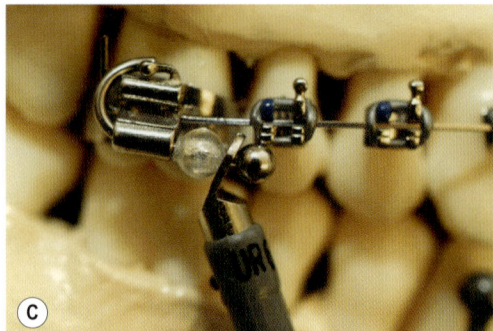

Fig. 24.2 Attachment of the Jasper Jumper appliance to the miniplate. (A) Routine placement on a model. (B) Placement of the distal portion of the appliance on the mesial end of the molar tube. (C) Addition of a ball stop for extra activation.

If more activation is needed, ball stops can be placed between the mesial end of the molar tube and the distal end of the Jasper Jumper (Fig. 24.2). If yet more activation is needed, the mandibular endings of the Jasper Jumper can be applied distal to the ball ends instead of mesial. The mandibular dental arch is not bonded during this stage.

FORSUS DEVICE

The same surgical procedure and plates are used as described for the Jasper Jumper.

To determine the correct size of the Forsus device, a special ruler is provided with the manufacturer's kit. The distal end of the ruler is placed to the distal part of the headgear tube of the maxillary molar and the mesial part is positioned to the distal part of the ball end of the miniplate. The appliance is applied to the headgear tube as instructed by the manufacturer with the only difference being that the rod that is supposed to be attached to the custom-made miniplates is applied by means of a ball-pin.

HERBST

The laboratory procedure for the fabrication of the conventional Herbst appliance should be performed very precisely because it does not allow lateral mandibular movements. When using this protocol (Herbst appliance in conjunction with miniplates), parallelism and precise placement of the Herbst appliance is crucial to successful treatment.

The body of the symphyseal plate for Herbst application has a triangular ledge that enhances the stability of the plate against turning forces. However, instead of ball ends, this design has circular heads that are designed to hold the anterior part of the Herbst appliance (see Fig. 13.1D). Screw and pivots of the Herbst appliance can be easily adapted to this part.

In order to reduce surgery time and increase the accuracy of plate positioning, three-dimensional models of the symphysis can be used to adapt the plates in readiness for fixation. Alternatively, and to avoid unnecessary radiation exposure, plates can be adapted during surgery.

The surgical procedure for application of the Herbst appliance is a little different to that described above. Under local anesthesia, the area of bone is exposed through a horizontal vestibular mucoperiosteal sulcus incision flap between the left and right first premolars. The miniplates are positioned with the mandible protruded. After releasing the mucoperiosteum, the Herbst appliance is screwed on the free ends of the miniplates. Plates are contoured manually with the first screw placed in the middle hole of the plate but not fully tightened. This allows jaw movements to be checked and the best position for the plate to be determined. While doing this, care is taken to prevent any lateral movement of the mandible. After achieving an harmonic position, the two free holes are then drilled (drill diameter, 1.5 mm) under saline irrigation; the miniplates are fixed through all three holes and the flaps closed as described above. Antimicrobial prophylaxis

is as above; the sutures are removed after 7 days and the Herbst is applied. Following the adaptation of the appliance, the opening and closing functions of the mouth should be checked.

CLINICAL PRESENTATIONS

CASE 1: JASPER JUMPER

A 14-year-old boy with Class II, division 1 malocclusion, horizontal (counterclockwise) growth pattern, a convex profile and Class II sagittal skeletal relationships caused by mandibular retrognathism sought treatment.

Following proper diagnosis and treatment planning, treatment started with rapid maxillary expansion using a fan-type expansion device (Fig. 24.3A,B). After maxillary expansion was completed, the maxillary dental arch was bonded and aligned. Six months later, the SS archwire was placed and cinched behind the first molar tubes (Fig. 24.3C). The expansion appliance was kept in the mouth for retention purposes. After the miniplates were placed and sutures removed, a Jasper Jumper was applied from the maxillary molar headgear tubes to the ball ends of the miniplates (Fig. 24.3D). After 6 months, a Class I canine and molar relationship was achieved on both sides (Fig. 24.3E). Following Class II correction, the mandibular teeth were bonded to solve the mild crowding of the mandibular dental arch, and Class II elastics were applied every night to control the risk of relapse.

A Class I dental relationship was achieved on both sides and the overjet and overbite were corrected to the normal values. Significant improvement was observed in the facial profile. The occlusal plane presented a clockwise rotation, which resulted in a slight increase of gingival exposure. Constriction of the mentalis muscle decreased with the overjet correction, which also improved the patient's profile.

CASE 2: FORSUS DEVICE

A 15-year-old boy presented with a Class II, division 2 malocclusion with horizontal (counterclockwise) growth pattern before initiation of treatment (Fig. 24.4A,C).

This patient was treated as in Case 1, above, but using a Forsus device. After leveling and alignment, the SS archwire was placed and cinched back. There was no need for expansion on the maxillary arch and, therefore, a transpalatal arch was placed to control posterior anchorage. The appropriate length of the Forsus module was attached to the maxillary molar headgear tubes and on ball ends of the miniplates (Fig. 24.4D). Jasper Jumper rods were used to adapt the Forsus appliance to the miniplates.

The Class II dental relationship had not improved by much at 8 months (Fig. 24.4E) although some improvement in the convex profile could be

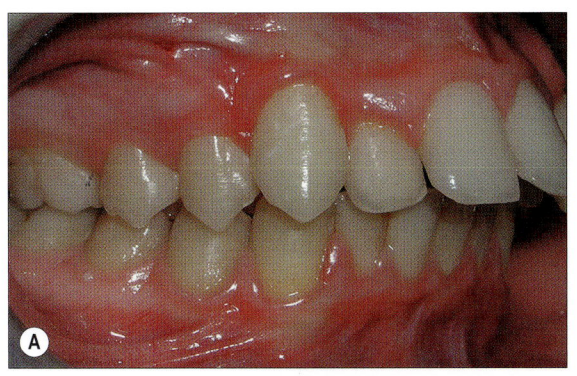
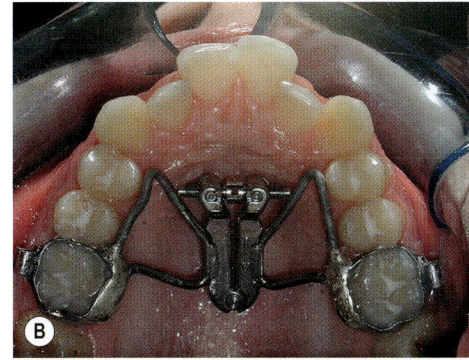
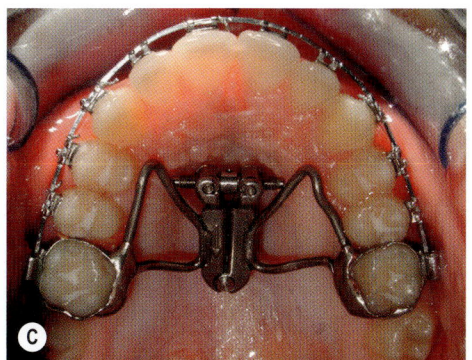

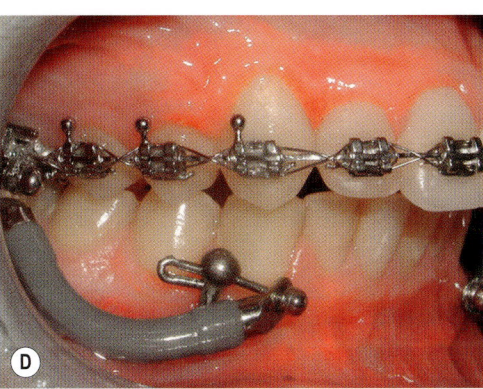
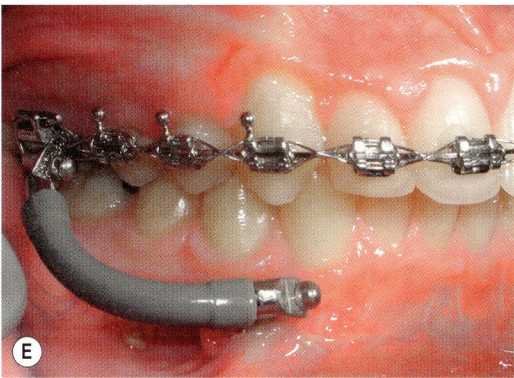

Fig. 24.3 Case 1: Jasper Jumper. (A) Pretreatment view of the occlusion. (B) Pretreatment occlusal view of the maxillary arch. (C) Occlusal view of the maxillary arch 6 months after bonding. The SS archwire and the Fan-type Hyrax appliance still remain in the mouth for retention purposes. (D) Jasper Jumper applied from the maxillary first molar headgear tubes to the lower ball ends of the chin plates. (E) Six months after fitting the Jasper Jumper and miniplates.

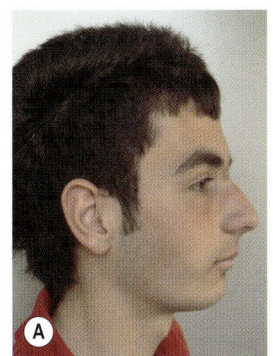
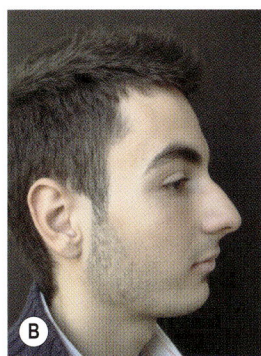

Fig. 24.4 Case 2: Forsus device. (A) Pretreatment profile. (B) Post-treatment profile. (C) Pretreatment lateral view of the occlusion. (D) Forsus device and miniplates in place. (E) Eight months after initiation of treatment. (F) Post-treatment lateral view of the occlusion.

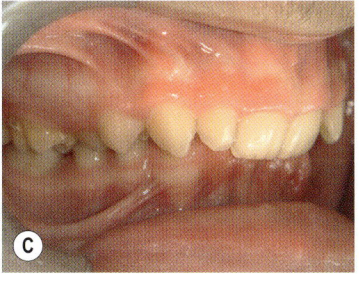
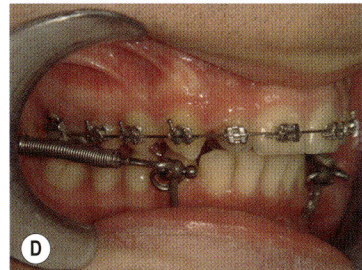
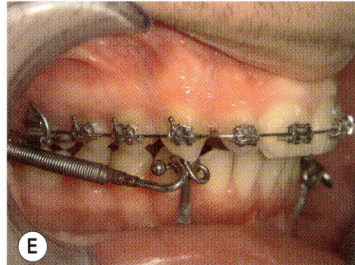
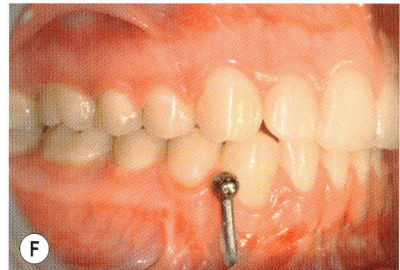

seen. To finalize treatment, the mandibular dental arch was bonded and aligned. Treatment continued with conventional Forsus application until Class I molar and canine relationships were achieved (Fig. 24.4B,F).

CASE 3: HERBST APPLICATION

A 14-year-old girl presented with Class II, division 1 malocclusion, Class II sagittal skeletal relationships and a convex profile caused by mandibular retrognathism, as well as a horizontal (counterclockwise) growth pattern (Fig. 24.5A,C).

A Herbst appliance was used in order to stimulate mandibular growth. Chromium–cobalt cast splints were fabricated for this purpose to include the maxillary first and second premolars and first molars, and a metal bar connecting the sides to each other was constructed 1 mm away from the palatal mucosa. The pivots of the Herbst appliance were soldered to the cast splints. The device was prepared accurately and attached to the miniplates in the chin area as described above (Fig. 24.5D).

The appliance remained in the mouth for 6 months (Fig. 24.5E) by which time the molars and canines were in Class I relationships and there was a significant improvement in the facial profile. After removal of the

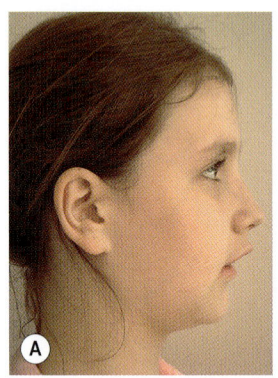
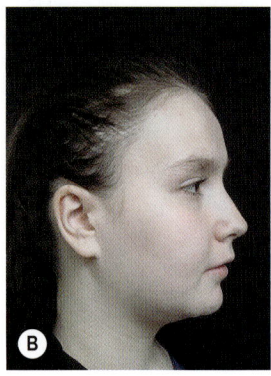

Fig. 24.5 Case 3: Herbst application. (A) Pretreatment profile. (B) Post-treatment profile. (C) Pretreatment lateral view of the occlusion. (D) Herbst appliance and miniplates in place. (E) Six months after initiation of treatment. (F) Post-treatment lateral view of the occlusion.

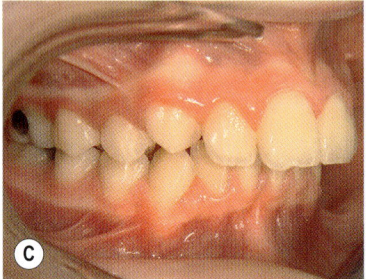
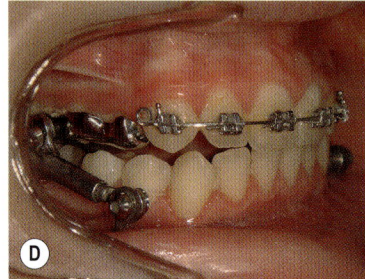
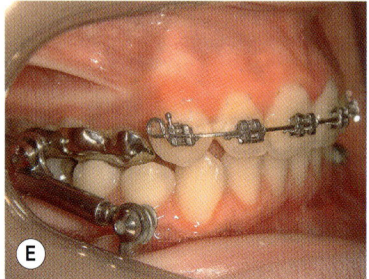
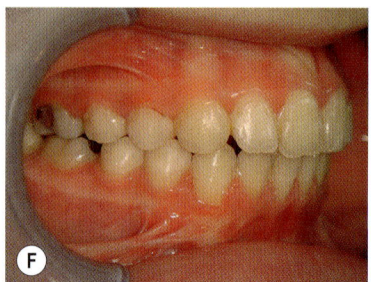

appliance, the maxillary and mandibular arches were bonded and the mild teeth malalignments were corrected. Following debonding, a significant improvement was evident in the profile and there was a good functional occlusion (Fig. 24.5B,F).

DISCUSSION

It is still unclear exactly how much skeletal effect is achieved with functional appliances whereas the dentoalveolar effects are much more evident; approximately 30% of the Class II correction achieved using fixed functional appliances has been attributed to skeletal response with 70% being dentoalveolar response.[1] Fixed functional appliances can create a 1–3 mm change in condylar growth or glenoid fossa remodeling.[3,4] The development of functional appliances that direct forces directly to the mandible and not through the dental arch is intended to maximize skeletal effects and improvements in soft tissue profile.

While fitting miniplates to the mandibular symphysis is quite easy, the positioning of the miniplate and attachment of the functional appliance needs to be very accurate, particularly for the Herbst, which allows little lateral movement of the mandible.

In groups of patients using the three appliances described above, skeletal and dental changes were assessed using lateral cephalometric radiographs obtained before and after treatment. The biggest group of patients (11) was treated with the Jasper Jumper, with only a few patients in the other two groups. This was insufficient for a statistical evaluation of the Forsus or Herbst but did provide some useful insights into what could be achieved and the treatment period needed.

The 11 patients treated with Jasper Jumpers were seen every 4 weeks to check oral hygiene and any problems related to the appliance. Patients found the appliances acceptable for comfort. During treatment, 50% of the Jasper Jumpers broke and were replaced. In addition, the appliances were renewed every 2 months because of the unpleasant odor from the vinyl cover. One patient developed peri-implantitis through poor oral hygiene and the mobile miniplates were removed. Another stopped for personal reasons. Treatment of the remaining nine patients continued and treatment was assessed after 6 months of treatment.

The cephalometric measurements in the Jasper Jumper group and the corresponding statistical evaluation revealed that only changes in the sella-nasion/palatal plane angle were significant (Table 24.1). The evaluations for the other two groups gave similar results.

However, statistically significant dental changes were observed in all the groups, mainly through alterations to the occlusal plane. More specifically, the occlusal plane/sella-nasion and the occlusal plane/palatal plane angles were increased significantly, while the occlusal plane/mandibular plane angle was significantly decreased. Similar changes have been reported with fixed functional appliances with conventional approaches rather than skeletal anchorage.[5]

All these changes resulted in posterior rotation of the mandible, maxillary incisor retroclination and extrusion, maxillary molar intrusion and distalization. Consequently, Class I molar relationship and overjet were corrected.

Miniplates fitted to the chin area seem to be suitable for the application of fixed functional appliances, except the Herbst. Although no miniplates were lost as a result of loading of orthopedic forces in the patients treated with the Jasper Jumper and Forsus, almost 50% of the plates in the Herbst group were lost during the first 6 months of loading. Consequently, treatment was only completed for two of the patients in this group. This confirms that this procedure is challenging and not suitable for rigid functional appliances such as the Herbst.

In all the groups, there was a remarkable decrease of overjet and correction of the Class II molar relationship. However, no significant increase in mandibular skeletal growth was seen in any patient. There are two possible reasons. First, the treatment period of 6 months may be insufficient for mandibular skeletal growth to occur. In addition, the changes in maxillary dentition that took place in a short period of time contributed to the quick correction of the dental discrepancy without leaving enough space for the mandibular skeletal correction. Second, mandibular skeletal growth and condylar adaptation simply do not occur as much as might be expected with fixed functional treatment regardless of the type of anchorage.

The approach described in this chapter using miniplates on the mandibular symphysis can be successfully utilized for the application of fixed functional appliances. However, more clinical studies with large study samples are needed to confirm its clinical effectiveness.

Table 24.1 Cephalometric measurements for patients treated with the Jasper Jumper

Measurements (°)	Pretreatment (SD)	Post-treatment (SD)	Difference (SD)	*p* value
SNA	82.29 (2.56)	81.57 (4.69)	0.71 (2.87)	0.492
SNB	75.86 (3.44)	76.00 (3.37)	−0.14 (1.22)	0.739
ANB	6.43 (3.31)	5.71 (3.25)	0.71 (2.43)	0.288
SN-Pog	78.14 (4.1)	77.57 (4.12)	0.57 (1.72)	0.458
SN–MP	35.29 (5.47)	35.57 (6.40)	−0.29 (2.14)	0.863
SN–PP	7.71 (2.06)	9.29 (2.06)	−1.57 (1.51)	0.042*
OP–SN	17.00 (5.03)	22.71 (5.77)	−5.71 (4.15)	0.028*
OP–MP	17.71 (3.3)	12.71 (2.75)	5 (3.51)	0.018*
PP–OP	9.86 (3.48)	13.43 (4.76)	−3.57 (2.76)	0.027*

A, A point; B, B point; MP, mandibular plane; N, nasion; OP, occlusal plane; Pog, pogonion; PP, palatal plane; SD, standard deviation, SN, sella-nasion.
*$p < 0.05$.

ACKNOWLEDGMENTS

We would like to thank Drs. Gühan Dergin and İmad M. Salih for performing the surgeries, and Dr. Cem Gazivekili for treatment of patients with the Jasper Jumper appliance.

REFERENCES

1. Creekmore TD, Radney LJ. Frankel appliance therapy: orthopedic or orthodontic? Am J Orthod 1983;83:89–108.

2. Kucukkeles N, Ilhan I, Orgun A. Treatment efficiency in skeletal Class II patients treated with the Jasper Jumper. Angle Orthod 2007;77:449–56.
3. Marsico E, Gatto E, Burrascano M. Effectiveness of orthodontic treatment with functional appliances on mandibular growth in the short term. Am J Orthod Dentofacial Orthop 2011;139:24–36.
4. Cozza P, Baccetti T, Franchi L, et al. Mandibular changes produced by functional appliances in Class II malocclusion: a systematic review. Am J Orthod Dentofacial Orthop 2006;129:599.
5. Weiland FJ, Ingervall B, Bantleon HP, et al. Initial effects of Class II malocclusion with the Herren activator, activator-headgear combination and Jasper Jumper. Am J Orthod Dentofacial Orthop 1997;112:19–27.

25 Overview of miniscrew implants in treatment of Class II malocclusion

Moschos A. Papadopoulos and Vasileios F. Zymperdikas

INTRODUCTION

Treatment of Class II malocclusion includes in general posterior movement of the maxillary dentition, anterior movement of the mandibular dentition or a combination of both; treatment can involve selective extraction of permanent teeth, either two maxillary premolars or two maxillary and two mandibular premolars (see Chapter 1).

In contrast to dental or orthodontic implants, miniscrew implants (MIs) are not osseointegrated but just mechanically retained in bone. They are easier to insert, can be used for anchorage without waiting for osseointegration and are removed at the end of treatment. Many types of tooth movement can be achieved using MIs for anchorage,[1] such as intrusion or uprighting of teeth, correction of open bite or deep bite, maxillary molar distalization and retraction of anterior teeth.

This chapter gives a brief overview of the use of MIs as temporary anchorage devices for the comprehensive treatment of Class II malocclusion. Other chapters in this section cover these systems in more detail.

NON-COMPLIANCE DISTALIZATION SYSTEMS USED WITH MINISCREW IMPLANTS

When MIs are used for the treatment of Class II malocclusion, they are usually combined with conventional fixed appliances or with non-compliance intramaxillary distalization systems to support distalization of the maxillary arch. They can also be combined with non-compliance intermaxillary devices to support mandibular advancement.

When MIs are used as anchorage reinforcement modalities, the provided anchorage can be hybrid (both bone-borne and tooth-borne) or pure skeletal (bone-borne) anchorage.

Examples of hybrid anchorage used in maxillary distalization include:

- the Distal Jet (Chapter 2) and its modifications using MIs for anchorage such as the skeletonized Distal Jet and the Implant Distal Jet
- the Pendulum appliance (Chapter 2) and its modification, the MI supported modified Pendulum appliance.

Examples of pure bone-borne anchorage systems used in maxillary distalization include:

- the Distal Jet and its modification by Bowman (Chapter 31)
- the Distal Screw (Chapter 32)
- the Pendulum B appliance (Chapter 33)
- the skeletal Pendulum-K appliance (Chapter 35)
- the bone-anchored Pendulum appliance (Chapter 36)
- the bone supported Pendulum appliance: similar to the bone-anchored system but a metallic bearing is placed in the anterior part of the Nance button, and TMA springs have a double-loop modification to control molar rotation[2]
- combination of MIs with pendulum springs
- the MI-supported distalization system (Chapter 29)
- the Advanced Molar Distalization Appliance (Chapter 30)

- the Beneslider (Chapter 33)
- the TopJet distalizer (Chapter 34)
- the palatal MI system with interchangeable units: two palatal MIs support a miniplate to which one of three detachable distalizing units fits for specific needs (see Chapter 23)
- the dual force distalizer: two palatal MIs anchor an acrylic plate with arms to which distalizating springs are attached
- the lever arm and MI system
- transpalatal arches (TPAs):
  - the MGBM system (Chapter 28)
  - the mesially extended TPA and MIs
  - intraosseous screw and TPA.

The forces needed for orthopedic correction are significantly higher than those needed for tooth movements and under such forces MIs can fail. Consequently, miniplates rather than MIs have been used as anchorage to support mandibular advancement (see Chapter 24). However, MIs have been used for this purpose with the Forsus Fatigue Resistant Device (see Chapter 46).

A brief description is given here of the non-compliance distalization systems listed above that are not covered in other chapters.

PENDULUM SPRINGS WITH A PALATAL MINISCREW IMPLANT

A modification of the original Pendulum appliance used a single MI (diameter, 3.8 mm; length, 9 mm) inserted in the anterior palatal region, laterally to the median palatal suture, combined with pendulum springs for molar distalization, thus eliminating the Nance acrylic button (Fig. 25.1).[3] A SS casting crown is fabricated on the MI to which two pendulum tubes are soldered bilaterally; these are used for the attachment of the TMA distalization springs (0.032 inch). The springs attached to lingual sheaths of the maxillary first molar bands deliver a distalization force of 300 g on both sides. When distalization is completed, the springs are replaced with 1.2 mm round SS wires, which are soldered between the abutment and the maxillary molar bands to retain the maxillary first molars in the acquired position during the subsequent phase of the distalization of the premolars and canines and retraction of the anterior teeth.

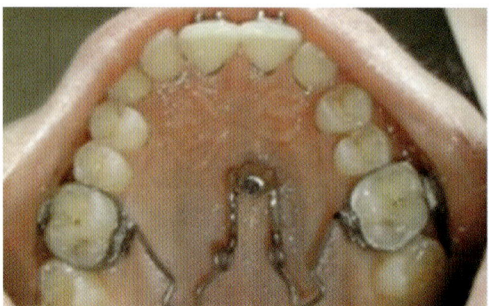

Fig. 25.1 Pendulum springs with a palatal miniscrew implant. (With permission from Oncag et al., 2007[3].)

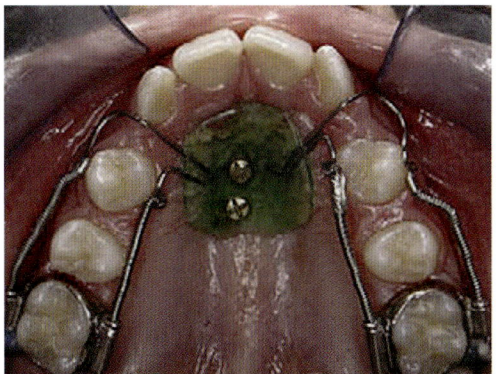

Fig. 25.2 The Dual Force Distalizer during maxillary molar distalization. (With permission from Oberti et al., 2009.[4])

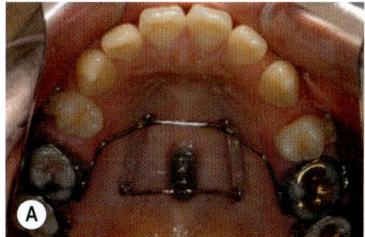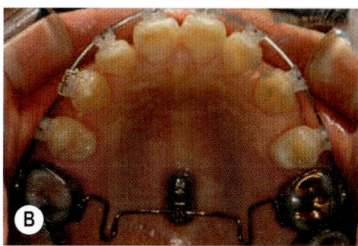

Fig. 25.3 The mesially extended transpalatal arch with miniscrew implants. (A) During active treatment. (B) Seven months after the start of treatment the device is removed and replaced with a modified transpalatal arch. (With permission from Kyung et al., 2009[5].)

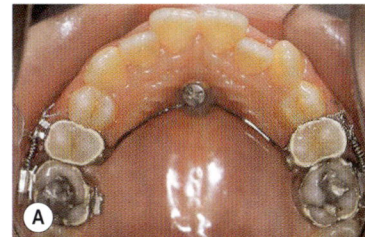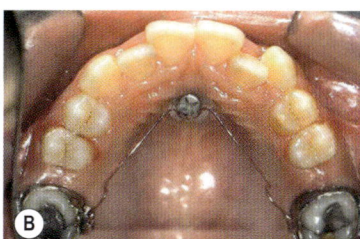

Fig. 25.4 A modified transpalatal arch with an intraosseous screw to support maxillary molar distalization. (A) The distalization system immediately after placement in the maxilla. (B) The modified Nance holding arch inserted after molar distalization is accomplished. (With permission from Gelgor et al., 2007.[7])

THE DUAL FORCE DISTALIZER

The dual force distalizer consists of an acrylic resin plate with four extension arms and two holes; it is anchored with two MIs inserted in the midpalatal suture on the anterior palatal region (Fig. 25.2).[4] Two arms of SS wires (0.028 inch) extend bilaterally on each side of the maxillary arch, one toward the buccal zone from the mesial aspect of the premolars and the other toward the palatal zone. Each arm is equipped with two stops and a Ni-Ti open coil spring and is placed into 0.045 inch tubes soldered on the vestibular and palatal sides of the first molar bands. The first stop is located mesially to the molar tube and is used to compress the coil spring in order to deliver the necessary distalization force of approximately 250–300 g, while the second stop is located distally to the molar tube to set a limit for the distalization of the first maxillary molar.

The patient is seen every month, and the coil springs are reactivated by placing a crimpable stop in the arms mesially to the coil spring. Distalization of the maxillary first molars is continued until a super-Class I is achieved. The appliance is left in place with the vestibular tubes removed and fixed appliances are bonded to the maxillary teeth to distalize the premolars and canines also to Class I occlusal relationships, as well as to retract the anterior teeth.

MESIALLY EXTENDED TRANSPALATAL ARCH WITH MINSCREW IMPLANTS

A mesially extended TPA (ME-TPA) combined with two MIs can provide absolute anchorage for the distalization of the maxillary first and second molars simultaneously after extraction of the third molars (Fig. 25.3A).[5] The MIs are placed in the median region of the midpalatal suture. A customized MI-supported S-sheath is cemented to the MI heads with flowable composite resin, and a removable sectional wire with two hooks bilaterally is placed into the sheath. A TPA, extended to the anterior region of the palate and equipped with two soldered hooks, is inserted in the lingual sheath of the maxillary molar bands. Elastics are used to connect the hooks of the TPA with the corresponding hooks of the S-sheath, producing as a consequence a distalization force. After a Class I relationship is accomplished, the ME-TPA is replaced with a modified TPA, which is connected again with the S-sheath in order to maintain the position of the distalized maxillary first molars and support the subsequent anterior teeth retraction (Fig. 25.3B).

INTRAOSSEOUS SCREW IN CONJUNCTION WITH A TRANSPALATAL ARCH

A modified TPA has also been used with an intraosseous MI to support maxillary molar distalization (Fig. 25.4A).[6,7] The MI was inserted in the anterior region of the midpalatal suture behind the incisive canal. The modified TPA was constructed with a U-bend (which should be in contact with the distal surface of the MI neck) and soldered to the maxillary first or second premolar bands. The TPA was then attached to the neck of the MI. Sectional arches and 0.036 inch Ni-Ti open coil springs were inserted buccally on both sides between the brackets of the maxillary first or second premolars and the corresponding first molars, producing a distalization force of 250 g to the molars. Patients were seen every 4 weeks for reactivation of the coil springs if necessary. After distalization of the maxillary molars to a super-Class I relationship, the modified TPA was replaced with another with two loops bilaterally for possible activations in case of anchorage loss, and again with a U-bend attached on the MI neck in order to provide further skeletal anchorage for the anterior teeth retraction with full fixed appliances (Fig. 25.4B). Use of this appliance in 25 patients resulted in 88% molar distalization and 12% reciprocal anchorage loss of the maxillary central incisors. The maxillary molar crowns tipped distally by 8.78°; the first premolars tipped mesially by 2.88°; and the maxillary incisors proclined by 1° and were moved forward 0.5 mm.[6] These changes were attributed to mesial tipping of the first premolars during molar distalization, the flexibility of the TPA and inadequate connection between the TPA and the MI, since there was only a single-point contact between them.

LEVER ARM AND MINISCREW IMPLANT SYSTEM

A lever arm and MI-supported system used for the distalization of maxillary molars consisted of two parts.[8] The lingual part comprised a conventional TPA (0.032 × 0.032 inch SS wire) attached to the palatal sheaths of the maxillary first molar bands and a MI inserted in the posterior region of the midpalatal suture. The buccal part comprised two lever arms made of SS wire (0.019 × 0.025 inch) attached to the bracket slots (0.032 × 0.032 inch) of the molar bands and two bilaterally positioned MIs, inserted in the inter-radicular space between the second premolars and the first molars on each side. By applying elastic chain modules between the MIs and the corresponding lever arms, a distal force of 150 g

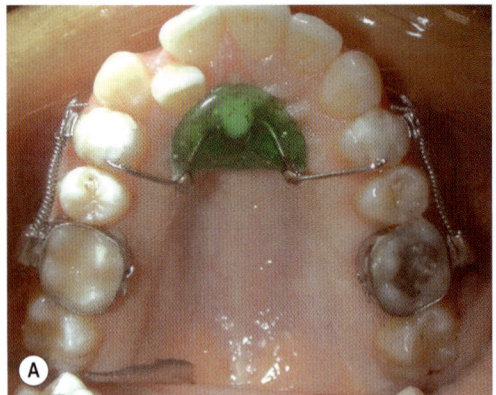
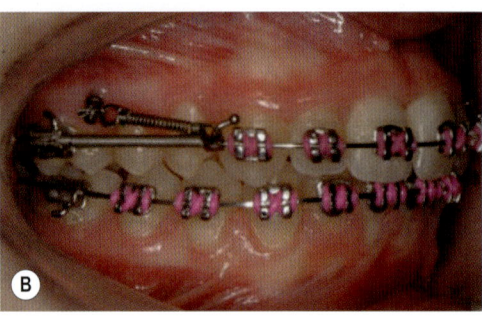
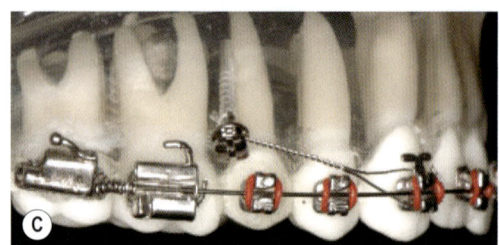

Fig. 25.5 Miniscrew implants (MI) to support appliances for maxillary molar distalization. (A) A MI in the anterior region of the midpalatal suture of the hard palate. (B) MIs buccally in the inter-radicular space between the second premolars and first molars and sliding jigs. (C) MIs in the inter-radicular space between the second premolars and the first molars. (With permission from Polat-Oszoy, 2008[9] (A), Young et al., 2007[1] (B) and Mizrahi and Mizrahi, 2007[10] (C).)

was applied buccally on each side, while between the midpalatal MI and the TPA a force of 300 g was applied palatally.

When a super-Class I was achieved, the buccal MIs were removed and fixed appliances were placed in order to align and level the maxillary teeth, while the TPA and the midpalatal MI remained in position to prevent relapse of the distal movement.

MAXILLARY DISTALIZATION WITH MINISCREW IMPLANTS IN COMBINATION WITH FIXED APPLIANCES

MIs can be used with various configurations in combination with conventional fixed appliances, for

- maxillary molar distalization alone
- distalization of the entire maxillary arch, either sequentially (molar distalization first and then anterior teeth retraction) or en masse
- anterior teeth retraction alone (usually after extractions of the maxillary first premolars).

For anterior teeth retraction, initial extraction of the first premolars provides the space into which the anterior teeth can be moved under the influence of MI-anchored systems.

Most clinicians use MIs with conventional fixed appliances for the distalization of the entire maxillary arch, either sequentially or en masse.

MAXILLARY MOLAR DISTALIZATION

MIs have been placed in various locations to support maxillary molar distalization (Fig. 25.5).

A MI in the anterior region of the midpalatal suture of the hard palate was used to support an acrylic Nance button (Fig. 25.5A).[9] The MI was embedded in the acrylic plate from which occlusal wires extended to bond to the maxillary first premolars bilaterally. After banding of the maxillary first molars and bonding of the first premolars, sectional arches and open coil springs were inserted between the first premolars and the first molars, delivering a distalization force of approximately 250 g on each side. At the end of distalization, the initial acrylic plate was removed with a bur to expose the MI, and a new Nance acrylic button was fabricated, again over the MI, to support molar anchorage during anterior teeth retraction.[9]

In addition, MIs implanted buccally in the inter-radicular space between the maxillary second premolars and first molars have been combined with sliding jigs to support molar distalization.[1] Each MI was connected through Ni-Ti coil springs to a sliding jig attached on the maxillary archwire, applying a distalization force to the maxillary first molars (Fig. 25.5B).

Furthermore, placement of MIs in the inter-radicular space between the second premolars and the first molars has also been used to provide indirect anchorage for the distalization of first and/or second molars.[10] Each MI was connected with a ligature tie to the canine, first or second premolar brackets, or to a hook soldered or bent onto the main archwire (Fig. 25.5C). The type of mechanics used depends on the eruption stage of the second molars. If the second molars are erupted, an open coil spring can be inserted between the first and second molars. Alternatively, an archwire incorporating an expansion loop can be used to distalize the second molars. In contrast, if the second molars are not erupted, a coil spring can be inserted between the second premolars and the first molars, or an expanding arch similar to the one used to distalize the second molars can be used to distalize the first molars.

SEQUENTIAL DISTALIZATION OF THE ENTIRE MAXILLARY ARCH

For a sequential distalization, two MIs are usually used and placed bilaterally between the roots of the second premolars and the first molars.

A two-component MI (C-implant, CIMPLANT, Seoul, Korea) was used with coil springs for the distalization of the maxillary posterior teeth, retraction of the maxillary anterior teeth and coordination of both arches for ideal occlusion.[11] Initially, the MIs were used with Class III elastics and fixed appliances in the lower arch to support uprighting of the mandibular molars (Fig. 25.6A). Then, fixed appliances were placed on the maxillary arch and the MIs were connected by means of Ni-Ti coil springs to sliding jigs attached on the maxillary first molars, which resulted in distalization of the maxillary first and second molars into a Class I relationship (Fig. 25.6B). This created a space between the maxillary first molars and second premolars that could be used for the retraction of the teeth anterior to molars. After molar distalization, the MIs were removed from between the roots of the second premolars and first molars and reinserted between the roots of the maxillary first and second molars. Immediately after MI relocation, a force of approximately 150 g was applied using Class I elastics connecting the MIs with hooks soldered on the maxillary archwire mesial to the canines for the retraction of the maxillary anterior teeth.

A similar two-step procedure used two MIs inserted bilaterally in the maxillary vestibular alveolar bone between the roots of the second premolars and first molars (Fig. 25.7).[12] After placing rectangular beta-titanium archwires, each MI was connected through a Ni-Ti coil spring or an elastomeric thread to the corresponding canine for the distalization of the posterior teeth, delivering a distalization force of approximately 200 g in each quadrant. The distalization of the posterior teeth created a small space

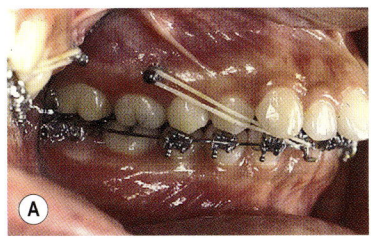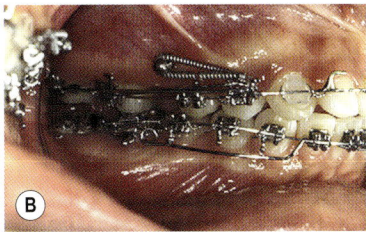

Fig. 25.6 Sequential distalization of the entire maxillary arch. (A) Miniscrew implants (MI) placed bilaterally between the maxillary second premolars and the first molars and application of Class III elastics from the MIs to soldered hooks mesial to the canines. (B) Coil springs attached bilaterally to the MIs and to the sliding jigs (attached on the maxillary first molars) for the distalization of the maxillary first and second molars into a Class I relationship. (With permission from Chung et al., 2010.[11])

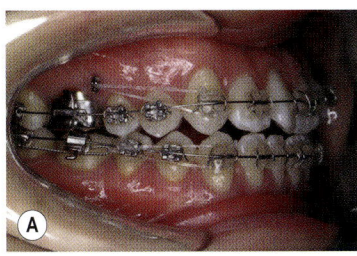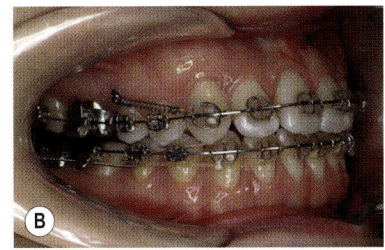

Fig. 25.7 Sequential distalization of the entire maxillary arch. (A) Initial leveling to gain space for the alignment of the anterior teeth. The distalizing force is applied from the miniscrew implants (MI) to the canines with elastics. (B) En masse retraction of the anterior teeth. The retraction force is applied from the MIs to the canines with coil springs. (With permission from Oh et al., 2011.[12])

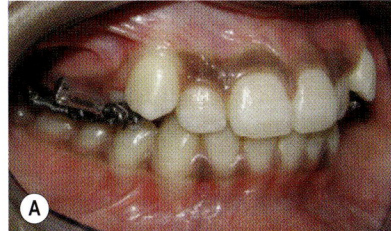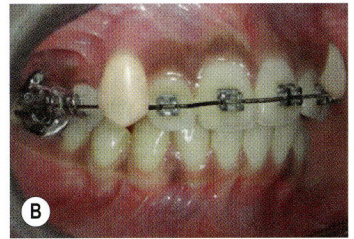

Fig. 25.8 Sequential distalization of the entire maxillary arch. (A) Lateral intraoral view showing the distalization system placed in the maxilla. (B) Progress lateral view showing premolar retraction after molar distalization and reinsertion of new miniscrew implants. (With permission from Doshi et al., 2011.[13])

mesial to the canine in each quadrant. After alignment, the six anterior teeth were tied together and a retraction force applied from the MIs to the canines or to short hooks attached on the archwire between the lateral incisors and the canines.

An alternative two-step procedure used two MIs inserted bilaterally in the inter-radicular space between the second premolars and first molars (Fig. 25.8).[13] The maxillary first and second premolars and first molars were banded and sectional wires with Ni-Ti coil springs extending from the maxillary first premolar to the corresponding first molar were placed on each side. Compressed coil springs between the second premolars and first molars delivered a continuous distalization force of 240 g per side, while a ligature wire was threaded to each MI neck and ligated to the first premolar bracket. As a result, the MIs provided indirect anchorage for the distalization of the molars. When a super-Class I relationship was accomplished, the MIs were removed and a second pair of MIs were inserted at an angle of approximately 30° mesial to the first molars. The insertion site not only permitted retraction of the premolars but also prevented the molars from moving mesially. Then the maxillary incisors and premolars were bonded and initial alignment was carried out. Subsequently, a

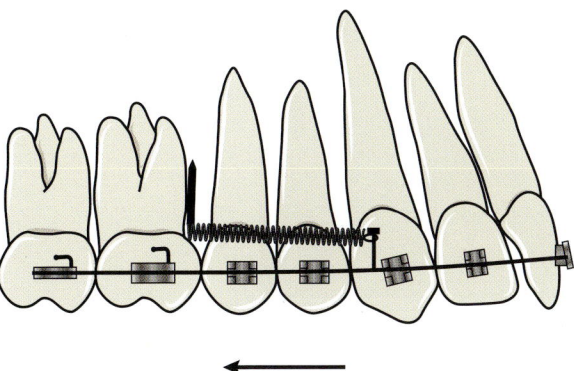

Fig. 25.9 En masse distalization of the maxillary arch achieved with miniscrew implants. (With permission from Yamada et al., 2009.[14])

stretched elastomeric module connected to the MIs was used to retract the premolars. Finally, the maxillary canines were also bonded and after alignment with a Ni-Ti archwire (0.016 inch) they were retracted as well.

EN MASSE DISTALIZATION OF THE ENTIRE MAXILLARY ARCH

Methods for en masse distalization of the entire maxillary arch use bilateral MIs for anchorage. MIs inserted bilaterally between the roots of the second premolars and first molars were combined with Ni-Ti coil springs or elastic chains.[14] After bonding and placement of a SS archwire (0.016 × 0.022 inch) on the maxillary arch, Ni-Ti closed coil springs or elastic chains were placed from the MIs to hooks attached on the maxillary archwire distal to the canines on each side, applying a distalization force of approximately 200 g (Fig. 25.9). The direction of the force was upward and backward and as parallel to the occlusal plane as possible. The molars were distalized without proclination of the anterior teeth, but this movement was not bodily since distal tipping also took place.

A similar treatment approach used MIs placed bilaterally in the buccal alveolar bone of the maxilla, 1 mm distal to vertical lines passing through the contact points of the first and second molars.[15] A SS archwire (0.016 × 0.022 inch) with hooks welded between the canines and the first premolars was placed in the upper arch. The welded hooks were fabricated short to avoid extrusion of the maxillary posterior teeth. Additional labial crown torque in the anterior region and an accentuated curve of Spee were given to the arch before placement. Then, power chains were attached between the MIs and the respective hooks bilaterally, producing a distalization force of 200 g per side.

A similar system used MIs inserted at the zygoma above the maxillary molars and the results obtained were considered to be a good alternative to conventional distalization with cervical headgears.[16] After placement of SS archwires (0.016 × 0.022 inch) on both arches, two sliding hooks were cinched with downward orientation between the maxillary lateral incisors and the canines. Two MIs with gold chains attached to their heads were inserted bilaterally in the maxillary buttress. The gold chains were connected through power threads to the corresponding sliding hooks, providing direct anchorage for anterior teeth retraction.

Another treatment approach concerning the correction of Class II deep bite, involves distalization of the maxillary arch with MI anchorage in combination with fixed appliances and bite blocks to increase the vertical dimension.[17] After bonding and initial aligning of both dental arches, two MIs were placed bilaterally in the inter-radicular space between the maxillary second premolars and first molars. After 2 months, resin bite blocks were bonded to the lingual surfaces of the maxillary central incisors, and later SS wires (0.016 × 0.022 inch) were inserted in both arches along with crimped hooks (length, 10 mm) attached bilaterally between the lateral

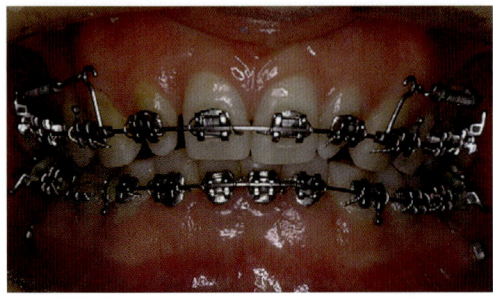

Fig. 25.10 Frontal view showing the beta-titanium alloy archwire with hooks and torquing bend, the miniscrew implants and the application of coil springs to retract en masse the maxillary dental arch. (With permission from Park et al., 2011.[17])

incisors and the canines. The distalization force was applied by Ni-Ti coil springs extending from the MIs to the corresponding hooks (Fig. 25.10). After 5 months, the maxillary posterior teeth were distalized but the maxillary second molars were extruded and tipped distally, which required these teeth to be bonded for uprighting during the subsequent final stage of treatment.

Treatment of skeletal gummy smiles in patients with Class II malocclusion is discussed in Chapter 38.

CONCLUSIONS

While MIs can be utilized efficiently as temporary anchorage devices in order to distalize maxillary molars or the entire maxillary dentition, the outcome of treatment depends greatly on the biomechanics used for molar distalization. When the force vector of the distalization system passes through or very close to the center of resistance of the molars, pure or almost bodily movement of the teeth is produced. Generally, this is mostly accomplished when the MIs are inserted in the palate, because this allows the application of forces parallel to the occlusal plane and close to the center of resistance of the molars. When MIs are inserted in the buccal area of the maxilla, the distalization forces are applied more occlusally and away from the center of resistance of the molars, leading to distal tipping of the molar crowns.

REFERENCES

1. Young KA, Melrose CA, Harrison JE. Skeletal anchorage systems in orthodontics: absolute anchorage. A dream or reality? J Orthod 2007;34:101–10.
2. Escobar SA, Tellez PA, Moncada CA, et al. Distalization of maxillary molars with the bone-supported pendulum: a clinical study. Am J Orthod Dentofacial Orthop 2007;131:545–9.
3. Oncag G, Akyalcin S, Arikan F. The effectiveness of a single osteointegrated implant combined with pendulum springs for molar distalization. Am J Orthod Dentofacial Orthop 2007;131:277–84.
4. Oberti G, Villegas C, Ealo M, et al. Maxillary molar distalization with the dual-force distalizer supported by mini-implants: a clinical study. Am J Orthod Dentofacial Orthop 2009;135:282.e1–5.
5. Kyung SH, Lee JY, Shin JW, et al. Distalization of the entire maxillary arch in an adult. Am J Orthod Dentofacial Orthop 2009;135:S123–32.
6. Gelgor IE, Buyukyilmaz T, Karaman AI, Dolanmaz D, Kalayci A. Intraosseous screw-supported upper molar distalization. Angle Orthod 2004;74:838–50.
7. Gelgor IE, Karaman AI, Buyukyilmaz T. Comparison of 2 distalization systems supported by intraosseous screws. Am J Orthod Dentofacial Orthop 2007;131:161.e1–8.
8. Lim SM, Hong RK. Distal movement of maxillary molars using a lever-arm and mini-implant system. Angle Orthod 2008;78:167–75.
9. Polat-Ozsoy O. The use of intraosseous screw for upper molar distalization: a case report. Eur J Dent 2008;2:115–21.
10. Mizrahi E, Mizrahi B. Mini-screw implants (temporary anchorage devices): orthodontic and pre-prosthetic applications. J Orthod 2007;34:80–94.
11. Chung KR, Choo HR, Kim SH, Ngan P. Timely relocation of mini-implants for uninterrupted full-arch distalization. Am J Orthod Dentofacial Orthop 2010;138:839–49.
12. Oh YH, Park HS, Kwon TG. Treatment effects of microimplant-aided sliding mechanics on distal retraction of posterior teeth. Am J Orthod Dentofacial Orthop 2011;139:470–81.
13. Doshi UH, Jamwal RS, Bhad WA. Distalization of molars using two stage mini-implants: a case report. J Orthod 2011;38:55–63.
14. Yamada K, Kuroda S, Deguchi T, Takano-Yamamoto T, Yamashiro T. Distal movement of maxillary molars using miniscrew anchorage in the buccal interradicular region. Angle Orthod 2009;79:78–84.
15. Jeon JM, Yu HS, Baik HS, Lee JS. En-masse distalization with miniscrew anchorage in Class II nonextraction treatment. J Clin Orthod 2006;40:472–6.
16. Munoz A, Maino G, Lemler J, Kornbluth D. Skeletal anchorage for Class II correction in a growing patient. J Clin Orthod 2009;43:325–31.
17. Park HS, Kim JY, Kwon TG. Treatment of a Class II deepbite with microimplant anchorage. Am J Orthod Dentofacial Orthop 2011;139:397–406.

INTRODUCTION

Class II division 1 malocclusions are described as having labially inclined maxillary incisors, increased overjet and a vertical overbite, which might vary from a deep overbite to an open bite. In contrast, Class II division 2 malocclusions show excessive lingual inclination of the maxillary central incisors overlapped on the labial by the maxillary lateral incisors. They always show a deep overbite with minimal overjet. There are two broad approaches for Class II correction: alteration of the skeletal base by surgical or orthopedic means or dental compensation, which involves masking the underlying skeletal discrepancy (if any) by dental movements.

This chapter discusses compensation mechanics using miniscrew implant (MI)-supported anchorage. Earlier chapters in this book have covered the general principles of MIs as anchorage and the biomechanics involved. Broadly speaking, the following typical dental movements are sought:

- distal movement of the maxillary teeth, either stepwise with molar first followed by rest of the teeth or en masse
- retraction of the maxillary anterior teeth into a premolar extraction space while maintaining the Class II molar relationship
- combination of retraction of the maxillary teeth and forward movement of the lower teeth.

Fig. 26.1 outlines the possible steps required, depending on the individual patient. The following will be discussed in this chapter:

- retraction of the maxillary anterior teeth while maintaining a Class II molar relationship

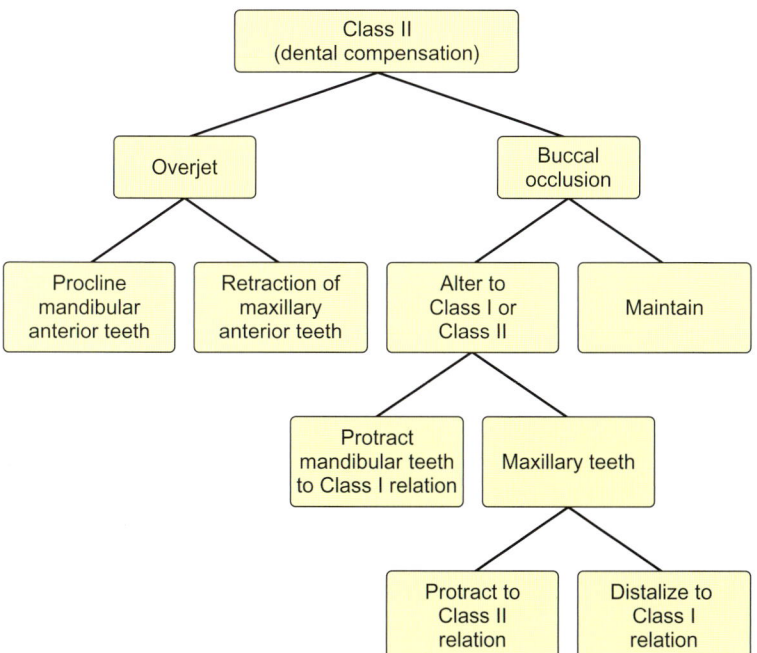

Fig. 26.1 Treatment objectives for compensating a dental Class II malocclusion.

- distalization of the posterior teeth
- molar protraction/mesialization.

RETRACTION OF THE MAXILLARY ANTERIOR TEETH

Treatment for the correction of Class II malocclusions in non-growing patients usually involves selective removal of permanent teeth, with subsequent dental camouflage to mask the skeletal discrepancy and provide a good facial balance. Extractions can involve two maxillary premolars or two maxillary and two mandibular premolars. The extraction of only two maxillary premolars and anterior teeth retraction is generally indicated when there is no crowding or cephalometric discrepancy in the mandibular arch. When retracting anterior teeth in a full cusp Class II malocclusion, anchorage control assumes profound importance because maintaining the posterior segment in place becomes very critical. A loss in molar anchorage can not only compromise correction of the anteroposterior discrepancy but also affect the overall vertical dimension of the face.[1]

The preferred location for MI placement is between the roots of the second premolars and first molars close to the mucogingival junction. An SS archwire (0.017 × 0.025 inch) and a force of 150–200 g are considered as optimum conditions for efficient retraction of the maxillary anterior teeth.[2,3] The biomechanics involved during en masse retraction of the anterior teeth with MI-assisted anchorage is illustrated in Fig. 26.2. In the second stage after space closure, continuation of the force from the springs, as is sometimes done for en masse distalization, can cause some intrusion and distalization of the entire arch. This is primarily because of increased friction between the archwire and the bracket. Therefore, the thicker the archwire, the greater the distalizing effect on the entire arch will be.

DISTALIZATION OF THE POSTERIOR TEETH

Sagittal movement of the dentition without extractions is often difficult and time consuming. Issues of unwanted tooth movements during distalization, which have to be corrected in a subsequent stage ("round tripping," see Chapter 2), can be avoided if MIs are used for skeletal anchorage.

MI-based anchorage can be lingually from the palate, buccally from the alveolar bone (between the roots), or from the zygomatic buttress.

MOLAR DISTALIZATION

Fig. 26.3 shows a simple buccal approach to distalize molars individually. The treatment plan demanded the creation of space by molar distalization before leveling and aligning the rest of the dentition. A push-coil spring from the MI inserted between the roots of the first premolar and canine linked to the molar with an SS wire (0.016 × 0.022 inch) bent passively from the MI to the auxiliary tube of the molar. Uprighting of the molar required the center of rotation to be closer to the root apex, leading in principle to greater tip-back of the crown and less root movement. This force system is illustrated in Fig. 26.3C–E.

Fig. 26.2 Biomechanics of en masse retraction of the anterior teeth with miniscrew implant anchorage. The force (*F*) exerted by the bilateral coil springs has two distinct components: a larger and predominantly retractive force (*r*) and a smaller intrusive force (*i*). There is also a clockwise moment (*M*) on the anterior segment as the total force passes below the estimated center of resistance (CR) of the anterior teeth. (A) Initial stage to close the extraction space. Significant M on the anterior segment causes tipping of the anterior teeth. (B) After space closure, the canine is in contact with the second premolar. The moment is reduced as the force from the spring is applied closer to the CR of the entire arch. Note the increase in the angulation of the total force relative to the occlusal plane.

Fig. 26.3 Molar distalization for a mesially tipped maxillary left first molar and to make space for eruption of an impacted maxillary left second premolar. (A) Immediately after miniscrew implant insertion and force application through a coil spring. (B) After molar distalization. (C) The force (*Fa*) applied from the MI through the push-coil pushes the molar distally, producing a moment (*Mf*) because *Fa* is not applied at the center of resistance (CR), causing the molar to tip around a point apical to the CR (approximately). (D) Once molar distalization is complete and a Class I relationship is obtained, the molar is included in the rest of the arch by placing continuous archwires, resulting in a couple (*Mc*) at the molar tube. (E) A couple creates a moment around the CR; therefore, although there is a moment to distalize the root, the same moment is also acting to mesialize the crown of the molar. This makes it imperative to have a passive distalizing force (*Fp*) on the molar too, which will ensure only root movement.

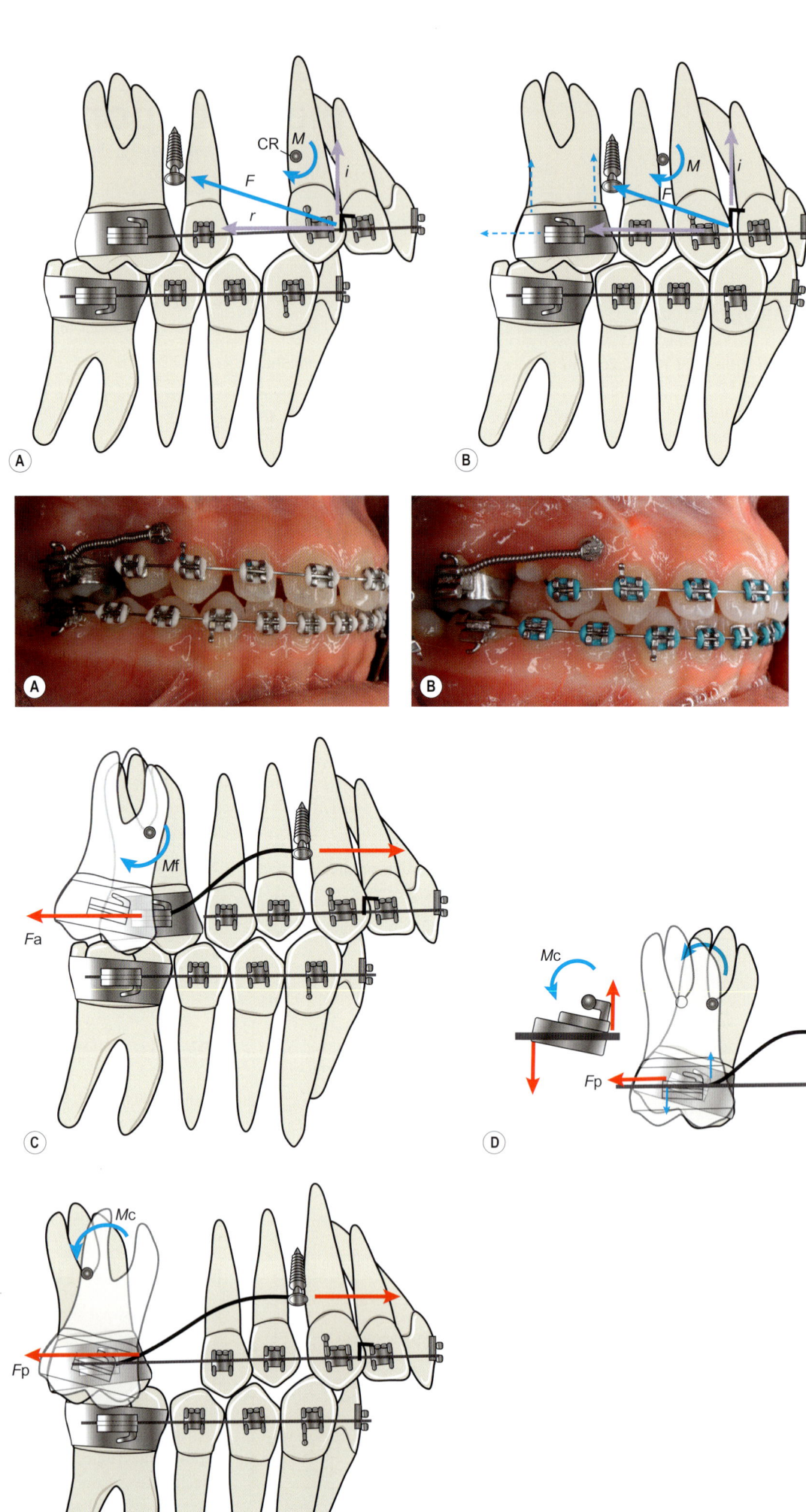

EN MASSE DISTALIZATION

Distalization of the maxillary arch by more than 2–3 mm cannot be achieved using an inter-radicular MI for anchorage. Placement of a MI, or miniplate, buccally above the mucogingival junction in the zygomatic bone is a feasible option but the surgery (particularly for miniplates) can be more extensive and there are more oral hygiene issues. Placement of MIs or implants in the palate is also an option (see Chapter 7). The mid-palatal suture area seems a particularly good placement site. Some clinicians favor the palatal area behind the incisive foramen while others prefer the paramedian region of the palate as there is more bone support.[4–8] One of the primary advantages of using palatal implants is the application of force closer to the center of resistance (CR) of the posterior teeth to achieve bodily translation with minimal tipping. In addition, there is no flaring or proclination of the anterior teeth and no mesial movement of the molar during retraction of the anterior teeth.

Distalization with MIs helps in efficient control of the vertical dimension by preventing the extrusion of the molars, thereby maintaining the mandibular plane angle (Fig. 26.4). A clockwise rotation of the mandibular plane can worsen the Class II malocclusion and make relapse more likely.

The vertical component of the total force can result in binding (or increase of friction) of the archwire to the brackets or tubes, thereby preventing sliding and resulting in the transmission of the force to the entire archwire and consequently greater amounts of distalization and intrusion. Small vertical changes at the posterior teeth can produce profound changes in the anterior area: 1 mm of intrusion at the posterior teeth can produce 3 mm of upward and forward movement at point gnathion and probably more at the chin.[9] Such a movement can be a critical factor for the correction of Class II relationships, particularly in high-angle relations. The occlusogingival position of the MI, or the use of power arms or crimpable hooks, can also be critical factors in defining the vertical component of the total force. With MIs placed higher up in the vestibule, the vertical component of the total force is significantly increased.

Patients with moderate to severe vertical facial patterns do not always have an anterior open bite, because often the incisors have been supra-erupted, compensating for the posterior vertical excess. Therefore, during orthodontic mechanotherapy, in addition to preventing extrusion of the maxillary and mandibular posterior teeth, it is equally important that the maxillary anterior teeth are intruded as they are retracted. This maximizes the upward rotation of the mandible as the incisal stop is moved further up. Without intrusion and control of the axial inclination of the maxillary anterior teeth, the patient is likely to have a longer face and a more downward and backward rotated mandible, exaggerating the Class II appearance.

LIMITATIONS OF DISTALIZATION

One of the limitations encountered in maxillary molar distalization is associated with the lack of space in the maxillary tuberosity area to move teeth distally. Extraction of maxillary third molars can provide sufficient space in the tuberosity area for teeth to move within the alveolar bone.

A further limitation can arise if the MI supporting the distalization can interfere with adjacent roots. To prevent such interference, MIs should be angulated superiorly, to give clearance between the MI and the root apex in coronal view; alternatively, roots can be tipped apart to create sufficient space before insertion of the MI.

MOLAR PROTRACTION/MESIALIZATION

Protraction of mandibular molars to correct a Class II molar relationship is biomechanically one of the most challenging scenarios. The mandibular molars are more difficult to move mesially because the mandible is made of thick cortical bone connected by coarse trabecular bone, and the molar roots are extremely wide buccolingually.[10] Conventional techniques not only cause mesial tipping of the molars but also lingual tipping of the anterior teeth, resulting in an increased overjet and worsening of the Class II profile (Fig. 26.5A). The large root surfaces of molars make their movement uncertain, while simultaneously they can cause unwanted tooth movements, such as lingual tipping of the incisors. Placement of a dental implant in the retromolar area for absolute anchorage has allowed effective closure of the space from a missing mandibular first molar.[11,12] The dental implants were strong enough to withstand the reactive forces and thus produced effective mesial movement of the mandibular molars without any lingual tipping of the incisors.[13,14]

Molar protraction usually involves pure forward bodily translation. If the line of force does not pass through the CR of the molar, there will be a tendency for the molar to tip forward during protraction. This may cause binding of the molar tube on to the archwire, resulting in bowing of the archform in the premolar area, which may lead to cessation of protraction or unwanted side effects on adjacent teeth (Fig. 26.5B). There are several methods to avoid these side effects during molar protraction with MIs:

- using thick SS archwire that almost fills the bracket slot: this reduces play between the molar tube and the archwire (Fig. 26.6A,D)
- using a rigid SS power arm or lever arm on the molar: the line of force from the MI passes through the CR of the molar (Fig. 26.6B)
- using regular sliding mechanics by engaging an elastic chain from the molar tube to the MI directly: after some protraction an uprighting spring has to be used to upright the molar (i.e. mesialize the root) and it is important to tie the molar to the MI with a ligature wire during uprighting to prevent distal movement of the crown (Fig. 26.6C,D)
- using a palatal MI (see Fig. 30.2): force can be applied at the CR of the molars, ensuring bodily movement with minimal side effects.

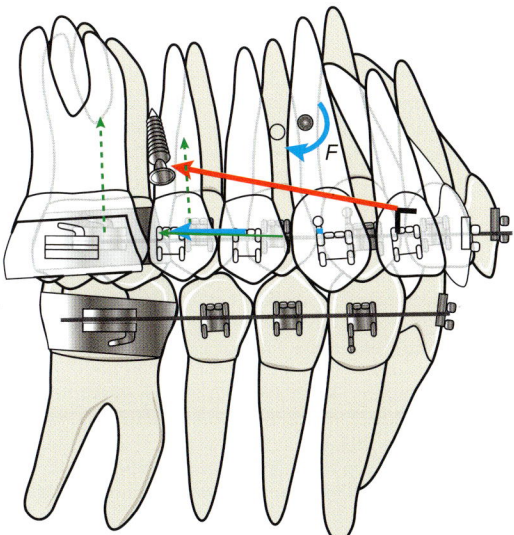

Fig. 26.4 En masse distalization of the entire arch using miniscrew implants (MIs) placed in the buccal alveolar bone. A single force (red) is applied bilaterally from the anterior segment to the MI. Horizontal and vertical components (in green) of the force tend to distalize and intrude the teeth. Stiff SS archwires will provide more effective distalization with fewer side effects than flexible archwires. The position of the MI will limit the amount of distalization as it could obstruct the roots.

Fig. 26.5 Conventional approach for molar protraction. (A) Although the anchorage of the anterior teeth is greater than the molar, the moments produced (blue) by an elastic chain (green) from the molar to the anterior segment. can cause rapid tipping of the anterior teeth. (B) If this is continued, the archwire can be distorted (deflected or bent). This can lead to stagnant tooth movement, poor control over the anterior teeth and the molar, and bite deepening.

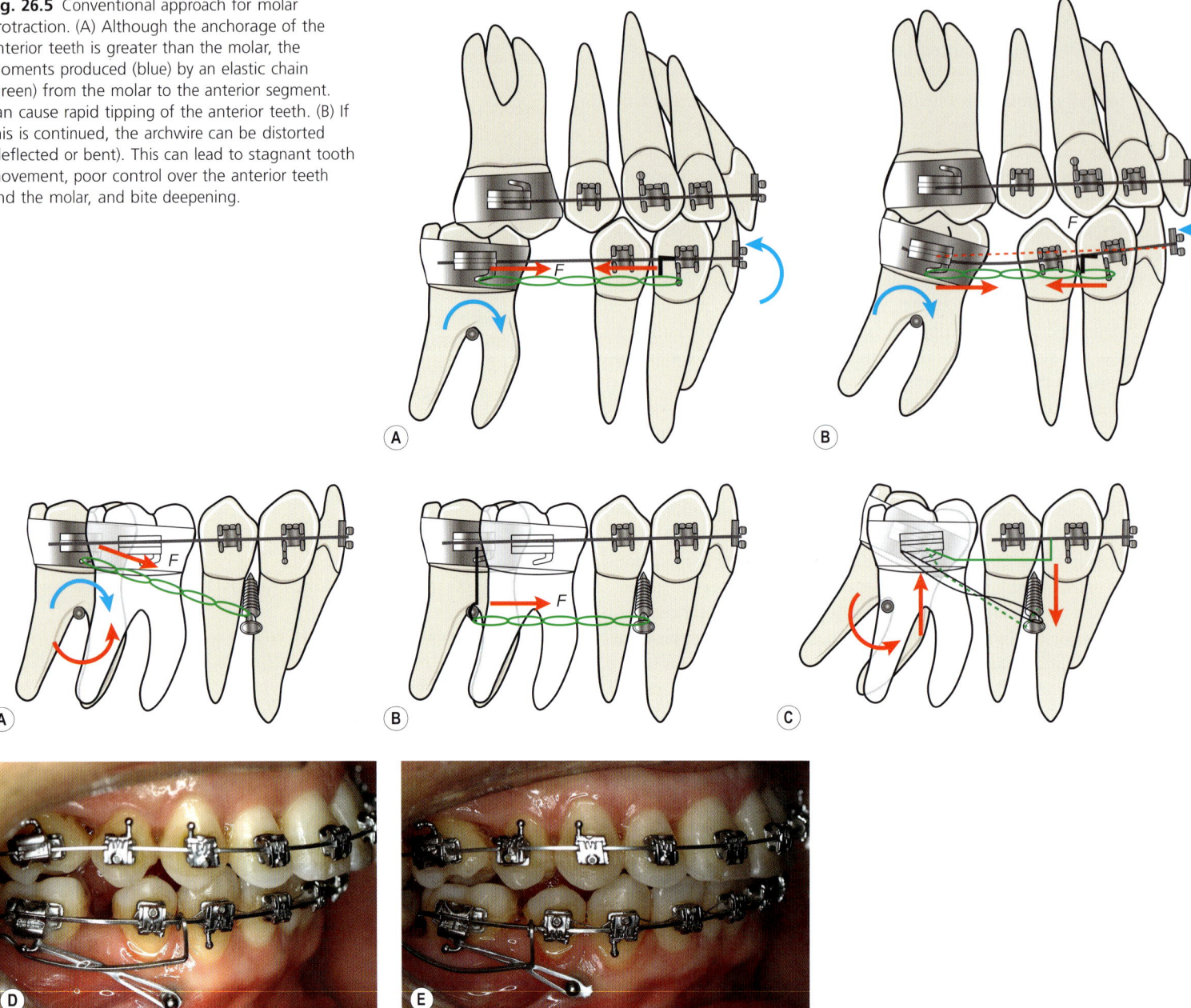

Fig. 26.6 Molar protraction without side effects from archwire distortion. (A) A stiff archwire avoids unwanted bending of the archwire during protraction, thereby effectively creating a countermoment (red) that prevents mesial tipping of the molar (blue). (B) An appropriately positioned power arm from the molar ensures bodily movement, as the force application (red) passes though the center of resistance of the molar. (C) Protraction divided into distinct phases; in the first the molar is tipped forward and subsequently, an uprighting moment (red) can be applied through an uprighting spring. The crown of the molar is prevented from tipping back by tying it to the MI with a ligature wire (black). (D and E) Clinical example of molar protraction as shown in (C).

REFERENCES

1. Upadhyay M, Yadav S, Nanda R. Vertical dimension control during en masse retraction with mini-implant anchorage. Am J Orthod Dentofacial Orthop 2010;138:96–108.
2. Upadhyay M, Yadav S, Nagaraj K, et al. Treatment effects of mini-implants for en-masse retraction of anterior teeth in bialveolar dental protrusion patients: a randomized controlled trial. Am J Orthod Dentofacial Orthop 2008;134:18–29.
3. Upadhyay M, Yadav S, Nagaraj K, et al. Dentoskeletal and soft tissue effects of mini-implants in Class II, division 1 patients. Angle Orthod 2009;79:240–7.
4. Kim HJ, Yun HS, Park HD, et al. Soft-tissue and cortical-bone thickness at orthodontic implant sites. Am J Orthod Dentofacial Orthop 2006;130:177–82.
5. Bernhart T, Vollgruber A, Gahleitner A, et al. Alternative to the median region of the palate for placement of an orthodontic implant. Clin Oral Implants Res 2000;11:595–601.
6. Miyawaki S, Koyama I, Inoue M, et al. Factors associated with the stability of titanium screws placed in the posterior region for orthodontic anchorage. Am J Orthod Dentofacial Orthop 2003;124:373–8.
7. Gracco A, Luca L, Cozzani M, et al. Assessment of palatal bone thickness in adults with cone beam computerised tomography. Aust Orthod J 2007;23:109–13.
8. King KS, Lam EW, Faulkner MG, et al. Vertical bone volume in the paramedian palate of adolescents: a computed tomography study. Am J Orthod Dentofacial Orthop 2007;132:783–8.
9. Kuhn RJ. Control of anterior vertical dimension and proper selection of extraoral anchorage. Angle Orthod 1968;38:340–9.
10. Roberts WE. Bone physiology, metabolism, and biomechanics in orthodontic practice. In: Graber TM, Vanarsdall RL Jr, editors. Orthodontics: current principles and techniques. St. Louis, MO: Mosby; 1994. p. 193–257.
11. Nagaraj K, Upadhyay M, Yadav S. Titanium screw anchorage for protraction of mandibular second molars into first molar extraction sites. Am J Orthod Dentofacial Orthop 2008;134:583–91.
12. Upadhyay M, Yadav S. Mini-implants for retraction, intrusion and protraction in a Class II, division 1 patient. J Orthod 2007;34:158–67.
13. Roberts WE, Marshall KJ, Mozsary PG. Rigid endosseous implant utilized as anchorage to protract molars and close an atrophic extraction site. Angle Orthod 1990;60:135–52.
14. Roberts WE, Nelson CL, Goodacre CJ. Rigid implant anchorage to close a mandibular first molar extraction site. J Clin Orthod 1994;28:693–704.

The Aarhus Anchorage System

Birte Melsen and Cesare Luzi

INTRODUCTION

This chapter illustrates the use of the miniscrew implants (MIs) of the Aarhus Anchorage System to enhance anchorage control in the treatment of different Class II malocclusions. The MIs can be used as direct or indirect anchorage depending on the treatment plan and the patient's anatomy.[1,2] Whenever possible, MIs are inserted through attached gingiva in order to minimize local irritation. Where this is not possible, one solution is to allow the MI to be covered with a wire or a ligature penetrating the mucosa. If indirect anchorage must be used, a MI with a bracket-like head is indicated. The load on the tooth linked to the MI is important as any lack of rigidity in the connection between the MI and the tooth can lead to loss of the MI.

TREATMENT PLANNING

Treatment planning can occur either through work-up of a three-dimensional visual treatment objective composed of an occlusogram combined with the tracing of a cephalometric radiograph or by simulating the desired tooth movements on virtual models. This is the stage where the clinician will determine the goal of treatment, which is often a compromise between what is possible and what is desirable.

When using an occlusogram, the orthodontist will have to:

- define the patient's symmetry line
- indicate the desired movement of the anterior teeth
- indicate a tentative transversal dimension of the arch in the premolar and molar regions
- choose the anterior arch form.

This will allow the clinician to:

- simulate tooth movements in all planes of space: when combined with the tracing of the cephalometric radiograph, the movement of the incisors in three planes in space can be visualized; when using virtual models instead of occlusal images of the study casts, three-dimensional simulations of all desired tooth movements can be performed
- define the active and reactive dental units
- evaluate the anchorage requirements.

Independent of the treatment approach planned, it is imperative to determine the desired displacement of the individual teeth or group of teeth. Only when the necessary tooth movements are defined it is possible to select the correct line of action for the forces. While treatment planning can to some extent be considered an art, the correct line of action for a specific tooth movement is based on science: the mathematics and an estimate of the center of resistance of the tooth/teeth based on biological evidence.

CLINICAL EXAMPLES OF TEMPORARY ANCHORAGE DEVICES FOR CLASS II CORRECTION

The following cases illustrate the use of temporary anchorage devices for molar distalization, retraction of the anterior segment in a degenerated dentition, extraction treatment for alleviation of anterior crowding and the use of intermaxillary forces in order to advance the mandible (e.g. with the Herbst appliance).

MOLAR DISTALIZATION

The only real indication for the distalization of the maxillary molars is a dental Class II or skeletal Class I (or very mild skeletal Class II in a growing individual) malocclusion without mandibular retrusion and associated with crowding of the maxillary arch.

CASE 1

A 14-year-old girl with good facial proportions presented with concerns about the position of her maxillary canines and their influence on her smile. The maxillary dental midline was deviated 3 mm to the left; she had a Class II dental occlusion with severe maxillary crowding and buccally displaced maxillary canines (Fig. 27.1AB). Radiography revealed aplasia of the mandibular third molars and partially impacted maxillary second molars. Extraction of the non-erupted second molars was performed in order to facilitate molar distalization and allow eruption of the third molars. Two MIs (thread length, 6.0 mm; diameter, 1.5 mm; Aarhus Mini-Implants, American Orthodontics, Sheboygan, WI, USA) were inserted bilaterally between the roots of the second premolars and the first molars and tightly ligated to the brackets of the first premolars with a 0.12 mm SS ligature to serve as indirect anchorage. A Pendulum appliance was inserted and the posterior beta-titanium springs were activated to achieve first molar distalization as well as to limit the mesial rotation (Fig. 27.1C,D). After 4 months, brackets were bonded on the maxillary incisors and a continuous archwire with two open coil springs was placed (bypassing the canines) bilaterally between the first premolars and first molars in order to prevent any mesial rotation generated by application of the force from the Pendulum springs on the palatal side (Fig. 27.1E,F). After 8 months, no anterior anchorage loss was registered and the molars were in a super-Class I relationship. The MIs were removed and a Nance button replaced the Pendulum appliance. Treatment was completed with continuous arch mechanics: an open coil spring was used to provide the space for the buccally blocked-out maxillary left canine and, at the same time, to correct the upper midline deviation. Intermaxillary elastics were used in the finishing phase to achieve proper intercuspation. Post-treatment radiography showed favorable eruption of the third molars. The result was satisfactory (Fig. 27.1G,H), but it could be argued that the patient could have been treated with two maxillary premolar extractions, in which case the use of MIs would have been superfluous.

RETRACTION OF THE ANTERIOR SEGMENT IN A DEGENERATED DENTITION

Many patients present with an increased overjet and overbite as a result of spontaneous migration of the anterior teeth, either following loss of lateral teeth and deepening of the bite or as a consequence of extrusion and flaring of maxillary incisors and simultaneous crowding in the mandibular arch due to lip pressure. These patients are characterized as Class

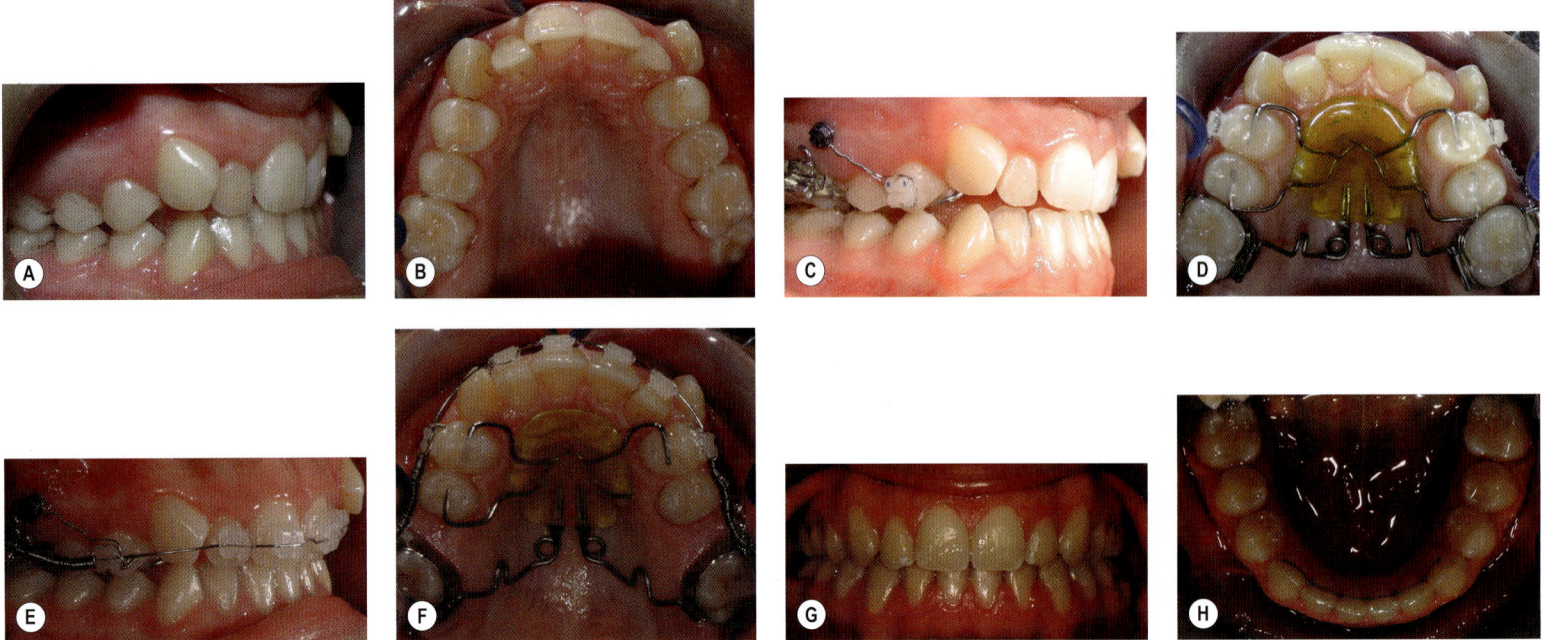

Fig. 27.1 Case 1: molar distalization for bilateral Class II malocclusion and high labial canines. (A,B) Pretreatment. (C,D) Miniscrew implants and a Pendulum appliance inserted. (E,F) Fixed appliances inserted on the maxillary dental arch and coil springs between the second premolars and first molars. (G,H) Post-treatment. (Treated by C. Luzi.)

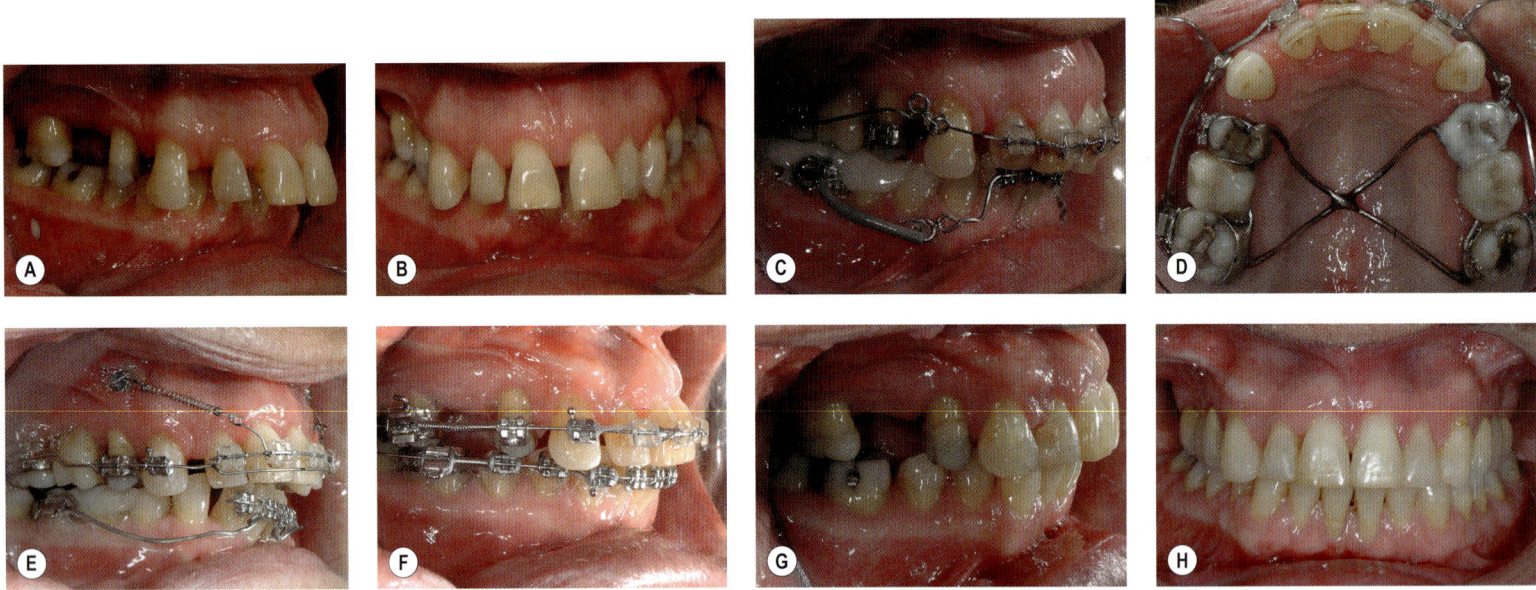

Fig. 27.2 Case 2: retraction of the anterior segment. (A,B) Pretreatment. (C,D) Retraction and intrusion of maxillary incisors with a three-piece mechanics. In the mandibular arch, three-piece mechanics is used for proclination, intrusion and midline correction. (E) During retraction and intrusion of the maxillary front segment against two mini-implants (one each on either side of the maxilla). (F) Finishing with straight wires. (G) The end of treatment. (H) After prosthetic reconstruction. (Treated by E. Serra under B. Melsen's supervision, School of Dentistry, Aarhus University.)

II and can benefit from skeletal anchorage since the lateral teeth cannot be loaded with the reactive force without iatrogenic or side effects.

CASE 2

A 49-year-old woman had experienced a gradually increasing overjet, flaring and spacing of the maxillary incisors, as well as deepening of her bite. She had impingement of the mandibular incisors to the lingual aspect of the maxillary incisors (Fig. 27.2A,B). The maxillary second premolars and first molars had been extracted previously. The second molars were rotated and slightly tipped mesially. The mandibular incisors were retroclined and presented with moderate crowding. The patient exhibited general bone loss but no bleeding at probing, and no pockets more than 4 mm were present.

During the first phase of treatment, the lateral segments were consolidated with a stiff anchorage appliance consisting of an iron-cross of SS wire (0.030 inch) and bands on the premolars and molars connected by SS wire (0.020 inch). In order to increase the occlusal feedback, thereby enhancing anchorage, composite teeth were inserted in the edentulous spaces and Triad occlusal onlays were placed on the mandibular lateral segments. After bonding, the maxillary incisors were leveled and retraction and intrusion were initiated with two curved cantilevers extending from the tube on the molars. In the mandibular arch, the incisors were intruded and proclined with two cantilevers extending from the molars and activated to correct the asymmetrical arch shape (Fig. 27.2C,D). Once the spacing between the incisors was closed and the deep bite partially corrected, the anchorage unit was slightly loosened and the retraction of the maxillary incisors was completed using skeletal anchorage. Two Aarhus MIs were inserted in the apical region mesial to the second molar, and the intrusion and retraction was performed using 50 cN coil springs extending from the MIs to the anterior segment, while the lateral segments were relieved from the transpalatal arches and leveled with a continuous arch bypassing the incisal unit of the anterior teeth (Fig. 27.2E). Finishing of the mandibular arch was carried out with straight wire mechanics (Fig. 27.2F).

At the end of the orthodontic correction (Fig. 27.2G), the patient was referred to the prosthodontic department for replacement of the missing teeth with two bridges (Fig. 27.2H). A 4-to-4 retainer was bonded in the mandibular arch, and once the bridges were inserted the patient received a 2 mm balanced splint to use at night. Careful instructions were given regarding periodontal control.

EXTRACTION TREATMENT FOR ALLEVIATING ANTERIOR CROWDING

Another approach for a crowded maxillary dental arch without a major component of mandibular retrusion involves extraction of two maxillary premolars.[3] Maximum maxillary posterior anchorage is necessary to minimize mesial movement of the maxillary molars and second premolars while retracting the anterior segment. Direct anchorage on MIs avoids placing any load to the posterior teeth of the maxillary arch, thus eliminating any undesired posterior shifts.

CASE 3

A 52-year-old woman was unhappy with the esthetics of her smile and was not interested in any therapeutic solution that would require maxillofacial surgery. She had a Class II malocclusion, severe crowding of the maxillary arch and mild crowding of the mandibular dental arch (Fig. 27.3A,B). Radiography revealed the absence of the mandibular third molars and a

severe osseous defect mesial to the right mandibular second premolar. The proposed treatment plan involved extraction of two maxillary premolars to alleviate crowding of the maxillary arch and to maintain the molars in the initial full Class II relationship. This could only be done with absolute anchorage control during the canine retraction and overjet reduction phases. Following segmental bonding of the maxillary arch, the second maxillary premolars were extracted (as they were considered more compromised than the first premolars from a restorative point of view) and two MIs (thread length, 6.0 mm; diameter, 1.3 mm) were inserted bilaterally on the upper buccal cortex between the roots of the first and second molars (Fig. 27.3C,D). Superelastic closed coil springs with 50 cN force were used bilaterally for the retraction of both canines and first premolars; power arms were used to obtain the necessary line of action of the force. A transpalatal arch was used for derotation of the second molars, and later on for the same purpose on the first molars. Once the canine retraction was completed, the maxillary incisors and the lower arch were bonded, leveling and alignment were completed and superelastic closed coil springs with 50 cN force were used together with sliding mechanics on a continuous SS rectangular posted full-size wire for overjet closure (Fig. 27.3EF). The reactive forces to the retraction of canines and incisors were loaded exclusively on the MIs, thus avoiding any possible anchorage loss and guaranteeing the final proper dental relationships (Fig. 27.3G,H). Following treatment, fixed bonded retainers were placed on both arches as permanent retention and the patient was sent for periodontal evaluation and a soft tissue graft for the recession present buccally on the maxillary right premolar. The initial buccal ectopic position outside the buccal cortex did not allow soft tissues to completely follow the orthodontic extrusion of the tooth.

Panoramic radiography indicated that the osseous defect between the mandibular right premolars was still present and the patient was instructed to maintain proper hygiene in that area.

INTERMAXILLARY FORCES TO ADVANCE THE MANDIBLE

Intermaxillary non-compliance appliances act in both maxilla and mandible in order to advance the mandible to a more forward position. (e.g. the Herbst appliance) (see Chapter 2).[4,5] All fixed bite-jumping devices have both skeletal and dental effects, with proclination of the mandibular incisors as an unwanted effect (see Fig. 2.15).[6,7] Although many attempts have

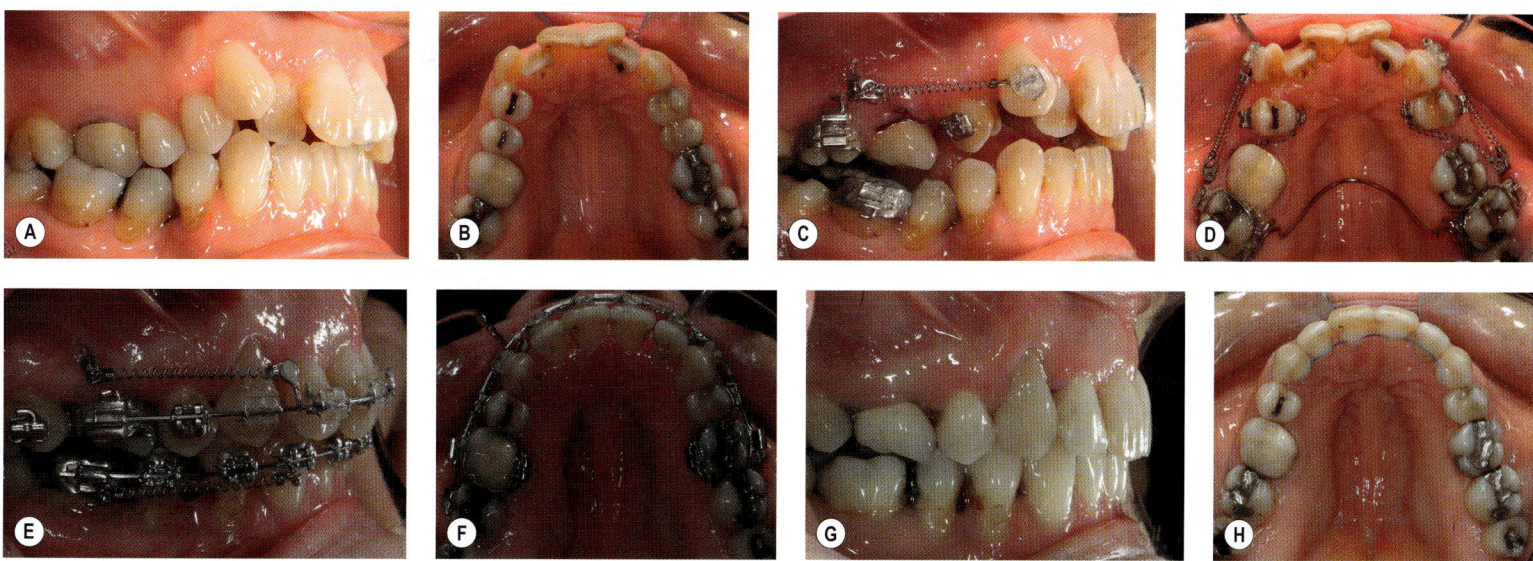

Fig. 27.3 Case 3: alleviation of anterior crowding with extractions. (A,B) Pretreatment. (C,D) Insertion of a transpalatal arch and two buccally positioned miniscrew implants. (E,F) The finishing phase. (G,H) Post-treatment. (Treated by C. Luzi under B. Melsen's supervision, School of Dentistry, Aarhus University.)

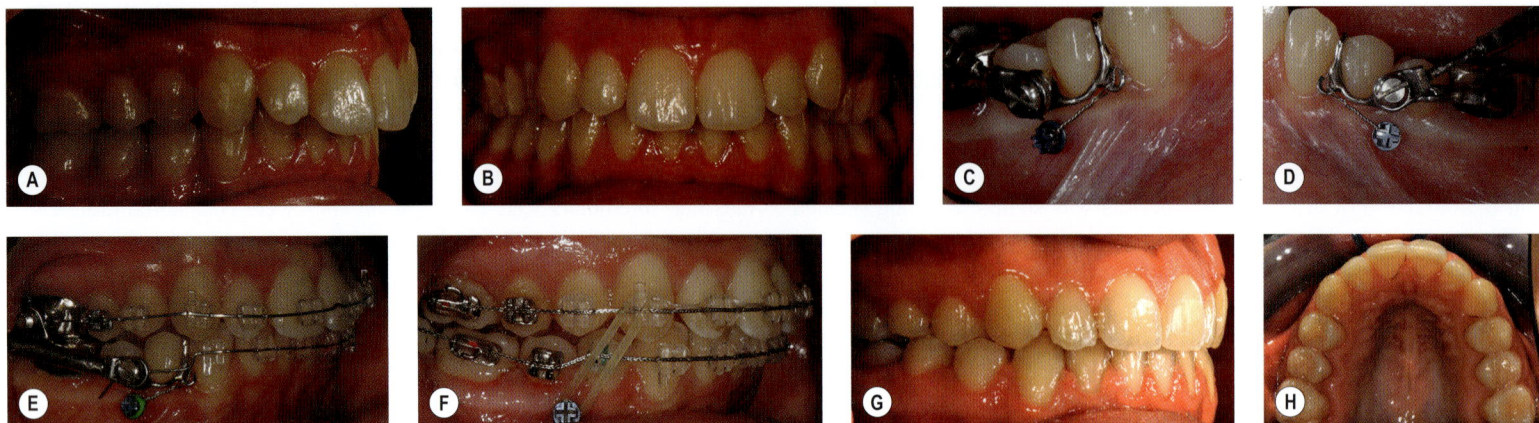

Fig. 27.4 Case 4: intermaxillary temporary anchorage with the Herbst appliance. (A,B) Pretreatment. (C,D) Insertion of a casted Herbst and two buccally positioned miniscrew implants. (E) Insertion of fixed appliances and leveling and alignment of both dental arches. (F) Herbst appliance removed and the finishing phase. (G,H) Post-treatment. (Treated by C. Luzi.)

been made to avoid mandibular incisor proclination (cast mandibular appliances, archwires with torque bends, brackets with selective torques), absolute anchorage control cannot be achieved and some amount of dentoalveolar compensation should be always expected.[8]

Temporary anchorage devices can be used in combination with bite-jumping appliances to maximize skeletal effects and reduce the side effect of incisor proclination. A combination of MIs and a modified Herbst appliance is described below.

CASE 4

A 14-year-old girl presented with a Class II, division I malocclusion with retrusive chin and a large overjet (Fig. 27.4A,B). Her maxillary dental arch was asymmetrical with a buccally displaced maxillary left canine and mild crowding; no space problems were present in the mandibular arch. Lateral cephalometric radiography revealed skeletal Class II sagittal relationships of the jaws from a retrusive mandible and normal vertical jaw relationships. The inclination of the mandibular incisors with regard to the mandibular plane (l1/GoMe) was 107°. The treatment plan involved mandibular advancement using a modified Herbst appliance. A casted Herbst was constructed on preformed reinforced bands equipped with two hooks bilaterally on the lower mesial part of the casted structure on the buccal side. Following insertion of the device, two Aarhus MIs (thread length, 6.0 mm; diameter, 1.5 mm) were inserted bilaterally in the lower buccal cortex between the roots of the first and the second premolars (Fig. 27.4C,D) and tightly ligated with a 0.12 mm SS ligature to the hooks of the Herbst appliance, thereby using the MIs as indirect anchorage to eliminate or reduce proclination of the mandibular incisors. Brackets were bonded on both arches and the teeth were leveled and aligned during the bite-jumping months (Fig. 27.4E). Once the Herbst was removed, 9 months after treatment start, full-arch bonding was completed and finishing wires were placed together with intermaxillary elastics to consolidate the intercuspation. The MIs were left in place and used as anchorage for the application of elastics in the mandibular arch (Fig. 27.4F) to prevent relapse and maintain a correct forward position of the mandible while the teeth were settling into the new occlusal relationships. The MIs and the fixed appliances were removed 20 months after initiation of treatment. The patient

received an upper retention plate for night use and a lower bonded fixed retainer. The final radiographs depicted improvement of the sagittal skeletal relationships and the final mandibular incisor inclination, which increased by 1° (l1/GoMe: 108°) compared with the start of treatment.

The use of temporary anchorage devices with Class II traditional devices such as the Herbst appliance and intermaxillary elastics can be standardized into future treatment protocols for Class II correction. Reducing dentoalveolar side effects on the mandibular arch can optimize treatment efficiency and success through increased skeletal response, enhanced profile improvement and better final dental relationships. Furthermore, it can reduce post-treatment relapse through solid ideal teeth intercuspation.

CONCLUSIONS

In addition to widening the spectrum of clinical orthodontic treatment, skeletal anchorage modalities can facilitate treatment, shorten treatment times and avoid side effects. Examples have been given of the use of temporary anchorage devices for direct and indirect anchorage for various approaches to Class II malocclusion.

REFERENCES

1. Melsen B. Mini-Implants: where are we? J Clin Orthod 2005;39:539–47.
2. Bae SM, Park HS, Kyung HM, et al. Ultimate anchorage control. Texas Dent J 2002;119:580–91.
3. Bryk C, White LW. The geometry of Class II correction with extractions. J Clin Orthod 2001;35:570–9.
4. Flores-Mir C, Ayeh A, Goswani A, et al. Skeletal and dental changes in Class II division 1 malocclusions treated with splint-type Herbst appliances: a systematic review. Angle Orthod 2007;77:376–81.
5. Jasper JJ, McNamara JA Jr. The correction of interarch malocclusions using a fixed force module. Am J Orthod Dentofacial Orthop 1995;108:641–50.
6. Barnett GA, Higgins DW, Major PW, et al. Immediate skeletal and dentoalveolar effects of the crown- or banded type Herbst appliance on Class II division 1 malocclusion. Angle Orthod 2008;78:361–9.
7. Martin J, Pancherz H. Mandibular incisor position changes in relation to amount of bite jumping during Herbst/multibracket appliance treatment: a radiographic–cephalometric study. Am J Orthod Dentofacial Orthop 2009;136:44–51.
8. Pancherz H, Ruf S, Erbe C, et al. The mechanism of Class II correction in surgical orthodontic treatment of adult Class II, division 1 malocclusions. Angle Orthod 2004;74:800–9.

The Spider Screw anchorage system 28

B. Giuliano Maino and Paolo Pagin

INTRODUCTION

This chapter discusses a system for the treatment of Class II malocclusion, with and without extractions, that combines sliding mechanics based on the bidimensional technique with miniscrew implants (MIs) as the only source of anchorage. The bidimensional technique is intended to give stronger torque control through the use of brackets with different horizontal slot sizes (0.018×0.025 inch in the incisors and 0.022×0.028 inch in the lateral segments). Using a single wire (0.018×0.022 inch), a total control of the anterior teeth is obtained while the wire can slide into the lateral segments (Table 28.1).[1]

THE MGBM SYSTEM

The MGBM system is designed to be used in growing patients as well as in adults with varying growth patterns; it is intended to be easy to use, of limited cost and a rapid procedure.

This chapter describes its use in distalization of the maxillary molars with and without extractions and in management of the vertical dimension.

DISTALIZATION OF THE MAXILLARY MOLARS WITHOUT EXTRACTIONS

The MGBM system comprises an anchorage unit and an active part; The anchorage unit is formed by a transpalatal bar bonded to the occlusal surfaces of the first premolars and with two long-neck Spider Screw K1 MIs (Fig. 28.1) (diameter, 1.5 mm; length, 10 mm; HDC, Sarcedo, Italy) positioned on the palatal side. The active part has two sectional SS wires (0.016×0.022 inch), two Ni-Ti coil springs of 200 g and, if the second molars are present, two sectional superelastic Ni-Ti (0.018×0.025 inch) wires.

The MIs are self-drilling and self-tapping, thus allowing them to be applied directly. The head has three slots and a transmucosal conical collar/

neck of two different heights (long or short) to use with thick or thin soft tissues (Fig. 28.1).[2]

Three phases of treatment are identified for monitoring progress, using the mandibular arch as reference against which to judge the movements of the maxillary teeth:

- phase 1: distalization of the maxillary molars to reach a "super-Class I" relationship
- phase 2: distalization of the premolars and canines
- phase 3: retraction of the incisors.

PHASE 1: DISTALIZATION OF THE MOLARS

If the second maxillary molars have not erupted, the first molars are distalized using sectional mechanics with the SS wire and an open Ni-Ti coil spring from the first premolar to the first molar. The coil spring is 10 mm longer than the space between the distal part of the bracket of the first premolar and the mesial extremity of the molar band. When the coil is compressed between the first premolar and the first molar, it is activated by 10 mm. The second premolar is not banded to facilitate the application of the coil (Fig. 28.2A).

The two MIs are inserted on the palatal side between the roots of the second premolars and the first molars or, if the interproximal space is large, between the first and the second premolars (Fig. 28.2A). The advantage of the latter position is that it allows spontaneous drift of the second premolars under the pull of the transeptal fibers. The insertion direction is about 30–40° with respect to the inclination of the palatal vault.

The transpalatal bar (0.036 inch SS wire) is bonded on to the occlusal surface of the maxillary first premolars and then connected to the MIs through a well-tightened metallic ligature (0.012 inch) (Fig. 28.2B). This way, the transpalatal bar prevents loss of anchorage and possible unwanted rotation, inclination and torsion effects on the premolars. To strengthen the anchorage to the palatal bar, acrylic resin can be added in a similar way to a Nance button so that it rests against the anterior part of the palate (Fig. 28.2B).

If the second molar has also emerged, treatment can be accelerated by integrating the MGBM protocol with the "simultaneous maxillary molar distalization system" (SUMODIS),[3] which has two distinct distalization components, one activated against the first molar and the other against the second molar (Fig. 28.2C–F). The component activated against the first molar has the same SS wire but with a precompressed coil spring positioned between the first premolar and the first molar. Before fixing the SS wire to the bracket of the first premolar, the wire is inserted in the lower section of a double sliding tube that is positioned adjacent to the bracket

Table 28.1 Characteristics of the brackets used for the bidimensional technique

	Dimension (inch)	Tip (°)	Torque (°)	Toe-in (°)
Maxillary arch				
Central incisors	0.018×0.025	5	12	0
Lateral incisors	0.018×0.025	9	8	0
Canines	0.022×0.028	7	0	0
Premolars	0.022×0.028	0	0	0
Molars	0.022×0.028	0	0	14
Mandibular arch				
Incisors	0.018×0.025	0	0	0
Canines	0.022×0.028	5	0	0
Premolars	0.022×0.028	0	0	0
Molars	0.022×0.028	0	0	0

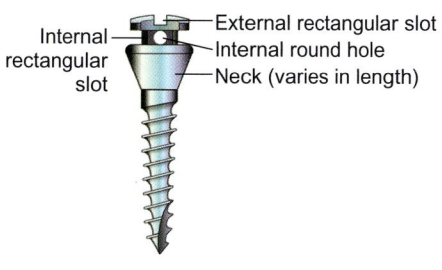

Fig. 28.1 The Spider Screw K1.

Fig. 28.2 Non-extraction treatment of Class II malocclusion. (A,B) Phase 1 distalization of the maxillary molars to reach a "super-Class I" relationship. (A) Positioning of the miniscrew implants (insertion angle on right). (B) The complete MGBM system. (C–F) Phase 1: modification of the MGBM protocol with the SUMODIS when the second molar has emerged. (C) The SUDOMIS system comprises a double sliding tube and a sectional Ni-Ti wire with stops (note that the tube on the second molar has been attached with a distogingival inclination). (D) The activated SUMODIS inserted on the maxillary arch. (E) The complete MGBM system with SUMODIS for the simultaneous distalization of the maxillary first and second molars. (F) End of phase 1, with the maxillary first molars in super-Class I relationship. (Adapted from Maino et al., 2007.[3])

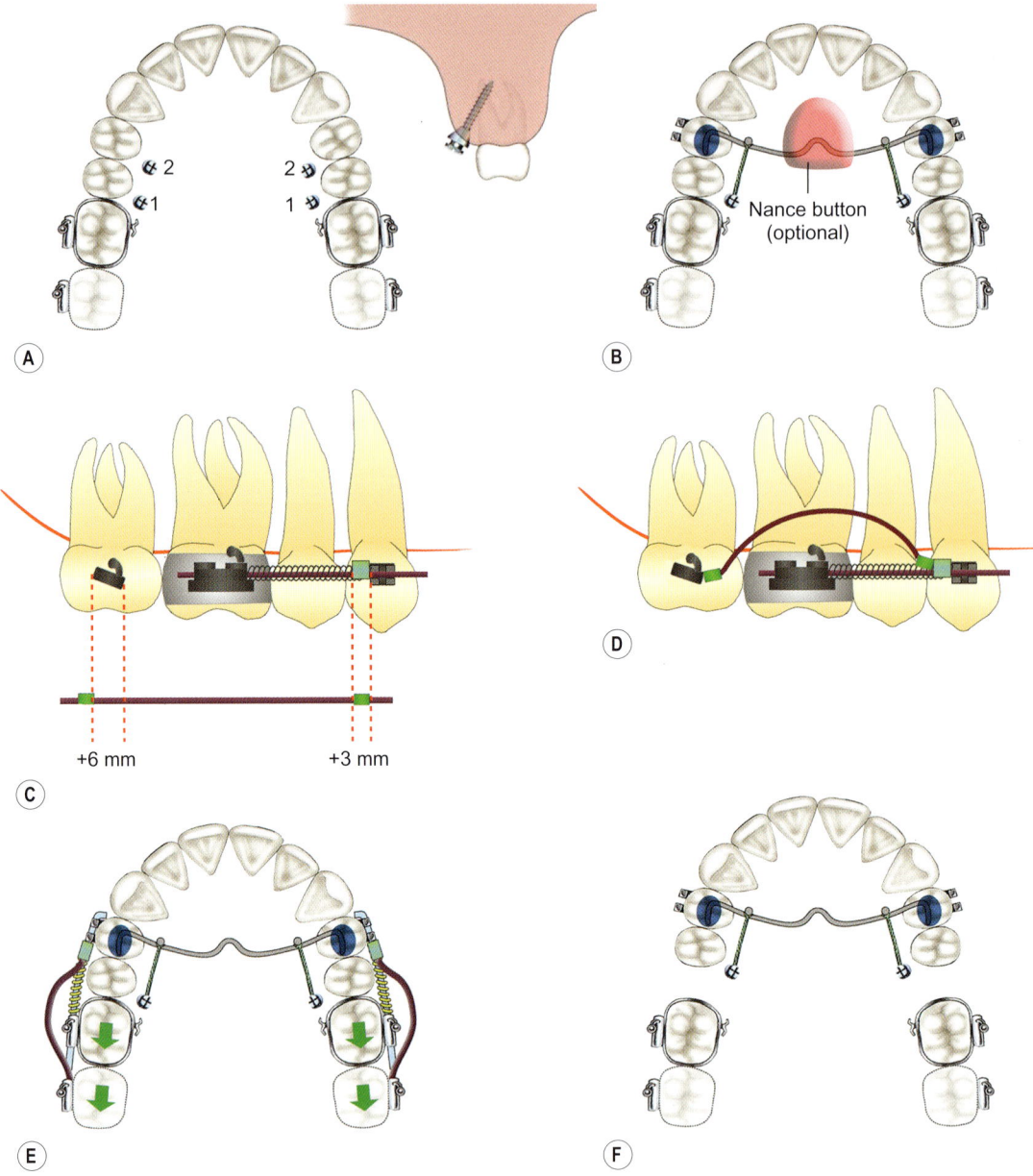

of the first premolar. The tube is blocked on one side by the precompressed coil and on the other by the bracket of the premolar. The second distal component is a sectional (0.018 × 0.025 inch) Ni-Ti wire with shape memory and excessive length on which a mesial and a distal stop are fixed (Fig. 28.2C). It is important that the tube is attached to the second molar with a distogingival inclination to counteract the distal crown tipping of the second molar that could occur because the Ni-Ti wire used to distalize that molar is not rigid. This is done by fixing a stop corresponding to the distal surface of the tube of the second molar and another at the level of the distal surface of the bracket of the first premolar; the distance between these two stops is approximately 9 mm longer than the distance between the mesial part of the tube on the second molar and the distal part of the double tube inserted on the sectional wire (Fig. 28.2C). This way, when the Ni-Ti wire is inserted into the tube of the second molar and into the upper part of the double sliding tube, it is raised into the buccal fold and is automatically activated by 9 mm (Fig. 28.2D).

Gradually, the sectional arch assumes its normal horizontal orientation, performing its distalization action at the level of the second molars at the same time as the distalization of the first molars (Fig. 28.2E). In the initial phase, a light force is applied to favor stabilization of the MIs. The simultaneous distalization is performed with a Ni-Ti wire of 160 g and a

superelastic coil of 200 g. At the end of phase 1, it is important to obtain a super-Class I molar relationship (Fig. 28.2F) in order to provide abundant space for the insertion of MIs in phase 2 in a position that will not interfere with the retraction of the second premolar (nor create problems if any small mesial movement of the MI happens).

PHASE 2: RETRACTION OF THE PREMOLARS AND CANINES

The transpalatal bar and the MIs in the palate are removed. Two MIs of 1.5 mm diameter (K1, 8/10 mm) are inserted bucally mesial to the first molars with a perpendicular or oblique direction to the cortical bone (Fig. 28.3A). The height of the insertion point in the buccal side is determined by biomechanical factors, whether or not an intrusive movement is needed for the molars and/or the incisors during the second and third phases of treatment. If intrusion is not needed, the MIs can be inserted low in the attached gingiva; if it is necessary, the MIs can be placed at the level of or slightly higher than the mucogingival line. Simultaneously, brackets can be applied to the entire maxillary arch. It is then possible to pass on to the alignment phase using superelastic Ni-Ti wire (0.016 × 0.022 inch) provided with stops positioned mesial to the first molars and hooks fixed

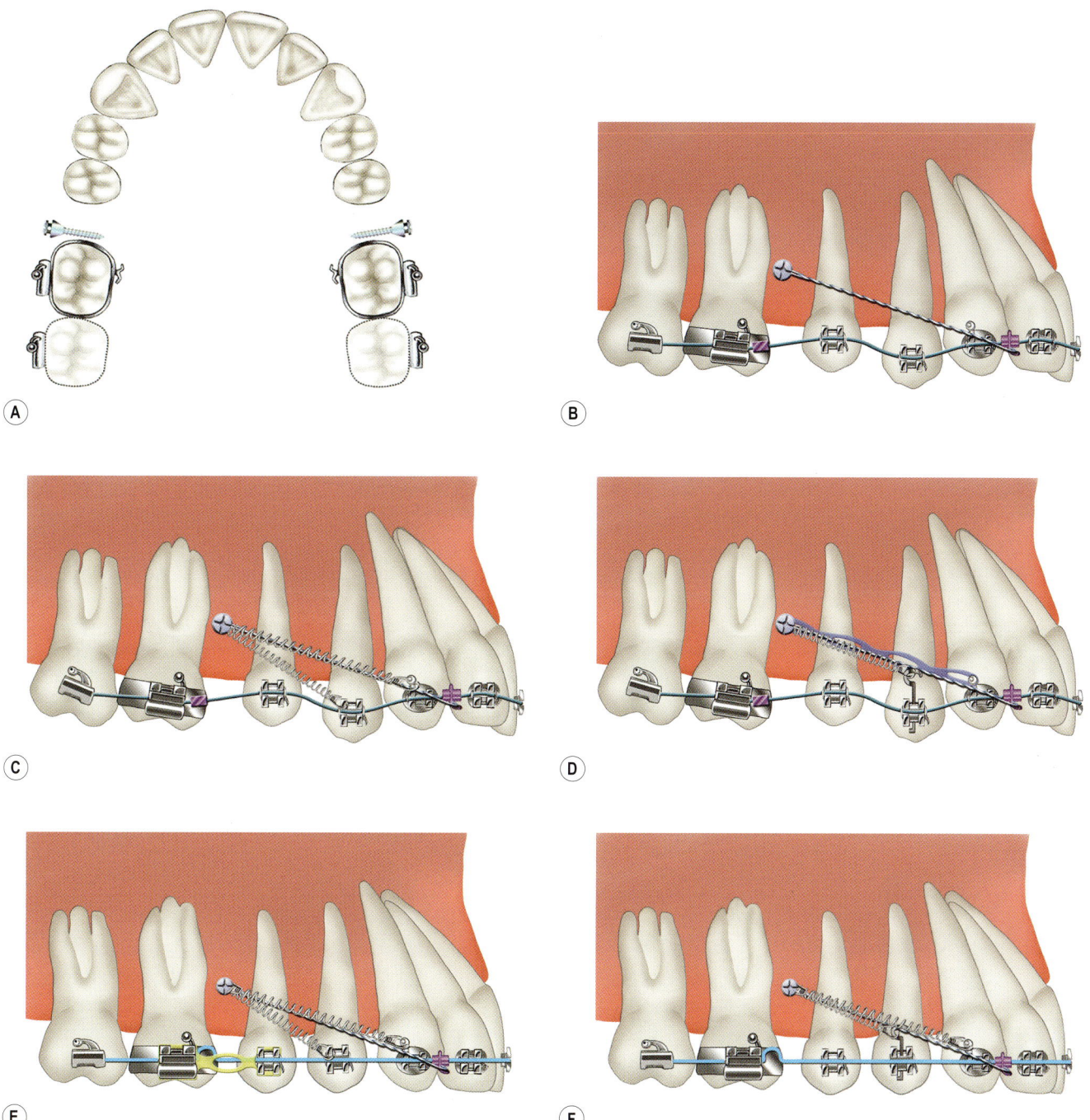

Fig. 28.3 Non-extraction treatment of Class II malocclusion. Phase 2: retraction of the premolars and canines. (A) Miniscrew implants (MIs) inserted after completion of molar distalization. (B) The alignment phase with Ni-Ti wire, a stop mesial to the first molars, a hook clamped on the archwire mesial to the canines and a metallic ligature between the MI and the hook. (C) Simultaneous alignment and distalization of the first premolars and canines during the alignment phase. (D) Simultaneous alignment and distalization of the first premolars and canines using power arms. (E) Simultaneous retraction of the first premolars and canines using direct anchorage. If needed, the second premolars are retracted using indirect anchorage. (F) Simultaneous retraction of the first premolars and canines using a power arm to retract the first premolar while minimizing the intrusive force.

mesial to the canines. If the molar has been correctly distalized into a super-Class I relationship, positioning of the stops can be slightly mesial to the first molars, which allows for a certain amount of mesial movement of the first molar, thus speeding up the alignment phase (Fig. 28.3B). A metallic ligature (0.012 inch) is applied from each of the MIs to the hooks clamped   to the archwire. This prevents mesial sliding of the first molars during the alignment phase, which may result in loss of the Class I relationship (Fig. 28.3B).

During the alignment phase premolars and canines can be moved distally during the alignment phase using light forces of about 50 g (Fig.

28.3C). Since the archwire is not rigid, it is possible to have better control of root inclination by positioning the distalization vector of the force closer to the center of resistance (CR) of the teeth using power arms inserted in the vertical slot of the brackets. The length of the power arm does not need to be excessive (6–8 mm) to avoid discomfort for the patient and decreased efficiency of tooth movement (Fig. 28.3D).

Once the alignment is complete, the SS wire (0.016 × 0.022 inch) is inserted with a stop mesial to the first molars and hooks mesial to the canines. The molars are stabilized with a metal ligature (0.012 inch) tightened between the MIs and the hooks. After 8 weeks for alignment, during which the reliability of the MIs is also checked, the forces of each of the

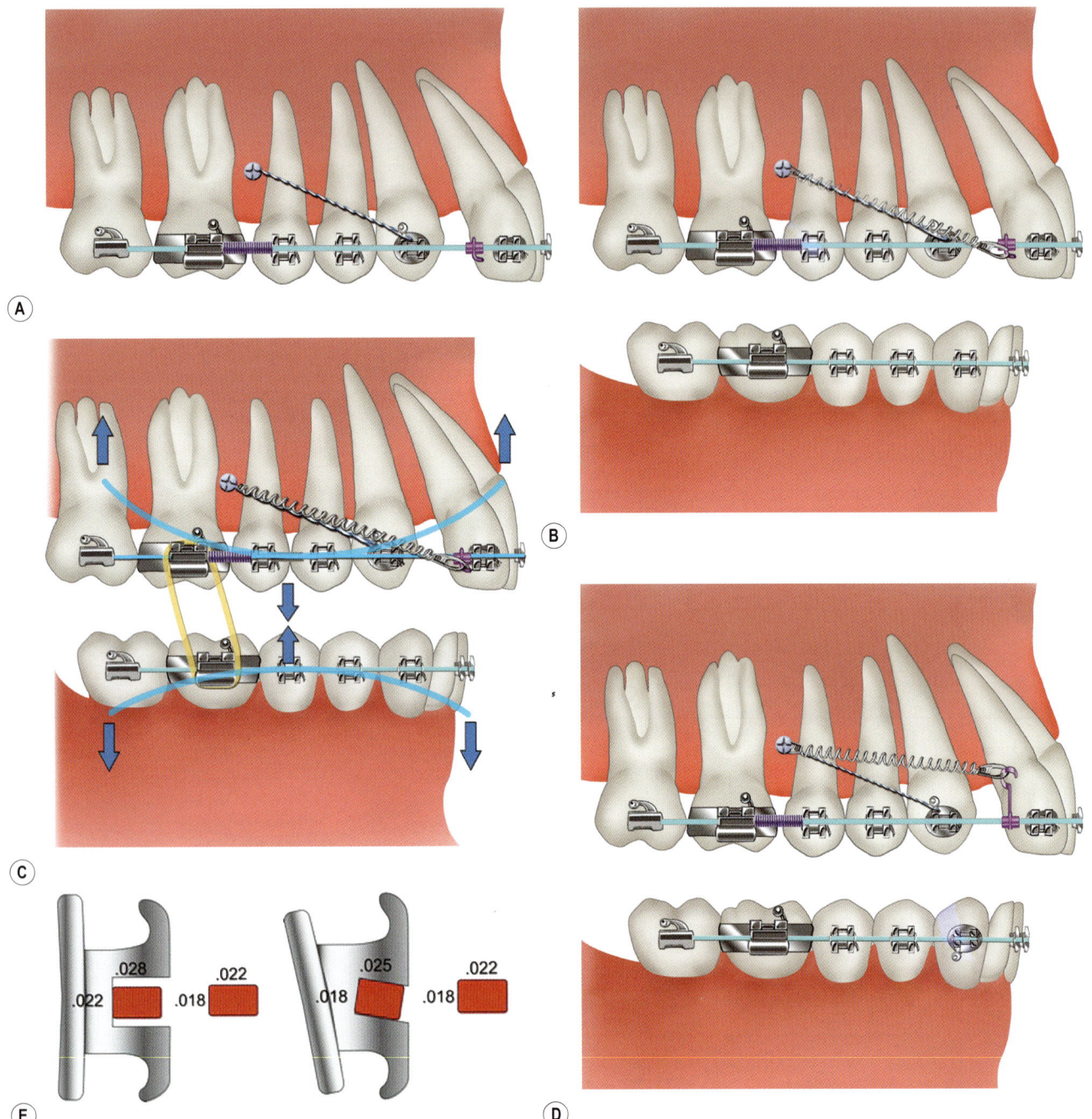

Fig. 28.4 Non-extraction treatment of Class II malocclusion. Phase 3 retraction of the incisors. (A) The closed coil spring between the first molar and second premolar prevents closure of the space between these two teeth. (B) The canines are ligated to the miniscrew implant (MI) with a metallic ligature and the incisors retracted with a coil spring linking the MIs to the hooks on the archwire. (C) Opening of the bite using an archwire with an exaggerated curve of Spee on the maxillary arch, a reversed curve on the mandibular arch and vertical elastics between the upper and lower molars. (D) Hooks with power arms clamped on the SS archwire minimize rotation of the occlusal plane. (E) Two different horizontal slot and a single wire used in Bidimensional Technique to produce a total torque control.

coil springs can be increased to 100–150 g. The simultaneous retraction of the canines and the first premolars is continued, with forces directed from the MI to the teeth applied from the vestibular side (direct anchorage) (Fig. 28.3E,F). The second premolar is not always retracted as sometimes it can reach the correct Class I position on its own.

If distal movement of the second premolar is required, Class I elastics using elastic chains attached to the first molars (indirect anchorage) can be initiated, from the buccal and if necessary also from the palatal side (Fig. 28.3E). Because of the stop on the archwire and the metal ligature between the MI and the hook clamped on the archwire mesial to the canine, the reaction force is transmitted to the MI and the first molar will remain in its position (Fig. 28.3F). To optimize the vertical control of the premolars, power arms are sometimes used. However, the use of power arms has

disadvantages, such as patient discomfort, interference with oral hygiene and sometimes a slowing of teeth movement.

PHASE 3: RETRACTION OF THE INCISORS

Phase 3 involves the retraction of the incisors using sliding mechanics. A SS wire (0.018 × 0.022 inch) with hooks distal to the lateral incisors is inserted along with a closed coil spring between the second premolar and the first molar to act as a space maintainer, keeping the space between the teeth constant and preventing possible contact of the mesial root of the first molar with the MI (Fig. 28.4A). A new metallic ligature wire (0.012 inch) is placed, this time from the MIs to the canines. Then, two 300 g Ni-Ti coil springs are positioned, one on each side, from the MIs to

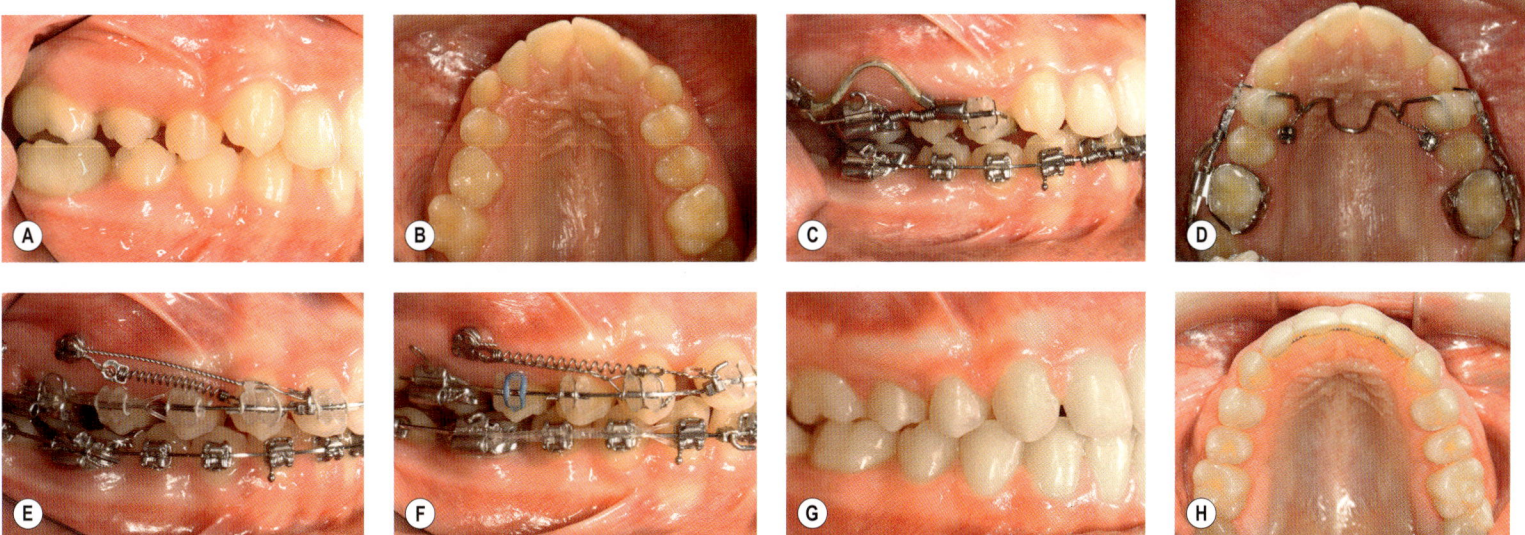

Fig. 28.5 A female patient treated with the MGBM system without extractions. (A,B) Pretreatment. (C,D). Phase 1 (distalization of the molars) in buccal view showing the SUMODIS (C) and occlusal view showing the transpalatal bar connected to the palatal miniscrew implants (MIs) through metallic ligature wires (D). (E) Phase 2: simultaneous retraction of the premolars and canines with buccally inserted MIs. (F) Phase 3: retraction of the incisors. (G,H) Post-treatment.

the crimped hooks on the archwire, and the en masse retraction of the incisors begins (Fig. 28.4B).

Because of the precise fit between the wire and the slot in the brackets of the incisors (0.018×0.025 inch), it is possible to accomplish the retraction of the incisors with full root control (bodily movement). On the other side, because of the larger dimension of the bracket slot in the lateral sectors (0.022×0.028 inch), the closure of the anterior spaces is accomplished with sliding mechanics. In adults, as well as in patients where the root length is greater than average, and whenever it is necessary to increase the torque control of the anterior teeth, it is possible to use an archwire with larger dimensions (e.g. 0.018×0.025 inch).

Many of the patients with Class II malocclusion to be treated without extractions present with a deep bite and so it is necessary to open the bite at the same time as retracting the incisors. The bite can be opened by intrusion of the maxillary or the mandibular incisors, extrusion of the molars or a combination of both.

To open the bite by intrusion of the incisors, an archwire with an exaggerated curve of Spee is inserted on the maxillary arch, with a reversed curve on the mandibular arch. Vertical elastics are used between the molars of the mandibular and maxillary arches to prevent any intrusion of the molars and consequent rotation of the occlusal plane (Fig. 28.4C).

A biomechanical alternative that minimizes rotation of the occlusal plane has two hooks with power arms clamped on to the SS archwire. This ensures that the force line from the MIs to the power arms is closer to the CR of the incisors, facilitating their en masse retraction (Fig. 28.4D). It is better not to use power arms of excessive length since this might slow down sliding of the wire through increased friction.

Fig. 28.5 presents in detail a patient treated with the MGBM system without extractions.

TREATMENT OF CLASS II MALOCCLUSION WITH EXTRACTIONS

PHASE 1

Phase 1 comprises extractions and MI insertion. Extraction of the two maxillary first premolars is indicated where there is excessive protrusion of the maxilla and/or a full Class II molar relationship where it is necessary to maintain maximum anchorage at the posterior teeth segment. Extraction

can be carried out after bonding of both the maxillary and mandibular dental arches to retain full control of the extraction space.

Correction of the molars should be carried out before MI insertion in order to ensure that the MIs will not interfere with the desired mesial movements of the molars. Once the definitive interarch molar relationship is established, treatment can proceed with MI insertion and retraction of the canines and the maxillary incisors.

Two MIs are applied directly in the vestibular region, usually in the interproximal space between the maxillary second premolars and the first molars. Anatomically, this usually offers greater space because it frequently corresponds to a concavity of the radicular surface mesial to the first molar. Alternatively, the MIs can be inserted in the interproximal space between the maxillary first and second molars. While this location is more efficient as it provides a longer distance between the MI and the canine during retraction, this longer distance has a greater curvature and so the elastic chains or coil springs can cause impingements or ulcers of the soft tissues.

The MIs are usually inserted at the mucogingival junction in a perpendicular direction, thus positioning the head of the MI a sufficient distance from the orthodontic appliance. This is biomechanically favorable and allows good oral hygiene. The perpendicular insertion plus the distance of the head of the MI with respect to the occlusal plane allows intrusion or extrusion movements of the molars to be carried out with ease, as well as intrusion of the incisors during retraction, according to the individual need. Where there is need to intrude the molars, it is preferable to apply the MIs 1 to 2 mm above the mucogingival line to have more space for maneuvers. Analogous to the description above for the non-extraction procedure, after the alignment phase, the position of the molars is stabilized with a stop mesial to the maxillary first molars on the SS archwire and a metallic ligature is applied from each of the MIs to hooks on the archwire.

PHASE 2

Distalization of the canines is carried out by applying a Class I force (i.e. using elastic chains) directly from the MIs to the canines (Fig. 28.6A). The force applied in this way combined with an exaggerated curve of spee and vertical elastics between the molars develops an intrusive component for the maxillary anterior teeth, which is useful for the correction of the deep bite that is often seen in most patients with Class II malocclusion (Fig. 28.4C).

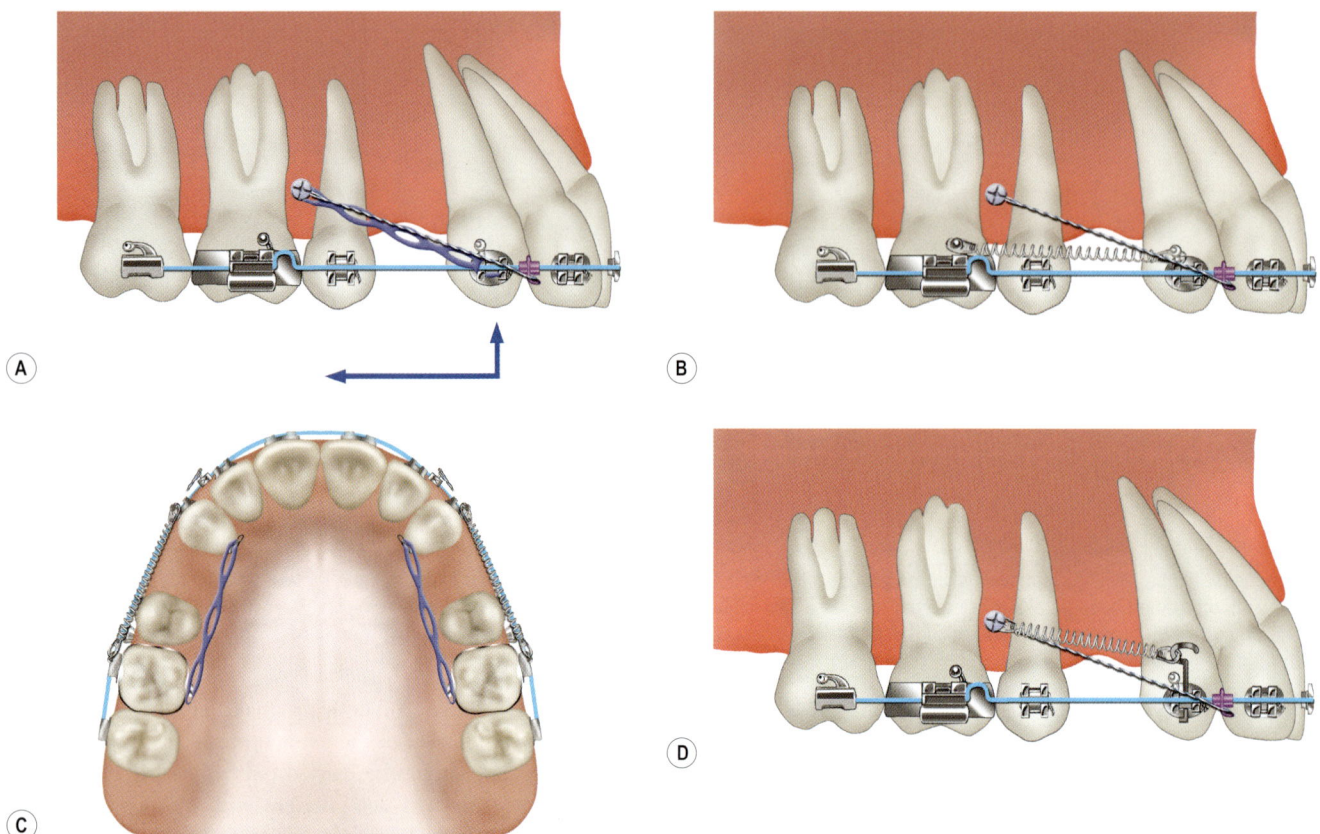

Fig. 28.6 Extraction treatment of Class II malocclusion. Phase 2 distalization of the premolars and canines. (A) Distalization of the canines by elastic chain between the miniscrew implants and the canines. (B,C) Indirect anchorage with a Class I force applied directly from the first molar to the canine (B) and from the palatal side (C). (D) Direct anchorage with application of forces to the power arm attached in the slot of the canine bracket.

Whenever intrusion of the anterior teeth is not needed, two biomechanical methods can be followed:

- indirect anchorage: Class I forces applied directly from the first molars to the canines from the buccal (Fig. 28.6B) and from the palatal side (Fig. 28.6C)
- direct anchorage: application of forces to a power arm attached in the slot of the canine bracket to move the point of force application on the canine higher, thus minimizing the vertical intrusive component (Fig. 28.6D).

PHASE 3

The retraction of the maxillary incisors is commenced once the canines have attained a Class I relationship. The canines are blocked with a metallic ligature wire (0.012 inch) to the MIs, and the en masse retraction of the incisors is performed using sliding mechanics as described above for the non-extraction procedure, using two coil springs of 300 g from the MIs to the hooks (Fig. 28.7A).

In deep bite, the procedure for intrusion of the incisors described above is followed (Fig. 28.7B–D). During this phase, the CR of the maxilla generally lies superior to or is coincident to the position of the MI,[4] and a Class I force from the MIs to the hooks will create rotation of the occlusal plane, with extrusion and palatal tipping of the incisors plus intrusion and distal tipping of the molars (Fig. 28.7E).[5] The intrusive component of the anterior teeth is needed in most cases to counteract the extrusive effect arising from the rotation of the occlusal plane. The precise coupling of the full thickness of the SS archwire (0.018 × 0.022 inch) in the bracket slot on the incisors (0.018 × 0.025 inch) limits the palatal tipping of the incisor crowns and allows controlled movement of their roots during retraction.

Another strategy to reduce any extrusive component of the incisors is to use the archwire with an exaggerated curve of Spee with indirect anchorage via the first molar to the clamped hook on the arch (Fig. 28.7F). Preservation of anchorage is ensured through the use of the SS ligature (0.012 inch) from the MI to the canine. At the discretion of the clinician, retraction of the anterior teeth can also be performed using archwires with anterior closed loops (Fig. 28.7G).

To reduce treatment time, it may be possible to retract the canines and the incisors simultaneously. In this case, we prefer that the canines always precede the movement of the incisors by a few millimeters, which allows them to reach a correct Class I relationship, as well as giving better management of any eventual Bolton discrepancies (Fig. 28.7H). In patients with some growth potential, particularly if differential growth of the mandible cannot be predicted accurately, an excess of anchorage can sometimes be observed during the closure phase. In this case, the MI can be removed, preferably after the canines have reached a Class I relationship.

CONTROL OF THE VERTICAL DIMENSION

Treatment plans need to be able to take into account variations in skeletal type and the bite type. In addition, response to therapy is not always as predicted and so the orthodontic approach should have versatility. This is one reason why the MGBM system routinely uses MIs from the palatal side for the distalization of the molars but from the buccal side for the retraction of the lateral teeth and of the incisors (see Figs 28.2E and 28.3A).

MIs in vestibular and posterior locations during phase 2 and 3 of treatment also allow the application of conventional direct anchorage biomechanics, thus avoiding problems from any instability of the MIs.

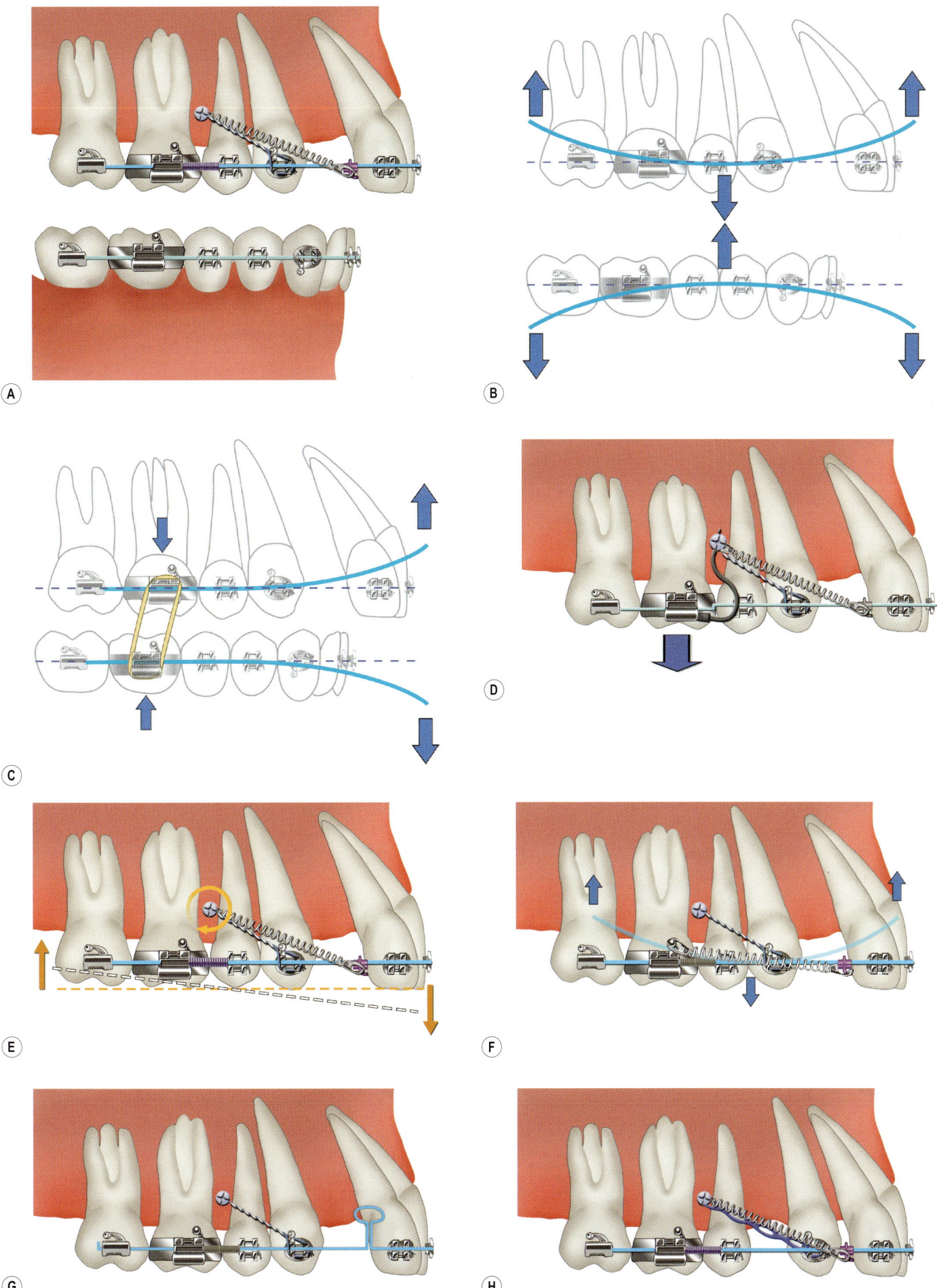

Fig. 28.7 Extraction treatment of Class II malocclusion. Phase 3 retraction of the maxillary incisors. (A) Retraction of the maxillary incisors. (B,C) Force vectors generated by an orthodontic archwire with an exaggerated curve of Spee on the maxilla and a slight reversed curve on the mandible, without (A) and with (B) vertical elastics between the maxillary and mandibular first molars. (D) Retraction of the maxillary incisors in deep bite with sliding mechanics and direct anchorage. (E) Occlusal plane rotation around the miniscrew implant during incisor retraction. (F,G) Retraction of the maxillary incisors with sliding mechanics and indirect anchorage (F) and with an archwire with anterior closed loops (G). (H) Simultaneous retraction of the canines and incisors, with the canine preceding the lateral incisor.

OPEN BITE

Excessive vertical dimension is characterized by evident open bite or by a tendency to open bite, and one of the most effective systems to control open bite is the intrusion of the molars. MIs offer the option of effective intrusion of the posterior teeth with good clinical control of the vertical dimension.

Various methods can be used for the intrusion of the molars, including two MIs in vestibular sites in different interproximal spaces, in ascending order of difficulty:

- between the first molars and the second premolars, when the second molars have not yet erupted
- between the first molars and the second premolars, when the second molars have erupted but there is insufficient space between the two molars
- between the first and second molars, which offers the advantage of moving the point of application of the intrusive force more distally, with more evident effects on the anterior part of the maxilla.

In general, the further the distance of the MI from the occlusal plane, the greater the biomechanical efficiency. Therefore, it is better to insert the MIs in higher sites.

If MIs are used as anchorage for the intrusion of the molars buccal tipping of the molar crowns must be controlled, since the applied force has a vestibular component with respect to the CR of the molars (Fig. 28.8). The following options are available:

- transpalatal bar between the first and/or the second molars (Fig. 28.8A): easiest to use, provides symmetrical molar intrusion but the bar must be solid enough and avoid impinging on the soft tissue of the palate

- palatal crown torque applied from a rectangular archwire: not very efficient and rarely effective as a single measure
- MIs in the inter-radicular spaces between the first and second molars on the buccal and palatal sides (Fig. 28.8B): use for severe open bite or if the intrusion required differs between sides
- MIs applied on the buccal side and in the palatal vault with or without a miniplate (Fig. 28.8C,D).

Two further approaches are useful for treatment of open bite. First, in the maxilla, Self-ligating Miniscrews (HDC, Sarcedo, Italy) can be coupled by wire to a miniplate, thus allowing optimal MI locations to be chosen while providing anchorage through the miniplate (Fig. 28.9). Second, where there is a need to maximize the counterclockwise rotation of the mandible in order to obtain closure of the bite and/or for esthetic improvement, intrusion of the mandibular molars can be carried out using two vestibular MIs and a rigid lingual arch. Orthodontic preparation of the interproximal space between the first and second mandibular molars is often necessary to allow insertion of MIs, and vestibular crown tipping on the maxillary arch must be controlled. The system includes the application of a stiff lingual arch (0.032 inch) soldered to the bands of the first molars and at sufficient distance from the soft tissues to avoid any tissue impingement.

DEEP BITE

Most Class II malocclusions are characterized by a deep bite, which can be managed by:

- distalization of the maxillary molars to Class I relationship: most common approach
- flattening of the curve of Spee, and in particular of the mandibular arch

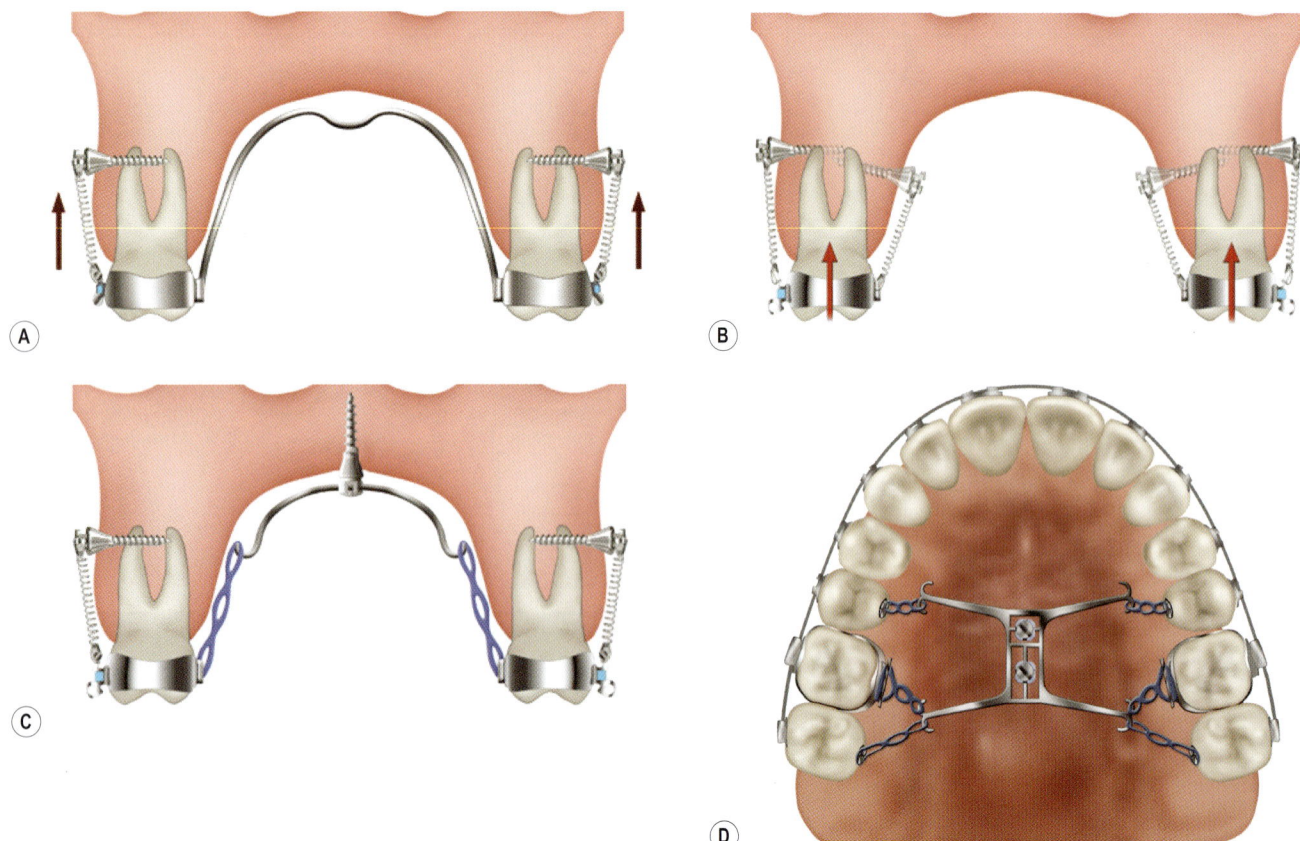

Fig. 28.8 Control of the buccal tipping of the molars. (A) Use of a transpalatal bar. (B) Use of miniscrew implants (MIs) in the inter-radicular spaces between the first and second molars on the buccal and palatal sides. (C,D) Application of MIs and miniplates in the palatal vault to intrude the maxillary molars (C) and second premolars (D).

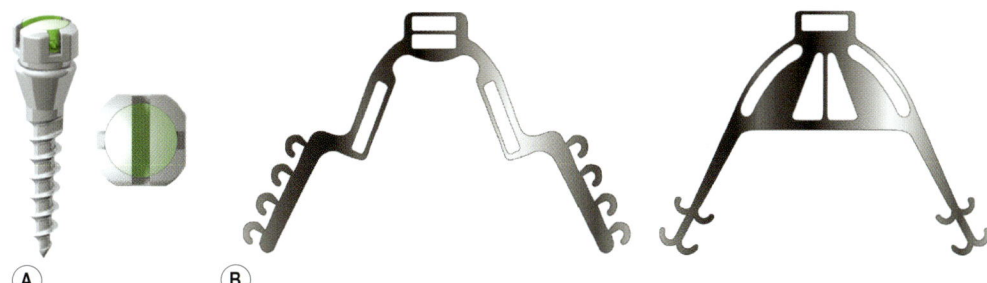

Fig. 28.9 The Self-ligating Miniscrew (A) and two types of miniplate for linkage (B). (HDC, Sarcedo, Italy.)

- intrusion of the maxillary incisors, degree determined by their visibility during speech and smiling
- extrusion of the molars.

Intrusion of the maxillary incisors is indicated only where there is a "gummy" smile or excessive visibility of the maxillary anterior teeth (>5 mm); otherwise intrusion of the mandibular incisors should be chosen. As this may not always completely resolve the problem, it is preferable to extrude the molars in growing patients with a hypo- or normodivergent facial type. The mandibular rotation that follows is compensated by subsequent condylar growth and so correction of deep bite can be obtained without excessive intrusion of the maxillary incisors and without damaging the patient's profile.[6,7]

The MGBM system with MIs on the vestibular side allows effective extrusion of the molars with an auxiliary device. A bend in the archwire (step-down) is added on the SS archwire between the second premolar and the first molar in order to control molar extrusion. A superelastic Ni-Ti wire (0.016 × 0.022 inch; 150 g) is inserted across the vertical slot of the Spider Screw (0.018 inch); the rectangular wire must be prepared for entry into the vertical slot by reducing its end and rounding it. The free end of the wire carries a crimpable stop before being inserted into the round tube of the molar band designed for housing the extraoral traction (see Fig. 28.7D). The amount of extrusion is controlled by making the step-down equal to the level of extrusion desired.

REFERENCES

1. Gianelly AA. Bidimensional technique: Theory and practice. New York: GAC International; 2000.
2. Maino BG, Bednar J, Pagin P, et al. The spider screw for skeletal anchorage. J Clin Orthod 2003;37:90–7.
3. Maino BG, Gianelly AA, Bednar J, et al. MGBM system: new protocol for Class II non extraction treatment without cooperation. Prog Orthod 2007;8:130–43.
4. Park YC, Lee KJ. Biomechanical principles in miniscrew-driven orthodontics. In: Nanda R, Uribe FA, editors. Temporary anchorage devices in orthodontics. St Louis, MO: Mosby-Elsevier; 2009.
5. Jung M, Kim T. Biomechanical considerations in treatment with miniscrew anchorage. Part I: The sagittal plane. J Clin Orthod 2008;42:79–83.
6. Bishara SE, Jakobson JR. Longitudinal changes in three normal facial types. Am J Orthod 1985;88:466–502.
7. Sleichter CG. Effects of maxillary bite plane therapy in orthodontics. Am J Orthod 1954;40:450–70.

29

The miniscrew implant-supported distalization system

Moschos A. Papadopoulos

INTRODUCTION

In addition to osseointegrated orthodontic implants that provide stationary anchorage, miniscrew implants (MIs) have been widely used clinically as temporary anchorage devices to support orthodontic movements. The miniscrew implant-supported distalization system (MISDS) was designed for the non-extraction treatment of Class II malocclusion in order to distalize maxillary molars in an invisible, non-compliant and efficient way.[1]

THE MINISCREW IMPLANT-SUPPORTED DISTALIZATION SYSTEM

The MISDS comprises an active and an anchorage unit. The active unit uses apically positioned wire tubes, Ni-Ti open coil springs and stop screws to provide the necessary force for molar distalization (Fig. 29.1F). The anchorage unit uses MIs positioned in the paramedian region of the palate for supporting anterior anchorage (in order to resist the anteriorly oriented reciprocal forces produced by the coil springs during the first phase of molar distalization) and for supporting posterior anchorage during the second phase of anterior teeth retraction. In contrast to conventional non-compliance devices (e.g. the Distal Jet or Keles Slider), spaces are created between all the posterior teeth rather than just between the maxillary first molars and second premolars. This is because the premolars and canines are able to drift distally under the pull of the transeptal fibers during the first phase of treatment.

The force exerted by the coil springs passes almost through or very close to the center of resistance of the maxillary molars, thus enabling an almost pure bodily molar distal movement with little or no distal molar crown tipping. Because the molars are forced to slide on and are guided through the wire-tube system, which is palatally positioned and runs parallel to the maxillary occlusal plane, no rotation of these teeth is anticipated during distalization.

THE ACTIVE UNIT

At the first appointment, bands are positioned on the first maxillary molars while an alginate impression is taken. The bands are transferred to the corresponding cast (Fig. 29.1A) for soldering of headgear tubes (inner diameter, 0.040 inch) palatally to the molar bands. The edge of the headgear tube extension opposite to the tube is trimmed prior to soldering to allow better contact with the bands. In order to force molars later on to slide on a line parallel to the dental arch, two pieces of straight laboratory orthodontic wires (diameter, 0.040 inch) are attached with plaster to the palate of the cast to run parallel to the occlusal plane at a distance of 2–3 mm from the mucosa to attach to the headgear tubes. This ensures that the tube extensions have proper contact with the bands (Fig. 29.1B). The tubes are then soldered to the molar bands using silver solder (Fig. 29.1C,D). A horseshoe-type palatal arch is formed from straight orthodontic wire (0.040 inch) with two symmetrical closed loops in the anterior region with their centers approximately 6–8 mm apart. These loops correspond to the insertion sites for the MIs. This palatal wire arch is checked on the cast for correct transversal dimension and length (Fig. 29.1E).

Two stop screws incorporating tubes (inner diameter, 0.040 inch) are inserted into the palatal arch from its distal end. The force module consists of two pieces of open Sentalloy coil springs (inner diameter, 0.044 inch; approximate length, 15 mm) that are inserted into the palatal arch from its distal ends following the insertion of the stop screws. The palatal archwire, along with the two stop screws and the two coil springs, is inserted into the headgear tubes from their mesial aspects. Two additional stop screws are inserted on the palatal archwire from its distal ends, which are then cut off so that the wires extend approximately 6–8 mm to allow distal movement of the maxillary molars. In order to control maximum distalization of the molars, the distal ends of the palatal archwire are bent to form small loops (Fig. 29.1F). This prevents the molars slipping out of the wire for any reason.

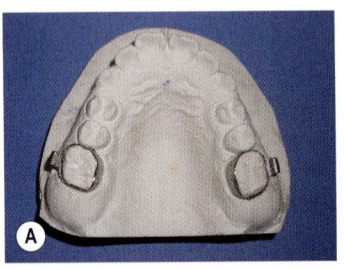
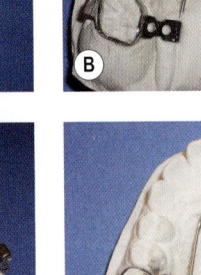
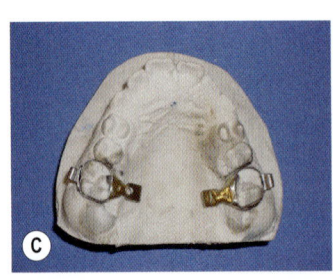
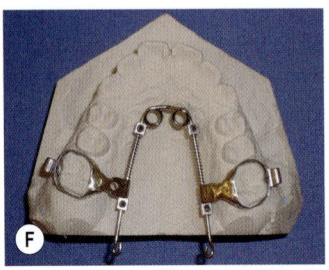

Fig. 29.1 Fabrication of the appliance. (A) Maxillary model cast with bands fitted on the first molars. (B) Positioning of two pieces of straight laboratory orthodontic wires on the palate through the headgear tubes. (C,D) Soldering of the tubes with the molar bands. (E) Positioning of the horseshoe-type palatal archwire on the maxillary model cast. (F) The miniscrew implant-supported distalization system after final adjustment and proper fitting on the maxillary cast. (F, from Papadopoulos, 2008.[1])

THE ANCHORAGE UNIT

Two self-drilling and self-tapping MIs (diameter, 2 mm; length, 8–10 mm; Aarhus Mini-Implant System, Medicon, Tuttlingen, Germany) are used. These are inserted paramedian in the anterior region of the palate, 3–9 mm posteriorly to the incisive foramen and 1–6 mm from the midpalatal suture. As the MIs will provide anchorage for both phases, the clinician needs to ensure that they are positioned so that they will not be in contact with the dental roots of the anterior teeth during their retraction. An initial clearance of 7–10 mm from the roots of the anterior teeth to avoid any contact during anterior teeth retraction is recommended.

CLINICAL PROCEDURE

The MISDS and the MIs can be inserted at the same appointment. The device is inserted in the patient's mouth and the insertion postion for the MIs is marked. The MIs are inserted using standard methodology. The MISDS is cemented on the maxillary molars and then fixed to the MIs with metallic ligatures (0.012 inch). To avoid plaque accumulation, a small amount of resin is added to each loop of the palatal archwire with the ends of the ligature wires. The MISDS is activated immediately with a light load. The stop screws distal to the headgear tubes are screwed approximately 5 mm to their distal aspect in order to prevent sliding of the tubes out of the palatal archwire upon distalization. The patient is seen every 4 weeks for further adjustments and reactivation of the appliance. The first maxillary molars usually take around 4–8 months to reach a Class I molar relationship. After molar distalization has been accomplished, the MISDS is used following a simple modification to support posterior anchorage (i.e. to retain maxillary molars in position) during the second phase of Class II treatement, including retraction of the anterior teeth and leveling and aligning the dental arches. This modification can be performed intraorally by simply removing the coil springs and screwing the stop screws in a position having contact with the mesial and distal aspects of each headgear tube (see Fig. 29.2H). Because this procedure avoids anchorage loss of the posterior dental unit in terms of mesial movement of the maxillary molars, it is only necessary to distalize the maxillary molars during phase one to a formal Class I relationship rather than a super-Class I. Following completion of treatment, the resin on the archwire loops is removed and the ligature wires are cut before removal of the MISDS. The MIs are removed by unscrewing the head of the MI. Local anesthesia may be needed only if there is any tissue covering the MI.

CASE PRESENTATION

An 11-year-old girl was referred for the chief complaint of protruding anterior teeth. She had a symmetric face, a convex facial pattern with a deep labiomental sulcus and a retruded mandible, a Class II, division 1 malocclusion of between half to three-quarters cusp molar and canine relationships, increased overjet (10 mm) and overbite (4 mm) and mild crowding of the anterior teeth. The maxillary midline was coincident with the facial midline, while the mandibular midline deviated 2 mm to the left. She had permanent dentition with no missing teeth or caries and good oral hygiene (Fig. 29.2A,B). There were no disturbances in mandibular movements and she had normal temporomandibular joint function.

Alveolar bone and root formation were within the normal limits. Cephalometric analysis of the lateral cephalometric radiographs using ViewBox version 3.1 (dHal, Athens, Greece) showed a skeletal Class II relationship associated with a prognathic maxilla and a slightly retrognathic mandible (Table 29.1). She had an average growth pattern with a slight tendency

Table 29.1 Cephalometric analysis during treatment

Variables	Normal values	T0	T1	T2
Sagittal relationships				
SNA (°)	81.3	83.6	84.1	83.6
SNB (°)	78.8	77.5	77.4	77.5
Facial angle (°)	83.9	88.3	89.7	88.5
ANB (°)	2.5	6.1	6.8	6.1
Wits appraisal (FOP) (mm)	0	3.9	4.2	4.6
NA-APg (°)	3.1	10.4	12.7	10.5
H angle (°)	12.3	21.0	16.9	21.3
Vertical relationships				
SN-SGn (°)	66.0	67.4	68.6	68.3
SN-NL (°)	7.1	5.0	5.4	3.9
SN-OcP (FOP) (°)	16.2	15.7	16.6	15.0
SN-ML (°)	32.3	30.7	31.5	31.3
Ar-Go-Me (°)	126.8	119.5	117.2	116.7
SGo:NMe (%)	65.5	66.9	66.7	66.9
Dental relationships				
1s-NL (°)	112	114.4	113.7	106.7
1i-ML (°)	92.5	104.8	103.5	107.3
1s-SN (°)	102	109.5	108.3	102.7
Lower incisor to A-Pg (mm)	1.4	2.4	1.4	2.5
Interincisal angle (°)	131.9	115.0	116.7	118.7
Soft tissue relationships				
Nasolabial angle (°)	110.7	111.6	108.9	102.2

T0, initiation of treatment; T1, after maxillary molar distalization; T2, after completion of total orthodontic treatment.

towards counterclockwise rotation and an upward inclination of the palatal plane. The incisors were protrusive and proclined in relation to the anterior cranial base and the mandibular plane. Soft tissue analysis showed a normal value for the nasolabial angle.

The patient did not want to wear any extraoral appliances and together with her parents requested full retraction of the maxillary anterior teeth without performing any extractions.

The treatment objectives were to distalize the first maxillary molars bilaterally by means of the MISDS in phase one and then, in conjunction with conventional full fixed orthodontic appliances, to retract and intrude the anterior teeth in the second phase. This would improve the interincisal angle relationship, achieve a stable, functional occlusion through the establishment of a well-intercuspated bilateral Class I canine and molar relationship, and improve lip competence and facial balance.

Treatment

Two MIs were inserted and the MISDS was placed as described above. The coil springs were compressed and the MIs loaded at the time of placement. The patient was instructed to maintain optimal oral hygiene. Cephalometric radiography confirmed that the MIs had clearance of approximately 7–10 mm from adjacent dental roots.

The patient was monitored every 4 weeks. After 6 months, the first maxillary molars were distalized to a Class I molar relationship (Fig. 29.2C,D). Spaces were created between all the posterior teeth. A further 3 months was allowed to enable the maximum drifting of the premolars and canines (Fig. 29.2E,F). However, it did become clear that almost all the

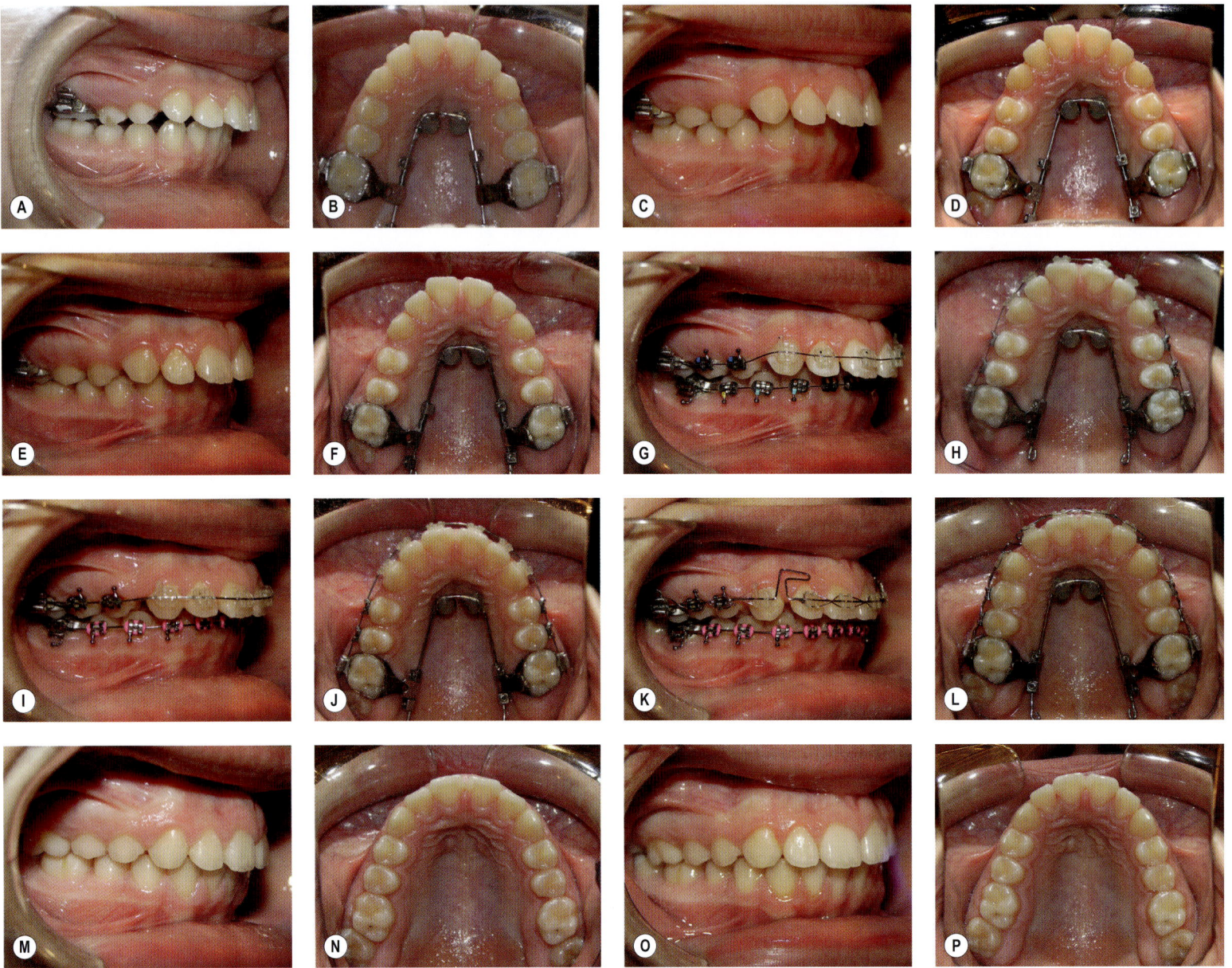

Fig. 29.2 An 11-year-old girl with Class II malocclusion. (A,B) Immediately after insertion of the miniscrew implant-supported distalization system (MISDS). (C,D) After molar distalization has been accomplished. Note the initial drifting of the premolars and canines. (E,F) Completion of drifting of the premolars and canines. (G,H) The MISDS converted to a skeletally anchored horseshoe-type palatal arch and used with a conventional full fixed orthodontic appliance. (I,J) Initial leveling and alignment completed. (K,L) Insertion of the SS retraction archwire. (M,N) Post-treatment. (O,P) Post-retention. (From Papadopoulos, 2008.[1])

drifting took place in the first 6 months and so this second waiting period was actually not needed.

A further radiographic evaluation revealed that the MIs were still stable and able to provide the required anchorage from their current position, and that there were no injuries to tooth roots. Only minimal non-significant cephalometric changes were seen (Table 29.1).

The second phase was commmenced by bonding a preadjusted edgewise appliance with Roth's prescription and 0.018 inch slot (Mini Master Series metallic and Silkon esthetic brackets; American Orthodontics, Sheboygan, WI, USA) and a superelastic Ni-Ti wire (0.012 inch) was inserted for initial alignment of the teeth. The MISDS was converted simply by pulling out the coil springs on both sides and screwing the stop screws into a position with contact to the mesial and distal aspects of each headgear tube. This creates a horseshoe-type transpalatal arch to provide the desired stationary anchorage for anterior teeth retraction and intrusion in conjunction with the conventional fixed appliances (Fig. 29.2G,H). In the second phase, the MIs were providing indirect anchorage to reinforce the posterior anchor teeth during anterior retraction.

After 2 months, Ni-Ti archwires (0.016 × 0.016 inch) were used for further teeth alignment in both arches (Fig. 29.2I,J), and after a further month SS archwires (0.016 × 0.022 inch) were used to finalize the alignment in both arches and to retract the maxillary canines into a Class I relationship. Two months later (i.e. 14 months after initiation of treatment), the teeth were fully aligned and a new SS retraction archwire formed individually with boot loops was used in the maxillary arch for en masse retraction and intrusion of the anterior teeth over another 2 months (Fig. 29.2K,L). The finishing phase used new SS archwires in both maxillary and mandibular dental arches for final alignment of the teeth and detailing the occlusion.

After 18 months of total treatment time, there was a good posterior intercuspation and a well-functioning and stable occlusion (Fig. 29.2M,N). The MISDS and MIs were removed and a lingual fixed retainer was bonded to the lingual surfaces of the lower anterior teeth extending from canine to canine. Maxillary retention was accomplished by means of a removable acrylic retainer. The patient was instructed to wear the retainers for 24 hours a day for 2 months and then at night only.

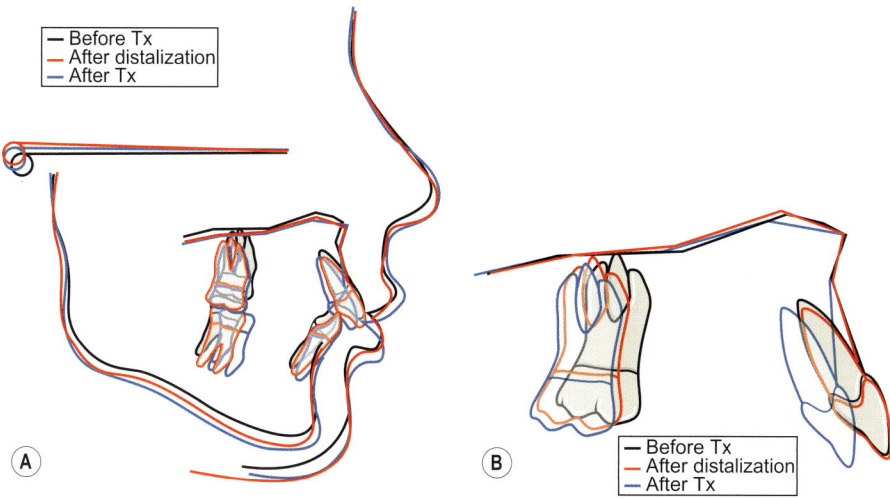

Fig. 29.3 Superimposition of the cephalometric tracings on the anterior cranial base (A) and on the maxillary plane (B), at treatment start before appliance insertion (black), after active molar distalization and subsequent drifting of the anterior teeth (red) and after completion of treatment and removal of all appliances (blue). (From Papadopoulos, 2008.[1])

Two years and five months after the end of active treatment, the occlusal relationships and the facial appearance of the patient remained stable and no relapse was evident (Fig. 29.2O,P).

Discussion

The treatment results were within the initial treatment goals and both the patient and her parents were very pleased with her final facial and dental appearance (Fig. 29.2M,N) and because no extractions had been needed and the girl did not need to wear any extraoral appliances or intermaxillary elastics.

Treatment achieved a bilateral Class I molar and canine relationship with optimal alignment of both maxillary and mandibular teeth, a well-intercuspated and stable occlusion and ideal overjet and overbite. The mild crowding, the midline deviation and the medial diastema were also corrected (Fig. 29.2M–P).

Root parallelism was confirmed on the post-treatment panoramic radiograph after debonding. Cephalometric analysis of the post-treatment lateral cephalometric radiograph after debonding showed maintenance of the skeletal Class II relationship as well as the sagittal skeletal position of the maxilla and mandible (Table 29.1). There were no, or only minimal, changes in growth pattern and the upward inclination of the palatal plane. The maxillary incisors were notably retracted while the mandibular incisors revealed a slight labial inclination. The interincisal angle was also slightly increased. Finally, soft tissue analysis showed a decrease of the nasolabial angle.

Superimposition of the cephalometric tracings shows the changes that occurred during treatment (Fig. 29.3). In total, there was a slight downward and forward positioning of the mandible due to normal growth (Fig. 29.3A). After maxillary molar distalization, a pure bodily distal movement of the first maxillary molar with a slight extrusion, but without distal tipping or extrusion, was evident, while no side effects of the "conventional" non-compliance distalization appliances (i.e. forward movement and proclination of the anterior teeth and distal molar crown tipping) were present (Fig. 29.3B). There was also a minimal distal movement and slight extrusion of the maxillary anterior teeth, which may reflect normal growth and remodeling of the maxillary alveolar bone. Further, after the completion of orthodontic treatment, the maxillary anterior teeth were retruded substantially without anchorage loss of the posterior teeth (i.e. mesial movement of the maxillary molars) (Fig. 29.3B).

These results were confirmed in a recent clinical trial that compared the skeletal, dental, and soft tissue effects of the MISDS and the bone-anchored Pendulum appliance (BAPA) using lateral cephalometric radiographs that were taken on the day of the insertion of the appliances and immediately after maxillary molar distalization was acomplished.[2] The maxillary molars were distalized successfully in both groups but nearly bodily distalization was observed only in the MISDS group, whereas significant distal tipping of the molars took place in the BAPA group. In addition, no statistically significant changes in the sagittal position of the maxilla and mandible, nor in the position of the maxillary incisors, were found in either group.

CONCLUSIONS

The case study presented in this chapter illustrates the effectiveness of the MISDS for treatment of Class II malocclusion with large overjet and overbite. The MISDS was used in the first phase to support anterior anchorage during molar distalization and, in the second phase, to support posterior anchorage for retraction and intrusion of the anterior teeth with conventional full fixed orthodontic appliances.

Comparisons of lateral cephalometric radiographs confirmed that there were none of the unwanted effects of forward movement and proclination of the anterior teeth, and distal molar crown tipping or rotation, as seen with conventional non-compliance appliances.

Treatment time was about 18 months since drifting of teeth takes place in the first 6 months while the molars are being distalized. The MIs remained stable despite being loaded with orthodontic forces continuously for the full treatment period.

The MIs must be inserted sufficiently far from roots of the adjacent teeth and safely placed to avoid any contact with the roots of the anterior teeth during the second phase of treatment.

The MISDS system has a number of advantages:

- it does not require patient cooperation
- it is not visible for the initial 4–6 months during maxillary molar distalization
- it can be used unilaterally
- it is simple to adjust for the specific needs of the individual patient
- it uses MIs for temporary and stationary anchorage to support both molar distalization and the subsequent anterior teeth retraction
- molar distalization occurs without distal tipping and/or rotation of molar crowns and without mesial movement and proclination of the anterior teeth
- the whole treatment can be provided chair-side.

REFERENCES

1. Papadopoulos MA. Orthodontic treatment of Class II malocclusion with miniscrew implants. Am J Orthod Dentofacial Orthop 2008;134:604, discussion 604–5.
2. Şar C, Kaya B, Ozsoy O, et al. Comparison of two implant-supported molar distalization systems. Angle Orthod 2013;83:460–7.

30

The Advanced Molar Distalization Appliance

Moschos A. Papadopoulos

INTRODUCTION

A number of systems have been developed to use miniscrew implants (MIs) as temporary anchorage devices to support orthodontic movements. Chapter 29 describes one such system, the miniscrew implant-supported distalization system (MISDS). While this system has many advantages, one disadvantage is the laboratory work needed for the fabrication of the appliance, and the consequent increased cost of treatment and delay in initiating treatment.

This chapter describes a novel MI-supported device, the Advanced Molar Distalization Appliance (AMDA), that has all the advantages of the MISDS but eliminates the need for laboratory work. The AMDA can be used for the efficient, invisible, non-compliant bilateral or unilateral distalization of maxillary molars (Fig. 30.1), as well as in conjunction with full fixed appliances for the subsequent retraction of the anterior teeth.[1]

THE ADVANCED MOLAR DISTALIZATION APPLIANCE

The AMDA (available soon by Dentaurum, Ispringen, Germany) is a prefabricated device anchored to the palate by MIs (Fig. 30.1A),[2] and comprising:

- a tubing system with encased compressed nickel-titanium (Ni-Ti) open coil springs to provide the necessary distalization force; in the conventional form this is used on both sides of the dental arch but can be activated unilaterally if needed
- conventional orthodontic bands on maxillary first molars equipped with lingual sheaths
- a horseshoe-type palatal archwire
- a palatal anchorage unit.

The design of the appliance unit and the use of palatal MIs to provide temporary and stationary anchorage for all phases of treatment avoids the unwanted problems of conventional non-compliance devices (see Chapter 2) such as molar rotation or distal crown tipping and forward movement and proclination of the anterior teeth. In contrast to conventional non-compliance devices, spaces are created between all the posterior teeth rather than just between the maxillary first molars and second premolars. This is because the premolars and canines are able to drift distally under the pull of the transeptal fibers, which also shortens overall treatment time.

THE TUBING SYSTEM

The tubing system (Fig. 30.1) runs on a horseshoe-type archwire and consists of two tubes sliding one into the other: an outer tube (approximate length, 10–12 mm; outer diameter, 3 mm) and an inner tube (approximate length, 8–10 mm; outer diameter, 2.3 mm). Compressed Ni-Ti open coil springs encased in each tubing system deliver a distalization force of approximately 300–350 g when fully activated. Two stop screws are incorporated in the tubing system, one at the mesial end of the inner tube and another at the distal end of the outer tube. Activation or deactivation of the force system takes place by screwing or unscrewing these stop screws. In addition, an SS extension wire (diameter, 0.9 mm; approximate total height, 10 mm) is attached to the external surface of the outer tube. It has an S-shape to allow height adjustment. The wire has a transpalatal type of ending (similar to a conventional transpalatal arch [TPA]) to facilitate insertion of the appliance into the lingual sheaths of conventional orthodontic bands cemented on the maxillary first molars.

The single tubing system version used for unilateral maxillary molar distalization (Fig. 30.1C) has an almost straight palatal archwire with one anterior loop for the insertion of a single MI, with an additional SS wire extension (diameter, 0.9 mm) soldered approximately 2 mm distal to the anterior loop and bonded to the occlusal surface of the first premolar for dental anchorage to avoid any rotational movements of the system during unilateral distalization.

Alternatively, for unilateral molar distalization a conventional AMDA relying only on skeletal anchorage can be used. In this case from the two bilateral tubing systems of AMDA only one is activated (Fig. 30.1B).

THE HORSESHOE-TYPE ARCHWIRE

The horseshoe-type SS archwire (diameter, 0.9 mm) is positioned on the palate at a distance of 1–2 mm from the mucosa and runs inside the inner tube of the tubing system (Fig. 30.1). The archwire is positioned approximately 10 mm apically to the occlusal surfaces of the maxillary molars, thus passing through or very close to their centers of resistance in order to facilitate an almost pure bodily molar distalization. Its position parallel to the occlusal plane forces the maxillary molars to slide on it and guides them distally without, or with minimal, rotation. Two symmetrical closed loops (or in a later version two movable metallic rings) are attached to the archwire to indicate the insertion sites for the MIs, as well as to secure the appliance onto the MIs.

THE ANCHORAGE UNIT

Two self-drilling and self-tapping MIs (suggested diameter 2 mm and length 8–10 mm) are used to anchor the AMDA and to resist the reciprocal forces during molar distalization and anterior teeth retraction. The MIs should have collars of varying lengths to allow a suitable size to be chosen for the individual's width of palatal mucosa. The MIs are placed in the

Fig. 30.1 The Advanced Molar Distalization Appliance (AMDA). (A) The horseshoe-type palatal archwire with the tubing systems for bilateral use. (B) The conventional AMDA for unilateral use relying only on skeletal anchorage with bilateral tubing systems of which only one is activated. (C) A single tubing system for unilateral use using both dental and skeletal anchorage. (A from Papadopoulos, 2010,[1] with permission of Bentham Science.)

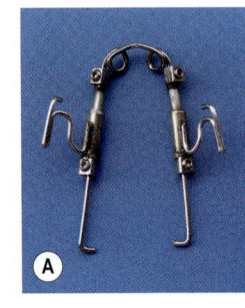
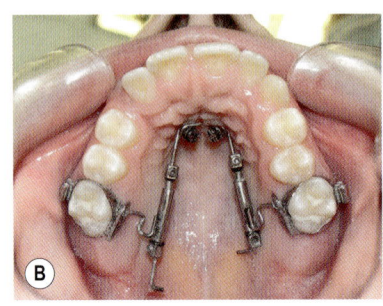
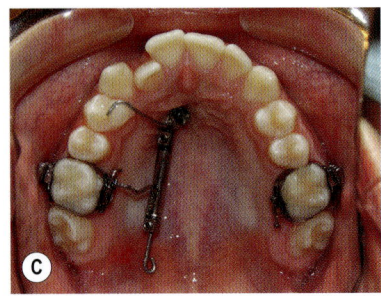

paramedian region of the palate 3–6 mm from the midpalatal suture and 3–6 mm posterior to the incisive foramen. The insertion of the two MIs at a distance of 3–6 mm posterior to the incisive foramen provides a safety clearance of approximately 7–10 mm between the MIs and the dental roots of the anterior teeth (depending on the root inclination of these teeth). This avoids contact of the MIs and these teeth during molar distalization, and, more importantly, during anterior teeth retraction.

CLINICAL PROCEDURE

PHASE ONE: MOLAR DISTALIZATION

The AMDA and MIs can be inserted in a single appointment by the orthodontist. Normal full infection control measures similar to those for extractions should be used, including sterilization of the MI kit.

Conventional orthodontic molar bands with lingual sheaths are cemented on the maxillary first molars. The AMDA is prefabricated and so some individual adjustments are only necessary, which can be carried out either directly in the patient's mouth or indirectly on the initial maxillary cast. The palatal archwire extensions are inserted in the lingual sheaths of the molar bands. Once the parallel positioning of the appliance and its width and height have been checked, the mesial stop screws are moved distally to fully compress the coil spring encased in the tubing system and the distal stop screws are screwed in place to stabilize the tubing systems on the archwire.

The final length of the palatal archwire is determined by marking its distal ends with a pencil, leaving approximately 8–10 mm extending out of the distal screw. With the appliance removed from the patient's mouth, the distal ends are cut off at the mark and a bend or loop is formed on each distal end to act as mechanical stop to prevent any distalization of the molars beyond this point and to avoid any tissue irritation. Alternatively or in addition, a small amount of light-cured resin can be added to the ends to ensure that the molars cannot slip out of the wire.

The appliance is then inserted into the patient's mouth, ensuring that it is parallel to the occlusal plane and the two symmetrical loops are 3–6 mm posterior of the incisive foramen. The wire extensions welded on the tubing systems are inserted into the lingual sheaths of the molar bands and secured in position with SS ligature wires.

MIs with appropriate collar length are inserted through the loops using the normal procedure. The head of the MI should be wider than the diameter of the loops to provide the appropriate stability to the system. However, in some cases, fixing of the AMDA with the MIs through SS ligature wires (diameter, 0.012 inch) might be necessary, particularly when MIs with smaller head dimensions are used. In some cases, SS ligature wires of a smaller diameter (0.012 inch instead of 0.040 inch) might be needed if the chosen MIs have smaller heads. A small portion of light-cure resin can be added to cover the top of each implant head plus the endings of the ligature wires and the loops of the palatal archwire to avoid plaque accumulation.

The AMDA can be loaded immediately with light orthodontic forces by unscrewing the distal screws to allow free distal sliding of the posterior part of the tubing system and thus distal movement of the maxillary molars. The mesial stop screws of the tubing systems (which are already moved and fixed distally) are not altered and so the compressed coil springs can begin to exercise their distalizing force. Distal movement of the maxillary molars can be enhanced through disocclusion of the posterior teeth using lower acrylic splints with posterior bite blocks or cemented build-ups.

Lateral cephalometric radiography can be used to check the installation immediately after placement, at the end of phase one and at a completion of treatment.

Patients are given clear instructions on how to maintain oral hygiene. They are monitored every 4 weeks for hygiene, for the stability of the MIs, and for further adjustments and reactivation of the appliance. Reactivation occurs by unscrewing the mesial stop screw, moving the anterior part of the tubing system more distally, thus squeezing the encased coil springs, and then rescrewing the stop screws in the new position. Any tendency for rotation of the maxillary molars can be countered by bending the wire extensions of the transpalatal archwire extensions welded to the tubing systems.

A treatment period of 4–8 months is usually needed for distalization of the first maxillary molars into a Class I molar relationship.

PHASE TWO: ANTERIOR TEETH RETRACTION

The AMDA is easily converted to a passive skeletally anchored horseshoe-type palatal arch providing indirect anchorage for the posterior teeth during a second phase of treatment to retract the anterior teeth and level and align the dental arches using a full fixed appliance. For this purpose, the distal stop screws are tightened to prevent any further molar distal movement and the mesial stop screws are moved distally and screwed in this position again, totally squeezing the coil springs encased in the tubing systems. This retains the first maxillary molars in their new positions and allows them to become the anchors to support the subsequent retraction of the anterior teeth.

In some cases, such as when the first maxillary molars are already rotated prior to the initiation of orthodontic treatment and the second molars are already erupted, rotation of first maxillary molars cannot be totally avoided during the active distalization phase through bend adjustments of the transpalatal archwire extensions of the tubing systems. In these cases the AMDA and the MIs are removed after retraction of the anterior teeth and, since there is no more need to support molar anchorage, a TPA is used until completion of treatment to correct this rotation.

REMOVAL OF THE APPLIANCE

The MIs are removed by unscrewing the head of the MI. Local anesthesia may be needed if there is any tissue covering the MI. The AMDA is removed by cutting the SS ligature wires that secure the transpalatal wire extensions to the lingual sheaths of the molar bands. The AMDA can then be removed from the sheaths in the normal way. Debonding of the conventional fixed orthodontic appliances (bands and brackets) and cleaning procedures are performed as usual.

CLINICAL APPLICATIONS

The AMDA can be used efficiently for the comprehensive treatment of Class II malocclusion. The following two case studies illustrate its use for bilateral and unilateral maxillary molar distalization.

CASE 1: BILATERAL MAXILLARY MOLAR DISTALIZATION

A 12-year-old girl was referred with a chief complaint of protrusion of the upper anterior teeth. She had a symmetric face and a convex facial profile with protruded lips, a retruded mandible and increased overjet (6 mm) and overbite (5 mm). She had permanent dentition, with the second permanent molars erupted, no caries and good oral hygiene. Both maxillary first molars, particularly the left one, were mesially rotated. Occlusal analysis revealed a Class II, division 1 malocclusion, with bilateral Class II molar relationships: three-quarters cusp on the right and full cusp on the left. She

Table 30.1 Cephalometric analysis during treatment

Variables	Normal values	T0	T1	T2	T3
Sagittal relationships					
SNA (°)	82.1	84.5	85.8	87.9	84.2
SNB (°)	80.2	80.3	78.9	79.7	79.7
Facial angle (°)	85.6	94.7	94.5	91.5	93.4
ANB (°)	1.9	4.2	6.9	8.2	4.5
Individual ANB (°)		5.1	6.1	6.9	5.3
NA-APog (°)	0.4	10.2	14.2	16.9	8.6
H angle (°)	11.3	17.4	10.9	21.7	20.2
Vertical relationships					
SN-SGn (°)	65.3	64.1	66.2	65.4	65.1
SN-NL (°)	6.8	4.8	5.7	5.5	4.1
SN-ML (°)	29.8	32.2	34.8	34.7	33.9
Ar-Go-Me (°)	124.4	135.8	132.3	137	136.2
SGo:NMe × 100 (%)	68.2	64.5	62.9	63.5	63.7
Dental relationships					
1s-NL (°)	112	122.4	115.6	106.9	110.8
1i-ML (°)	92.7	94.5	92.2	95.1	98.7
1s-SN (°)	104	117.6	109.9	101.3	106.7
Lower incisor to A-Pg (mm)	1.2	4.1	2.6	3.8	5.3
Interincisal angle (°)	132.3	117.6	123.1	128.9	120.7
Soft tissue relationships					
Nasolabial angle (°)	112	93.2	105.3	99.8	99.7

T0, initiation of treatment; T1, after maxillary molar distalization; T2, after completion of anterior teeth retraction; T3, immediately after completion of total orthodontic treatment.

had spaces in her upper anterior teeth, which were also proclined, and there was a mild crowding in the lower anterior teeth. Maxillary midline was coincident with the facial midline, while the mandibular one deviated 2 mm to the left.

Functional analysis revealed no disturbances of mandibular movements and normal temporomandibular joint function.

The initial panoramic radiograph showed that the third molars were present, no teeth were missing and alveolar bone and root formation were within normal limits. Cephalometric analysis of the lateral cephalometric radiographs using ViewBox version 3.1 (dHal, Athens, Greece) showed skeletal Class II relationships associated with a prognathic maxilla and an orthognathic mandible (Table 30.1). Analysis of vertical skeletal relationships showed a slight tendency towards a vertical growth pattern with a corresponding clockwise rotation of the mandible and an upward inclination of the palatal plane. Analysis of dental relationships revealed protrusive incisors, as well as proclination of the upper and lower incisors in relation to the anterior cranial base and the mandibular plane, respectively. Finally, soft tissue analysis showed a decreased nasolabial angle.

The patient did not want to wear any extraoral appliances and together with her parents requested orthodontic treatment without any extractions.

The treatment objectives were to distalize the first maxillary molars bilaterally and then to correct overjet and overbite by retracting and intruding the maxillary anterior teeth, to improve the interincisal angle relationship, correct the midline deviation and achieve a stable, functional occlusion as well as improve lip competence and facial balance.

Treatment

Two MIs were placed in the paramedian region of the palate and the AMDA fitted; it was activated and correct placement confirmed radiographically as described above (Fig. 30.2A,B). Since both first and second molars had to be moved simultaneously, and in order to enhance distal movement of these teeth, a removable acrylic splint with posterior bite blocks was also inserted to disocclude the posterior teeth. The patient was instructed to wear this splint 24 hours a day including meals and to remove it only for cleaning.

After 4 months, the splint with bite blocks was removed as the maxillary molar cusps no longer interfered with the mandibular molar cusps.

After 7 months, both first and second maxillary molars were distalized bilaterally and the first maxillary molars had a Class I molar relationship (Fig. 30.2C,D). The maxillary premolars and canines had also drifted to an almost Class I relationship. Further radiographic evaluation confirmed that the MIs were stable and would not interfere with retraction of the anterior teeth.

The second phase was commenced by bonding a preadjusted edgewise appliance with Roth's prescription and 0.018 inch slot (Silkon esthetic brackets; American Orthodontics, Sheboygan, WI, USA), and a Ni-Ti archwire (0.012 inch) was inserted for initial alignment of the teeth (Fig. 30.2E). The AMDA was converted to a horseshoe-type TPA as described above (Fig. 30.2F).

After another month, Ni-Ti wires (0.016 inch) were used for teeth alignment in both arches. Two months later, Ni-Ti archwires (0.016 × 0.016 inch) were placed and elastic chains were also inserted on the maxillary arch in order to start the en masse retraction of the maxillary anterior teeth. One month later, SS archwires (0.016 × 0.016 inch) were inserted to further align both dental arches and for the continuation of the en masse retraction of the maxillary anterior teeth. After a further month (i.e. 12 months after initiation of treatment), the retraction of the anterior teeth was completed (Fig. 30.2G,H).

At that time, a slight increase in mesial rotation of the maxillary first molars was observed despite adjustment of the transpalatal-type wire extensions of the AMDA during treatment. Therefore, it was decided to remove the AMDA and the MIs and insert a TPA to correct the rotations.

After 3 months, the molar rotation had been corrected and SS archwires (0.016 × 0.016 inch) with reverse curves of Spee and asymmetric elastics were inserted to fully align the dental arches, correct the midline deviation and further correct the deep bite (Fig. 30.2I,J). Four months later, new SS archwires were used for final alignment of the teeth and detailing the occlusion.

The fixed appliances were removed 5 months later (i.e. after 24 months of total treatment time), following establishment of a nice posterior intercuspation and a well-functioning and stable occlusion (Fig. 30.2K,L).

After debonding, a lingual fixed retainer was bonded to the mandibular anterior teeth extending from canine to canine. Maxillary retention was accomplished by means of a removable acrylic retainer. The patient was instructed to wear the retainer 24 hours a day for 2 months and then at night only.

Treatment Results

The treatment results were within the initial treatment goals and both the patient and her parents were very pleased with her final facial and dental appearance (Fig. 30.2K,L) and because treatment did not involve extraoral appliances, intermaxillary elastics or extractions. Treatment took 24 months and achieved a bilateral Class I molar and canine relationship with optimal alignment of both maxillary and mandibular teeth, a well-intercuspated and

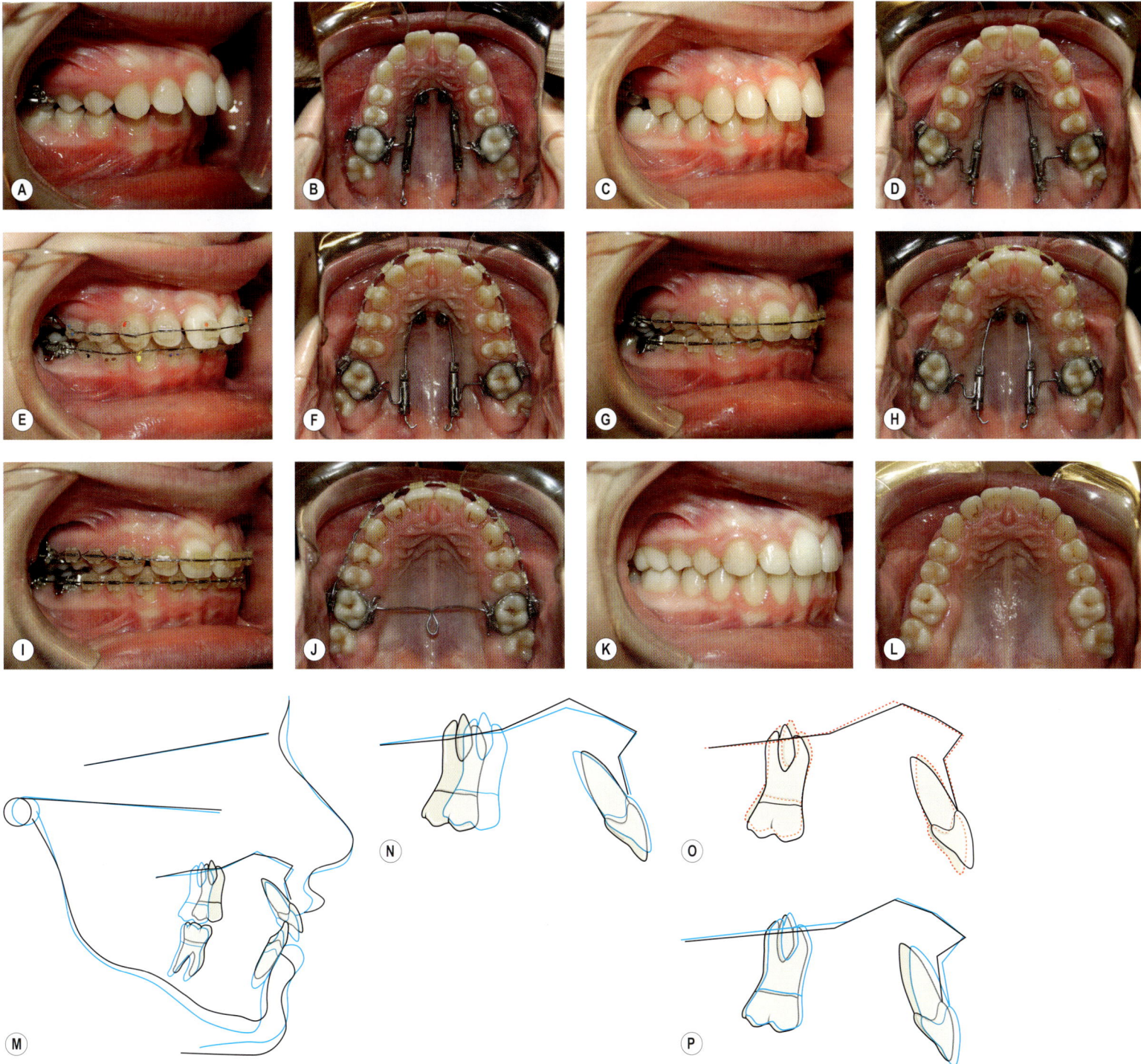

Fig. 30.2 Case 1: unilateral maxillary molar distalization. (A,B) Pretreatment views immediately after insertion of the Advanced Molar Distalization Appliance (AMDA). (C,D) Molar distalization completed. Note the initial drifting of the premolars and canines. (E,F) Insertion of conventional full fixed orthodontic appliances and conversion of the AMDA to a skeletally anchored horseshoe-type transpalatal arch. (G,H) Retraction of the maxillary anterior teeth. (I,J) Correction of molar rotation. (K,L) At end of treatment following removal of the fixed appliances. (M,N) Superimposition of the cephalometric tracings to show changes from before treatment start (black line) to end of active molar distalization (blue line) on the anterior cranial base (M) and the maxillary plane (N). (O,P) Superimposition of the cephalometric tracings on the maxillary plane to show changes from after active molar distalization (black line) to retraction of the maxillary anterior teeth (red line) (O) and from after retraction of the maxillary anterior teeth (blue line) to completion of treatment and removal of all appliances (black line) (P). (A–G from Papadopoulos, 2010,[1] with permission of Bentham Science.)

stable occlusion and ideal overjet and overbite. The mild crowding, the midline deviation and the medial diastema were also corrected (Fig. 30.2K,L). Root parallelism was confirmed radiographically.

Cephalometric Analysis after Distalization

After distalization, the first maxillary molars were moved almost bodily without distal tipping, while the anterior teeth did not procline at all; instead they were slightly retruded. Further, during the subsequent retraction of the anterior teeth, the maxillary molars, which served as anchors during this phase, remained almost totally stable, while the anterior teeth retruded substantially. Skeletal Class II relationships were maintained as were the sagittal skeletal positions of the maxilla and mandible (Table 30.1). There was a slight increase in vertical growth pattern. The maxillary incisors were notably retracted, while the mandibular incisors had a slight lingual inclination. The interincisal angle was also significantly increased. There was an increase in nasolabial angle.

Superimposition of the cephalometric tracings on the anterior cranial base from before treatment start and after active molar distalization (and subsequent passive drifting of the anterior teeth; Fig. 30.2M) showed a slight downward positioning of the mandible due to movement of maxillary molars into a more distal position, forcing the bite to open. The corresponding superimposition on the maxillary plane (Fig. 30.2N) showed a pure bodily distal movement of the first maxillary molars with a slight extrusion but without distal tipping, as well as slight retrusion and extrusion of the anterior teeth.

Cephalometric Analysis after Anterior Teeth Retraction

A comparison of the situation after the anterior teeth retraction phase with that at the end of molar distalization showed maintenance of the skeletal Class II relationships, while both the maxilla and mandible were moved slightly anteriorly (Table 30.1). Vertical growth pattern remained almost stable. The maxillary incisors were further retracted, while the mandibular incisors had a slight labial inclination. The interincisal angle was also significantly increased. Soft tissue analysis showed a decrease in the nasolabial angle. Trace comparisons confirmed that the first molars remained stable in position while the anterior teeth were retracted and slightly extruded (Fig. 30.2O).

Cephalometric Analysis at End of Treatment

A comparison of the final result with that before treatment start showed maintenance of the skeletal Class II relationships as well as of the sagittal skeletal positions of the maxilla and mandible (Table 30.1). There was a slight increase in vertical growth pattern, the maxillary incisors were significantly retracted, the mandibular incisors slightly proclined and the interincisal angle was slightly increased. Finally, there was an increase in nasolabial angle.

Superimposition of the cephalometric tracings on the maxillary plane after anterior teeth retraction and after completion of treatment revealed that the position of the first molars remained unchanged, while the anterior teeth were further intruded and slightly retruded (Fig. 30.2P).

CASE 2: UNILATERAL MAXILLARY MOLAR DISTALIZATION

A 14-year-old boy was referred with a complaint of a crossbite by the upper right lateral incisor. He had a symmetric face and a slightly convex facial profile. He had a complete permanent dentition with the second permanent molars already erupted in both arches, good oral hygiene and no caries. Occlusal analysis revealed a one-half cusp Class II molar relationship on the right and a Class I on the left side. There was a crossbite between the right upper and lower lateral incisors, a normal overjet of 6 mm, an overbite of 3 mm and a slight maxillary midline deviation of 1 mm to the left. In addition, there was 3 mm crowding on the maxillary anterior teeth and a mild crowding on the mandibular anterior teeth. Functional analysis revealed no disturbances of the mandibular movements and normal temporomandibular joint function.

The initial panoramic radiograph showed that the third molars were present, and no teeth were missing. Cephalometric analysis of the pretreatment lateral cephalometric radiograph showed skeletal Class I relationships associated with a slight prognathic maxilla and an orthognathic mandible (Table 30.2). There was a slight tendency towards a vertical growth pattern with a corresponding clockwise rotation of the mandible and a downward inclination of the palatal plane. There was also a slight retroclination of the upper incisors in relation to the anterior cranial base and proclination of the lower incisors in relation to the mandibular plane,

Table 30.2 Cephalometric analysis during treatment

Variables	Normal values	T0	T1	T2
Sagittal relationships				
SNA (°)	82.1	84.3	83.2	83
SNB (°)	80.2	80.6	79.7	81.8
Facial angle (°)	85.6	96	95.4	99.2
ANB(°)	1.9	3.7	3.5	1.2
Individual ANB(°)		4.8	4.4	4.1
NA-APog (°)	0.4	5.5	4.1	−0.5
H angle (°)	11.3	17.9	17.4	15.9
Vertical relationships				
SN-SGn (°)	65.3	65.2	65.7	64.2
SN-NL (°)	6.8	9.4	6.7	4.8
SN-ML (°)	29.8	31.1	31.4	30.1
Ar-Go-Me (°)	124.4	116.6	122.8	123.5
SGo:NMe X 100 (%)	68.2	65.4	66.7	67.8
Dental relationships				
1s-NL (°)	112	110.3	111.6	116
1i-ML (°)	92.7	96	96.7	102.5
1s-SN (°)	104	100.9	104.8	111.3
Lower incisor to A-Pg (mm)	1.2	0.3	0.4	1.8
Interincisal angle (°)	132.3	132	127.2	116.1
Soft tissue relationships				
Nasolabial angle (°)	112	101.6	100.5	101.8

T0, initiation of treatment; T1, after maxillary molar distalization; T2, immediately after completion of total orthodontic treatment.

while the interincisal angle was normal. Finally, there was a decreased nasolabial angle.

The patient and his parents wanted a treatment plan that did not involve extraoral appliances or extractions.

The treatment objectives were to distalize the right first maxillary molar into a Class I relationship, to maintain the Class I relationship of the left first molars and then to correct the crossbite between the right upper and lower lateral incisors, the anterior crowding in both arches and the midline deviation, plus to achieve a stable, functional occlusion by establishing a well-intercuspated bilateral Class I molar and canine relationship.

Treatment

Treatment was started with the placement of the single-tube configuration of AMDA (Fig. 30.1C) on the right side of the palate. Skeletal anchorage was provided by a single MI inserted through the anterior loop of the AMDA, while additional dental anchorage was provided by bonding the extension wire on the occlusal surface of the right maxillary first premolar (Fig. 30.3A,B). The AMDA was activated and correct placement confirmed radiographically, as described above. Light-cured resin was applied to the top of the implant head to avoid plaque accumulation.

A removable acrylic splint with posterior bite blocks was also inserted to disocclude the posterior teeth in order to enhance simultaneous distal movement of the first and second molars and to facilitate correction of the crossbite of the right maxillary lateral incisor (Fig. 30.3C). The patient was instructed to wear this splint 24 hours a day including meals, and to remove it only for cleaning.

After 3 months, the extension wire bonded on the occlusal surface of the right maxillary first premolar was cut in order to facilitate distal drifting of the right first premolar and canine (Fig. 30.3D). During the following

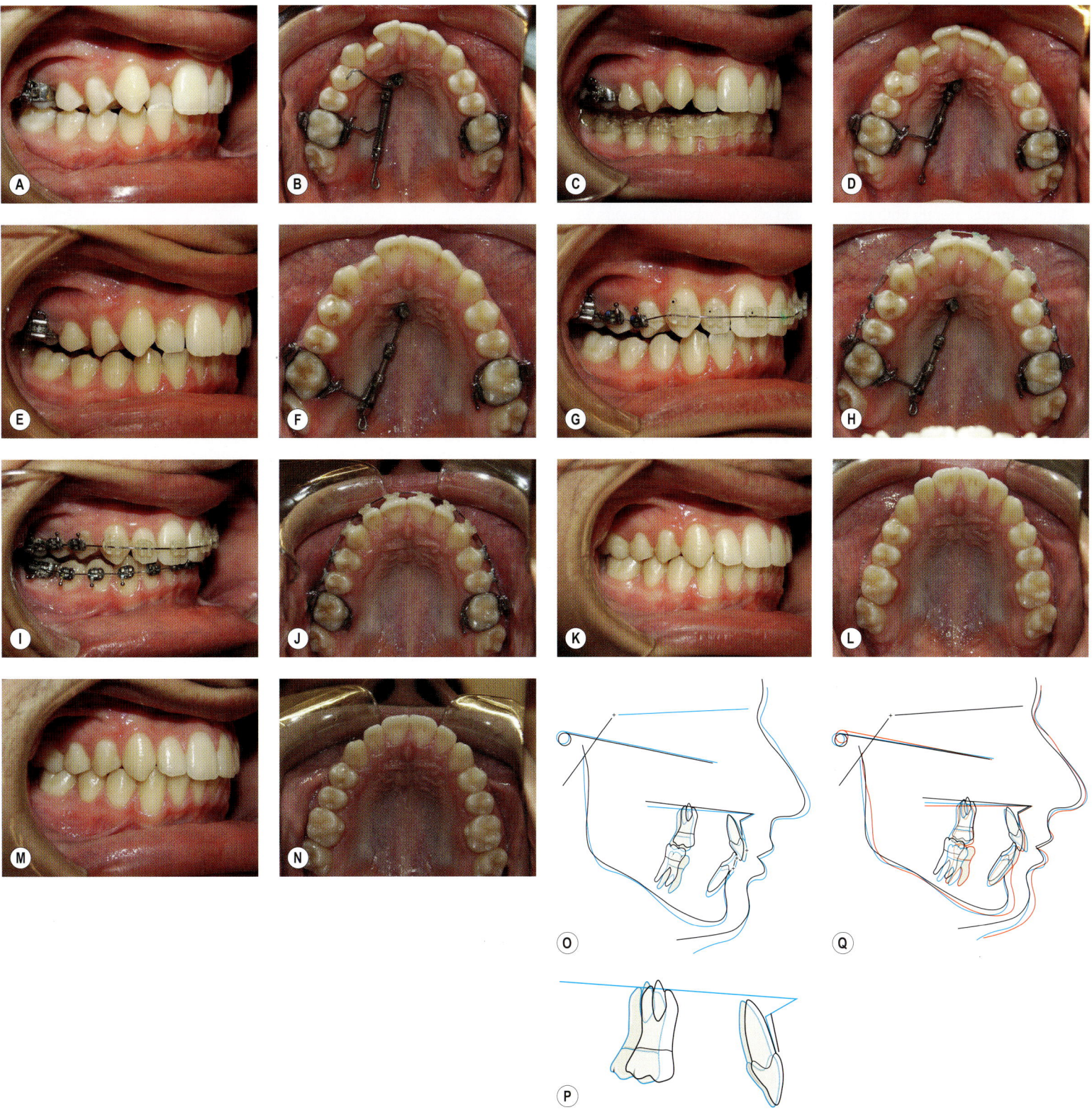

Fig. 30.3 Case 2: unilateral maxillary molar distalization. (A,B) Immediately after insertion of the unilateral Advanced Molar Distalization Appliance (AMDA). (C,D) After extension wire bonded on the occlusal surface of the first premolar. (E,F) After unilateral molar distalization has been completed. Note the initial drifting of the premolars and canines and the labial movement of the lateral incisor. (G,H) Insertion of conventional full fixed orthodontic appliance on the maxillary arch and conversion of the unilateral AMDA to a passive skeletal anchored device. (I,J) Insertion of conventional full fixed orthodontic appliance on the mandibular arch. (K,L) Following removal of the fixed appliances. (M,N) One year after the removal of the fixed appliances. (O,P) Superimposition of the cephalometric tracings to show changes from before treatment start (black line) to end of active molar distalization (blue line) on the anterior cranial base (O) and the maxillary plane (P). (Q) Superimposition of the cephalometric tracings on the maxillary plane before treatment (black line), after molar distalization (blue line) and after completion of treatment (red line).

appointments, spontaneous drifting of the right premolars and canines could be seen plus spontaneous opening of the space between the right maxillary canine and central incisor, proclination of the right lateral incisor and spontaneous correction of the crossbite.

Seven months after start of treatment, the tip of the right maxillary lateral incisor was positioned slightly more labially to the tip of the right mandibular lateral incisor and the crossbite had vanished. The cusps of his posterior maxillary teeth no longer interfered with those of the mandibular teeth. The lower splint with the posterior bite blocks was removed.

After a further month, both right first and second maxillary molars were distalized while the first maxillary molars presented a Class I molar relationship on both sides (Fig. 30.3E,F). The maxillary premolars and canines had also drifted distally, the space for the right lateral incisor was enlarged and the spontaneous labial movement and proclination of the lateral incisor was further improved.

Further radiographic evaluation confirmed that the MIs were stable and would not interfere with retraction of the anterior teeth.

Eight months after start of treatment the molar relationship was Class I; distal drifting of the right premolars and canines had occurred and the anterior crossbite was slightly corrected. A fully bonded preadjusted edgewise appliance with Roth's prescription and 0.018 inch slot (Mini Master Series metallic and Silkon esthetic brackets, American Orthodontics) and a Ni-Ti archwire (0.012 inch) was inserted for initial alignment of the teeth (Fig. 30.3G,H). The AMDA was converted to a passive skeletal anchorage device as described above.

One month later, a Ni-Ti archwire (0.016 inch) was inserted on the maxillary dental arch, and after another month (i.e. 10 months after initiation of treatment) the AMDA and MIs were removed and a Ni-Ti archwire (0.016 × 0.016 inch) was inserted for further alignment of the maxillary dental arch.

Eleven months after treatment start, the lower dental arch was bonded, a Ni-Ti archwire (0.012 inch) was inserted for initial alignment in the lower arch, and a SS archwire (0.016 × 0.016 inch) was inserted in the upper arch (Fig. 30.3I,J). At that point, the slight mesial rotation of the right maxillary first molar had been corrected.

Two months later, a Ni-Ti archwire (0.016 × 0.016 inch), and after another month a SS archwire (0.016 × 0.016 inch) were used for further alignment of the lower dental arch.

Fifteen months after initiation of treatment, SS archwires (0.016 × 0.016 inch) with reverse curves of Spee were inserted to fully align both dental arches and detail the occlusion.

The fixed appliances were removed 5.5 months later (i.e. 20.5 months from treatment start). The anterior crossbite had been corrected and a good posterior intercuspation and a well-functioning and stable occlusion had been established (Fig. 30.3K,L).

After debonding of the fixed appliances, a lingual fixed retainer was bonded to the mandibular anterior teeth extending from canine to canine. Maxillary retention was accomplished with a removable acrylic retainer. The patient was instructed to wear the retainer 24 hours a day for 2 months and then only at night. The patient followed these recommendations and 18 months after debonding his occlusal relationships as well as his facial appearance remained stable with no evident relapse (Fig. 30.3M,N).

Treatment Results

The treatment results were within the initial treatment goals and both the patient and his parents were very satisfied with his final facial and intraoral (Fig. 30.3K,L) appearance, particularly because this had been achieved without extraoral appliances or extractions.

Treatment took 20.5 months to achieve a Class I molar and canine relationship on the right side of the maxillary dental arch, while relationships were unaffected on the contralateral side. The crossbite between the upper and lower right lateral incisors, the midline deviation and the anterior crowding were also corrected, while an optimal alignment of both maxillary and mandibular teeth, and a well-intercuspated and stable occlusion were obtained. Ideal overjet and overbite were also achieved (Fig. 30.3K,L). There was a great improvement in the patient's smile and facial esthetics. Root parallelism was confirmed radiographically.

Cephalometric Analysis after Distalization

After distalization, the right first maxillary molar had moved almost bodily without distal tipping, while the anterior teeth did not procline at all; instead they were very slightly retruded. During the subsequent phase of distal movement of the right maxillary canines and premolars, the maxillary molars, which served as anchors, and the anterior teeth remained almost totally stable.

Skeletal Class I relationships and the sagittal skeletal positions of the maxilla and mandible were maintained (Table 30.2). There was a slight decrease of the vertical growth pattern, moving close to average values. The inclination of maxillary incisors was slightly increased towards labial, while the inclination of the mandibular incisors remained almost unaffected. The interincisal angle was slightly decreased. There was a slight decrease in nasolabial angle.

Superimposition of the cephalometric tracings on the anterior cranial base from before treatment start and after active molar distalization (Fig. 30.3O) showed a slight downward positioning of the mandible resulting from the movement of maxillary molars to a more distal position, forcing the bite to open. The corresponding superimposition on the maxillary plane (Fig. 30.3P) revealed a pure bodily distal movement of the right first maxillary molar without distal tipping, as well as a slight retrusion and extrusion of the anterior teeth.

Cephalometric Analysis at End of Treatment

A comparison of the final result with that before treatment start showed strengthening of the skeletal Class I relationships, maintenance of the sagittal skeletal position of the maxilla and a slightly more forward position of the mandible (Table 30.2). There was a further decrease of the vertical growth pattern towards average. The inclination of maxillary and mandibular incisors was slightly increased towards labial, while the interincisal angle was decreased. The nasolabial angle was maintained.

Superimposition of the cephalometric tracings on the maxillary plane after molar distalization and after completion of treatment showed that the position of the first molars and the anterior teeth remained unaffected (Fig. 30.3Q).

CONCLUSIONS

The construction and application of the AMDA is based on careful consideration of the issues related to the use of non-compliance distalization appliances with orthodontic implants. Features include:

- use of self-drilling and self-tapping MIs to make insertion easier for the patient and a process that can be carried out by the orthodontist
- MI dimensions of 2 mm diameter and 8–10 mm length to give ideal stability
- MIs with varying collar length to allow a choice of length to suit the patient's mucosal thickness
- two MIs to provide effective skeletal anchorage
- the paramedial region of the palate (3–6 mm from the midpalatal suture and 3–6 mm posterior to the incisive foramen) as the safest site for MI insertion

- a palatal force system with the line of force application passing as close as possible to the center of resistance of the maxillary molars
- the open Ni-Ti coil springs encased in the tubing system to reduce issues of plaque accumulation and irritation of the tongue.

The AMDA can be used for either bilateral or unilateral maxillary molar distalization without the need of extractions, as illustrated in the two cases.

The cephalometric evaluations described above confirm that the AMDA achieves the desired tooth movements without the side effects of other distalization systems, such as anchorage loss and molar tipping. The two cases illustrate its effectiveness in bilateral treatment as well as for unilateral distalization without side effects on the contralateral side.

A unique advantage of the AMDA is that it can be easily converted chair-side to a skeletal anchored horseshoe-type transpalatal arch to support subsequent treatment with a conventional full fixed orthodontic appliances.

The advantages of the AMDA can be summarized as:

- can be used for the complete non-compliance correction of Class II malocclusion, initially to distalize the maxillary molars and later to retract the anterior teeth
- prefabricated design eliminates complicated laboratory procedures
- insertion is easily carried out in one appointment by the orthodontist
- activation is initiated immediately after its insertion
- appliance is invisible during distalization of maxillary molars
- no side effects of distal molar tipping
- no anchorage loss of anterior teeth during active distalization
- distal drifting of posterior teeth and the incisors during molar distalization, which reduces the total treatment time
- conversion of the AMDA to a horseshoe-type palatal arch is simply performed intraorally

- no anchorage loss of the molars is anticipated during anterior teeth retraction
- can be used bilaterally or unilaterally
- closed tubing system protects from excessive distalization if the patient misses an appointment
- the AMDA can be used for a broad spectrum of orthodontic problems requiring maximum anchorage on the maxillary dental arch.

There are also some disadvantages:

- it may cause discomfort, especially during swallowing and speech
- there can be difficulties in maintaining optimal oral hygiene
- irritation of the tongue or palatal soft tissues can occur
- bodily movement of the maxillary molars may cause a mandibular downward rotation and thus worsen Class II jaw relationships; therefore, this system should be used with caution in patients with a vertical growth pattern or open bites.

The AMDA can be used for the efficient, invisible, non-compliant bilateral or unilateral distalization of maxillary molars, as well as in conjunction with full fixed appliances for the subsequent retraction of the anterior teeth (i.e. for the comprehensive treatment of Class II malocclusion).

REFERENCES

1. Papadopoulos MA. The "Advanced Molar Distalization Appliance": a novel approach to correct Class II malocclusion. Recent Pat Biomed Eng 2010;3:6–15.
2. Papadopoulos MA. German patent 10 2006 033 774; US patent 7,785,102.

INTRODUCTION

The Distal Jet appliance was developed to apply distalizing forces (through a couple) close to the center of resistance of a molar to reduce the degree of tipping that is an unwanted effect of many devices (see Chapter 2).[1] The Distal Jet appliance serves two purposes: molar distalization without patient compliance and subsequent conversion to a modified Nance holding arch to maintain molar position after distalization. Compared with other devices, the Distal Jet produces the least amount of molar tipping, minimal extrusion of maxillary teeth and negligible changes in mandibular plane angle, lower anterior face height, while expanding and rotating if preadjusted.[2,3] However, like other idstalizers it still exhibits the issue of anchorage loss. Once the initial distalization has been achieved, the molars must be maintained in their new position or they will move mesially. At this stage, it is preferable to select methods that are simple, comfortable, versatile, esthetic, hygienic, easy to comply with, cost effective, self-limiting and with few undesirable side effects, and yet are predictable, effective and efficient.

The Bowman modification, or Horseshoe Jet (Sybron AOA Laboratory, Racine, WI, USA) (Fig. 31.1) simplifies the conversion to a holding arch by replacing the original tube-and-piston construction with a more rigid, solid tracking; the coil springs are not removed.

DEVELOPMENT OF THE HORSESHOE JET

Initial attempts to use minscrew implant (MI) anchorage with the Distal Jet involved inserting MIs through holes in the acrylic button into the anterior palate or placing the MIs between the premolars in the palatal alveolus and tied them to the supporting arms of the appliance attached to the premolars.[4]

Reducing the Distal Jet into a 'horseshoe' eliminated the acrylic button (Fig. 31.2A).[5] Initially, implants were inserted either anterior to the horseshoe framework and luted together with light-cured flowable composite or they were placed posteriorly and tied to the wire with SS ligatures. However, no consideration was given to the issue of MI tipping and so anchorage was lost unpredictably.[5,6]

To prevent mesial loss of anchorage, it became clear that skeletal anchorage needed to be separated from dental anchorage. Consequently, the appliance was further simplified by eliminating the supporting arms to the premolars, leaving only the horseshoe wire (Fig. 31.2B,C).[7–9] There are then no reciprocal forces from the coil springs acting on the teeth anterior to the molars. Pure skeletal anchorage is used to push the molars distally and the rest of the maxillary teeth are left completely unfettered. Any tipping of the MIs (Fig. 31.2C) is inconsequential apart from the fact that they should not be used as a Björk implant for cephalometric investigations.

Ideally, a MI should be used in a way that can be tested easily for integrity and easily removed if it fails, with replacement of a new MI at a different location. The final Horseshoe Jet design[9,10] can be supported by nearly any type of MI, inserted in any number of locations (e.g. anterior or palatal alveolus) and connected to the horseshoe wire by luting with bonding adhesive or tied with ligature wire. The appliance can be adjusted fore and after by unlocking the stop screws and moving the wire back and forth to avoid impinging on the anterior palate or to increase the working length for more distalization.

CLINICAL PROCEDURE

Orthodontic molar bands are seated on the first molars and a pick-up impression is taken. Full fixed preadjusted brackets (e.g. Butterfly System;

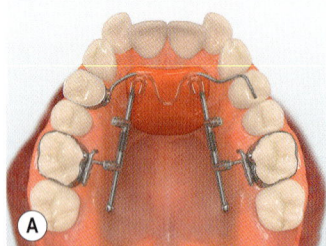 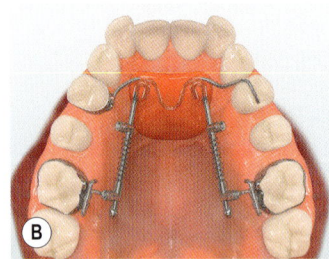 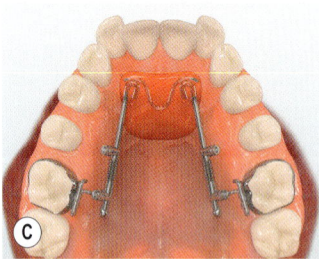

Fig. 31.1 Modified Distal Jet. (A) The Bowman modification is a laboratory modification in which the tube-and-piston construction has been replaced with simple tracking wires for better geometry and rigidity. Bands or bonded occlusal rests and a Nance acrylic button provide anchorage. Mesial locks are slid posteriorly to compress the coil spring. The appliance is activated every 4–6 weeks for 6–9 months. Distal stop screws are unlocked a quarter turn to initiate the process. (B) The distal stop screws are tightened at the end of distalization to stop the process. Note: premolars have followed molars as transseptal fibers were stretched. (C) Simple transition to a modified Nance holding arch required only sectioning the premolar support arms at the acrylic button.

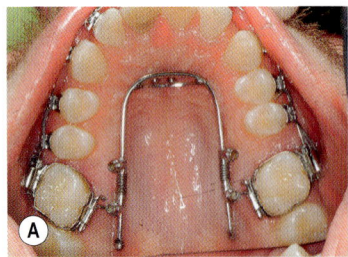 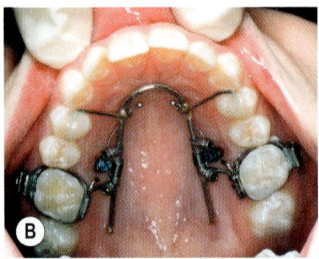 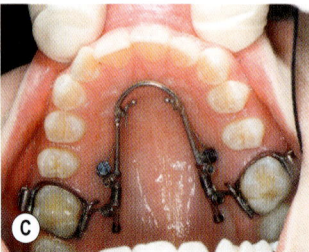

Fig. 31.2 The Horseshoe Jet appliance. (A) The original design with only skeletal anchorage. The tracking wire is abutted against two miniscrew implants (MIs) inserted in the anterior palate. (B,C) The simplified Horseshoe Jet and MIs (Note: the premolar supporting arms should not be used) (B); as molars are pushed distally, the premolars follow, moving past the MIs, which tip mesially (C).

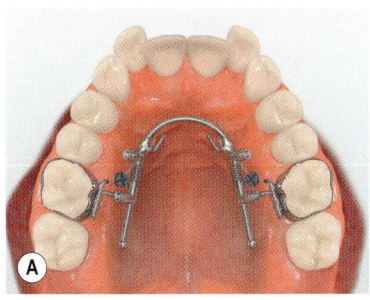 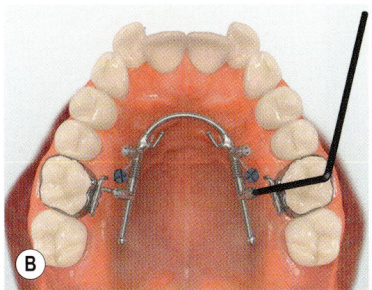 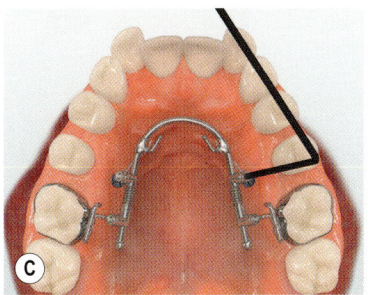 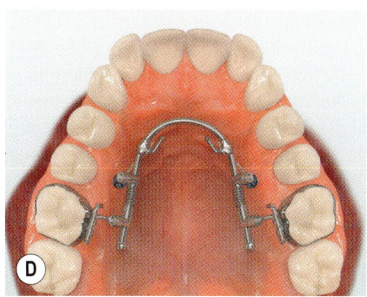

Fig. 31.3 The final modified Horseshoe Jet. (A) The appliance attached to miniscrew implants (MIs) between the first molars and second premolars. SS ligatures tie the MIs to hooks on the anterior part of the tracking wire. The mesial stop screw is moved posteriorly to compress the coil spring and locked into place. (B) The distal stop screw is unlocked a quarter turn to permit distalization. (C) At the conclusion of distalization, the mesial stop screw is moved back to compress the coil spring and prevent food impaction. The tracking wire is now held in place by both pairs of arch locks and steel ligation to the MIs. (D) The Horseshoe Jet serves as indirect skeletal anchorage for retraction of the remaining maxillary teeth with preadjusted appliances.

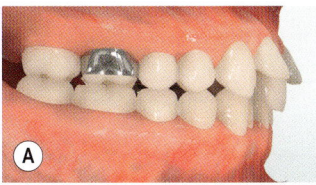 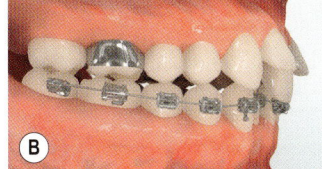 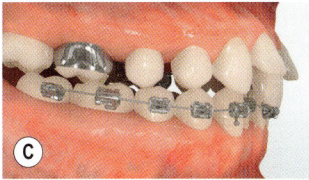

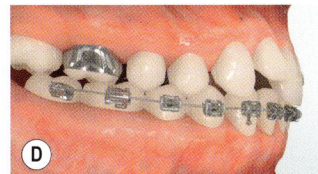 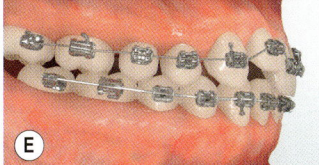 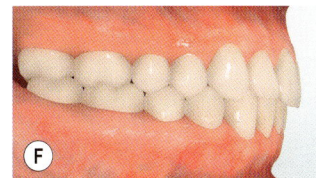

Fig. 31.4 Treatment of a Class II, division 2 malocclusion. (A) Maxillary Horseshoe Jet inserted and supported by two miniscrew implants. (B) Mandibular preadjusted appliance placed. (C) Molar distalization with pure skeletal anchorage to prevent unintended anterior anchorage loss. (D) A super-Class I molar relationship achieved; the premolars have drifted posteriorly under the influence of the transseptal fibers. (E) A maxillary preadjusted appliance is then applied and the Horseshoe Jet is locked down to serve as indirect skeletal anchorage for the retraction of remaining maxillary teeth. (F) The final result.

American Orthodontics, Sheboygan, WI, USA) are placed on only the lower arch to initiate leveling and alignment. The plaster cast with bands is sent to the laboratory for fabrication of the Horseshoe Jet. After the appliance is constructed, a trial fit is done.

Self-drilling MIs of nearly any head design can be used (e.g. 1.5–2.0 mm diameter and 6–8 mm length). Insertion of MIs follows a standard procedure: the position of MI insertion is indicated by the small bleeding point where local anesthetic is infiltrated. The preferred site is in the palatal alveolus between the first molar and second premolar and approximately 5–8 mm apical to the gingival margin. As the root of the second premolar is typically oriented buccally, this is an ideal insertion site for use with the Horseshoe Jet as the premolars will move past the screws.

The Horseshoe Jet is then cemented into place and SS ligatures are doubled over for added strength and tied tightly from the MIs to hooks on the anterior part of the tracking wire (Fig. 31.3). The distal stop screws are unlocked by a one-quarter turn only, just to permit distal movement along the tracking wire. Each mesial stop screw is unlocked and moved posteriorly, compressing the superelastic open coil springs on the wire, and then locked in position (Fig. 31.3). The patient is seen over 5–10 months at 4-week intervals to reactivate the device (recompress the springs). If the tracking wire comes into contact with the tissues of the anterior palate, the mesial stop screws are loosened, the tracking wire moved posteriorly to provide clearance and the device religated and reactivated.

As the molars are pushed distally, the premolars begin to follow under the pull of the transseptal fibers (Fig. 31.2C). Since the MIs are inserted at an angle to the alveolus, and because the root of the second premolar is angled buccally, there should be no interference. The MI may begin tipping mesially[6] and the second premolar may move distally, adjacent to the tip of the MI. In most cases, the MI will end up transposed between the second and first premolars at the conclusion of distalization (Fig. 31.2C).

Once the molars have been distalized, the distal stop screws are locked to prevent further movement (Fig. 31.3C). The Horseshoe Jet is now converted to MI-supported indirect anchorage for retraction of the rest of the maxillary teeth (i.e. acting as transpalatal arch with MI support).

CASE EXAMPLES

Three examples illustrate the use of the Horseshoe Jet. In the first, the appliance is used for a Class II, division 2 malocclusion (Fig. 31.4). In the second, it is used for a Class II, division 1 subdivision malocclusion (Fig. 31.5) and in the third it is used in a Class II, division 2 malocclusion (Fig. 31.6).

CONCLUSIONS

The development of the Horseshoe Jet has addressed many of the concerns regarding molar distalization. Use of pure skeletal anchorage appears to be the only way to avoid unwanted anchorage loss resulting from reciprocal forces. The simplification of the process with the Horseshoe Jet has improved the predictability of molar distalization for Class II malocclusion. The advantages of the Horseshoe Jet can be summarized as:

- one appliance serves two purposes: molar distalization and subsequent retraction
- simple conversion to MI-anchored lingual arch
- dual locks to avoid anchorage slippage
- coil springs remain in place
- force applied via a couple near tooth center of resistance
- completely adjustable anteroposteriorly

Fig. 31.5 An 11-year-old girl with a Class II, division 1 subdivision malocclusion. (A) The Horseshoe Jet with two miniscrew implants inserted. (B) At completion of distalization, upper braces and sliding retraction was initiated with indirect skeletal anchorage support. (C) Torquing auxiliary inserted to improve incisor position. Treatment was completed in 23 months.

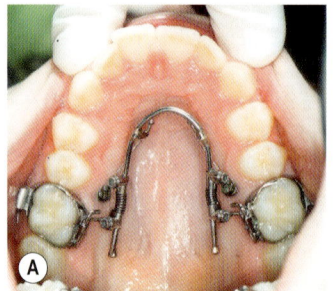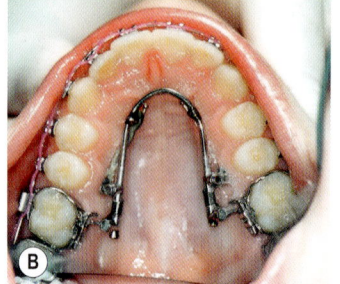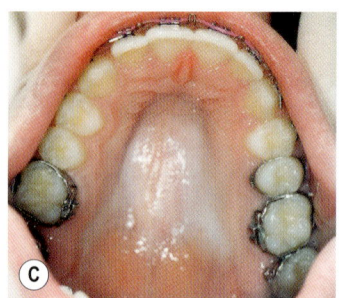

Fig. 31.6 An 11-year-old girl with a Class II, division 2 malocclusion. (A) The Horseshoe Jet is inserted with miniscrew implants (MIs) at an angle between the upper first molars and second premolars. (B) Steel ligatures are tied from the MIs to hooks on the tracking wire to provide anchorage support for molar distalization. (C) Upper brackets are added at completion of distalization. (D) Sliding space consolidation is supported indirectly by MIs via the Horseshoe Jet. (E) Space closure complete and the Horseshoe Jet removed. (F) Final results in 25 months.

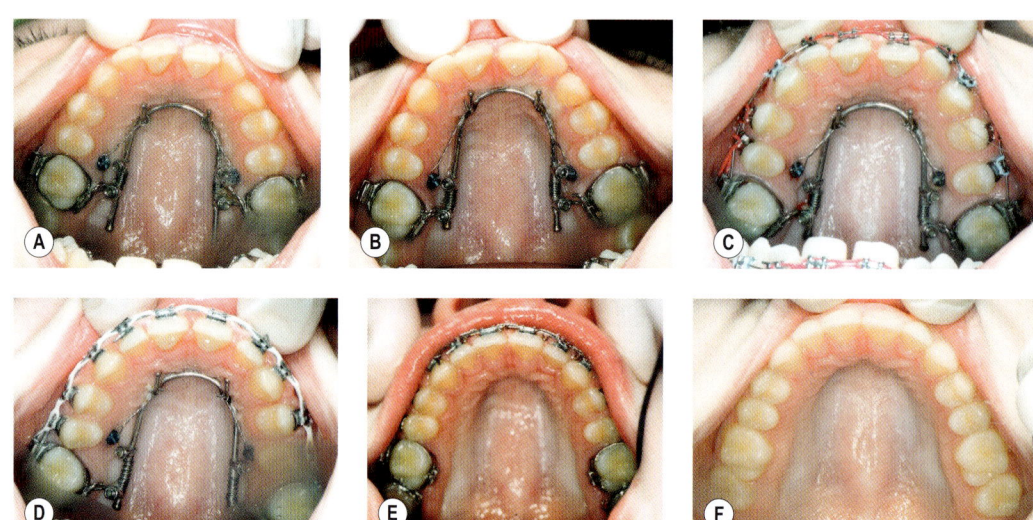

- pure skeletal anchorage
- no anterior dental support
- no acrylic button needed so more hygienic, less tissue impingement
- nearly any type of MI can be used
- option for multiple MI insertion sites
- no need to remove and reposition MI
- largest inter-radicular sites for MI insertion
- no root interference
- no incisive papilla injection
- fewer issues with tongue playing with MIs and food impaction
- no contra-angle handpiece MI driver needed
- direct driver access for insertion
- no concerns with midpalatal suture
- no analogue impression caps for MIs
- appliance not 'keyed' or locked to MIs
- less MI loss rate in palatal tissues
- compress springs to distalize uni- or bilaterally
- self-limiting appliance.

REFERENCES

1. Carano A, Testa M. The Distal Jet for upper molar distalization. J Clin Orthod 1996;30:374–80.
2. Bolla E, Muratore F, Carano A, et al. Evaluation of maxillary molar distalization with the Distal Jet. Angle Orthod 2002;72:481–94.
3. Ferguson DJ, Carano A, Bowman SJ, et al. A comparison of two maxillary molar distalizing appliances with the Distal Jet. World J Orthod 2005;6:382–90.
4. Velo S, Rotunno E, Cozzani M. The implant Distal Jet. J Clin Orthod 2007;41:88–93.
5. Kinzinger GSM, Diedrich PR, Bowman SJ. Upper molar distalization with a miniscrew-supported Distal Jet. J Clin Orthod 2006;40:672–8.
6. Liou EJ, Pai BC, Lin JC. Do miniscrews remain stationary under orthodontic forces? Am J Orthod Dentofacial Orthop 2004;126:42–7.
7. Bowman SJ. Thinking outside the box with mini-screws. In: McNamara JA Jr, Ribbens KA, editors. Microimplants as temporary anchorage in orthodontics [Craniofacial Growth Series]. Ann Arbor, MI: University of Michigan; 2008. p. 327–90.
8. Ludwig B, Baumgartel S, Bowman SJ, editors. Mini-implants in orthodontics: innovative anchorage concepts. Berlin: Quintessence; 2008.
9. Bowman SJ. Distal Jets refined: Bowman modification and Horseshoe Jet. AOAppliances 2008;11:1–5.
10. Bowman SJ. Class II combination therapy: molar distalization and fixed functionals. In: Nanda R, Kapila S, editors. Current therapy in orthodontics. St. Louis, MO: Elsevier-Mosby; 2009. p. 115–36.

32

The Distal Screw: a modified Distal Jet

Mauro Cozzani, Mattia Fontana, Anna Menini, Marco Pasini, Robert Ritucci and Francesco Zallio

INTRODUCTION

Issues of anchorage loss that are inherent with the original Distal Jet appliance can be avoided by using intraosseous instead of dental anchorage with the Distal Screw, a modified Distal Jet. Anchorage is obtained by using miniscrew implants (MIs) as temporary anchorage devices. As these MIs are not osseointegrated, they do not guarantee absolute anchorage and so the Distal Screw retains the palatal button of the classical anchorage set-up.

THE DISTAL SCREW

The main characteristic that differentiates the Distal Screw from the original Distal Jet is the use of a steel plate with two to five holes that is inserted in the Nance button (Fig. 32.1). The holes are large enough to receive the MIs and the larger number of holes permits the clinician to choose the best insertion site and to replace the MI in a different place in case of failure. Since bone anchorage is utilized, the premolar anchorage arms of the conventional Distal Jet are not needed.[1]

A bayonet bend in the arm incorporating the coil spring allows the point of force application to be closer to the center of resistance of the teeth. The telescopic arms are parallel to their insertion parts on the first molar lingual sheaths; this allows the distalization of the maxillary first molars to follow the natural arch form and avoids an excessive increase in intermolar width.

Compared with the Distal Jet, the Distal Screw is less bulky and also permits spontaneous premolar distalization under the pull of the transeptal fibers,[2] which can decrease treatment time.

At the end of the active distalization phase, the appliance can be used to support anchorage for the distalization of the premolars and canines (Fig. 32.2) as well as for bite opening. It cannot be used for anterior teeth retraction because the acrylic resin Nance button would impede their movement. Consequently the Distal Screw must be removed before the retraction of the maxillary incisors.

CONSTRUCTION OF THE APPLIANCE

Orthodontic bands are fitted on the maxillary first molars and an impression is taken with alginate. The impression with the bands positioned in it is sent to the laboratory for the construction of the appliance.

Plaster casts are prepared with the molar bands positioned. A steel plate is adapted to the palate vault and blocked out on the cast with some wax.

The preformed back-end telescopic arms are bent to form a 90° angle, about 8 mm away from the lingual sheath of the molar band (Fig. 32.3A), and adjusted so that they will not contact the underlying soft tissues. The arms must extend a few millimeters mesially to the steel plate so that they form a 5° angle with the line passing along the fossae of the posterior teeth (Fig. 32.3B).

A telescopic pipe is cut and positioned on the arms to allow for easy movement without binding. The anterior end of the pipe is bent to ensure adequate retention in the Nance button. When the two pipes (on the left and right sides) are positioned and adapted, they are blocked with wax (Fig. 32.3C). The acrylic resin button is prepared avoiding any resin blocking the holes in the steel plate.

All elements of the appliance are assembled with the spring activation device and a 240 g Ni-Ti coil spring positioned on the tube and a stop screw for the coil spring positioned on the arms.

The tubes are inserted on the wire arms and the appliance is checked on the plaster cast. A temporary metallic ligature is used to prevent the two parts from moving apart during cementing in the patient's mouth (Fig. 32.3D).

CLINICAL APPLICATION

The maxillary molar bands are cemented in place. The appliance is checked in the patient's mouth to verify its adaptation and stability before being fixed in position.

Usually, one MI per palatal side is inserted through a guide hole drilled with a handpiece and the MIs are tightened using either a hand-tightened screwdriver or a slow-speed handpiece. The appliance is activated by cutting the metallic ligatures.

Once the first maxillary molars have reached their correct position, the appliance can be used to support anchorage for premolar and canine retraction. The coil spring is cut and removed, the pipe at the distal end of the arm is brought into position and blocked with the stop screw and the telescopic arm is squeezed with Weingart pliers to ensure its fixation.

CASE PRESENTATION

A 12-year-old girl presented with a bilateral dental Class II malocclusion in her permanent dentition, protrusive maxillary incisors, deep bite and a hypodivergent growth pattern (Fig. 32.4A,B; Table 32.1).

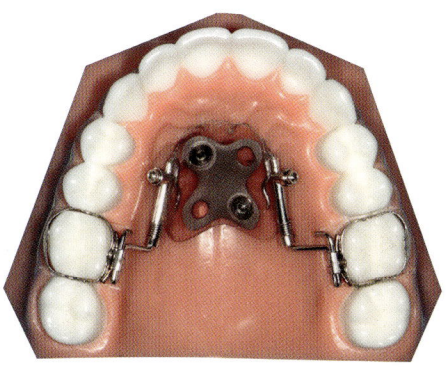

Fig. 32.1 Distal Screw positioned on a plastic model. Bone anchorage is used and so the premolar anchorage arms of the conventional Distal Jet have been removed.

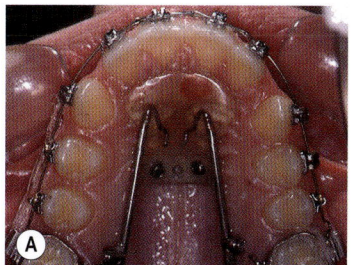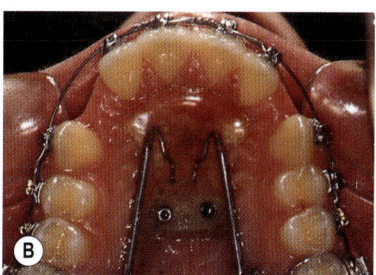

Fig. 32.2 At the end of the active distalization phase, the Distal Screw can be used as anchorage for the distalization of the premolars and canines, before (A) and after (B) distalization.

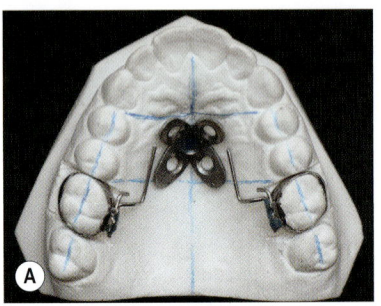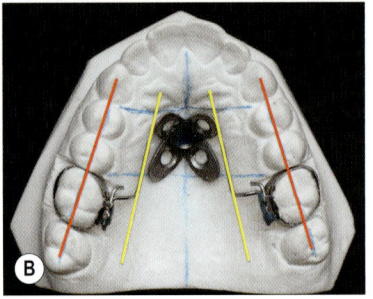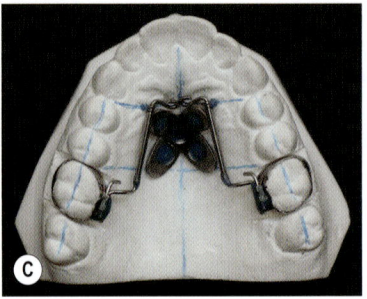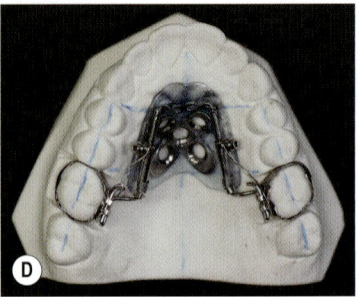

Fig. 32.3 Construction of the appliance. (A) Telescopic arm is bent to form a 90° angle about 8 mm away from the lingual sheath of the molar band and adapted to avoid contact with the underlying soft tissues. (B) The arms (yellow line) form a 5° angle with the line passing along the fossae of the posterior teeth (red line). (C) The two tubes are positioned and adapted and then blocked with wax. (D) The appliance is checked on the cast and a metallic ligature is used to hold the two parts together during cementing in the patient's mouth. (Courtesy of Mr Andrea Bertelli.)

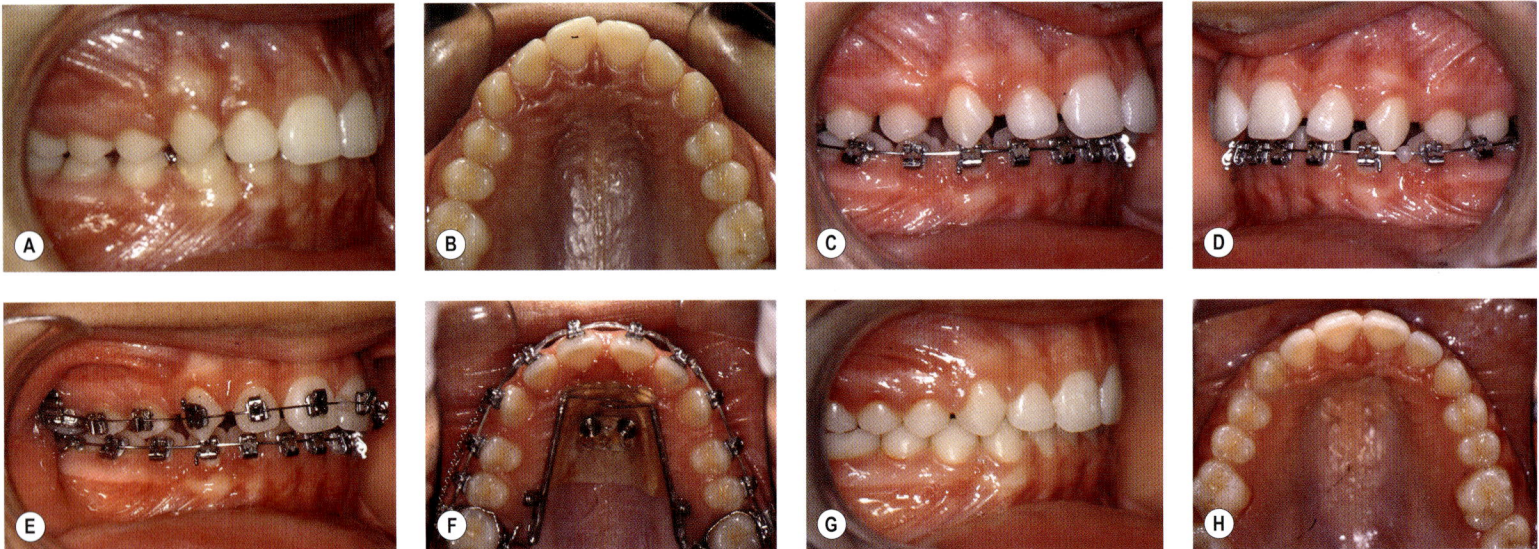

Fig. 32.4 Treatment of bilateral dental Class II malocclusion with the Distal Screw. (A,B) Pretreatment. (C,D) Immediately after completion of maxillary molar distalization. (E,F) After insertion of fixed appliances. (G,H) After completion of treatment and removal of all appliances.

Table 32.1 Cephalometric analysis during treatment			
Variables	**Normal (mean ± SD)**	**T1**	**T2**
Sagittal skeletal relations			
Maxillary position, SNA (°)	82 ± 3.5	76	76
Mandibular position, SNPg (°)	82 ± 3.5	74	74
Sagittal jaw relationship, ANPg (°)	2 ± 2.5	2	2
Vertical skeletal relations			
Maxillary inclination, SN/ANS-PNS (°)	8 ± 3.0	11	11.5
Mandibular inclination, SN/Go-Gn (°)	33 ± 2.5	29	27.5
Vertical jaw relation, ANS-PNS/Go-Gn (°)	25 ± 6.0	18	16
Dentobasal relations			
Maxillary incisor inclination, +1-ANS-PNS (°)	110 ± 6.0	110	107
Mandibular incisor inclination, −1-Go-Gn (°)	94 ± 7.0	100	100
Mandibular incison compensation, −1-A-Pg (mm)	2 ± 2.0	3	1
Dental relations			
Overjet (mm)	3.5 ± 2.5	5.5	4.0
Overbite (mm)	2 ± 2.5	5.0	4.0
Interincisal angle (°)	132 ± 6.0	133	136

T1, before the insertion of the Distal Screw; T2, after removal of all appliances.

A non-extraction treatment plan was considered appropriate using a Distal Screw for molar distalization together with fixed appliances. The Distal Screw was cemented and fixed. Appliances were inserted at the same time in the mandibular arch in order to prepare it for possible anchorage support with Class II elastics. The distalizing phase to Class I molar relationship took about 12 months. At this point there were spaces between all posterior maxillary teeth and the maxillary canine had moved distally (Fig. 32.4C,D).

The Distal Screw was deactivated and fixed appliances were inserted in the maxillary arch for alignment and retraction of the anterior teeth (Fig. 32.4E,F).

At the end of treatment, there was good alignment in both arches and molar and canine bilateral Class I relationships had been achieved (Fig. 32.4G,H) (Table 32.1). Total treatment time was approximately 30 months.

CONCLUSIONS

Distalization is more effective prior to the eruption of the maxillary second molars, and if it is carried out before the mandibular second premolars have emerged, this allows the leeway space to be exploited. Although molar distalization is not recommended in patients with increased facial divergence or skeletal open bite, the Distal Screw can be used because it produces an almost bodily movement of the molars with no significant vertical changes.

The Distal Screw has a number of advantages:

- it is a non-compliance method that is generally accepted by patients because it is invisible when they talk or smile
- it is less bulky and less time consuming than the Distal Jet
- it uses skeletal anchorage with MIs in the median and paramedian region of the palate, which is an area that is easily accessible, easy to maintain a good oral hygiene and less likely to interfere with vessels, nerves or roots of teeth
- it does not require radiographic evaluation for MI placement or surgical guides as the modified Nance button acts as a guide
- treatment time is reduced because there is no anchorage loss of the anterior teeth and the maxillary first and second premolars can drift distally spontaneously
- maxillary molars are moved almost bodily with a minimum degree of crown tipping
- there is no significant change in the vertical dimension
- first premolar and canine retraction, as well as incisor intrusion, can be accomplished using the skeletonized Nance button as anchorage.

REFERENCES

1. Carano A, Testa A, Bowan J. The distal jet simplified and updated. J Clin Orthod 2002;36:586–90.
2. Cozzani M, Zallio F, Lombardo L, et al. Efficiency of the distal screw in the distal movement of maxillary molars. World J Orthod 2010;11:341–5.

33

The Beneslider and Pendulum B appliances
Benedict Wilmes

INTRODUCTION

The Beneslider and Pendulum B appliances are designed to take advantage of direct anchorage using miniscrew implants (MIs) as temporary anchorage devices for maxillary molar distalization.[1-3] Both are fixed to the top of the MIs with exchangeable abutments, part of the Benefit system (PSM, Tuttlingen, Germany) (Fig. 33.1). The Beneslider device is better for bodily distal movement of the maxillary molars whereas the Pendulum B seems to be more appropriate when the maxillary molars need to be uprighted and/or derotated while being distalized.

CLINICAL APPLICATION

One or two Benefit MIs are inserted in the anterior median region of the palate near the third palatal rugae using standard techniques. A predrilled pilot hole may be needed. MI insertion can be carried out using a handpiece adapted to a commonly used contra-angle. It is advisable to choose MIs with a wider diameter for higher stability. Coupling of two MIs in the line of force in the sagittal direction will minimize the risk of MI tipping or failure. If one MI is used, the recommendable dimension is 2.3×11 mm; if two MIs are inserted, the anterior one should be 2.0×11 mm and the posterior 2.0×9 mm.

The Beneslider appliance comprises two activation locks, two open springs and two Benetubes (Fig. 33.2). Bands with lingual sheaths are bonded to the maxillary molars and Benetubes are inserted in the molar sheaths. A Beneplate with a 1.1 mm SS wire in place is then adapted to the curvature of the palate and connects the MIs with the molars. Depending on the insertion site and angle of the MIs, the Beneplate body may need to be bent as well. The Beneplate wire should be parallel to the occlusal plane if the molars have to be distalized horizontally. By changing the angulation of the Beneplate wire, the molars can be intruded or extruded during distalization (Fig. 33.3).

The Beneplate is then connected to the MIs with two fixing screws using a small hand driver or a contra-angle. If the Beneslider is based on just one MI, the abutment with a wire in place (Fig. 33.2C) is used instead of

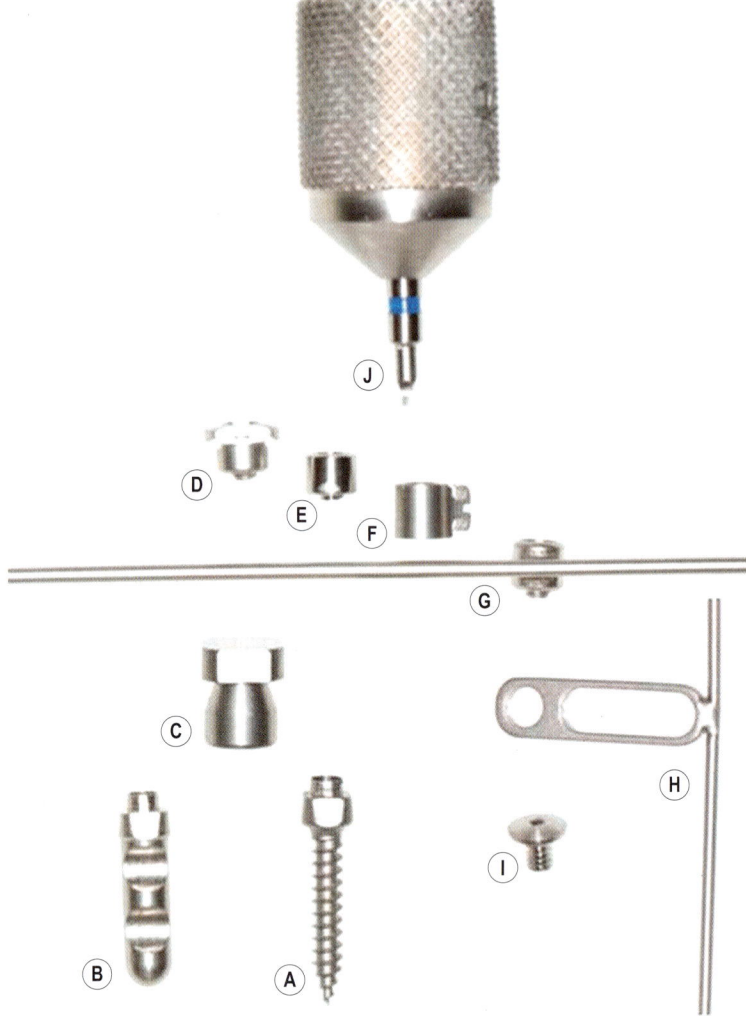

Fig. 33.1 The Benefit system. A, Miniscrew implant; B, laboratory analogue; C, impression cap; D, slot abutment; E, standard abutment; F, bracket abutment; G, abutment with a wire in place (1.1 or 0.8 mm); H, Beneplate with a wire in place (1.1 or 0.8 mm); I, fixing screw for the Beneplate; J, screwdriver for fixation of the abutments/Beneplates.

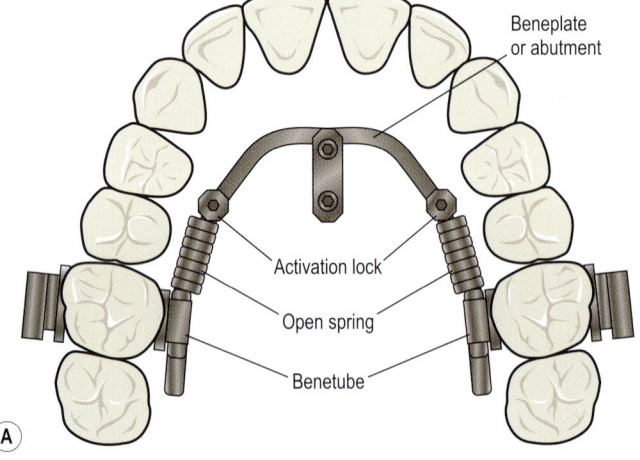

Beneplate or abutment

Activation lock

Open spring

Benetube

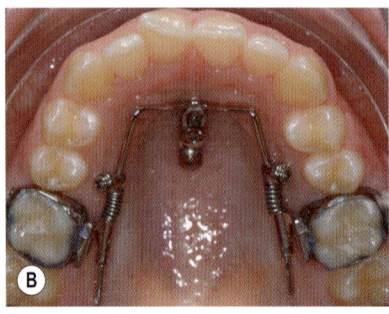

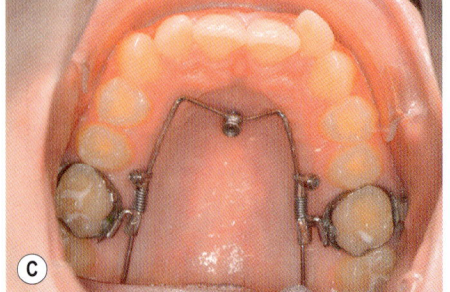

Fig. 33.2 (A) The Beneslider comprises two activation locks, two open springs and two Benetubes. (B) Beneplate with two miniscrew implants. (C) Beneplate with one miniscrew implant. In both, an abutment is used with a 1.1 mm wire.

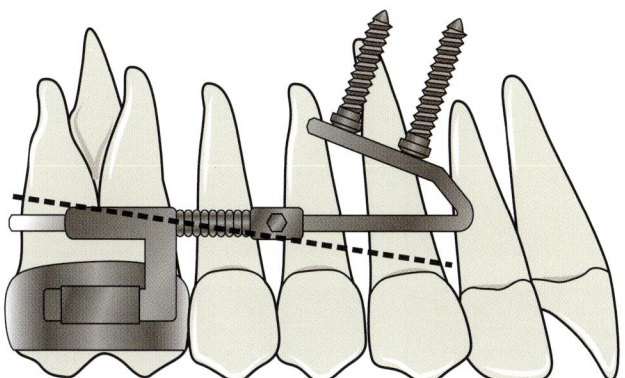

Fig. 33.3 Proper guidance of the molars is achieved using a 1.1 mm SS wire through the center of resistance of the teeth. If the molars have to be distalized horizontally, the Beneplate wire should be parallel to the occlusal plane. By changing the angulation of the wire, the molars can be intruded or extruded simultaneously to the distalization process (dashed line, in this case intrusion).

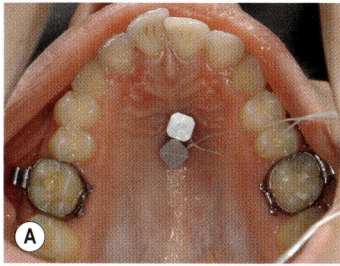
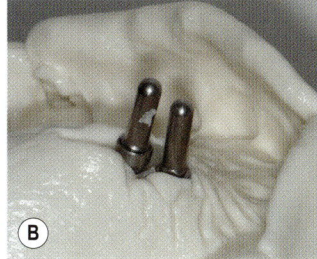
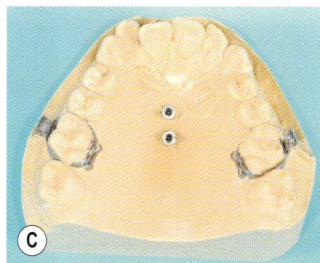

Fig. 33.4 Adaptation of the appliance in the laboratory. (A) Impression caps are plugged on top of the miniscrew implants. (B) After taking an silicon impression, laboratory analogues are plugged into the impression caps. (C) Plaster cast with molar bands and laboratory analogues (when extraoral bending of the Beneslider is preferred).

the Beneplate. The Beneslider is completed by two open coils and two activations locks. Molar distalization force is achieved by pressing of the activation locks against the coil springs. In young adolescents, 240 g springs are used. If the second molars are fully erupted, 500 g springs are recommended.

Both the Beneslider and the Pendulum B appliance can be bent and adapted intraorally. To shorten the chair-side time, impressions can be taken and adaptation of the appliances can be carried out in the laboratory on a plaster cast (Fig. 33.4).

CASE EXAMPLES

THE BENESLIDER

A 16-year-old boy with a full Class II occlusion and maxillary anterior crowding was initially treated with a headgear but he refused to wear it sufficiently. In order to avoid extraction of two premolars, molar distalization was performed using a Beneslider. Figure 33.5 outlines the treatment steps. The treatment time was 10 months for the invisible distalization and 15 months with brackets in place.

THE PENDULUM B APPLIANCE

Pendulum B mechanics are employed if frictionless mechanics is preferred and/or the molars should be uprighted or derotated simultaneously to the distalization.

A 39-year-old man with a Class II malocclusion and upper and lower anterior crowding presented for treatment. Four premolars had been extracted when he was a child (Fig. 33.6). After 6 months of treatment with the Pendulum B appliance, the distalization effect was appropriate in this patient (approximately 5 mm) (Fig. 33.6D,E). This was followed by leveling and retraction of the anterior dentition using fixed appliances and a power chain (Fig. 336F). Panoramic radiography after retraction of the anterior dentition confirmed good bodily distalization of the molars. The

total treatment time was 14 months (6 months distalization and 8 months leveling and retraction of the anterior dentition) (Fig. 33.6G,H).

DISCUSSION

Both the Beneslider and the Pendulum B are effective appliances for maxillary molar distalization without any side effects in terms of anchorage loss of the anterior dentition.

The distalization effect (approximately 5 mm) achieved with Beneslider mechanics is adequate when compared with other distalization devices.[1] There is very little first molar tipping, which can be attributed to the fact that the line of force is near the estimated center of resistance of the molar and correct guidance is delivered by the SS wire.[1]

The Benefit MIs were inserted in the anterior palate in the region of the midpalatal suture in all patients, including adolescents. The MI insertion method provided sufficient stability and did not adversely affect maxillary growth. Use of MIs to support maxillary distalization in 178 patients showed major MI tipping in only seven (a failure rate of 3.9%). The maximum insertion moments of the MIs ranged from 8 to 25 Ncm, which can be regarded as adequate to achieve a sufficient primary stability for MIs of diameter 2.0 or 2.3 mm.

The question of whether there might be an impairment of transversal maxillary growth was investigated by Asscherickx et al.[4] using Orthosystem implants in beagle dogs. In this case, they saw transversal growth inhibition, although only in one parameter. However, the MIs used in this study had a greater diameter plus a rougher surface to stimulate osseointegration. Our clinical observations have not revealed any tendency for reduced transversal growth of the maxilla. If desired, the MIs could be inserted lateral to the suture. No clinical problems were observed even when the posterior MI appeared to penetrate the nasal cavity.

Maxillary molar distalization takes approximately 3 months until distalization of the molars is visible. This is partly because there is a simultaneous distal migration of the premolars under the pull of the transseptal fibers. Employing indirect anchorage devices (using premolars) leads to

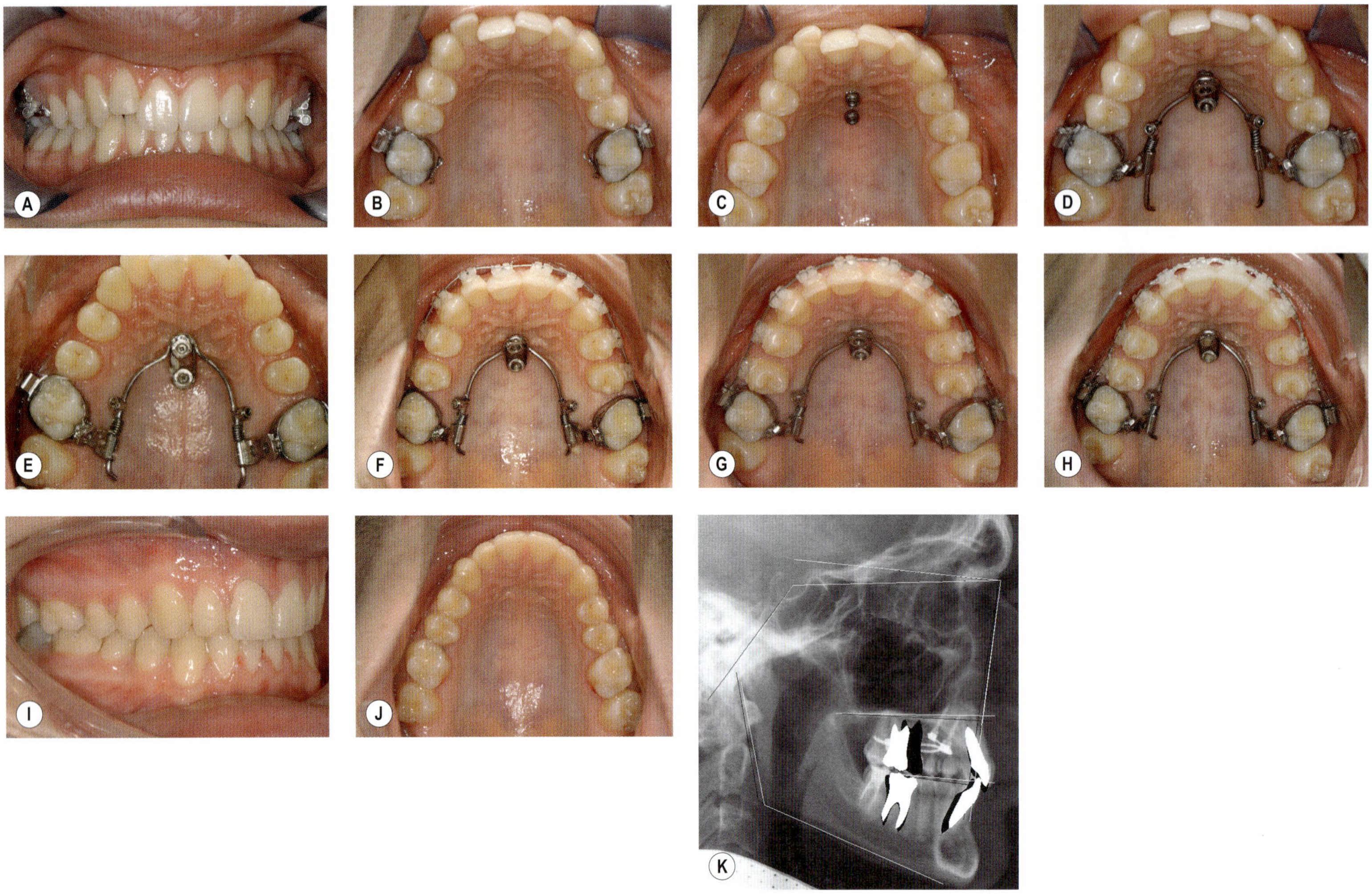

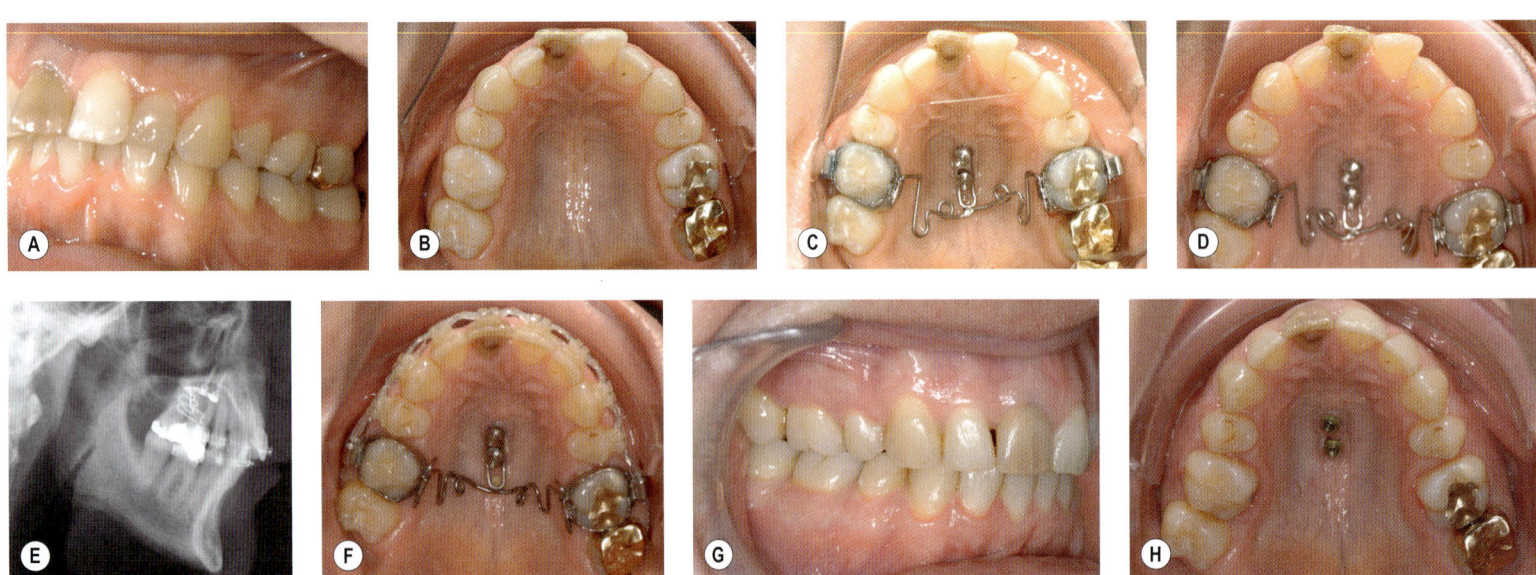

Fig. 33.5 Full Class II occlusion, maxillary anterior crowding and deep bite treated with the Beneslider. (A,B) Pretreatment. (C) Two Benefit miniscrew implants in place. (D) Beneslider in place with posterior coupling using a headgear tube since Benetubes were not available at the time. (E) After 10 months of follow-up. (F) Situation after bonding of brackets. Bite opening is achieved by bonding of resin "bite turbos" at the palatal surfaces of the upper central incisors. (G) One month after bonding: application of an intrusion overlay in the lower arch. (H) Four months after bonding, leveling is finished. Retraction of the anterior dentition with a SS wire (0.016 × 0.22 inch) and a power chain. The Beneslider is now used for anchorage of the molars. (I,J) Treatment end. (K) Superimposition of cephalometric radiographs before and after distalization: maxillary molars were distalized approximately 7 mm.

Fig. 33.6 Class II malocclusion and upper and lower anterior crowding treated with the Pendulum B appliance. (A,B) Pretreatment. (C) To avoid tipping and severe rotation during distalization, Pendulum mechanics preactivated by uprighting and antirotation bends. (D) Distalization effect after 6 months with the Pendulum B appliance; many spaces can be seen in the posterior region. (E) Cephalometric radiograph showing the distalization effect (approximately 5 mm) after 6 months of treatment. (F) After leveling and aligning, the anterior dentition was retracted with a power chain. During this retraction phase, the Pendulum B appliance was reactivated properly for molar anchorage purposes. (G,H) After debonding.

the reverse effect of mesial migration of the premolars (anchorage loss), which create spaces between the second premolars and the first molars that may appear to be the result of distalization of the first molars.

CONCLUSIONS

A MI system with exchangeable abutments offers a variety of different mechanics; for example, either a Beneslider or a Pendulum B can be used for maxillary molar distalization. If bodily distal movement of maxillary molars is needed, the Beneslider provides very effective and easy mechanics. If maxillary molars have to be distalized and simultaneously uprighted or derotated, the Pendulum B is suggested.

REFERENCES

1. Wilmes B, Drescher D. Application and effectiveness of the BENEslider: a device to move molars distally. World J Orthod 2010;11:331–40.
2. Wilmes B, Drescher D, Nienkemper M. A miniplate system for improved stability of skeletal anchorage. J Clin Orthod 2009;43:494–501.
3. Wilmes B, Drescher D. A miniscrew system with interchangeable abutments. J Clin Orthod 2008;42:574–80.
4. Asscherickx K, Hanssens JL, Wehrbein H, et al. Orthodontic anchorage implants inserted in the median palatal suture and normal transverse maxillary growth in growing dogs: a biometric and radiographic study. Angle Orthod 2005;75:826–31.

34

The TopJet distalizer

Heinz Winsauer

INTRODUCTION

Three molar distalizers using purely bone-borne anchorage via miniscrew implants (MIs) are currently in use: the Beneslider, with elements of the Distal Jet and the Keles Slider (Chapter 33); the miniscrew implant-supported distalization system (Chapter 29) and its development, the Advanced Molar Distalization Appliance (Chapter 30), and the TopJet, which is connected to a palatal arch and thus offers a friction-free distalizing force.[1,2] The TopJet was the first "ready-to-use" appliance for molar distalization.

THE TOPJET DISTALIZER

The TopJet distalizer consists of a distalizing open coil spring power module, an adjustment module housed biaxially in a twin tube and a prefabricated transpalatal arch (TPA) in seven different sizes (Fig. 34.1).

THE POWER MODULE

The power module is a cylinder containing an open Ni-Ti coil spring that extends a plunger. It is connected to the MI in the anterior palate with the C-clip at the plunger's front end. At the power module's rear end, a parachute safety thread holds the open coil spring compressed during insertion by means of a "crimped" golden-colored pearl (Fig. 34.1A). This thread is cut and removed along with the pearl to start distalization.

THE ADJUSTMENT MODULE

The adjustment module comprises a tube with four slots housing an extendable plunger. For individual adjustment in length, this plunger can be extended towards the TPA to allow fitment to different sizes of palate. The T-shaped connector with crimpable wings at the rear end of the plunger enables a secure connection to the TPA. This joint provides a hinge along the axis of the TPA–wire but also some resistance against molar tipping in the vertical axis. Four circumferential rubber elastics are sequentially wedged into the four available slots during the initial and subsequent activation. The mechanics of molar distalization with the TopJet are summarized in Fig. 34.2. For reactivation of the power module, the twin tube is pushed towards the MI's head to recompress the open coil spring.

THE TRANSPALATAL ARCH

Seven prefabricated TPAs are available and the size is chosen to correspond to the patient's maxillary intermolar fossae distance. This can be measured either directly in the patient's mouth or on a plaster cast. The U-shaped portions of the TPA can increase the distance between the MI insertion point and section-D of the TPA to provide a minimum distance of 14 mm for placement of the TopJet. If this distance is longer, the TopJet can be elongated as described above. The T-connector embedded in section-D is kept firm and cannot slide on the TPA. Even in unilateral molar distalization, a TPA with bilateral U-shaped bends is preferred as section-E allows easy adjustment of the TPA's height. The classical Goshgarian-type TPAs end with a double-back bend to allow molar torque for correction of molar inclination. As long as molar torque is not needed, section-A of the TPA, which is a single wire with retention notches that is fixed with light-cure resin into the fenestrated lingual sheaths of the molar bands, is sufficient to withstand rotation and tipping movements of the molars during distalization.

The distalizing force of the TopJet is transferred through the TPA to the connected molar(s). As the force is delivered close to the center of resistance of the molars and the TPA prevents rotation of the molars, a friction-free bodily molar distalization is expected. If the distalizing force is applied in the middle between the molars, both molars are distalized equally. Pure unilateral distalization would require a distalizing force passing through the center of resistance of the molar. Since the T-connector is connected

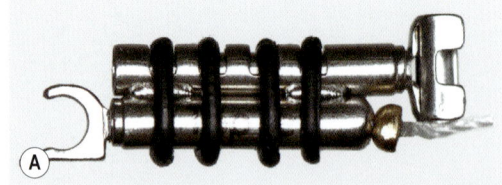
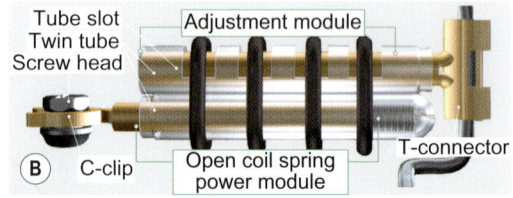

Fig. 34.1 The TopJet molar distalizer. (A) Before activation, the golden pearl and the securing thread keep the open Ni-Ti coil spring compressed. (B) After activation, the C-clip is connected to the miniscrew implant head; the pearl and thread are removed and the T-connector is attached to the transpalatal arch.

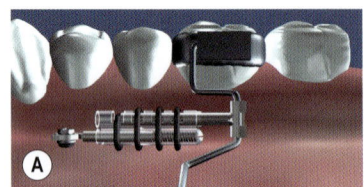
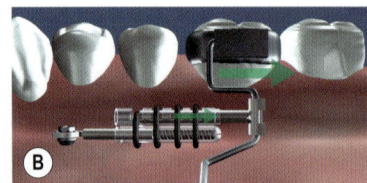
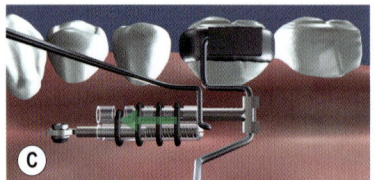
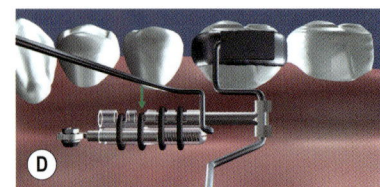

Fig. 34.2 Distalization mechanics of the TopJet. (A) TopJet in place, securing thread removed and open coil spring still compressed. (B) Coil spring decompressed; twin tube, adjustment module, transpalatal arch and molars have been moved distally. (C,D) For reactivation, the twin tube is pushed towards the screw head with a fork probe or a hooklet probe (C) until the next rubber elastic falls into the slot (D) to keep the plunger of the adjustment module in its new, extended position. This procedure recompresses the coil spring and restarts distalization.

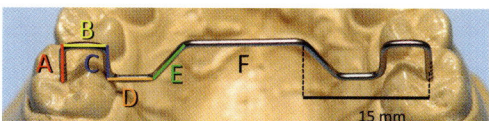

Fig. 34.3 The prefabricated transpalatal arch (TPA) with its sections A–F (before placement in the palate). Section-A is placed into the Goshgarian lingual sheath; section-B positions the TopJet in or near the center of resistance of the molar; section-C elongates the distance between screw head and TPA; section-D attaches the T-connector to the TPA; section-E allows adjustment of the TPA in height; section-F is predetermined by the anatomical size of the palate. The individual TPA length corresponds to the intermolar fossae distance.

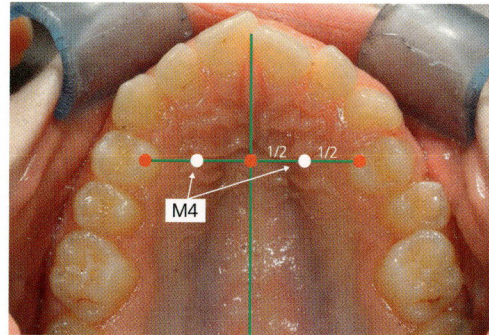

Fig. 34.4 The bilateral M4 sites on the transverse line through the palatal cusps of the first premolars half way to the midpalatal suture.

to the TPA, part of the distalizing force will act on the contralateral molar. This can be of advantage when slight distalization of the contralateral molar is desired. In this case, bilateral retention is required for stability after the end of the distalization in order to prevent relapse. Otherwise, the contralateral molar will relapse while the extended TopJet keeps the distalized molar in position. Differing from other appliances, unilateral molar distalization with the TopJet needs no more than one MI (see Fig. 34.7 below). Alternatively, if any contralateral distalization is not required, a second MI inserted on the contralateral side may be connected with a ligature to the TPA to retain the distance. An elastic chain between the MI and TPA will even mesialize molars, if needed, on this side while the buccal teeth are distalized on the other side (push–pull appliance).

TOPJET VERSIONS

The TopJet has a length of 14 mm, a diameter of 2.4 mm and is a prefabricated compact distalizer. There are three TopJet versions: the TopJet 250 and TopJet 360, which produce forces of 250 and 360 cN, respectively, and the TopJet plus 8, which is an 8 mm elongated version of the appliance.

The TopJet 360 is indicated for the en masse distalization of premolars and second molars. After insertion of the MI, the TopJets 360 or 250 are connected to them and fully activated respectively with 360cN or 250cN. If less force is required, an initial reduction of the distalizing force can be ensured by lifting the stopper elastics that have dropped into the tube slots during the insertion or reactivation process. This is done one at a time, so that the twin tube can slide backwards while decompressing the coil spring (Fig. 34.3). The same procedure can be applied if less power is desired in the course of treatment with the TopJet 250 or 360 and its actual version (see below). The extra-long version (plus 8 mm) is indicated in large maxillae or for distalizing the second molars.

CLINICAL APPLICATION

INSERTION PROCEDURE

Step 1: Insertion of the Miniscrew Implants

The TopJet is anchored with self-drilling MIs (e.g. Dual-Top Jet Screws; Jeil Medical, South Korea). A thread length of 7 mm is required, with a smooth neck varying between 3 and 7 mm depending on gingiva thickness. The MIs are inserted on the transverse line through the palatal cusps of the first premolars, half way to the midpalatal suture, the so-called M4 site (Fig. 34.4). In order to pass through the palatal mucosa at this position, the MI is initially placed perpendicular to the surface of the bone, somewhat medial to the final required position, and inserted for four or five turns. It is then uprighted over a few turns and is ultimately screwed into the bone in a strict vertical direction (perpendicular to the occlusal plane) with no more than three turns per second until the head is in the desired position.

Step 2: Insertion of the Transpalatal Arch

Conventional molar bands equipped with fenestrated lingual sheaths are banded on both maxillary first molars. The prefabricated TPA section-A is adjusted to fit passively into the lingual sheaths with adequate distance from the palatal mucosa. To enable the desired expansion during distalization, the TPA is routinely activated transversally 2–4 mm per side before its final insertion. The fenestrated lingual sheaths facilitate the application of light-cure resin to stabilize the inserted TPA.

Step 3: Insertion of the TopJet

The securing thread of the TopJet is unrolled. This thread prevents the patient from accidentally swallowing the appliance and also holds the open coil spring compressed to ensure that it remains passive during insertion. The TopJet is securely held in place with self-locking forceps, and the C-clip is moved toward the groove of the MI's head and clipped on to it with Weingart pliers (Fig. 34.5A–C). The piston in the adjustment module is then extended towards the TPA with a fork probe in order to connect the piston's T-connector to section-D of the TPA (Fig. 34.6A). During this extension, one or two elastics fall into the slot(s) of the adjustment module's twin tube (Fig. 34.2D), thus preventing the piston from sliding back into the tube. If the piston has been pulled out too far, it can easily be pushed back by lifting the appropriate elastic. Using pliers (TopJet pliers or a modified angle Tweed plier), the upper and lower flaps of the T-connector are closed tightly around the TPA (Fig. 34.6B). Light-cure resin is used to fill the gaps around the T-connector and the median portion of the C-clip. This provides a stable connection in terms of rotation and angulation at the C-clip and a hinge axis-like joint at the T-connector, allowing bodily movement of the molars. The MI head and the C-clip are also covered and secured with light-cure resin, while avoiding any resin contacting the mucosa. This provides a stable yet reversible connection in terms of rotation and angulation for the TopJet. Insertion of the MIs and the TopJet is painless and usually takes less than 20 minutes.

Once the appliance, including the TPA, has been secured, the safety thread is pulled slightly laterally and cut between the golden pearl and the power module (Fig. 34.6C). This releases the closed Ni-Ti coil spring and the patient should notice a light pressure on the maxillary molars.

CLINICAL CONSIDERATIONS

If not reactivated, the TopJet can produce a distalization of 5.6 mm. At that distance, the force of the open coil spring decreases to 50 cN. However, in order to efficiently distalize the molars, the appliance will need to be reactivated at intervals. This can be achieved in 2 mm increments (i.e. the distance between two rubber elastics). Using a fork probe or hooklet probe, the twin tube is pulled forward towards the anchorage MI,

Fig. 34.5 Easy, fast and safe clip-on (A–C) and clip-off (D–F) of the C-shaped connector.

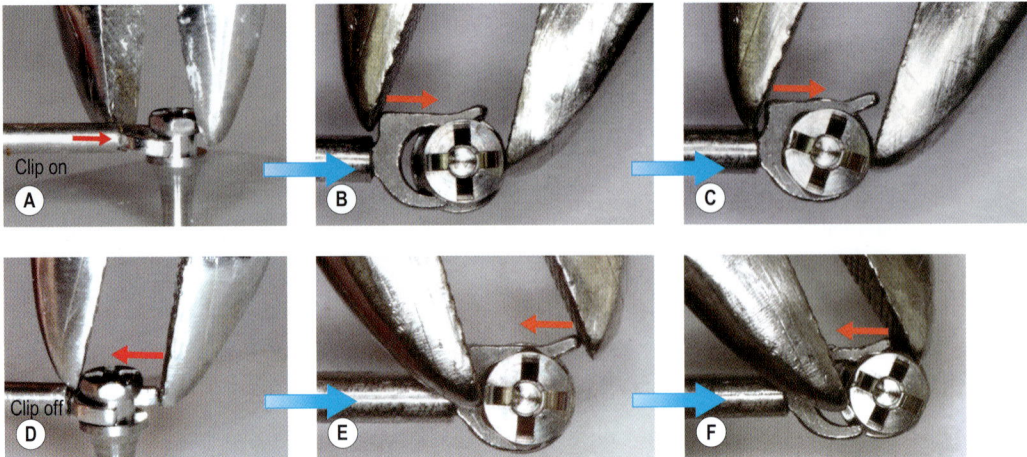

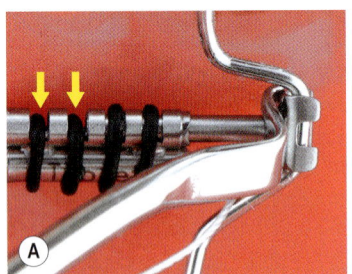
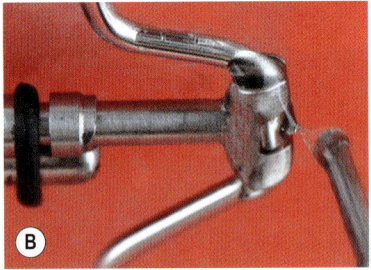
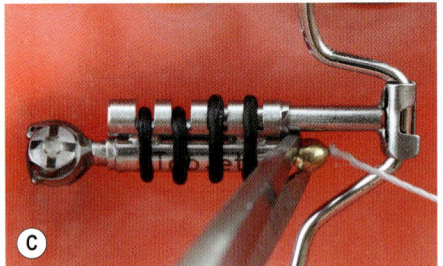
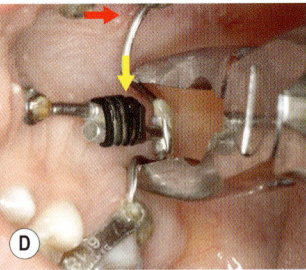

Fig. 34.6 Connecting the TopJet to the transpalatal arch (TPA). (A) The plunger in the adjustment module is extended towards the TPA with a fork probe. When the T-connector has reached section-D of the TPA, one or two elastics fall into the slots, thus preventing the adjustment plunger from sliding back. (B) The upper and lower flaps of the T-connector are closed tightly around the TPA with pliers and light-cured resin is used to fill the gaps around the T-connector. This provides a stable hinge axis-like joint granting bodily movement of the molars. (C) To activate the TopJet, the safety thread is cut between the golden pearl and the power module. (D) If there is soft tissue irritation, section-E has to be bent slightly downward.

which compresses the open coil spring encased in the power module, re-establishing the distalization force; when the elastic has fallen into its recess, the piston within the adjustment module can be locked (Fig. 34.2CD). If the elastics have been lost, a stop can also be created by slightly compressing the corresponding arch between the slots behind the piston (irreversible stop). In total, a maximum molar distalization of 14 mm is possible if all four increments are used to reactivate the appliance.

A period of 2 to 3 months is required for bodily movement and en masse distalization of up to three molars per side. During this time, the second and first premolars start to drift distally under the pull of the transeptal fibers. A gap mesial to the first molars will appear. After 3 to 5 months of molar distalization, premolar and canine brackets are used to gain space in the anterior region. Because the posterior palate becomes narrower and inclines towards inferior, extensive distalization may be accompanied by palatal soft tissue irritation caused by the TPA. In this case, section-C of the TPA has to be bent slightly inwards and section-E upwards for immediate relief (Fig. 34.6D). After sufficient distalization, the twin tube is released backwards by lifting up the appropriate elastic (the stopper elastic) to deactivate the compressed coil spring. The residual force of 50 cN will prevent relapse.

In addition to spontaneous premolar distal movement during molar distalization, the premolars can be retracted with segmented arches to accelerate treatment progress. If further (en masse) retraction of the anterior teeth is required, the necessary retraction force can be counteracted either by increasing the distalization force accordingly (reactivation of the TopJet) or by crimping the plunger at the anterior end of the cylinder to create a rigid anchorage.

REMOVAL OF THE TOPJET

Composite is removed from the MI head and a Weingart plier is placed between the mesial C-clip extension of the TopJet and the MI head, pushing back the clip without applying any pressure on the MI (Fig. 34.5D–F). The anterior part of the TopJet can then be raised, which breaks the composite cover at the posterior end of the T-connector, and the flaps opened to release the TopJet.

After the removal of the TopJet, the prefabricated TPA is removed. Usually, section-A of the TPA extends through the lingual sheath by about 2 mm. The covering resin is broken away and the ends of the TPA are pushed mesially with the Weingart plier. If this is not possible, the TPA can be cut with a water-cooled mini-diamond bur while being secured with a needle holder, and the remaining segments can be pulled out.

CLINICAL APPLICATIONS

CASE 1: UNILATERAL DISTALIZATION

An 11-year-old boy presented with a low-angle growth pattern, bialveolar protrusion of the maxillary and mandibular anterior teeth and normal sagittal relationships (ANB, 2°; Wits appraisal, 0 mm). He had unilateral Class II of half a premolar width on the right side with an upper midline shift to the left of 2 mm, as well as minor crowding of the maxillary incisors (Fig. 34.7A,B). Treatment plan was a unilateral distalization of the right maxillary teeth to create space, to correct the upper midline and to retrocline the maxillary incisors. A MI (length, 12 mm; diameter, 2 mm) was used to

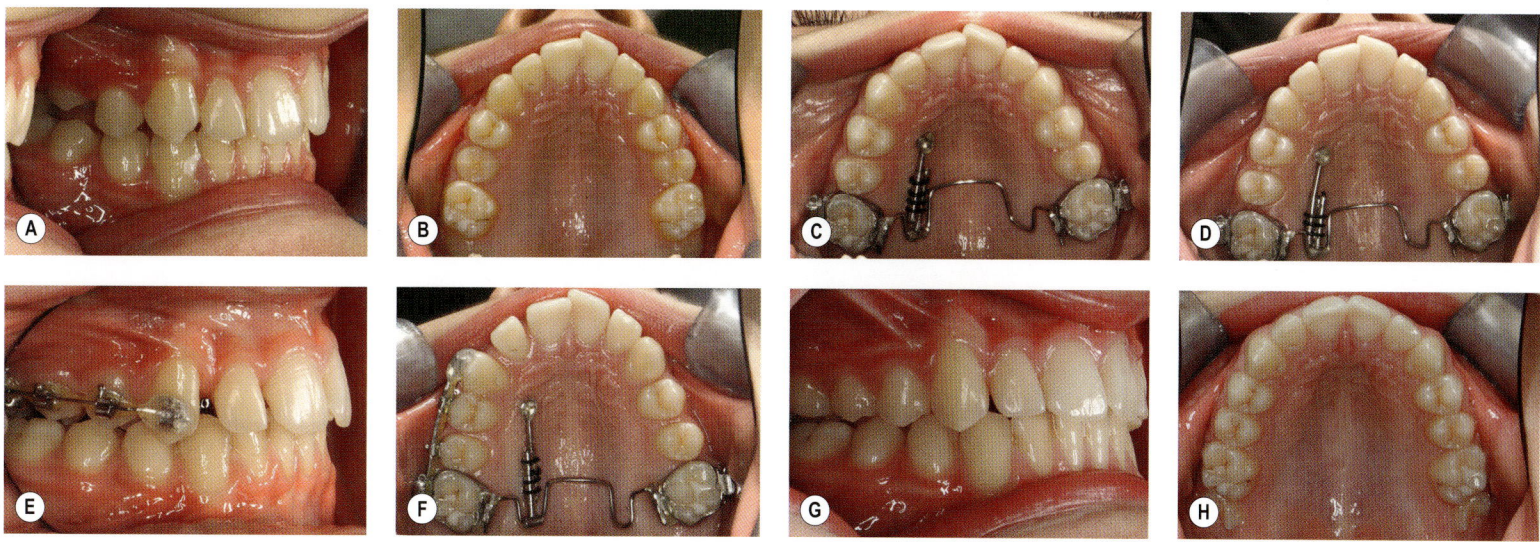

Fig. 34.7 Case 1: unilateral distalization. (A,B) Pretreatment. (C) TopJet immediately after insertion. (D) Unilateral space creation after 2.5 months of distalization. (E,F) End of distalization after 7 months. (G,H) Post-treatment after strict unilateral distalization and orthodontic treatment with two sets of aligners.

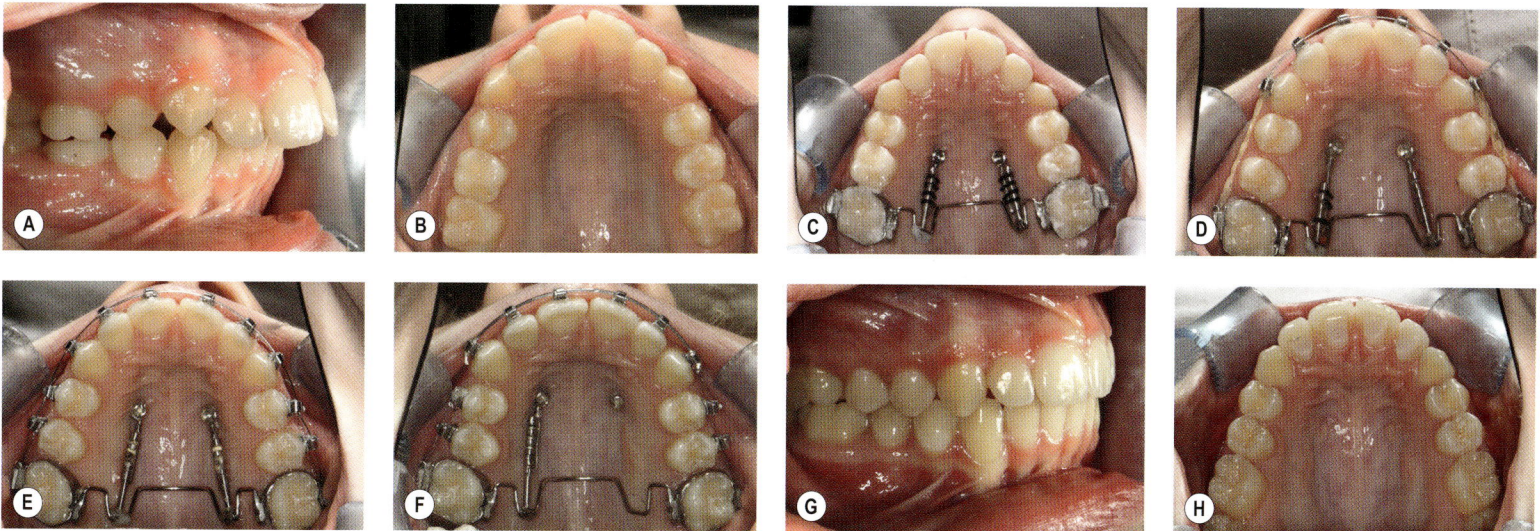

Fig. 34.8 Case 2: bilateral distalization. (A,B) Pretreatment. (C) Insertion of the TopJet distalizers. (D) Creation of space in the premolar region, en masse retraction of the upper incisors with elastic chains. (E) Insertion of full fixed appliances; TopJet remained in place for further distalization. (F) Further distalization required on the right side, left side finished. (G,H) Post-treatment.

anchor a TopJet 250 on the right side (Fig. 34.7C). After 10 weeks, a total of 3 mm of space between the maxillary right molar, the second and first premolar and the canine had been achieved (Fig. 34.7D). Brackets were bonded on the right maxillary canine and the first and second premolar, and these teeth were then distalized with an elastic chain (Fig. 34.7E,F). After 9.5 months, the MI and the TopJet were removed. The maxillary right first molar reached an overcorrected Class I relationship (one-third a premolar width), and the upper midline corrected spontaneously. No tipping or rotation of the maxillary right molar occurred during distalization. The rest of the teeth of the maxillary and mandibular arch were treated with two sets of aligners (Copyplast, Scheu Dental, Iserlohn, Germany). Overall treatment time was 22 months (Fig. 34.7G,H). The presence of the third right maxillary molar did not prolong treatment time.

CASE 2: BILATERAL DISTALIZATION

A girl aged 11.5 years presented with bilateral Class II malocclusion of one-half a premolar width, bialveolar protrusion and a vertical growth pattern: a classic indication for premolar extractions (Fig. 34.8A,B).

Extraction of four premolars was suggested but because her parents were opposed to extractions, an attempt at bilateral non-compliant distalization of the maxillary posterior teeth was agreed. Two MIs and two TopJet 250 were installed without any other appliances (brackets) (Fig. 34.8C). Seven months later, both first molars were in a Class I relationship. For overcorrection, the TopJets stayed in place for another 5 months, and the patient also wore Class III elastics to distalize the mandibular posterior teeth (Fig. 34.8D–F). Finally, the distalizers and the MIs were removed and the treatment was finished with fixed appliances and positioners. In order to keep the vertical dimension, bite ramps were placed on the maxillary incisors. At completion of treatment, a perfect Class I occlusion and retrusion of the incisors with sufficient overbite was achieved (Fig. 34.8G,H). Although maxillary third molars were present, pure bodily distalization of first molars was achieved.

DISCUSSION

There are now several prefabricated distalizers available in addition to the TopJet (versions of the Beneslider and the miniscrew implant-supported

Fig. 34.9 Current version of the TopJet.

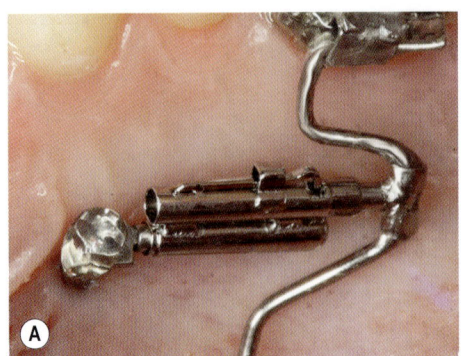

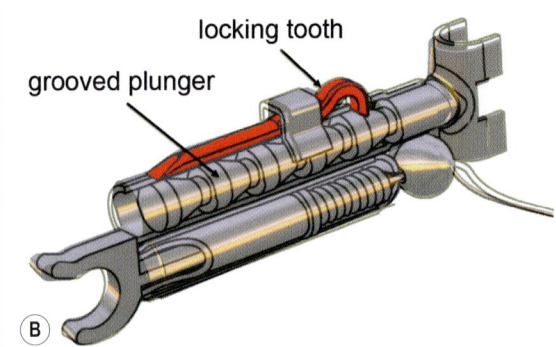

distalization system, plus the Advanced Molar Distalization Appliance); all need only some small adjustments of their wire elements either on the casts or in the patient's mouth in order to be used directly for molar distalization. They have a number of advantages:

- partially or completely prefabricated
- use conventional molar bands with standard lingual sheaths
- can be inserted chair-side in one session
- can be reactivated stepwise
- offer the possibility for spontaneous movement (drifting) of the premolars and canines
- can be used for anterior tooth retraction.

The TopJet has a number of additional advantages:

- the unique clip-on/clip-off mechanism enables an easy, secure, fast, reliable and reversible connection
- the telescopic adjustment mechanism enables individual palatal length adaptation using an automatic locking system
- removal and reinsertion are easy
- the MIs are placed bilaterally (unilateral MI is possible) in the anterior palate in an area presenting the greatest bone height
- friction-free bodily molar distalization occurs
- the TPA does not permit rotation of the molars during distalization.

In contrast, the new Beneslider requires anchorage in the midpalatal suture while the Advanced Molar Distalization Appliance requires more complex adjustment at fitting. Both also have some friction during distalization and some minor rotations can occur, although the latter can be counteracted by means of adjustable bends on the wire extensions of the tubing system.

In general, complications with the TopJet are rare but palatal soft tissue irritation can occur, particularly at the later stages of distalization, but this can be relieved by adjusting section-C and section-E of the TPA. MI loss is seen in less than 2% of the patients.[3]

ACTUAL VERSION OF THE TOPJET

It has been shown that the rubber elastics tended to accumulate plaque. For hygienic reasons, these rubber elastics have been replaced in the new version of the TopJet by a ratchet mechanism with a locking tooth (Fig. 34.9A) and the extendable plunger has been replaced by an extendable grooved plunger. This modification allows easy activation and deactivation in the clinical setting (Fig. 34.9B).

CONCLUSIONS

The TopJet is a prefabricated fixed non-compliance molar distalizer with a unique and easy clip-on/clip-off mechanism and elegant telescopic adjustment to fit palate dimensions. Insertion is easy, secure and quick, taking a single appointment of 20–30 minutes. The connnection of the TopJet to the TPA is reliable and stable, but still easy to disengage. The insertion procedure can be carried out by an orthodontic practitioner. Reactivation of the appliance is easy, fast and safe. The TopJet 360 (360 cN) can even distalize premolars and molars en masse without unwanted effects. These advantages make the TopJet feasible for the everyday practice as a time-saving and ready-to-use appliance.

REFERENCES

1. Winsauer H, Muchitsch P, Winsauer C, et al. The TopJet: a convenient appliance for routine bodily molar distalization. J Clin Orthod 2013;in press.
2. Winsauer H, Vlachojannis J, Winsauer C, et al. Körperliche Distalisation der Molaren-mitdem TopJet-Konzept. Inf Orthod Kieferorthop 2011;43:197–204.
3. Winsauer H, Vlachojannis J. Letter to the editor. Inf Orthod Kieferorthop 2010;42:211.

INTRODUCTION

The original Pendulum K appliance required dental anchorage. This introduced reactive side effects, predominantly protrusion of the anterior teeth (see Chapter 2).[1-3] The skeletal Pendulum-K appliance incorporates miniscrew implants (MIs) for anchorage and thus avoids these issues. To fabricate the appliance, components were selected due to their compact design and ease of clinical use.[4] These prefabricated components are available from manufacturers.[5]

THE SKELETAL PENDULUM-K APPLIANCE

The prefabricated components of the Pendulum-K, which is commercially known as the Skeletal Frog Appliance (Forestadent, Pforzheim, Germany), are customized in the laboratory. These components are comprised of a distalization screw, a SS or TMA preformed transpalatal arch (TPA) (0.032 inch) and a hex adjustment key for intraoral activation of the screw in the sagittal direction (Fig. 35.1). The TPA can be removed from the screw housing and used separately. The appliance is activated at the anterior end of the screw, allowing the adjustment key to be inserted sagittally into the hex, thus providing an easy method of activation intraorally during treatment.

CLINICAL APPLICATION

MINISCREW IMPLANTS

The Pendulum-K appliance is supported by two MIs that are placed in the anterior palate slightly mesial to the line connecting the first premolars,

or, if there are missing canines or mesial drift of the premolars, behind the most posterior palatal rugae. The MIs should be no more than 3 mm from the median suture to ensure an area with adequate bone thickness.[6-8]

CHOOSING THE ABUTMENTS

Initially, the Pendulum-K appliance was anchored to the MIs through an acrylic resin Nance button. However, this had an issue of maintaining oral hygiene, so an adapted abutment was developed from the Ortho-Easy system (Forestadent, Pforzheim, Germany). This would allow direct connection between the MIs and the appliance (Fig. 35.2). Alternatively, the skeletal Pendulum-K can be connected to the Benefit system (PSM Medical Solutions, Tuttlingen, Germany) (see Fig. 33.6) or any other MI-system offering abutments.

TAKING THE ALGINATE IMPRESSION

After the abutments have been checked in the mouth, any adjustments are made to improve attachment to the device. The abutments are then filled with petrolatum to provide a better fit. The molar bands are selected and the abutments are placed on the MI heads (Fig. 35.2B). During alginate preparation, the patient holds the abutments in position. Prior to the impression, it is suggested to put a dab of alginate on each abutment.

LABORATORY FABRICATION PROCEDURE

The molar bands and the abutments are embedded in the alginate impression and fixed into position. A transfer MI is inserted into each coping, and the impression is poured with high-strength dental stone. This ensures

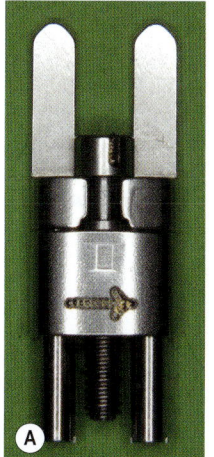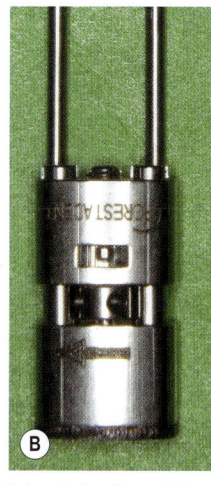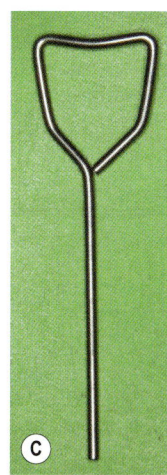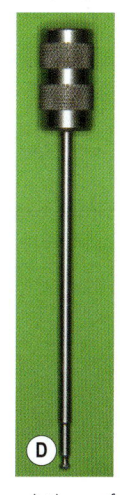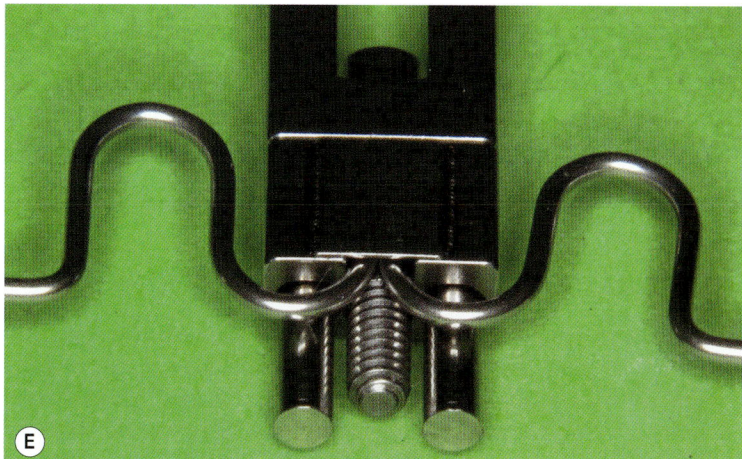

Fig. 35.1 Components of the skeletal Pendulum-K appliance. (A,B) Two variations of the distalization screw. (C,D) Two variations of the adjustment key for frontal or lateral activations. (E) Preformed transpalatal arch inserted in the adjusted slot of the screw.

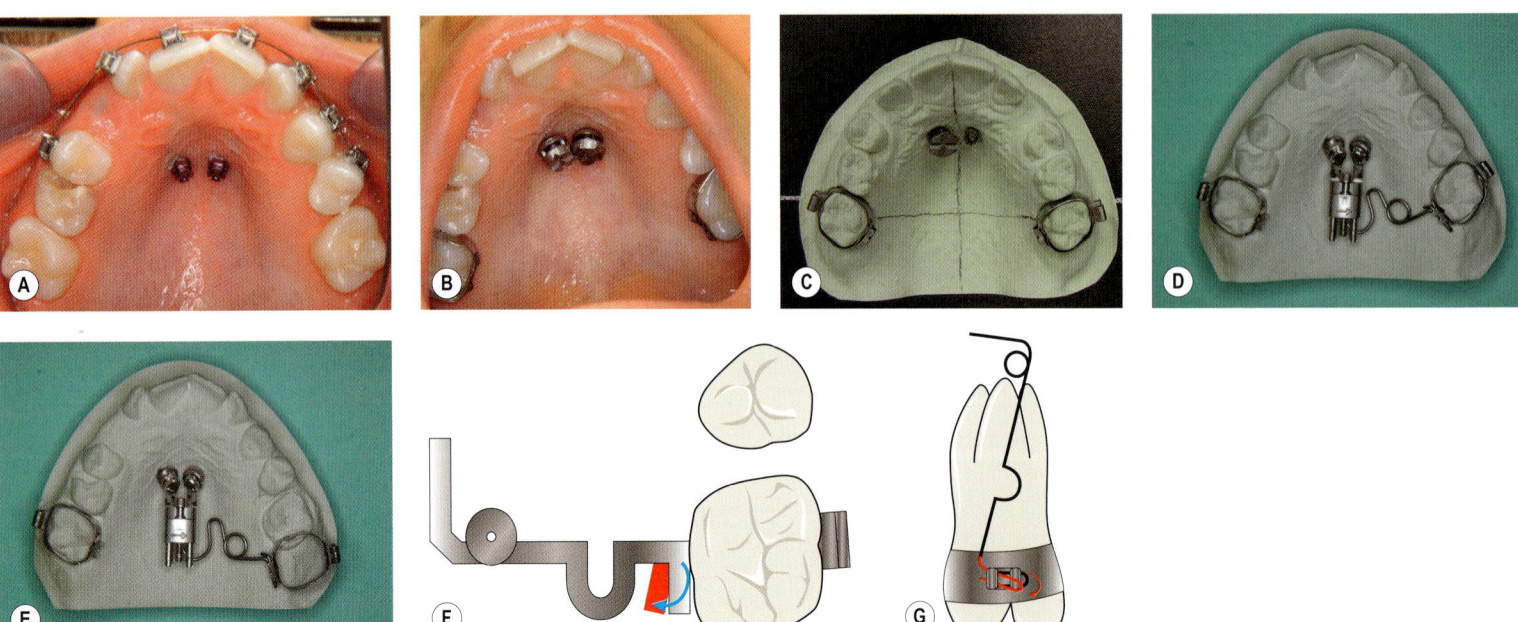

Fig. 35.2 (A) The miniscrew implants (MIs) in situ. (B) Abutments and molar bands in situ before undertaking the impression. (C) Working model of high-strength dental stone with an abutment and the molar bands. (D) Finished laboratory work with passive fitting of the transpalatal arch to the molar bands. (E) Finished laboratory work with distal activation of the transpalatal arch. (F) Toe-in bend of approximately 5–10° to derotate the molars. (G) Uprighting activation of approximately 15–20° to avoid distal tipping of the molars.

that the two MI heads on the cast correspond to the exact intraoral position (Fig. 35.2C). The abutments are removed from the impression, fitted over the MI heads and integrated into the appliance as coupling elements. Afterwards, the abutments are soldered to the tabs of the distal screw, on the working cast. The TPA is customized and inserted passively in the lingual sheaths of the molar bands (Fig. 35.2D).

PREACTIVATING THE PALATAL ARCH

The skeletal Pendulum-K uses TMA wire with the K-Pendulum prescription instead of a prefabricated SS arch. Each wire is bent into a double spring based on the Kinzinger concept (Fig. 35.2D). The end-sections have to be initially set up with three different bends:

- a distal activation (about 2N) (Fig. 35.2E)
- a toe-in bend to produce an antirotation effect (Fig. 35.2F and 35.3)
- an upright activation to counteract the tipping moment (Figs 35.2G).

Hence, the skeletal Pendulum-K appliance has the same biomechanical control as the dental K-Pendulum. The application of the distal force, which should be approximately 200 g, can be measured with a Correx gauge.

INTRAORAL MOUNTING OF THE APPLIANCE

The preactivated appliance is attached to the molars, while the abutments are fixed with glass–ionomer cement or with a ligature wire to the MIs of the Ortho-Easy system. When the Benefit system is used, the abutments are screwed. After insertion, the abutments completely cover the MI heads. As the appliance has only metallic parts, it is rigid and stable, while the elimination of an interconnecting Nance button ensures easier maintenance of oral hygiene.

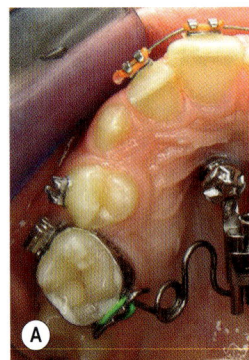
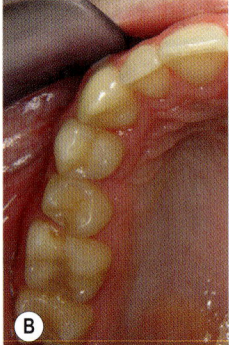
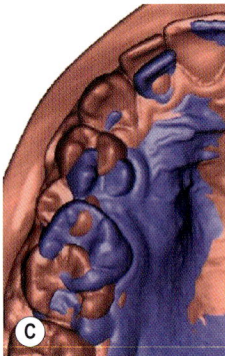

Fig. 35.3 (A) A toe-in bend is necessary to derotate the molars during distalization. (B) Intraoral situation at the end of treatment. (C) Superimposition of the start and finished 3D-casts.

CLINICAL CONSIDERATIONS

According to Walde,[1,4] activation of the screw every 4–5 weeks (by turning the screw three to five times) is adequate to achieve a distalization of 1–2 mm per month. A full 360° activation of the screw body opens the appliance 0.4 mm longitudinally. Alternatively, the appliance can also be activated with a quarter turn every 3 days by the patient him- or herself or a carer.

CASE EXAMPLE

Fig. 35.4 illustrates activation and clinical application of the skeletal Pendulum-K appliance.

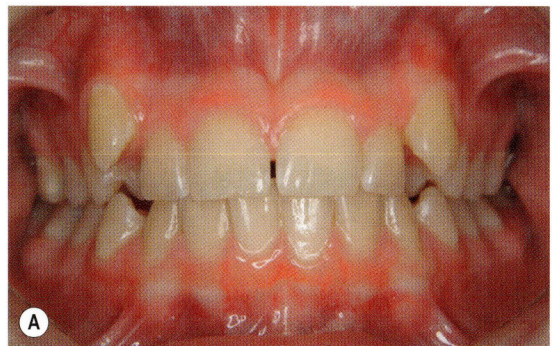
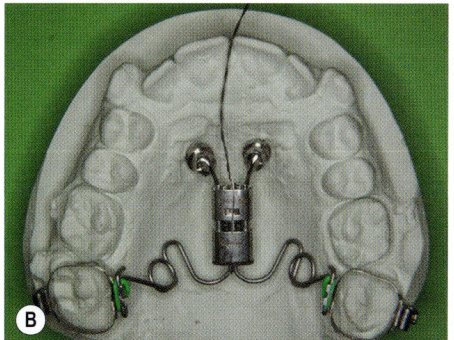
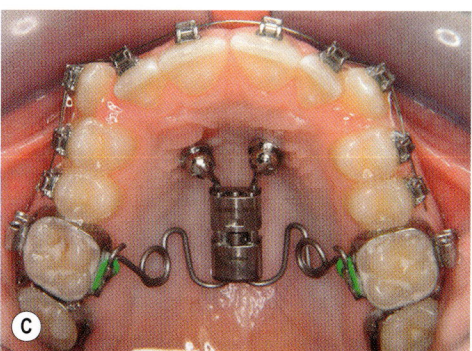
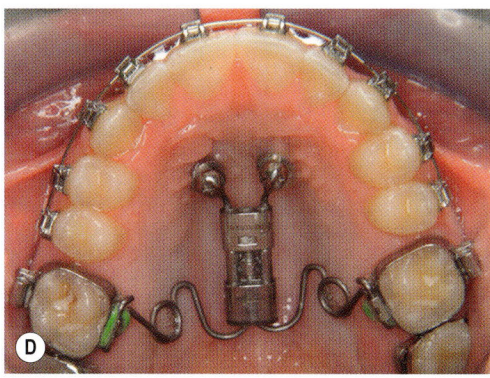
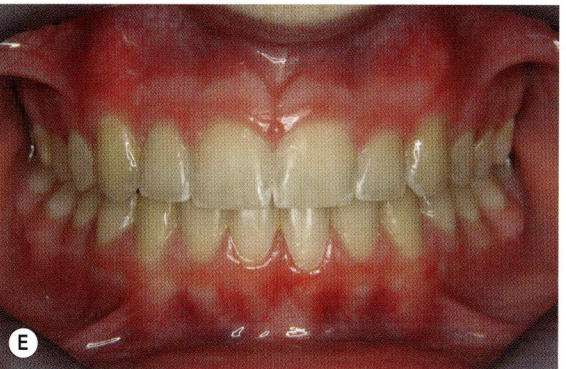

Fig. 35.4 The skeletal Pendulum-K appliance to treat a patient with Class II molar relationships and ectopic maxillary canines. (A) Pretreatment. (B) Preactivated pendulum springs on the model cast: toe-in bend, uprighting activation, and additional activation for distalization. (C) Occlusal view immediately following insertion of the preactivated appliance and its fixation on the miniscrew implants. (D) Occlusal view after 4 months of treatment. (E) Frontal view post treatment.

CONCLUSIONS

The skeletal Pendulum-K appliance has proven to be an efficient maxillary molar distalization device with significant clinical results. The adaptation from the dentally anchored appliance enables effective molar distalization and simultaneous leveling and alignment of the maxillary dental arch without reactive side effects.

REFERENCE

1. Kinzinger G, Fuhrmann R, Gross U, et al. Modified pendulum appliance including distal screw and uprighting activation for non-compliance therapy of Class-II malocclusion in children and adolescents. J Orofac Orthop 2000;61:175.
2. Kinzinger GS, Wehrbein H, Diedrich PR. Molar distalization with a modified pendulum appliance–in vitro analysis of the force systems and in vivo study in children and adolescents. Angle Orthod 2005;75:558.
3. Kinzinger G, Syree C, Fritz U, et al. Molar distalization with different pendulum appliances: in vitro registration of orthodontic forces and moments in the initial phase. J Orofac Orthop 2004;65:389.
4. Walde KC. The simplified molar distalizer. J Clin Orthod 2003;37:616.
5. Ludwig B, Glasl B, Kinzinger GS, et al. The skeletal frog appliance for maxillary molar distalization. J Clin Orthod 2011;45:77.
6. Lombardo L, Gracco A, Zampini F, et al. Optimal palatal configuration for miniscrew applications. Angle Orthod 2010;80:145.
7. Ludwig B, Glasl B, Bowman SJ, et al. Anatomical guidelines for miniscrew insertion: palatal sites. J Clin Orthod 2011;45:433.
8. Gracco A, Lombardo L, Cozzani M, et al. Quantitative evaluation with CBCT of palatal bone thickness in growing patients. Prog Orthod 2006;7:164.

The bone-anchored Pendulum appliance

Beyza Hancıoglu Kircelli and Zafer Ozgur Pektas

INTRODUCTION

The original Pendulum appliance had two main parts: the active TMA springs, delivering a light and continuous distal force to the maxillary first molars, and a large palatal acrylic resin Nance button that provided anchorage through attachment to teeth (see Fig. 2.8). The intramaxillary appliance generated a distal and intrusive force to the maxillary molars and a reciprocal mesial and extrusive force to the anchoring premolars. The active TMA springs produced a broad swinging arch or pendulum type of force from the midpalate to the molars.

The major concern regarding the Pendulum appliance is the anchorage loss of the anterior teeth in terms of forward movement (see Chapter 2). With forces applied on the molars, the reactive forces are received by the anchoring premolars and mucosa of the palatal vault. Therefore, the reactive forces emerging on the anterior anchorage segment create a mesial tipping and extrusion of the premolars, and consequently incisor proclination and increase of the overjet. This effect is in contradiction to the goals of treatment of Class II malocclusion at most times, particularly where there is already an increased overjet or crowding of the maxillary dental arch. In order to overcome the problem of anterior anchorage loss, in 2006, Kircelli et al.[1] modified the original Pendulum appliance by using miniscrew implants (MIs) under the Nance button to create the the bone-anchored Pendulum appliance (BAPA). A further modification combined the pendulum springs with palatal osseointegrated implants.[2]

CLINICAL APPLICATION

The BAPA is a modified Pendulum appliance that is anchored to the palatal bone by MIs, preferably two, which are located under an acrylic resin Nance button. Pendulum springs of TMA wire (0.032 inch) are fabricated and activated in the same way as with the original Pendulum appliance.

Two MIs (diameter, 2.0 mm; fixation screw length, 8 mm; IMF intermaxillary, Stryker, Leibinger, Germany) are inserted in the paramedian region of the anterior median palatal suture, 7–8 mm posterior to the incisive foramen and 3–4 mm lateral to the median line (see Fig. 36.2B, below).

After soft tissue healing, impressions and casts are obtained. The MI heads are blocked out with wax on the cast, and the appliance is constructed according to Hilgers' descriptions,[3] excluding the auxiliary wires for dental anchorage. The appliance is checked in the mouth and the springs are activated parallel to the median palatal suture. The acrylic resin plate is connected to the MI heads using cold-curing, methyl methacrylate-free acrylic resin (Ufi Gel hard, Voco, Cuxhaven, Germany). Finally, the activated TMA springs (Ormco Corp, Glendora, CA, USA) are inserted into the lingual sheaths on the first molar bands (Fig. 36.1).

Patients should be instructed carefully on oral hygiene and regular use of a mouthwash. The soft tissues are checked at each appointment, when the springs can also be reactivated if necessary.

REMOVING THE APPLIANCE

The only difficulty that may be experienced in removing the BAPA is in detaching the acrylic resin plate from the MI head. A carbide bur with an

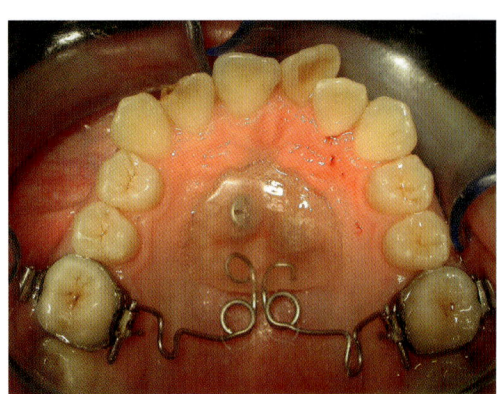

Fig. 36.1 The bone-anchored Pendulum appliance in place.

aerotor under copious irrigation can be used. To facilitate this detachment, it is suggested that the resin plate is made no thicker than 2 mm over the MI head and the grooves on the top of the MIs are filled with a thin layer of wax. Alternatively, the Nance button can be fabricated without acrylic resin coverage of the MIs.[4]

CASE PRESENTATION

A 12-year-old girl was referred with crowding of her teeth (Fig. 36.2). She had a skeletal Class I relationship (ANB angle, 2.1°) with dental Class II molar and canine relationships. She had an average growth pattern, with a Frankfort–mandibular plane angle of 27° and a sella/nasion–mandibular plane angle of 34°. She had 7 mm crowding in the maxillary arch and mild crowding in the mandibular arch. The maxillary canines were erupted buccally. The maxillary dental midline was shifted 2 mm to the right side. She had a normal overjet and overbite of 3.7 mm and 2.3 mm, respectively. Maxillary and mandibular incisor inclinations were within the normal limits. Her profile was well balanced (lower lip to E-plane, 0.9 mm).

The treatment plan was to distalize the first molars in the maxillary arch to achieve a Class I molar and canine relationship and to gain space for the alignment of the maxillary crowding and correction of the midline shift. In the mandibular arch, proximal stripping of the mandibular incisors was planned to gain the appropriate space needed for alignment of the mild crowding. Since the maxillary and mandibular incisors presented normal inclinations and the profile was well balanced, molar distalization would be undertaken using the BAPA (Fig. 36.2C).

Maxillary molar distalization took 7 months to achieve a super-Class I molar relationship on both sides. In addition, the first and second premolars drifted distally to a Class I relationship. Because of this spontaneous distalization, partial alignment of the maxillary anterior crowding was achieved and even the midline discrepancy was spontaneously corrected (Fig. 36.2D,E).

The second phase of treatment used full fixed appliances. During the uprighting process of the distally tipped molars and premolars, the BAPA was left in place to reinforce anchorage of the newly distalized molars. Overall treatment lasted approximately 22 months. After finishing, flattened and dead soft 8-braided wire (Bond-a-Braid, Reliance Orthodontics, Itasca, IL, USA) was bonded to each tooth from canine to canine in both maxillary and mandibular arches for retention purposes (Fig. 36.2F,G). In

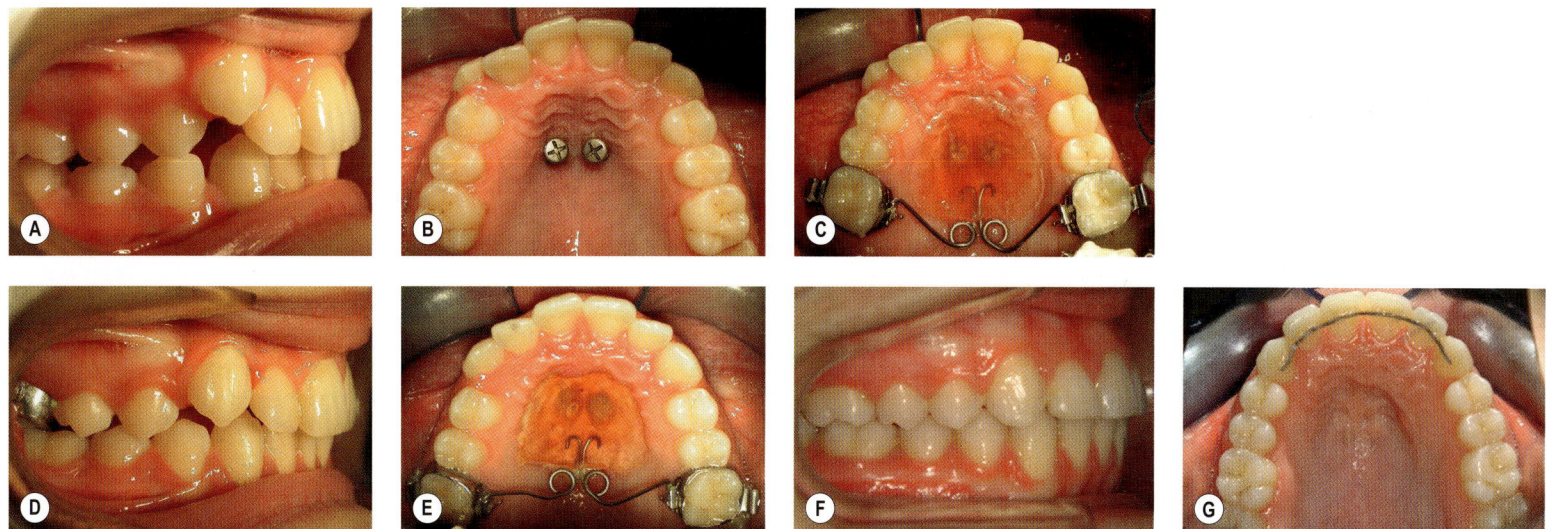

Fig. 36.2 Treatment of a 12-year-old girl with skeletal Class I relationships with dental Class II molar and canine relationship. (A,B) Pretreatment. (C) The bone-anchored Pendulum appliance in place. (D,E) After maxillary molar distalization, with distal drift of the premolars along with the first molars to a Class I relationship and the spontaneous alignment of the canines. (F,G) Post-treatment.

addition, for the first 6 months after debonding, transparent thermoplastic vacuum-molded retainers were recommended to be worn at night.

DISCUSSION

The BAPA seems to be an effective intraoral maxillary molar distalization appliance. Kircelli et al.[1] reported a mean maxillary first molar distalization of 6.4 mm in approximately 7 months, with the second and first premolars drifted distally a mean of 5.4 and 3.8 mm, respectively. This simplifies and shortens treatment. Anterior crowding can be, at least partially, corrected spontaneously during molar distalization, with an average of 13.9 and 6.2 mm of space gain after molar distalization in the total maxillary dental arch and in the anterior segment, respectively.[1] As the BAPA is identical to the original Pendulum appliance apart from the method of anchorage, maxillary molar tipping could be expected to occur. Studies using MI-supported Pendulum appliances show various degrees of molar tipping, from 9.1 to 14.4°.[1,2,4,5] A systematic review has evaluated the effectiveness of the distalization of molars with distalizers supported by temporary skeletal anchorage compared with tooth-borne anchorage.[6] Greater molar distal tipping was seen with the devices supported by temporary skeletal anchorage, which the authors suggested might be a consequence of the greater pressure exerted on the molars in this method. We also consider that the increased tipping is linked to the greater amount of distalization achieved. This is supported by studies showing more distal tipping with a greater molar distalization.[6,7] This link could have two causes. First, clinicians may prefer to use devices supported by temporary skeletal anchorage for patients who need more extensive molar distalization. Second, anchorage loss, through space opening between the diverging molars and the second premolars, in a tooth-supported system may occur earlier in distalization and so the process would be terminated earlier, thus limiting the amount of molar tipping. A comparison of the original Pendulum appliance with the BAPA in a group of 39 patients indicated that 4.8 mm of molar distalization and 9.1° of molar tipping was achieved in 6.8 months with BAPA therapy, while 2.7 mm of molar distalization and 5.3° of molar tipping was evident after 5.1 months of treatment with the tooth-anchored appliance (Table 36.1). This supports the idea that the greater distal movement of maxillary molars may cause more distal tipping of their crowns.

Table 36.1 Comparison of treatment changes between the bone-anchored Pendulum appliance and the conventional Pendulum appliance

Variables	Bone anchored (mean ± SD)	Conventional (mean ± SD)	*p* value[a]
No. in group	22	17	
Age of patients (years)	13.6 ± 2.1	13.6 ± 2.0	
Distalization time (months)	6.8 ± 1.7	5.1 ± 0.9	0.010
1st molar (mm)	4.8 ± 1.8 distal mv.	2.7 ± 1.7 distal mv.	0.025
1st molar (°)	9.1 ± 4.6 distal tip.	5.3 ± 3.8 distal tip.	0.008
2nd premolar (mm)	4.1 ± 2.1 distal mv.	2.3 ± 2.1 mesial mv.	0.000
2nd premolar (°)	9.9 ± 5.2 distal tip.	3.8 ± 2.7 mesial tip.	0.000
1st incisor (mm)	1.2 ± 1.7 retrusion	0.1 ± 1.7 protrusion	0.035
1st incisor (°)	1.7 ± 2.9 retroclination	0.9 ± 2.4 proclination	0.034

mv, movement; tip, tipping; SD, standard deviation; BAPA, bone-anchored Pendulum appliance; CPA, conventional Pendulum appliance.
[a]Significance from independent t-test.
Source: from Polat-Ozsoy et al., 2008.[5]

Distalization with tipping is significant because some of the space created can be lost during molar uprighting when full fixed therapy is initiated. However, the BAPA can be left in place immediately after distalization and it will then be able to maintain molar position when a continuous archwire is applied to upright the molars. Thus, molar position can be maintained when leveling and retracting the first premolars and canines. This concept of "active anchorage" is helpful to cope with the anchorage concerns when distalizing maxillary molars.[8] Overcorrection of the molar relationships could also be used to support molar anchorage during full fixed therapy, particularly if distal tipping exists. In this context, the BAPA can be used to move maxillary molars to a super-Class I relationship to overcome the anchorage loss that takes place during the leveling and anterior teeth retraction phase of treatment.

Some skeletal and soft tissue effects have been observed with the BAPA; the cant of the palatal plane remained unchanged but the mandibular plane rotated by 0.98° in a clockwise direction after molar distalization.[1]

Clockwise rotation can be attributed to the fact that maxillary molars move distally into the wedge of occlusion as well as to cusp interferences. Although clinically insignificant, point A moved anteriorly by 0.6 mm. This might occur through a modeling process with reciprocal forces acting on the anterior plate causing bone apposition at the A-point. Further studies should be conducted to test this hypothesis. No significant differences were observed regarding the upper and lower lip positions relative to the esthetic line after molar distalization with the BAPA.[1]

COMPREHENSIVE TREATMENT OUTCOMES

Cephalometric outcomes following distalization of the maxillary molars using the BAPA have been assessed.[9] In the first distalization stage, the maxillary first molars moved distally 4.6 mm and the second and first premolars drifted distally 2.9 and 2.2 mm, respectively. At the end of the comprehensive treatment, statistically significant mesial movement of the molars (2.8 mm) and the second premolars (1.7 mm) was observed. The maxillary first molars exhibited significant distal tipping (13.0°) during the first phase of treatment, but they were effectively uprighted in the second phase with fixed orthodontic appliances. Approximately 61% of the molar distalization obtained in the first phase of treatment was lost during the second phase of treatment; however, the Class I molar relationship was maintained. The mesial movement detected at the end of the comprehensive treatment in this study could not be totally attributed to relapse of distalization since continuing eruption of the maxillary molars in a forward and downward direction was taking place and this may have contributed to the mesial molar movement.[9]

In patients with growth potential, the mandible outgrows the maxilla and thus the mandibular first molars move anteriorly in most patients. Consequently, despite the mesialization of the maxillary molars, maintenance of the new Class I molar relationship at the end of fixed appliance therapy is probably achieved by dentoalveolar compensation and continued normal anterior mandibular growth.

CONCLUSIONS

The BAPA presents an efficient, convenient and cost-effective Pendulum appliance modification. It is a reasonable choice for non-compliant treatment of Class II patients presenting with a horizontal or average growth pattern in routine clinical practice. It is particularly useful for borderline situations where there is usually a need to extract the maxillary premolars. The major drawback of the appliance is the significant distal tipping of the molar crowns, which occurs along with molar distalization. In addition, minor mandibular posterior rotation should be taken into account when using the BAPA.

When deciding an individual treatment plan, it must be considered that more than half of the amount of the new maxillary position achieved by intraoral molar distalization will be lost. It is obvious, therefore, that the mandibular growth pattern is very important to maintain the achieved Class I molar relationship, and patients who present a vertical growth pattern may not be good candidates for treatment by intraoral molar distalization with the BAPA.

REFERENCES

1. Kircelli BH, Pektaş ZO, Kircelli C. Maxillary molar distalization with a bone-anchored pendulum appliance. Angle Orthod 2006;76:650–9.
2. Oncag G, Seckin O, Dincer B, et al. Osseointegrated implants with pendulum springs for maxillary molar distalization: a cephalometric study. Am J Orthod Dentofacial Orthop 2007;131:16–26.
3. Hilgers JJ. The pendulum appliance for Class II non-compliance therapy. J Clin Orthod 1992;26:706–14.
4. Escobar SA, Tellez PA, Moncada CA, et al. Distalization of maxillary molars with the bone-supported pendulum: a clinical study. Am J Orthod Dentofacial Orthop 2007;131:545–9.
5. Polat-Ozsoy O, Kircelli BH, Arman-Ozcirpici A, et al. Pendulum appliances with 2 anchorage designs: conventional anchorage vs bone anchorage. Am J Orthod Dentofacial Orthop 2008;133:339.
6. Fudalej P, Antoszewska J. Are orthodontic distalizers reinforced with the temporary skeletal anchorage devices effective? Am J Orthod Dentofacial Orthop 2011;139:722–9.
7. Antonarakis GS, Kiliaridis S. Maxillary molar distalization with noncompliance intramaxillary appliances in Class II malocclusion. Angle Orthod 2008;78:1133–40.
8. Byloff FK, Kärcher H, Clar E, et al. An implant to eliminate anchorage loss during molar distalization: a case report involving the Graz implant-supported pendulum. Int J Adult Orthodon Orthognath Surg 2000;15:129–37.
9. Kircelli BH, Pektas ZO, Karan S, et al. Evaluation of the changes associated with bone-anchored pendulum appliance after the completion of comprehensive orthodontic treatment. Turkish J Orthod 2008;21:13–24.

Non-extraction treatment of Class II malocclusion using miniscrew implant anchorage

George Anka and Moschos A. Papadopoulos

INTRODUCTION

Correction of Class II malocclusion with a non-extraction and non-compliance protocol may be performed either through maxillary molar distalization using temporary anchorage devices such as miniscrew implants (MIs) and/or through mandibular advancement using intermaxillary non-compliance appliances.[1]

When planning to treat Class II malocclusion without extractions, an important issue to be considered is how far the patient's maxillary molars can be distalized. Implantation of MIs is not a problem in adults unless there is periodontal involvement. However, when fixed intermaxillary non-compliance appliances are used for mandibular advancement, distalization of maxillary molars is limited.

This chapter discusses two non-extraction and non-compliant approaches for the correction of Class II malocclusion using MIs as temporary anchorage devices and intermaxillary non-compliance devices.

MAXILLARY MOLAR DISTALIZATION

When a tooth or a group of teeth needs to be moved, the preferable movement is bodily without tipping. Two factors need to be taken into consideration: the center of resistance (CR) of that particular tooth, or group of teeth, and the location of the MI from which the forces will be applied. In the maxilla, as the number of teeth to be moved increases, the CR is moving upward and towards the cranial base (Fig. 37.1). This issue of balancing the location of the MI and the force application required has led clinicians to favor indirect force application, where the force is applied indirectly to the MI using an auxiliary or a hook.

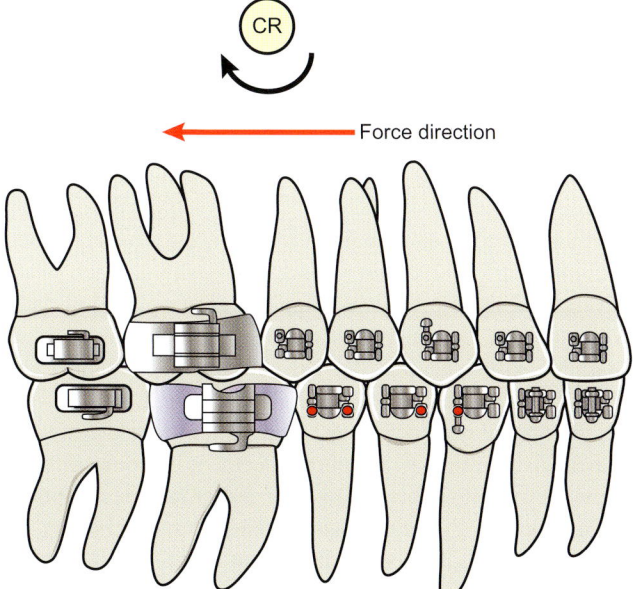

Force direction

Fig. 37.1 Biomechanics of the en masse distalization of the maxillary arch.

Another issue to be considered is the type of molar distalization approach needed, sequential or en masse:

- sequential distalization: initially the first and second molars are distalized, then the premolars and then the anterior teeth
- en masse distalization: the whole maxillary arch is distalized as one rigid block.

Choice between the approaches relates to the CR of the tooth or teeth to be distalized. As the force in en masse distalization is always located below the CR of the maxillary teeth, the occlusal plane always tips with a clockwise rotation in a downward direction (Fig. 37.1). In contrast, sequential distalization can avoid or minimize this tipping but at the cost of increased treatment time.

The final position of the molars and the inclination of the occlusal plane at the end of treatment should be considered and should be based on pretreatment imaging, with an awareness of what is suitable for that patient in terms of occlusal plane manipulation. Factors that need to be considered include in detail the position of the occlusal plane in relation to the condylar pathways, the form and health of both condyles, the morphology and cusp height of the posterior teeth, canine and anterior guidance and the patient's wishes. The presence of third molars (as buds or erupted) may also limit the amount of maxillary molar distalization, but their removal to facilitate first molar distalization is controversial. When the second molars have not yet fully erupted, distalization of the first molars with a continuous force (e.g. using elastic chains and MIs) will also push the second molar buds distally. However, this movement is uncontrolled and so their final position is uncertain. Routine panoramic radiography is necessary to ensure that molar distalization approaches control second or third molar uprighting and eruption in a position that will not cause significant problems in the future.

Several other issues need to be considered. Assuming that the third molars are absent, the first and second maxillary molars can theoretically be distalized about 8 to 9 mm, enabling an anterior teeth retraction of approximately 3–4 mm without any extractions. However, when the maxillary anterior teeth are moved distally, their roots may touch the palatal side of the corresponding alveolar bone and this can lead to root resorption. Root resorption of the central incisors may also take place if their roots are positioned too close to the anterior palatine foramen (incisive foramen). The extent to which any arch length discrepancy can be resolved without extractions must also be considered, including the degree of pretreatment protrusion, the specific goals of treatment and whether expansion of the dental arch is possible in order to gain space. Approximately 16–18 mm could be provided by distalization. In addition, if a transversal expansion of 10 mm is possible, the 6 mm gain in arch length will provide an additional 12 mm, giving a total of 30 mm of space that can be used to resolve arch length discrepancy without extractions of teeth.[2]

A realistic treatment plan should depend on the characteristics of each individual patient while taking into consideration these anatomical issues.

THE TRANSPALATAL ARCH PLUS HOOKS DEVICE

A transpalatal arch (TPA) with hooks soldered or attached to it (TPA-PH device) provides an easy force application system via elastic chains

(Fig. 37.2). The design and construction of the device depends on the final occlusal plane position required.

The TPA is fabricated from an SS wire (diameter, 1 mm) and is soldered to the bands of the first maxillary molars (Fig. 37.2A). The first molars are used to anchor the appliance since these teeth dictate the type of occlusion and are of significant importance when maneuvering the dental arch in three dimensions (Fig. 37.2B).

A full-size or close to full-size main archwire with closing loops is inserted in the bracket slots of the maxillary teeth (e.g. 0.017 × 0.025 inch archwire for 0.018 inch bracket slots) (Fig. 37.2C). Both ends of the archwire have additional loops that are essential to control any tipping of the second molars that might take place during distalization. In addition, omega loops positioned mesial to the first maxillary molars are used to control sequential or en masse distalization through linkage to the corresponding attachments of the molar tubes.

Once the treatment plan has been prepared, the exact design of the TPA-PH and the insertion position for MIs can be decided.

Optional Designs

There are three available designs of the TPA-PH device (Fig. 37.2D–F). The A design is simple and more easily accepted by the patient (Fig. 37.2A,D). It has hooks to facilitate placement of elastics from the MIs to the device. The length of the hooks can be adjusted depending on the biomechanics needed (e.g. bodily distalization, distalization and intrusion for open bite (Fig. 37.2G) or distalization and extrusion for deep bite (Fig. 37.2H).

The B design differs from the A design only in the number and position of MIs used: the B design uses a single MI positioned on the midline of the palate (Fig. 37.2D,J), while the A design uses two MIs positioned inter-radicularly on either side of the palate (Fig. 37.2E).

With the B design, the force direction cannot be changed and so control and manipulation of the occlusal plane is restricted. Where a differential force application is needed to distalize the maxillary right and left molars asymmetrically, the C design is recommended (Fig. 37.2F,I). This design uses a combination of a miniplate (Beneplate, PSM Medical Solutions, Tuttlingen, Germany) and two MIs with caps to secure the miniplate. The miniplate incorporates an extended wire (diameter, 1.1 mm) that is soldered at its distal end. Two hooks are bent at both ends of this wire, which can be positioned in different positions on the palate according to the biomechanical needs of the patient.[3]

Insertion Position for Miniscrew Implants

The preferred location for inter-radicular MIs is the alveolar bone area between the roots of the maxillary first molars and second premolars, where there is a wide interdental root space. The MIs are inserted, on average, 5–7 mm from the cervicogingival line, although 11 mm distance may be needed in some patients, depending on the alveolar bone volume and the position of the maxillary sinus. Occasionally the maxillary sinus extends too far down to make insertion of MIs feasible. If there is not adequate alveolar bone for the implantation of MIs, the midline of the anterior area of the palate can be used (Fig. 36.2I,J). In young adults, the midpalatal suture is not fully ossified and placement in the paramedian region, about 3–6 mm away from the midpalatal suture, is recommended.

MANDIBULAR ADVANCEMENT USING INTERMAXILLARY NON-COMPLIANCE APPLIANCES

In Class II with mandibular deficiency, the treatment of choice is the advancement of the mandible to a more forward position in order to improve the skeletal discrepancy, the E-line (esthetic line) and thus the facial appearance. These treatment goals can be achieved through the use of intermaxillary non-compliance appliances.

The Forsus Fatigue Resistant Device with Direct Push Rod (FFRD-DPR; 3M Unitek, St. Paul, MN, USA) is a spring type (flexible) jumping appliance (see Fig. 37.4D, below). This and other types of flexible intermaxillary non-compliance appliances can provide a gentle way to gradually advance the mandible in a more forward position with more protection for the temporomandibular joint than is possible with the rigid appliances, which create this advancement instantly.[4]

When using intermaxillary non-compliance appliances, it is possible to distalize the maxillary molars in addition to the main effect of advancing the mandible. However, the applied force system usually produces unwanted labial tipping and proclination of the mandibular incisors. To counteract this effect, it is recommended tthat brackets with negative torque values are used for the mandibular anterior teeth. Alternatively, MIs implanted in the posterior region of the mandible may be very effective in preventing this proclination of the anterior mandibular teeth.

DISTALIZATION OF MANDIBULAR MOLARS

In many Class II patients, there is a certain amount of arch length discrepancy that has to be resolved, usually through distalization of all maxillary and mandibular teeth and/or some expansion of the dental arches.

LINGUAL ARCH PLUS HOOKS DEVICE

Mandibular molars can be distalized using a modified lingual arch in combination with MIs for indirect force application, the so-called Lingual Arch Plus Hooks (LA-PH) device (Fig. 37.3). This incorporates two cantilevers that are soldered on the buccal surfaces of the mandibular first molar bands and extend to the area of the first premolars. The mesial ends of these cantilevers are bent to form hooks, which are used to apply the distalization forces from the MIs. This system facilitates differential force application in order to control the vertical dimension of the molar movement depending on the specific needs. Depending on the point of force application, on the hooks or on the distal aspect of these cantilevers, molar intrusion (Fig. 37.3C) or extrusion (Fig. 37.3D) can take place simultaneously to the distalization of mandibular molars.

The MIs are inserted inter-radicularly on the buccal side of the alveolar process between the roots of the first molars and second premolars, near the mucogingival junction and usually about 8 mm below the cervicogingival line. If there is insufficient space, more space can be created by leveling and aligning the mandibular dental arch, an alternative site can be selected or miniplates can be considered for anchorage. Some women have a high mandible plane angle, which makes inter-radicular implantation difficult.

The system requires that the mandibular first molars are already aligned within the arch, and that left and right molars are parallel to each other. Therefore, conventional fixed orthodontic appliances are placed initially in order to level and align the mandibular dental arch so that the roots of the teeth are parallel, sufficient space for MI placement is available and left and right first molars are also parallel to each other. The LA-PH device is bonded with the lingual arch acting as a rigid fixation of the molars, thus allowing their distalization as a group. Placement of hooks directly on the main archwire to start molar distalization earlier may be an option, but it should be avoided as it is usually associated with molar tipping.

There are some limitations concerning the extent of molar distalization in the mandible as in the maxilla. The main limitations include the bone of the mandibular ramus and the soft tissues in front of it. The distance of

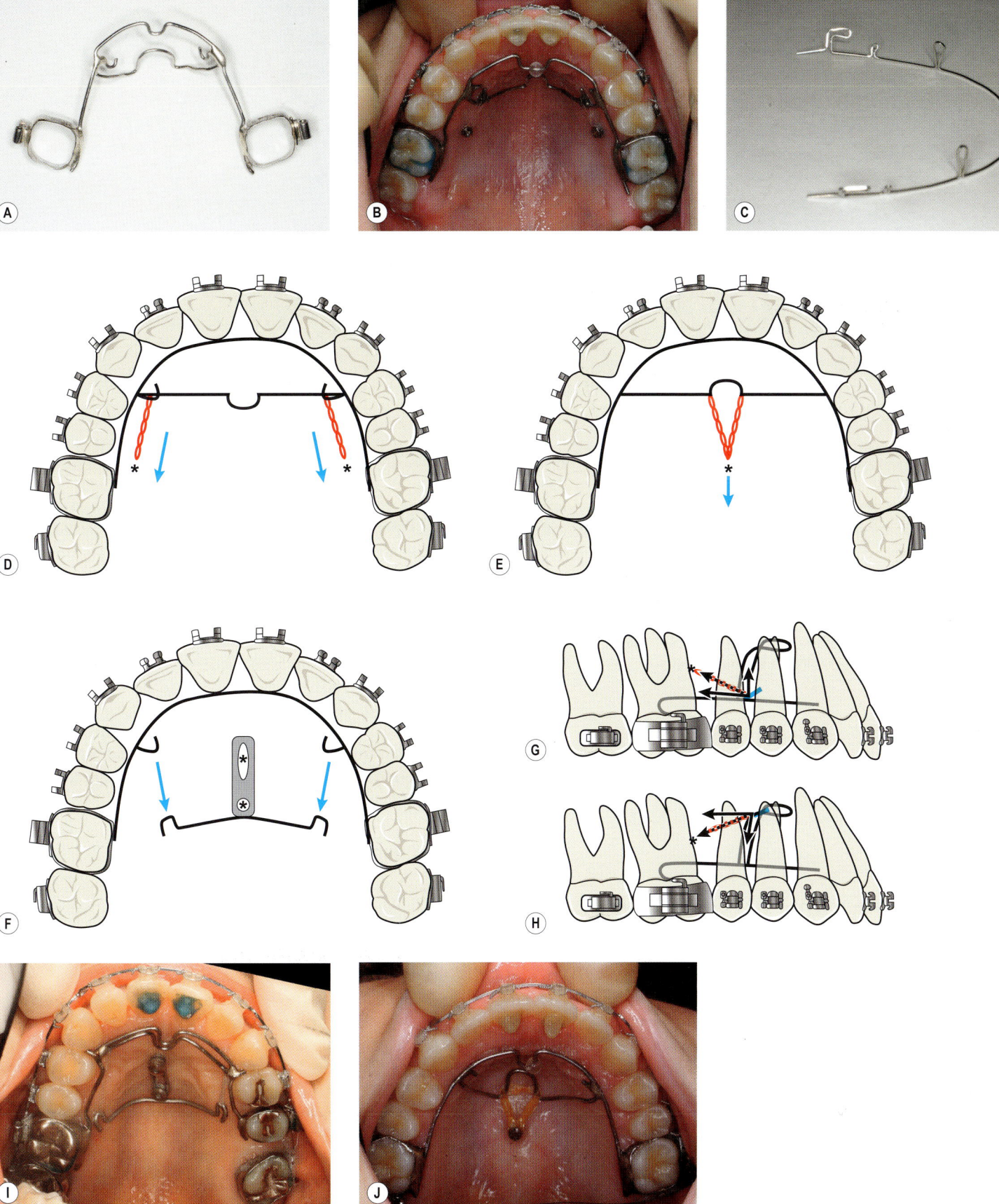

Fig. 37.2 The Transpalatal Arch Plus Hooks device. (A,B) The standard device. (C) The maxillary archwire with closing loops used for molar distalization. (D-F) The three designs: A design (D) B design (E) and C design (F). (G,H) The Transpalatal Arch Plus Hooks device as it is used for maxillary molar intrusion (G), and maxillary molar extrusion (H). (I,J) The C design supported by two miniscrew implants (I) and the B design supported a single one on the midpalatal suture (J).

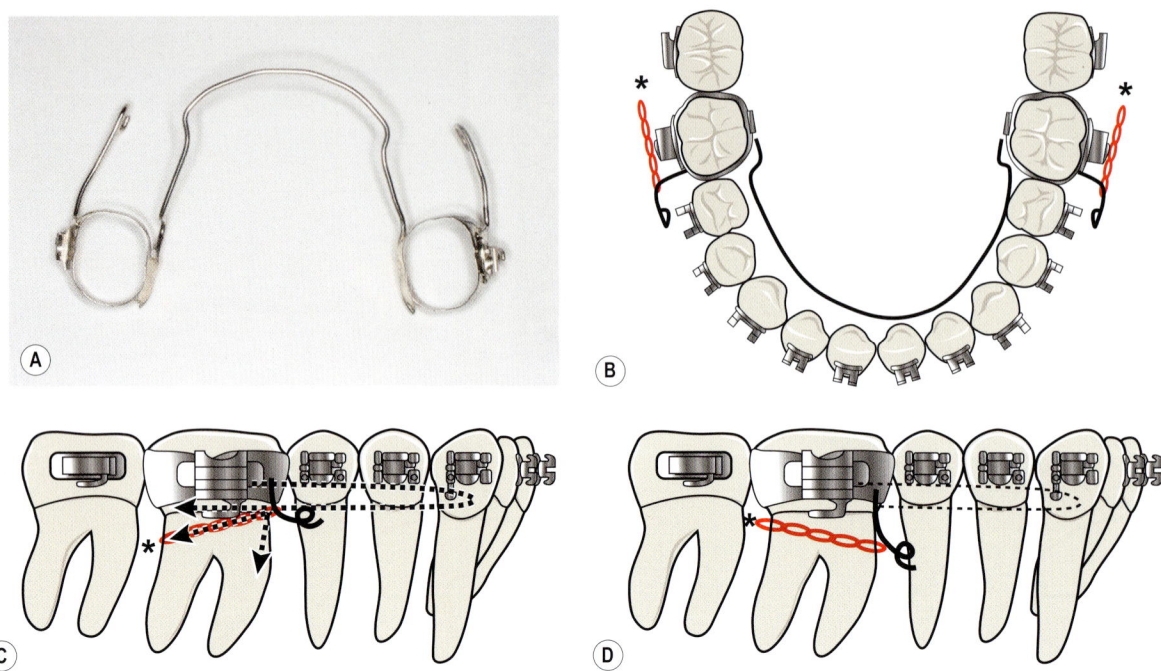

Fig. 37.3 The Lingual Arch Plus Hooks device. (A) Construction of the device. (B) Placement. (C) Biomechanics in mandibular molar distalization and intrusion. (D) Biomechanics in mandibular molar distalization and extrusion.

the distal surface of the second molars from the surface of the ramus soft tissues increases with age; consequently, mandibular molar distalization is less effective in young patients. The use of laser devices to cut the soft tissues distally to the second molars, particularly in young patients, may provide some millimeters of space, but this should be performed very carefully in order to avoid creation of gingival pockets, which would facilitate food impaction and periodontal inflammation.

CLINICAL EXAMPLES

Two cases are presented that the treatment approaches described above have been used: a patient presenting a Class II, division 1 malocclusion with maxillary protrusion and a patient with Class II malocclusion, subdivision left.

CASE 1: CLASS II, DIVISION 1 MALOCCLUSION WITH MAXILLARY PROTRUSION

A 14-year-old boy presented with a chief complaint of maxillary protrusion, which did not allow proper lip closure. He had a symmetric face and a convex facial pattern with a deep labiomental sulcus and a retruded mandible. He could only close his lips by straining the orbicularis oris muscle complex. He had a bilateral Class II molar relationship (Fig. 37.4A,B), an overjet of 10 mm and an overbite of 7 mm. He had an arch length discrepancy of 7 mm in the maxilla and 11 mm in the mandible. The boy showed little interest in maintaining his oral hygiene, which was a reason to have as short as possible treatment time.

Prior to the initiation of treatment, three-dimensional CT was performed in order to determine the amount of movements needed to correct Class II into Class I molar relationship. The results indicated that the maxillary molars had to be distalized 6 mm on each side, resulting in a total movement of 12 mm. Together with the 7 mm of arch length discrepancy in the maxillary arch, this meant that a total of 19 mm of space was needed in order to correct the Class II relationship. Each molar needed to be distalized approximately 9.5 mm, which is considered very difficult to achieve. Although the

patient had passed his growth peak, intermaxillary non-compliance appliances could be used to take advantage of the remaining growth of the mandible. It was, therefore, decided to use the FFRD-DPR in order to advance the mandible to a more forward position, gaining a maximum of 4 mm toward mesial. This would decrease the need for maxillary molar distalization to a total 11 mm (19 mm less 2 × 4 mm), a distalization of 6.5 mm per side, which is considered a moderate molar movement.

Expansion of the maxillary dental arch was also planned in order to gain some additional space to further decrease the need for pure maxillary molar distalization. Finally, since the patient presented with a deep bite, an increase of the vertical dimension by opening the bite would be advantageous, and so retraction of the maxillary teeth was planned, with some extrusion of the maxillary molars.

Treatment Course

Following insertion of conventional fixed appliances, a Hyrax appliance was used to expand the maxilla (Fig. 37.4C). An FFRD-DPR exerting a force of 180 g per side was used for 1 year (Fig. 37.4D). During this period, a TPA-PH device modification was used, where the elastic chain was used to generate a force to distalize and extrude the molars simultaneously (Fig. 37.4E). Two MIs were inserted in the palatal alveolar bone between the roots of the first molars and the second premolars and the elastic chain was strapped around the anterior omega loop of the TPA, exerting a force of 300 g. On the frontal part of the TPA, a pearl was used to provide non-compliant tongue position training, as well as to enable the patient to position his tongue away from the anterior teeth, which could decrease the distalization capacity of the device. Tongue myofunctional training was also prescribed but the patient was not cooperative.

The TPA-PH device, the MIs and the fixed appliances were removed after 2 years of total treatment time, when a good posterior intercuspation and a well-functioning and stable occlusion were established (Fig. 37.4F,G).

Superimposition of the cephalometric tracings before and after treatment and cephalometric analysis show that the bite was opened after treatment, as a result of a clockwise rotation of the occlusal plane as well as of the mandible (Fig. 37.4H). This clockwise rotation positioned the mandible further backwards but this was counteracted by the FFRD-DPR,

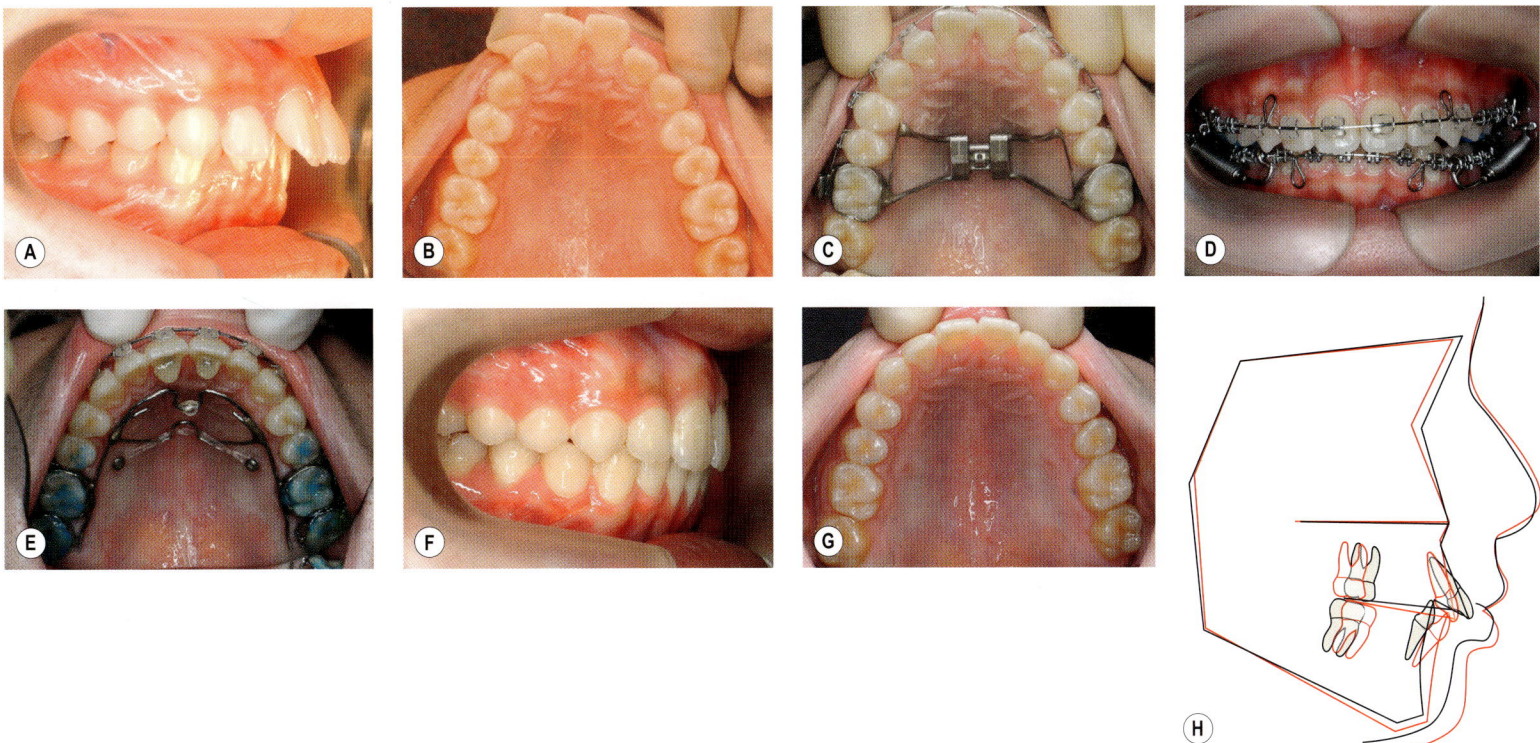

Fig. 37.4 Case 1: Class II, division 1 malocclusion with maxillary protrusion. (A,B) Pretreatment. (C) Occlusal view of the maxillary arch following application of fixed appliances and a Hyrax expansion device. (D) Application of the Forsus Fatigue Resistant Device with Direct Push Rod. (E) Application of the Transpalatal Arch Plus Hooks device for molar distalization and extrusion. (F,G) Post-treatment. (H) Superimposition of the cephalometric tracings before (black) and after treatment (red) on the sella–nasion line.

which also advanced the mandible to a more forward position after treatment.

The maxillary left molar was distalized 2.4 mm and the right 4.6 mm. This distalization was enough to correct the Class II malocclusion since the remaining discrepancy was corrected through the mandibular advancement produced by the FFRD-DPR (Fig. 37.4D) (Table 37.1). In order to avoid relapse of the deep bite under the heavy forces of the masticatory muscles, composite build-ups were bonded on the palatal sides of the maxillary central incisors (Fig. 37.4E). The size of these build-ups was kept to minimum in order just to prevent the relapse and not to actively intrude the anterior teeth.

Treatment Results

The extraoral and intraoral treatment results (Fig. 37.4G,H) were good in spite of the lack of cooperation from the patient during treatment. The patient and his parents were very satisfied with the treatment outcome.

After completion of treatment, a lingual fixed retainer was bonded on the mandible and a maxillary removable clear plastic retainer was given to the patient for retention purposes. Despite instructions, the patient did not attend routine check-ups.

CASE 2: CLASS II MALOCCLUSION, SUBDIVISION LEFT

A 26-year-old woman presented with a chief complaint of crowding of her anterior teeth and lack of confidence because of her malocclusion. Although she was charming, she did not like to smile and tried to prevent exposure of her anterior teeth.

She had a Class II malocclusion, subdivision left (a Class I molar relationship on the right side and a Class II on the left side), moderate to severe

Table 37.1 Cephalometric evaluation

Variables	Before treatment	After treatment
Facial angle (°)	84.8	86.7
Convexity (°)	0.8	0.9
A-B plane (°)	–5.1	1.0
Y-axis (°)	62.9	62.9
FH to SN (°)	7.4	6.8
SNA (°)	77.7	80.3
SNB (°)	75.7	80.5
ANB (°)	2.0	–0.2
N-Pg to SN (°)	77.4	79.9
Nasal floor to SN (°)	7.9	6.2
Nasal floor to FH (°)	0.4	–0.6
ML to SN (°)	29.0	30.2
ML to FH (°)	21.6	23.4
Ramus plane to SN (°)	94.3	94.8
Ramus plane to FH (°)	86.8	88.1
Gonial angle (°)	114.7	115.3
U1 to SN (°)	119.6	105.1
U1 to FH (°)	127.1	111.9
L1 to ML (°)	95.7	97.6
Interincisal angle (°)	115.7	127.1
OP-SN (°)	12.8	14.1
OP-FH (°)	5.4	7.4

crowding of the maxillary anterior teeth, moderate crowding of the mandibular anterior teeth and deviation of the mandibular midline to the left (Fig. 37.5A–C).

The patient expressed her desire to receive an orthodontic treatment that would not alter her facial appearance. After discussing some alternatives, including the use of intermaxillary non-compliant devices or the use of

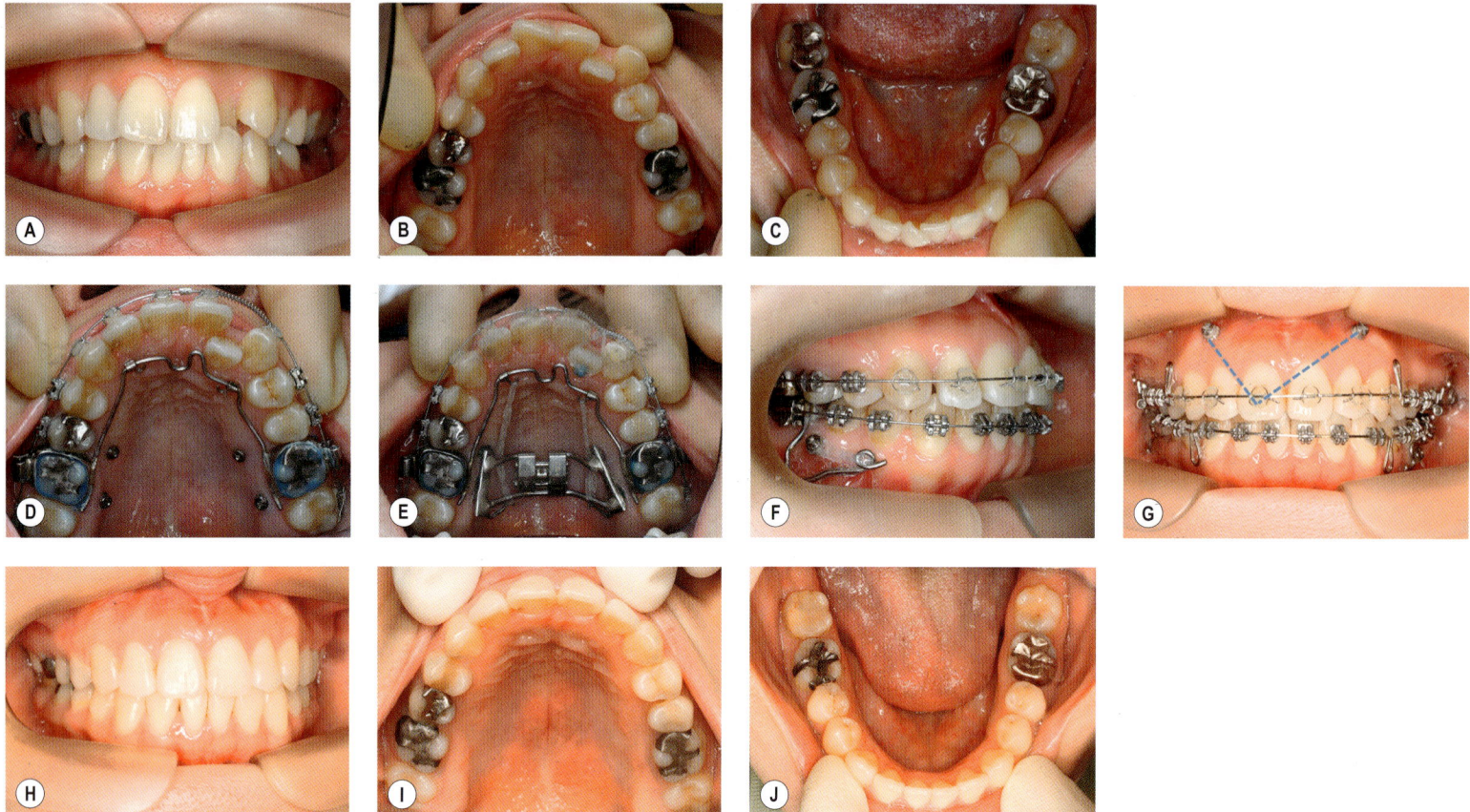

Fig. 37.5 Case 2: Class II malocclusion, subdivision left. (A–C) Pretreatment. (D) The maxillary arch showing the insertion position of the four miniscrew implants (MIs) and of the modified Transpalatal Arch Plus Hooks device. (E) The maxillary arch showing the bone-borne Hyrax expansion device attached to the MI heads and elastic chains for distalization of the maxillary molars. (F) Placement of the Lingual Arch Plus Hooks device, insertion of the MIs and the application of elastic chains for distalization of the mandibular molars. (G) Insertion position of the two MIs for anterior teeth intrusion. (H–J) Post-treatment.

lingual appliances, the following non-extraction treatment approach was agreed and executed.

Treatment Course

Following placement of conventional fixed appliances, a modified TPA-PH device was placed in the maxilla in order to distalize the maxillary molars (Fig. 37.5D).

Expansion of the maxillary arch was necessary to resolve crowding. However, because the midpalatal suture was already ossified, it was decided to use a Hyrax appliance (Fig. 37.5E) anchored on four MIs (two on each side of the palate) (Fig. 37.5D) and not a tooth-borne device. The maxillary sinus was positioned downward and very close to the roots of the maxillary teeth, probably a result of chronic maxillary sinusitis, which made MI placement very difficult. Because of the deficient bony support, it was decided to use the bone-anchored Hyrax device already in place to apply the distalization forces during the expansion procedure by incorporating hooks on its distal aspect. Thus, both the expansion and the distalization devices were constructed and inserted in such a way as to facilitate both distalization and expansion of the maxillary dental arch (Fig. 37.5D,E). Two elastic chains were used on each side of the palate, attached to the hooks of the Hyrax appliance and to the hooks on the anterior part of a TPA-PH, producing a distalization force of approximately 250 g per side. An expansion of 8 mm in the area of the first molars was achieved.

Following placement of fixed appliances on the mandibular arch and initial alignment, a standard LA-PH device was used in combination with two MIs inserted between the roots of the first molars and the second

premolars in order to correct anterior crowding by distalizing the mandibular molars (Fig. 37.5F). Elastic chains were attached between the MIs and the hooks of the LA-PH. The force generated was 200 g per side. Full-size archwires were used during mandibular molar distalization. Distalization of the mandibular molars was necessary to avoid labial proclination of the mandibular incisors, resulting in an anterior crossbite and an adverse effect on facial appearance. Because of the slight open bite tendency, intrusion of the molars was also performed during distalization, while myofunctional treatment was also prescribed.

Some degree of canting of the occlusal plane was detected during the orthodontic treatment when the patient was smiling. The canted occlusal plane was caused probably by the asymmetric positions of the maxillary and mandibular dental arch. Smile was also affected by the constriction of the risorius muscle on the right corner of her mouth, making it asymmetrical. In addition, an asymmetric gummy smile was detected during treatment, since gingival exposure of the right side of her mouth was more pronounced. To eliminate this problem, myofunctional therapy, facial massage and training were prescribed, while progressive intrusion of the maxillary incisors was also performed. This was done by intrusion of the anterior teeth using anchorage of two MIs in the frontal area of the maxillary alveolar bone between the roots of the lateral incisors and the canines (Fig. 37.5G). These measures were successful in correcting both the gummy smile and the canted occlusal plane.

Treatment Results

After 1 year and 8 months of treatment, a bilateral Class I molar and canine relationship with optimal alignment of both maxillary and mandibular teeth was obtained, plus a well-intercuspated and stable occlusion. Ideal overjet and overbite were also achieved. Anterior crowding of both arches and midline deviation were also corrected (Fig. 37.5H–J).

The post-treatment extraoral photographs showed no significant change of the patient's profile, as she had wished. The treatment results achieved were within the initial treatment goals and the patient was very satisfied with her final dental and facial appearance, particularly because no extractions and no significant soft tissue profile changes were performed.

After completion of treatment, the patient rediscovered her confidence and started to smile again without any psychological restrictions.

CONCLUSIONS

Non-extraction Class II correction can now be performed using intermaxillary non-compliance appliances and MIs even in adults. Further, the combined use of MI-supported treatment and expansion of the maxillary arch may at least theoretically provide sufficient space to resolve arch length deficiency. The use of MI-anchored devices can facilitate camouflage orthodontic treatment of patients with orthognathic problems, who previously had to be treated surgically. However, it should be noted that, when providing a camouflage treatment, only the teeth and the corresponding alveolar bone are moved in order to restore oral function, esthetics and self-esteem for the patient; there is no change to modify the underlying skeletal structures. Therefore, clinicians should remain aware of the limitations of such treatments, as well as of the biological limitations that govern tooth movements.

Patients' expectations of treatment outcomes and treatment times vary and this must be taken also into consideration. While the use of MI-anchored devices can enable complex situations to be treated without extractions and in a more predictable way, a longer treatment time is usually needed, which is sometimes beyond the expectations of patients.

Finally, not all Class II patients can or should be treated by non-extraction approaches. In some cases, such as in severe Class II malocclusion or with increased arch length discrepancies, extraction of teeth still remains a treatment option not only to achieve but also to retain an appropriate treatment result.

REFERENCES

1. Papadopoulos MA, editor. Orthodontic treatment for the Class II non-compliant patient: current principles and techniques. Edinburgh: Elsevier-Mosby; 2006.
2. Anka G, Aonuma M. TAD (temporary anchorage device) use in distalizing molars. Tokyo Orthod J 2009;19:169–78.
3. Wilmes B, Drescher D, Nienkemper M. A miniplate system for improved stability of skeletal anchorage. J Clin Orthod 2009;43:495–501.
4. Anka G. Management of non-compliant Class II, division 1 extraction cases with jumping appliance Forsus DPR: a suggestion of the use of Gurin lock and anterior fixed bite plate. Ortodontia 2004;9:122–33.

Treatment of skeletal origin gummy smiles with miniscrew implant-supported biomechanics

James Cheng-Yi Lin, Leslie Yen-Peng Chen, Eric Jein-Wein Liou and S. Jay Bowman

INTRODUCTION

Improving the "smile line" is one aspect of esthetic enhancement that may benefit from orthodontic treatment. The excessive exposure of gingival tissue upon smiling, the gummy smile, may, in fact, be a patient's chief complaint.[1] Since gingival display can be caused in a number of ways, proper diagnosis is critical prior to embarking upon any resolution (Table 38.1).[2–4] Although surgical approaches may be effective for some etiologies, this is not always acceptable to patients, and this has stimulated interest in alternative treatment methods.

The use of tooth movements supported by miniscrew implant (MI) anchorage has become more refined and widely accepted. This chapter describes an innovative non-orthognathic approach using MI-supported biomechanics, with or without alveoloplasty (periodontal plastic surgery), to resolve the skeletal origin gummy smile in adults.

DIAGNOSIS

A number of factors need to be considered in the management of skeletal origin gummy smile.[5]

- Skeletal Class II malocclusion and vertical growth pattern, as opposed to skeletal Class III malocclusion or horizontal growth pattern, is associated with a gummy smile and can be deemed as the representative facial morphology.
- Retrusive mandible, excessive anterior maxillary height, labially inclined maxillary incisors and upper lip, plus a significant overjet and overbite, are obvious in patients with a gummy smile. The cant of the palatal plane is not a factor. The actual length of upper lip is usually the same or longer than normal, but the ratio of upper lip length to anterior maxillary height is often reduced.

Table 38.1 Possible etiology and treatment strategies of excess gingival display (gummy smile)

Origin	Etiology	Treatment strategy
Dental	Plaque- or drug-induced gingival enlargement	Gingivectomy/gingivalplasty
	Altered/delayed passive eruption	Mucogingival surgery combined with alveoloplasty (re-establish ideal biological width)
	Retroclined maxillary incisors	Torque control
Skeletal	Vertical maxillary excess	Orthognathic surgery + orthodontic treatment
Muscular	Hyperactivity of the elevator muscle of upper lip (hypermobile lip)	Lip surgery Cartilage spacer/silicone laid; V-Y cheiloplasty; Botulinum toxin type A injection
	Short upper lip length (philtrum length)	Botulinum toxin; myotomy of the levator labii superioris muscle
Combination	Combination etiologies	Combination treatment

- Gingival exposure during maximum posed smile (measured from the gingival margins to the lower border of the upper lip), clinical crown lengths and pocket depths of the maxillary anterior teeth, activity of the elevator muscles of the upper lip, philtrum length, age, sex, as well as individual craniofacial features must also be considered.

Wu et al. recommend the following four diagnostic measurements to facilitate diagnosis.[5] With all of these, the patient's age, sex and personal preference will be modifying factors that need to be considered.

- *Amount of maxillary incisor display with the upper lip at rest.* This should ideally be 2 mm and is used as a reference to avoid overintruding the maxillary anterior teeth.
- *The clinical crown lengths and periodontal pocket depths of the maxillary central incisors.* The length of a maxillary central incisor is typically 9.5–11.2 mm for pleasing tooth proportions.[6,7] The pocket depths of healthy incisors should be no more than 3 mm. These measurements are important (1) to determine if the excessive gingival display is a result of altered passive eruption and/or gingival inflammation, (2) to estimate how much maxillary anterior intrusion is required, and (3) to determine the optimal clinical crown lengths and relative gingival margins of the other maxillary anterior teeth by using the maxillary central incisor as a reference.
- *The distance between the gingival margins of maxillary anterior teeth and upper lip in the maximum posed smile.* More than a 2 mm continuous band of gingival exposure during maximum posed smile may be considered as excessive. This measurement is also important in determining if the gingival display is muscular in origin if the patient exhibits normal clinical crown lengths and pocket depths of maxillary anterior teeth.
- *The distance between the palatal plane and tip of maxillary incisor edge.* The average value of the upper incisor–palatal plane (U1–PP) cephalometric variable is 31.0 ± 2.34 mm. Patients may simply be "long in the tooth" compared with the palatal plane.

Commonly, patients with a skeletal origin gummy smile have a combination of the last two criteria. The first two measurements are used to determine if there are other etiological factors contributing to the excessive gingival display.

CLINICAL APPROACH

MINISCREW IMPLANTS

The LOMAS orthodontic MI system (Lin/Liou OrthodonticMini Anchor System, Mondeal Medical Systems, Tuttlingen, Germany) comprises a series of self-tapping and self-drilling titanium alloy MIs (diameters, 1.5, 2.0 and 2.3 mm; lengths, 7.0, 9.0, 11.0 and 13.0 mm).[8–10] The variety of sizes and designs allows flexibility in insertion site and biomechanics. Two designs of MI head are available: the Hook screw and the Quattro screw.

Table 38.2 Four types of miniscrew implant-supported treatment biomechanics for skeletal origin gummy smile correction

Biomechanics	Anterior implant sites and MI size	Posterior implant sites and MI size	Force delivery
Type 1 direct anchorage with alveoloplasty (Case 1)	Interseptum bone between upper 1&2 (Hook screw L, 9.0 mm; D,1.5 mm) Interseptum bone between upper 2&3 (Hook screw L, 9.0 mm; D, 1.5 mm)	Interseptum bone between upper 5&6 (Quattro screw L, 9.0 mm; D, 2.0 mm) Infrazygomatic crest (Quattro screw L, 9.0–11 mm; D, 2.0 mm) Alveolar ridge without teeth (Hook/Quattro screw L, 9.0–11 mm; D, 1.5–2.0 mm)	Intrusion–retraction forces: coil springs/power chains
Type 2 indirect anchorage with alveoloplasty (Case 2)		Interseptum bone between upper 5&6 (Quattro screw L, 9.0 mm; D, 2.0 mm) Infrazygomatic crest (Quattro screw L, 9.0–11 mm; D, 2.0 mm) Alveolar ridge without teeth (Hook/Quattro screw L, 9.0–11 mm; D, 1.5–2.0 mm)	Intrusion forces: segmented level arms (0.017 × 0.025″ TMA wires) Retraction forces: coil springs/power chains
Type 3 indirect anchorage without alveoloplasty (Case 3)		Interseptum bone between upper 5&6 (Quattro screw L, 9.0 mm; D, 2.0 mm) Infrazygomatic crest (Quattro screw L, 9.0–11 mm; D, 2.0 mm) Alveolar ridge without teeth (Hook/Quattro screw L, 9.0–11 mm; D, 1.5–2.0 mm)	Intrusion forces: segmented level arms (0.017 × 0.025″ TMA wires) Retraction forces: coil springs/power chains
Type 4 direct anchorage without alveoloplasty (Case 4)	Interseptum bone between upper 2&3 (Screw size L, 6.0 mm; D, 1.6 mm)	Interseptum bone between upper 6&7 (Screw size L, 8.0 mm; D, 1.6 mm)	Intrusion forces: power chains

D, diameter; L, length; MI, miniscrew implant.

The Hook screw features a simple hook on the top of the MI head, similar to a molar hook, for the application of forces (e.g. elastic chain, thread or coil springs). The Quattro screw has a head with a rectangular slot and an edgewise tube (0.018 × 0.025 inch or 0.022 × 0.028 inch) to permit the insertion of rectangular segmented wires to utilize indirect anchorage while elastic chains or superelastic coil springs can be attached at the same time. This allows the MI to serve two purposes.

TREATMENT BIOMECHANICS

The authors have developed four types of MI-supported biomechanics to treat skeletal origin gummy smile (Table 38.2):

- *type 1*: direct MI anchorage with alveoloplasty (e.g. Case 1)
- *type 2*: indirect MI anchorage with alveoloplasty (e.g. Case 2)
- *type 3*: indirect MI anchorage without alveoloplasty (e.g. Case 3)
- *type 4*: direct MI anchorage without alveoloplasty (e.g. Case 4).

There are four issues to consider when selecting which type to use in a particular clinical situation.

- Is there sufficient inter-radicular space to safely insert the MI between the roots of teeth? This is particularly significant when MIs are to be placed in the anterior alveolus for direct anchorage support of intrusion forces.[11]
- Will the MIs produce severe irritation of the lip and/or vestibular mucosa?
- Do the clinical crowns of the teeth to be intruded exhibit favorable height to width ratio?
- Would any excess and/or irregular bony protuberances above the maxillary anterior teeth be noticed, thereby being indicative of requiring post-orthodontic alveoloplasty?

CASE EXAMPLES

The following case examples illustrate the four types of MI-supported biomechanics.

CASE 1: DIRECT ANCHORAGE WITH ALVEOLOPLASTY FOR EXCESS GINGIVAL EXPOSURE DURING SMILING

A 26-year-old woman presented with the chief complaint of excess gingival exposure during smiling (Fig. 38.1A). She exhibited more than 7 mm of gingival exposure in her posed smile, along with a convex profile, an acute nasolabial angle, retrognathic chin, short upper lip and a degree of lip incompetence. She had a Class II canine and molar relationship, 11 mm of overjet, a 4 mm overbite and multiple missing teeth (Fig. 38.1D,E). The clinical crown lengths of the maxillary central incisors and other anterior teeth were all obviously shorter than normal values. The gingival margins of all maxillary anterior teeth stayed almost at the same level. The pocket depths of the maxillary anterior teeth were between 1.0 and 3.0 mm, with no gingival inflammation. Cephalometric analysis indicated skeletal Class II relationships, while the U1–PP distance (39.0 mm) was significantly larger than the norm. It was determined that her excessive gingival display had both skeletal and dental origin, while any contribution of the muscular system could not be determined.

As part of informed consent, two treatment options were discussed with the patient. The first option included traditional orthodontic treatment in combination with Le Fort I osteotomy to "impact" or shorten the height of the maxilla, thereby reducing the gingival display in the posed smile. The second option involved no orthognathic surgery but used MI-assisted direct anchorage to produce intrusive forces to the maxillary dentition. This would, in turn, reduce the amount of gingiva exposed during smiling. After reviewing the risk–benefits of both options, the patient gave her informed consent to the more conservative and less invasive method.

Treatment was initiated with fixed preadjusted appliances to level and align the dentition. After 5 months, two Quattro MIs (diameter, 2 mm; length, 7 mm) were inserted into the bilateral alveolar ridges and two Hook MIs (diameter, 1.5 mm; length, 9 mm) were placed into the alveolar bone between the maxillary lateral incisors and canines above the root apices.

Immediately after MI insertion, a retraction force of approximately 200 g was applied through power chains connected from the bilateral

Fig. 38.1 Case 1: direct anchorage with alveoloplasty. (A,D,E) Pretreatment showing excess gingival exposure during smiling. (F,G) LOMAS miniscrew implants (MIs) inserted for retraction and intrusion of the maxillary anterior teeth with power chains extending from the MIs to hooks on the upper archwire. (H) Overjet and overbite before treatment. (I) Intrusion and retraction of the maxillary anterior teeth at 15 months of treatment. (B,J,K) Final treatment result. (L) Superimposition of the pretreatment (black line) and post-treatment (red line) cephalometric tracings. (C) Post-retention view. (M) Superimposition of the post-treatment (red line) and post-retention (black line) cephalometric tracings.

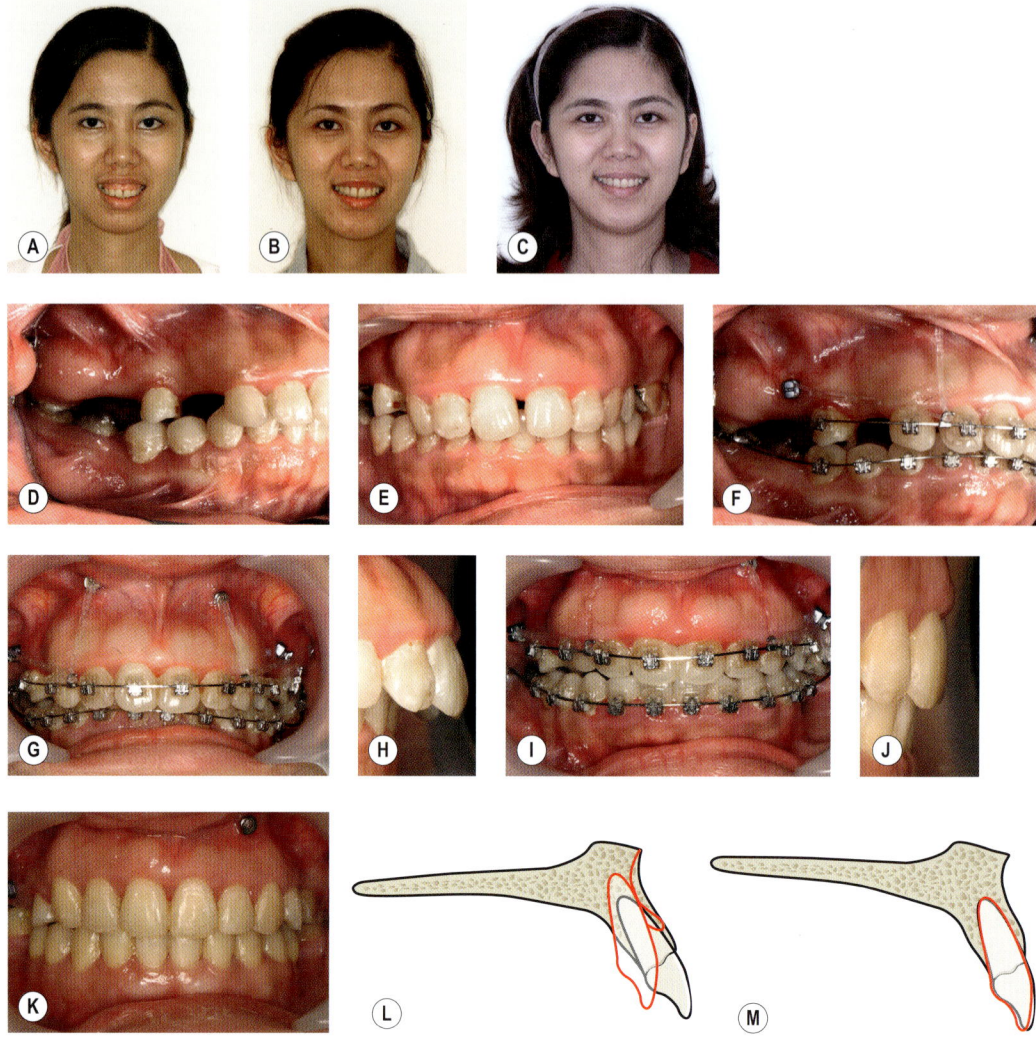

posterior MIs to hooks on the upper archwire, positioned between the laterals and canines. An intrusive force of 50 g was also applied from the anterior MIs to the same hooks (Fig. 38.1F,G). The intent was to both intrude and en masse retract the maxillary dentition to correct the Class II relationship and improve the smile line.

Fifteen months later, the patient's original severe gummy smile and overjet were substantially improved. Unfortunately, the clinical crown lengths of the maxillary anterior teeth had decreased as the teeth were intruded or "buried" in the gingiva, which was an unintended (but anticipated) side effect (Fig. 38.1H). In addition, an excess protuberance of alveolar bone near the gingival margin was noted both intraorally and in a lateral cephalometric radiograph (Fig. 38.1I). Because of these iatrogenic changes, alveoloplasty was recommended to eliminate the excess alveolus and improve the clinical crown length. Specifically, the gingival margins of the maxillary anterior teeth were coordinated with the lower border of the upper lip in her posed smile.

After periodontal procedures had taken place, a dramatic esthetic improvement in the patient's smile was obvious when compared with her pretreatment photographs (Fig. 38.1B,J,K). The gingival margins of the maxillary anterior teeth were coordinated with the lower border of the upper lip in her smile. Her original gummy smile had been corrected without undergoing orthognathic surgery.

Superimposition of the cephalometric tracings demonstrated significant retraction and intrusion of the maxillary teeth (Fig. 38.1L), while the U1–PP was reduced from 39.0 to 34.5 mm. Despite substantial tooth movement, only minor root resorption of the maxillary incisor apices was noted in the post-treatment periapical radiographs. Total treatment time was 20

months to resolve the patient's chief complaints and to achieve the "orthognathic-like" treatment effects.[4]

After 45 months of post-treatment retention, the facial profile, smile line and occlusion were favorable despite a slight amount of labial movement of the maxillary incisors (Fig. 38.1C,M).

CASE 2: INDIRECT ANCHORAGE WITH ALVEOPLASTY FOR SIMULTANEOUS REDUCTION IN GUMMY SMILE AND VERTICAL DIMENSION

A 21-year-old woman did not like her protrusive profile and excess gingival display when smiling. She exhibited a convex profile, acute nasolabial angle, retrusive chin, short upper lip length and a mentalis strain upon lip closure. More than 3 mm of gingival display was apparent in her posed smile. She had bilateral Class I canine and molar relationships, mild anterior bimaxillary crowding without periodontal involvement, and 2 mm overjet and overbite (Fig. 38.2A,D). The clinical crown lengths of her maxillary central incisors and of other anterior teeth were normal, but the gingival margin of the maxillary right lateral incisor was uneven. The probing depths of the periodontal pockets of the maxillary anterior teeth were no more than 3 mm, and the gingiva was healthy. She had skeletal Class II relationships, a significantly obtuse mandibular plane, a retrognathic chin and flared mandibular incisors. Both maxillary and mandibular incisors and molars were substantially erupted. The etiology of the excessive gingival display appeared to be skeletal in origin (U1–PP, 36.5 mm) (Table 38.3).

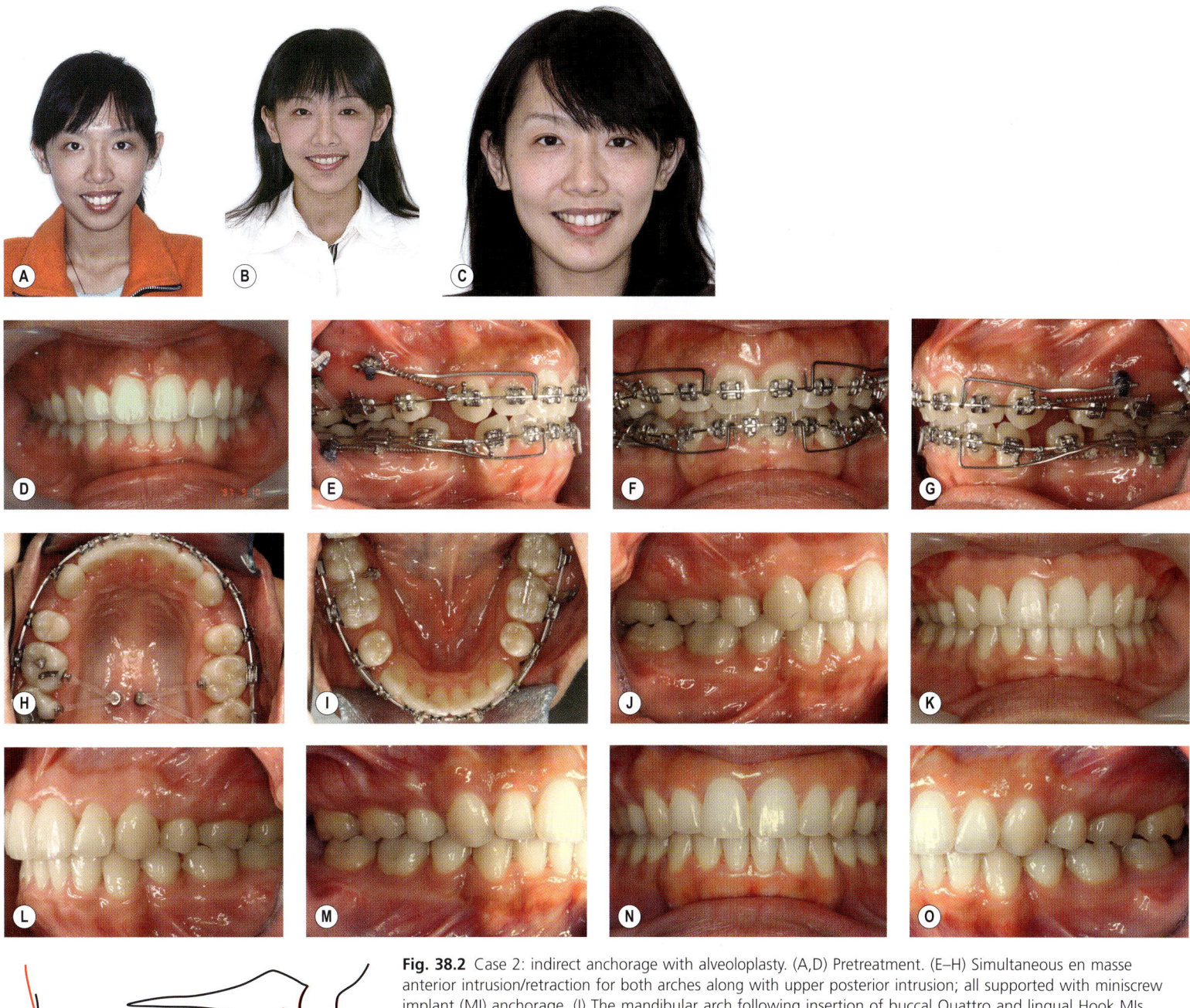

Fig. 38.2 Case 2: indirect anchorage with alveoloplasty. (A,D) Pretreatment. (E–H) Simultaneous en masse anterior intrusion/retraction for both arches along with upper posterior intrusion; all supported with miniscrew implant (MI) anchorage. (I) The mandibular arch following insertion of buccal Quattro and lingual Hook MIs. (B,J,K,L) Post-treatment. (C,M,N,O) Post retention views. (P) Superimpositions of the pretreatment (black line) and post-treatment (red line) cephalometric tracings on the anterior cranial base.

The patient was diagnosed with a Class I malocclusion with underlying Class II skeletal relationships, a hyperdivergent long-face pattern, a retrognathic chin and a gummy smile resulting from vertical maxillary excess.

The treatment objectives were (1) to improve the gingival display, (2) to improve the facial appearance by maximum retraction of the anterior teeth, (3) to reduce the lower anterior facial height, and (4) to permit autorotation of the mandible to improve the chin projection.

Two treatment options were presented to the patient: an orthodontic/orthognathic surgical approach, and a non-surgical approach using MI-anchored mechanics to produce "orthognathic-like" treatment effects. At the conclusion of informed consent, the patient chose the non-surgical alternative.

Indirect MI anchorage mechanics were used in both dental arches for three reasons: (1) the gummy smile, vertical dimension and mandible autorotation could be addressed simultaneously; (2) simultaneous intrusion and retraction forces could be applied from the same MIs; (3) increased mandibular autorotation was anticipated to improve the retruded chin position.

Table 38.3 Case 2: cephalometric data

Variables	Pretreatment	Post-treatment
SNA (°)	80	79.5
SNB (°)	72.5	73
ANB (°)	7.5	6.5
MPA (°)	49	46
U6-PP (mm)	27.5	25.0
U1-PP (mm)	36.5	32.5
L6-MP (mm)	39.0	39.0
L1-MP (mm)	52.0	50.0

MP, mandibular plane; PP, palatal plane.

Both dental arches were bonded with preadjusted fixed appliances for initial leveling and alignment. Four first premolars were extracted to provide space to permit retraction of the anterior dentition in order to reduce bimaxillary protrusion. In addition, all third molars were also extracted.

Four months later, six MIs were placed in the maxillary arch and two in the mandibular arch: two Quattro MIs (diameter, 2.0 mm; length, 7 mm) bilaterally between the roots of the maxillary second premolars and first molars; two Hook screws (diameter, 1.5 mm; length, 9 mm) in the buccal alveolus between the maxillary first and second molars; two Hook screws (diameter, 2.0 mm; length, 7 mm) in the paramedian palatal area (2 mm from the midpalatal suture) near an imaginary midline between the maxillary first and second molars; and two Quattro screws (diameter, 2.0 mm; length, 9 mm) in the buccal oblique ridge between the mandibular first and second molars.

All MIs were loaded 2 weeks after their insertion. Sectional, intrusive lever arms (0.017 × 0.025 inch TMA wire) were inserted into the rectangular tubes of the Quattro screws in both arches. In addition, Ni-Ti closed coil springs were attached to the heads of the Quattro MIs and stretched to hooks on the canines. The combination of forces applied from these MIs was designed to provide simultaneous maxillary en masse anterior retraction and intrusion.

Additional maxillary posterior intrusion was produced by attaching elastic chains from the Hook screws (between the first and second molars) to the main archwire and also from the palatal Hook screws to the lingual buttons on the maxillary molars (Fig. 38.2E–H).

Although significant intrusion of the maxillary posterior teeth and mandibular autorotation were noted 15 months after treatment start, chin projection was still not prominent and more was desired. Consequently, two Hook MIs (diameter, 1.5 mm; length, 9 mm) were inserted bilaterally, oriented obliquely into the lingual alveolus between the mandibular first and second molars. Immediately after MI placement, lower posterior intrusion was initiated by attaching power chains from the buccal Quattro MIs to the lingual Hook MIs, laid across segments of SS wires (0.016 × 0.022 inch) that had been bonded across the occlusal surfaces from the mandibular first to second molars (Fig. 38.2I).

After 24 months of treatment, the original skeletal gummy smile was substantially improved through the large amount of simultaneous intrusion and retraction of the maxillary anterior teeth. Unfortunately, the clinical crown lengths of the maxillary anterior teeth had been decreased and some iatrogenic bony protuberances were noticed in the labial alveolus as well as in lateral cephalometric radiographs. Alveoloplasty was performed to improve the sclinical crown lengths.

Post-treatment photographs (after 28 months of orthodontic treatment) revealed a Class I occlusion with normal overbite/overjet, along with improvement of the patient's profile and smile (Fig. 38.2B,J,K,L).

Superimposition of the cephalometric tracings confirmed significant retraction and intrusion of the maxillary and mandibular anterior teeth, which were accompanied by a significant amount of intrusion of the maxillary posterior teeth (Fig. 38.2P). The entire maxillary dentition appears to have been retracted and intruded, much like that achieved by orthognathic surgery. The mandibular molars were moved mesially into the extraction sites but without extrusion. The U1–PP improved from 36.5 to 32.5 mm; U6–PP changed from 27.5 to 25.0 mm, and the mandibular plane decreased 3.0°. The chin projection was improved by the counterclockwise rotation of the mandible. Thirty-three months after completion of treatment, there was minimal change in incisor position (Fig. 38.2C,M,N,O).

CASE 3: INDIRECT ANCHORAGE WITHOUT ALVEOLOPLASTY FOR PROTRUSIVE MAXILLARY ANTERIOR TEETH AND A GUMMY SMILE

A 16-year-old girl presented with chief complaints of protrusive maxillary anterior teeth and a gummy smile. She had a convex profile, protrusive upper lip, recessive chin, lip incompetence and mentalis muscle strain. She also had 6 mm of gingival display in her full smile and the maxillary midline was coincident to her facial midline (Fig. 38.3A).

Her lower dental midline deviated 2 mm to her right side; the molar relationship on the right side was Class II and on the left side was Class I (Fig. 38.3C). The overjet was 6 mm, while the overbite was 3 mm. Both the maxillary and mandibular dental arch forms were ovoid and symmetrical with mild anterior crowding. The space deficiency was 2.0 mm in the maxillary arch and 4.0 mm in the mandibular arch. The clinical crown lengths of the maxillary central incisors and of the other anterior teeth were within the normal range; however, their gingival margins were uneven. The probing depths of periodontal pockets of the maxillary anterior teeth were between 2.0 and 3.0 mm.

Panoramic radiography showed the presence of all third molars, a missing mandibular right first molar and mesial tipping of the mandibular right second molar. Analysis of the lateral cephalometric radiograph revealed skeletal Class II relationships, an obtuse ANB angle, a steep mandibular plane, a retrognathic mandible and vertical maxillary excess (U1–PP, 35.6 mm) (Table 38.4). Soft tissue analysis demonstrated an acute nasolabial angle and protrusive upper and lower lips.

The patient was diagnosed with a skeletal Class II mandibular retrognathism with steep mandibular plane, vertical maxillary excess and dental Class II, division 1, subdivision malocclusion.

The treatment objectives were (1) to relieve the anterior crowding, (2) to correct the lower dental midline, (3) to achieve Class I molar on the left and Class II molar on the right side, and (4) to improve lip posture, gummy smile and chin projection.

The treatment plan suggested was a non-surgical approach featuring closure of the mandibular right edentulous space, as well as extraction of the maxillary first premolars and of the mandibular left first premolar. Both direct and indirect anchorage would be derived from MIs. Retraction and intrusion of both dental arches was anticipated along with substantial mandibular autorotation.

Quattro screws (diameter, 2.0 mm; length, 9 mm) were inserted into the infrazygomatic crests of the maxilla and in the oblique ridges of the mandible to support bimaxillary en masse retraction and intrusion using cantilever arms, Ni-Ti closed coil springs, a transpalatal arch and a lingual holding arch as follows (Fig. 38.3D–K).

■ *Low-friction TMA archwires (0.017 × 0.025 inch) with lingual root torque for the anterior teeth.* Lingual root torque was applied to reduce lingual tipping of the incisors during retraction. Crimpable hooks were attached to the archwire about 3 mm distal to the

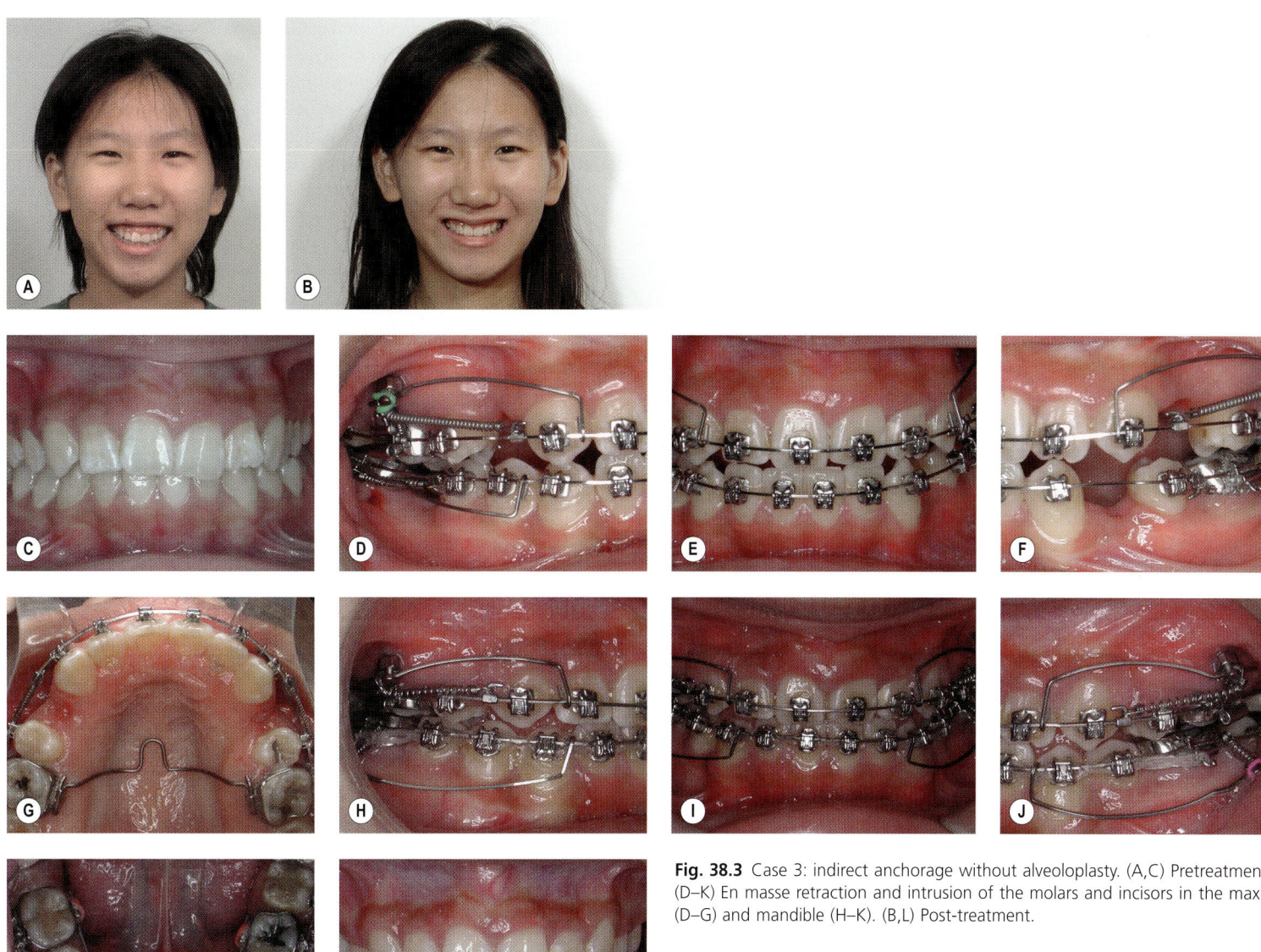

Fig. 38.3 Case 3: indirect anchorage without alveoloplasty. (A,C) Pretreatment. (D–K) En masse retraction and intrusion of the molars and incisors in the maxilla (D–G) and mandible (H–K). (B,L) Post-treatment.

brackets on the maxillary and mandibular canines and superelastic closed coil springs were stretched posteriorly to the MIs.

■ *TMA cantilever arms (0.019 × 0.025 inch) with 110° of tip-back bends.* Removable and adjustable sectional arms were inserted into one of the tubes in the heads of the Quattro screws and then hooked over the main archwire between the laterals and canines. These arms employed indirect anchorage derived from the MIs to produce light intrusive forces on the anterior teeth.

■ *Medium force Ni-Ti closed coil springs.* Closed coil springs were attached from the MIs to crimpable hooks on the main archwire to produce en masse sliding retraction of the anterior teeth. Additional springs were stretched perpendicularly from the MIs to the archwire for posterior intrusion.

■ *TMA transpalatal and lingual holding arches (0.032 inch).* A transpalatal arch and a lower lingual arch were constructed from TMA wire featuring double backs for insertion into the lingual sheaths of the first molars. The double-back portions of these removable arches were bent with 6° of mesial angulation and 10° of buccal root torque to prevent the molars from "rolling out" during simultaneous posterior intrusion and en masse retraction.

Table 38.4 Case3: cephalometric data		
Variables	**Pretreatment**	**Post-treatment**
SNA (°)	80	79
SNB (°)	72	72
ANB (°)	8	5
MPA (°)	46	44
U1-SN (°)	103	94
IMPA (°)	97	96
U6-PP (mm)	23.7	19.7
U1-PP (mm)	35.6	28.1

MP, mandibular plane; PP, palatal plane; IMPA, incisor mandibular plane angle.

After 27 months, the treatment objectives were achieved. More specifically, the patient's facial profile, lip posture, gummy smile and chin projection were all improved (Fig. 38.3B,L). The maxillary incisor clinical crown length and the probing depth of their periodontal pockets were similar before and after treatment. No alveoloplasty was performed. The post-treatment cephalometric analysis demonstrated that U1–PP was reduced from 35.6 to 28.1 mm; U6–PP was improved from 23.7 to 19.7 mm, and the mandibular plane decreased 2.0° (Table 38.4). Cephalometric superimpositions revealed an "orthognathic-like" treatment effect, including vertical shortening of the entire maxillary dentoalveolar process, substantial maxillary and mandibular anterior retraction and intrusion. These changes resembled the effects of LeFort I maxillary impaction surgery, maxillary and mandibular anterior segmental osteotomy, and counterclockwise rotation of the mandible.

CASE 4: DIRECT ANCHORAGE WITHOUT ALVEOLOPLASTY FOR SIMULTANEOUS REDUCTION IN GUMMY SMILE AND VERTICAL DIMENSION

A 12-year-old girl presented after more than 2 years of orthodontic treatment including premolar extractions that had been performed elsewhere. She had a mildly convex profile, an acute nasolabial angle, a retrusive chin, normal upper lip length, lip incompetence and a mentalis strain upon lip closure. More than 5 mm of gingival display was apparent in her posed smile. She had bilateral Class I canine and molar relationships; the extraction spaces were still evident, and the maxillary anterior teeth had been extruded and tipped lingually (Fig. 38.4A,C). The clinical crown lengths of the maxillary central incisors and other anterior teeth were normal with no periodontal burdens, despite poor oral hygiene. She had a Class I relationship, an obtuse mandibular plane and a retrognathic chin. The etiology of the excessive gingival display appeared to be skeletal and dental in origin.[12]

Orthodontic treatment focused on the following issues: (1) completion of extraction space closure with root parallelism, (2) management of the vertical dimension during future facial growth, (3) improvement in the overbite/overjet, (4) reduction of the lip incompetency, and (5) application of biomechanics not dependent upon patient compliance. Ideally, treatment would have used Tweed biomechanics of setting anchorage, intruding the incisors during space closure, controlling vertical dimension and producing counterclockwise rotation of the occlusal plane anchored by J-hook highpull headgear. However, as this patient had already endured the typical timeframe for a course of orthodontic treatment, she was uninterested in complying with headgear, and even oral hygiene was problematic. Consequently, it was decided to employ direct anchorage derived from MIs in both dental arches to support all these planned teeth movements.

A mandibular lingual arch was installed and MIs (diameter, 1.6 mm; length, 8 mm) were inserted between the mandibular first and second molars. Elastic separators were stretched from the first molar tubes to the MIs to provide posterior intrusive force (transmitted through a continuous rectangular steel archwire) in order to maintain the vertical dimension and counteract any extrusion resulting from Class II elastics wear.

MIs (diameter, 1.6 mm; length, 6 mm) were also inserted between the roots of the maxillary central and lateral incisors (Fig. 38.4D–F). These were used for direct anchorage support of elastic forces to intrude the maxillary anterior teeth. Retraction and intrusion of the anterior dental segment was accomplished using an asymmetrical TMA T-loop with accentuated curve of Spee (0.017 × 0.025 inch).[13] The combination of these biomechanics was intended to control the vertical dimension and occlusal plane. Despite the use of the rectangular wire for retraction, there was no improvement in the incisal angulation. Consequently, an anterior root torquing auxiliary was utilized to facilitate lingual root torque for the incisors. Upon removal of her appliances, the patient wore a custom positioner 24 hours a day for 1 week to accentuate "settling" of her occlusion, followed by overlay retainers.

The resulting elimination of this patient's chief complaint of gummy smile without employing a J-hook headgear (Fig. 38.4B,G) was accentuated by the improvement in her facial profile and lip incompetency, even

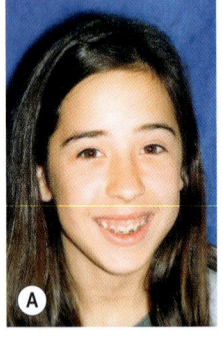
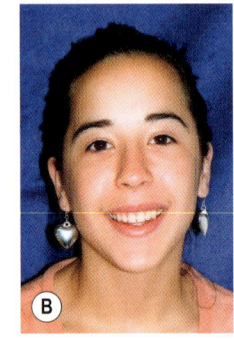
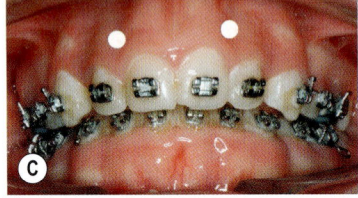
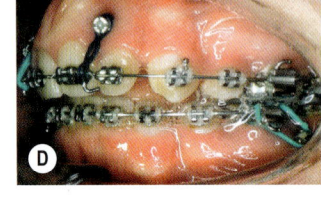
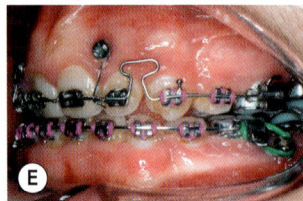
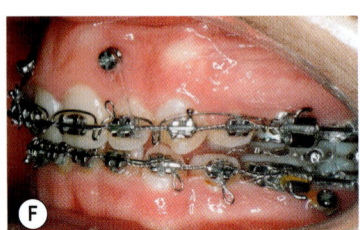
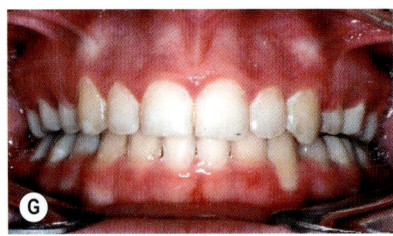
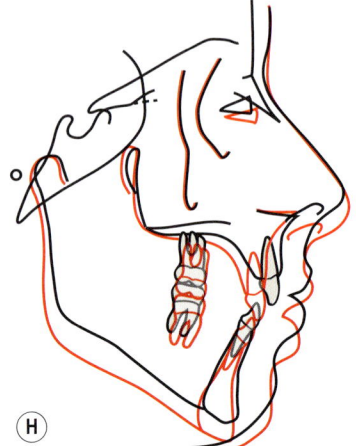

Fig. 38.4 Case 4: direct anchorage without alveoloplasty. (A,C) Pretreatment (after more than 2 years of orthodontic treatment with premolar extractions performed elsewhere). (D–F) Insertion of two miniscrew implants (MIs) in the maxillary anterior alveolus and closed loop mechanics, as well as after insertion of two MIs between the lower molars. (B,G) Post-treatment. (H) Superimposition on the anterior cranial base of the pretreatment (black line) and post-treatment (red line) cephalometric tracings.

considering the continued facial growth she exhibited during treatment (Fig. 38.4H).

DISCUSSION

Although orthognathic surgery was a treatment option to reduce vertical maxillary excess and the associated gummy smile for all the patients described in this chapter, all elected to pursue non-surgical approaches. This decision was based, at least in part, on concerns that the nasal alar base tends to widen with Le Fort I impaction procedures and that jaw surgery carries some risk of serious sequelae, such as excessive hemorrhage, infection, loss of tooth vitality, periodontal problems, plus the risks inherent with anesthesia. In contrast, orthodontic treatment, including the insertion of MIs, offered fewer risks and potential side effects. The disadvantage is that it requires substantially more time for the correction to occur.

Two of the patients required alveoloplasty procedures to eliminate iatrogenic bony protuberances that were produced by substantial incisor intrusion and retraction. The risks associated with these periodontal surgical procedures are substantially less than those associated with orthognathic surgery. Two patients did not require alveoloplasty. Individual variations of bone physiology may play an important role in deciding whether short clinical crowns necessitating alveoloplasty will result from these types of biomechanics.

Two of the patients had sufficient inter-radicular space to permit safe placement of MIs between the roots of the maxillary teeth to provide direct anchorage for simple power chains to hooks on the base archwire for both intrusion and retraction. For the other two patients, alternative sites for MI placement were needed (e.g. between the roots of maxillary second premolars and first molars for Case 2, or in the infrazygomatic crests of the maxilla for Case 3) to provide indirect anchorage for intrusion using sectional mechanics.

Although non-surgical correction of skeletal origin gummy smiles appears to be quite effective for certain patients, such as the ones described here, clinicians should be cautious in deciding if a patient would benefit from this approach, avoid overly optimistic expectations and carefully evaluate any potential for relapse. In some instances, different retention strategies, such as overcorrection, slow intrusive movement to allow for neuromuscular adaptation, longer retention periods, active retention methods, and perhaps some periodontal surgical procedures (intrasulcus incision or alveoloplasty), should be employed.

There are also probable limitations to the amount of retraction/intrusion that is possible. For example, the cortex bone of the incisive canal may be the biological boundary for such types of tooth movement and impacting that bone could result in external apical root resorption.[14]

CONCLUSIONS

Soft tissue and smile esthetics are often major concerns for patients. While the surgical–orthodontic approach has often been the only recommended solution for skeletal origin gummy smiles, for a number of reasons orthognathic surgery is not always acceptable for patients. The new non-surgical alternative proposed here combines MI-anchored orthodontic treatment and alveoloplasty to simulate an orthognathic-like treatment effect. The advantages of this new approach include:

- avoiding the risks inherent to orthognathic surgery
- simple and reliable orthodontic biomechanics
- no substantial discomfort compared with surgery
- cost effective
- no change in alar base or the midface, which can accompany surgery.

It appears that orthodontists now have a viable option to orthognathic surgery for patients presenting with a gummy smile since more predictable, effective and efficient tooth movements are possible using MI anchorage.

REFERENCES

1. Hugh O, Johnston C, Hepper P, et al. The influence of maxillary gingival exposure on dental attractiveness. Eur J Orthod 2002;24:199–204.
2. Sarver DM, Proffit WR, Ackerman JL. Diagnosis and treatment planning in orthodontics. In: Graber TM, editor. Orthodontics: current principles and techniques. 3rd ed. St. Louis: Mosby; 2000. p. 65–109.
3. Silberberg N, Goldstein M, Smidt A. Excessive gingival display: etiology,diagnosis, and treatment modalities. Quintessence Int 2009;40:809–18.
4. Liou EJW, Lin JCY. The appliances, mechanics, and treatment strategies toward orthognathic-like treatment results. In: Nanda R, editor. Temporary anchorage devices in orthodontics. St. Louis, MO: Elsevier; 2008. p. 167–97.
5. Wu H, Lin J, Zhou L, et al. Classification and craniofacial features of gummy smile in adolescents. J Craniofac Surg 2010;21:1474–9.
6. Chiche GJ. Proportion, display and length for successful esthetic planning. In: Cohen M, editor. Interdisciplinary treatment planning, principle, design, implementation. Chicago, Berlin: Quintessence; 2008. p. 1–48.
7. Sarver D. Principles of cosmetic dentistry in orthodontics: Part 1. Shape and proportionality of anterior teeth. Am J Orthod Dentofacial Orthop 2004;126:749–53.
8. Lin JCY, Liou EJW. A new bone screw for orthodontic anchorage. J Clin Orthod 2003;37:676–81.
9. Lin JCY, Liou EJW, Yeh CL. Intrusion of over-erupted maxillary molars with miniscrew anchorage. J Clin Orthod 2006;40:378–83.
10. Liou EJW, Lin JCY. The Lin/Liou Orthodontic Mini Anchor System (LOMAS). In: Cope JB, editor. OrthoTADs: the clinical guide and atlas. Dallas, TX: Under Dog Media; 2007. p. 213–30.
11. Poggio PM, Incorvati C, Velo S, et al. "Safe zones": a guide for miniscrew positioning in the maxillary and mandibular arch. Angle Orthod 2006;76:191–7.
12. Lin JCY, Yeh CL, Liou EJW, et al. Treatment of skeletal-origin gummy smiles with miniscrew anchorage. J Clin Orthod 2008;42:285–96.
13. Hilgers JJ, Farzin-Nia F. Adjuncts to bioprogressive therapy: the asymmetrical "T" archwire. J Clin Orthod 1992;26:81–6.
14. Mimura H. Treatment of severe bimaxillary protrusion with microimplant anchorage: treatment and complications. Aust Orthod J 2008;24:156–63.

39 Altering the smile line with miniscrew implant-supported biomechanics

James Cheng-Yi Lin, Eric Jein-Wein Liou, S. Jay Bowman and George Anka

INTRODUCTION

Although orthodontics involves more than simply improving patients' smiles, the esthetic display of teeth is certainly one of the primary motivating factors for seeking orthodontic treatment. Challenges in using appropriately controlled mechanics to improve proper function while producing favorable esthetics have been enhanced with the availability of miniscrew implant (MI) anchorage. This chapter describes the management of the vertical dimension by either decreasing gingival display via intrusion or by improving the smile line via extrusion.

INCREASING INCISOR DISPLAY

Insufficient maxillary incisor display may result from a variety of factors (e.g. short face heights, anterior open bites) (Table 39.1).[1] If the etiology is primarily skeletal in nature, then combined surgical–orthodontic treatment is often suggested. As an alternative, a successful non-surgical treatment to improve smile line used a modified lip bumper, rapid palatal expansion and elastics.[2] The case below illustrates the use of MI-supported biomechanics to provide a non-surgical option.

CASE 1: IMPROVING SMILE LINE ACCOMPANYING SHORT FACE HEIGHT

A 28-year-old woman presented with a chief complaint of insufficient display of the maxillary incisors. She exhibited a straight profile, obtuse nasolabial angle, short upper lip length and a mildly prominent chin button. Less than 20% of the clinical crown length of the maxillary incisors could be seen in her full smile. Intraoral examination demonstrated a Class I relationship with favorable periodontal health. However, multiple posterior teeth were missing and she had a fractured dental bridge (Fig. 39.1A,D). Cephalometric analysis revealed that the insufficient incisor display was a result of maxillary vertical deficiency (Table 39.2).

Two treatment options were offered: (1) traditional orthodontic treatment in combination with Le Fort I osteotomy, including downgrafting, to increase maxillary height, and (2) MI-based orthodontic mechanics to extrude the maxillary dentition (Fig. 39.1H–O). The intent of dental extrusion was to increase the lower anterior face height and to increase incisor display during smiling.

The patient provided her informed consent to the more conservative method after the risks and benefits had been discussed.

Treatment Progress

Treatment was initiated using fixed preadjusted appliances (0.022 inch) for leveling and alignment. After 6 months, the fractured upper left bridge was removed and replaced with a temporary resin bridge, which was constructed with elongated crowns. This "bridge" served as a "bite opener" to assist in increasing the patient's vertical dimension. "Propping open" the bite facilitated the extrusion of the maxillary dentition (except of the bridge abutments).

Two weeks later, a thermal Ni-Ti wire (0.016 × 0.022 inch) was inserted into the edgewise slots of all brackets, except those on the maxillary central incisors, where the wire was laid just apical to the gingival tie wings of the brackets to initiate sequential extrusion of the maxillary anterior teeth (Fig. 39.1H,I). To control the reciprocal forces on the lateral incisors (i.e. anchoring the extrusion of the central incisors), intermaxillary elastics (50 g) were hooked from the lateral incisors down to one LOMAS Hook MI (diameter, 2 mm; length, 9 mm; Mondeal Medical, Tuttlingen, Germany), which had been inserted, angled apically, in the mandibular symphysis below the roots of the mandibular central incisors.[3]

At the next visit, the upper wire was positioned apical to the lateral incisor brackets to extrude them (Fig. 39.1J,K). The elastics were also moved sequentially to the next teeth down the line. The patient was also asked to wear "up-and-down" intermaxillary elastics from the maxillary to mandibular first molars (Fig. 39.1H–O). The intent of the combined anterior and posterior elastics was to extrude the anterior teeth but also to counteract the reciprocal intrusive forces on the posterior teeth, thereby altering the facial profile and improving the smile line.

Table 39.1 Possible etiologies and treatment strategies for insufficient maxillary incisor display

Origin	Etiology	Treatment strategy
Dental	Short clinical crown length	Increase clinical crown length using crown, veneer, periodontal surgery
	Flared maxillary incisors	Orthodontic torque and/or retraction
Skeletal	Vertical maxilla deficiency	Maxillary downgrafting with Le Fort I osteotomy
Muscular	Hypoactivity of the elevator muscle of the upper lip	Smile trainer
	Long upper lip length	Lip lift surgery
	Aging	Face lift
Combination	Combination etiologies	Combination treatments

Table 39.2 Case 1: cephalometric data

Variables	Pretreatment	Post-treatment
SNA (°)	84	83.5
SNB (°)	80.5	78
ANB (°)	3.5	5.5
MPA (°)	27	31
U1-SN (°)	108	99.5
IMPA (°)	99	99.5
U6-PP (mm)	23.0	25.0
U1-PP (mm)	27.5	31.0
L6-MP (mm)	30.0	32.5
L1-MP (mm)	37.0	38.5

MP, mandibular plane; MPA, mandibular plane angle; PP, palatal plane; SN, sella-nasion; IMPA, incisor mandibular plane angle.

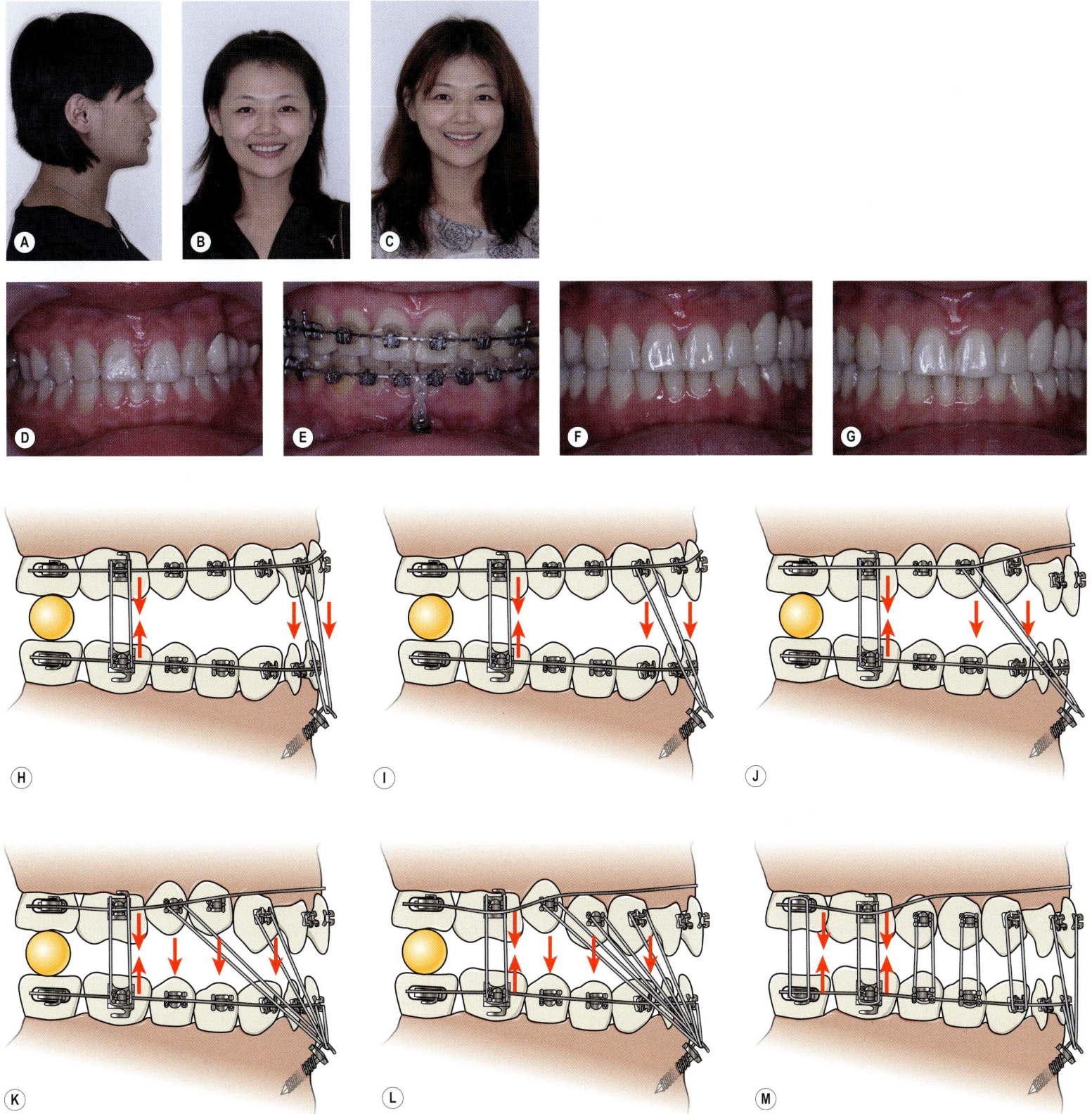

Fig. 39.1 Case 1: improving smile line accompanying short face height. (A,D) Pretreatment. (H–O) Biomechanics for sequential extrusion of the maxillary dentition from anterior to posterior teeth in order to improve the maxillary vertical deficiency and increase anterior dental display. (H,I) A posterior bite block is used to prop open the anterior bite in order to facilitate extrusion of the anterior teeth. The archwire is initially placed just apical to the central incisors to extrude them. Elastics are worn from the maxillary lateral incisors to a miniscrew implant (MI) inserted in the mandibular symphysis and also from upper to lower molar. (J,K) The archwire is placed apical to the canine bracket and then on the first premolar bracket to continue the extrusion process. Elastics are also moved to the next adjacent tooth distal to the one to be extruded. (L,M) The process of individual tooth extrusion continues to the first molar, then "up-and-down" elastics are worn on every tooth. (N,O) Increasing the extrusion of the upper incisors and deepening the overbite can be achieved using elastics from the anterior teeth to the MI inserted in the symphysis. (E) To satisfy the patient's desire for even more incisor display, the anterior teeth were further extruded using elastics from the canines to the mandibular MI while simultaneously intruding the mandibular incisors with elastic chains from the same MI. (B,F) Post-treatment after 24 months of treatment. (P) Overall superimposition on sella–nasion line demonstrates the intended changes: extrusion of the maxillary dentition, increase in lower anterior face height and clockwise rotation of the mandible. (C,G) At 18 months after treatment completion.

Continued

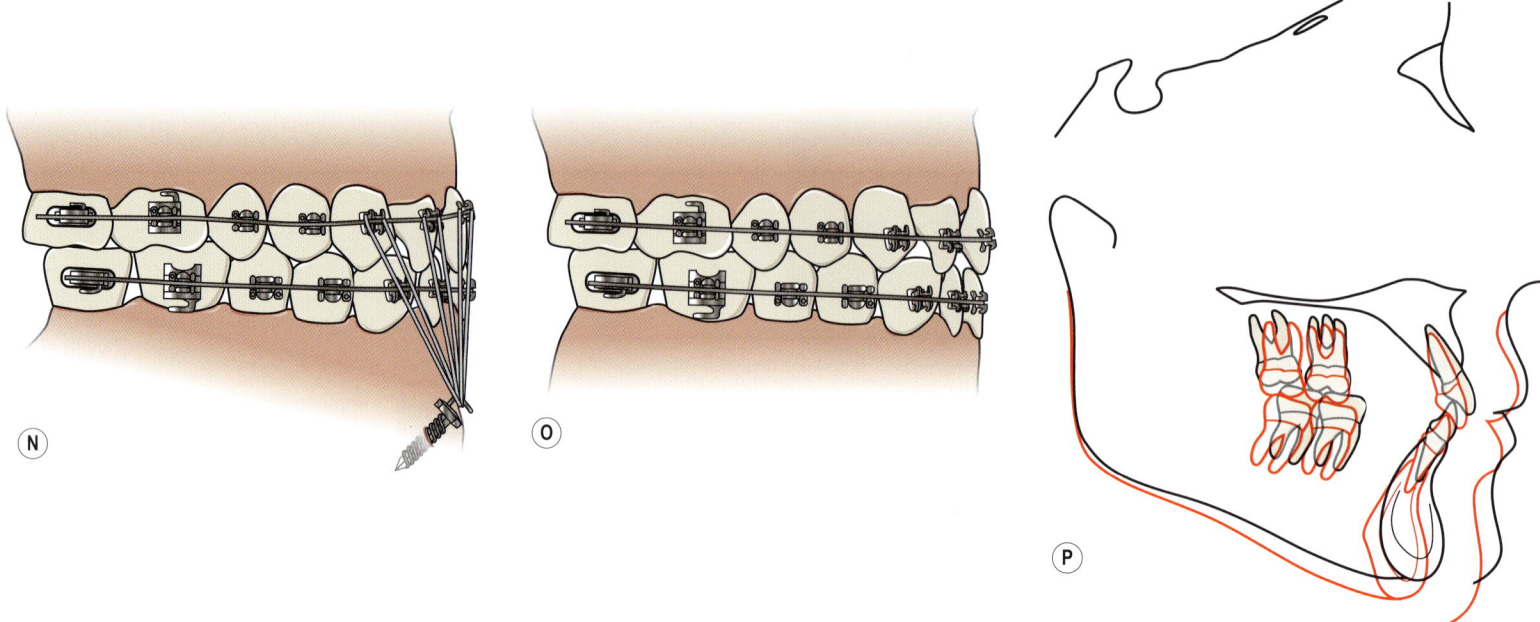

Fig. 39.1, cont'd

After 11 months of treatment, the temporary resin bridge was sectioned to permit some movement of the abutments. Three months later, the patient requested an even greater increase of incisor display. In order to achieve this goal, the mandibular anterior teeth were intruded using elastic chains extended from the MI positioned on the symphysis directly to the lower archwire, while simultaneously extruding the maxillary incisors with an additional intermaxillary elastic worn to the same MI (Fig. 39.1L,M,E).

Twenty months after the start of treatment, the patient's original insufficient incisor display had been dramatically improved without orthognathic surgery. Final cephalometric data are shown in Table 39.2.

After completion of orthodontic treatment, prosthetic replacements for the missing teeth were placed (Fig. 39.1F).

Treatment Results

After 24 months of orthodontic care, there were clear improvements in facial and smile esthetics: substantial maxillary incisor display was achieved, which answered the patient's original complaint (Fig. 39.1B,F,P).

Cephalometric superimposition revealed significant positional change of the maxillary dentition, similar to that produced in LeFort I downgrafting (Fig. 39.1P). Interestingly enough, the mandibular teeth exhibited some extrusion despite the intrusive forces applied from the MI in the symphysis. The patient's chin projection became less prominent as a result of the clockwise rotation of the mandible and the increased lower anterior facial height. These positive changes appear to be stable 18 months after the completion of treatment (Fig. 39.1C,G). Nevertheless, the stability of these types of change in the vertical dimension has been a subject of debate.[4,5]

The same biomechanics were applied in the following case, which illustrates further the insertion location of the Hook MI in the symphysis.

INCREASING INCISOR DISPLAY IN ANTERIOR OPEN BITE

Some patients with anterior open bite exhibit also a so-called "reverse smile line," which could benefit from not only posterior intrusion but also from some limited anterior extrusion to close the bite and improve smile esthetics. In other instances, the process of orthodontic leveling and alignment may inadvertently create or exacerbate an anterior open bite by unintended extrusion of posterior teeth: "propping open the bite."

CASE 2: OPEN BITE AND POOR SMILE

A woman presented with a chief complaint of an open bite and "upside-down smile," which could be improved with simultaneous intrusion of the posterior and extrusion of the anterior teeth (Fig. 39.2A,C–E).

Treatment Progress

Two Aarhus MIs (length, 6 mm; American Orthodontics, Sheyboygan, WI, USA) were inserted between the roots of the maxillary first molars and second premolars to provide direct anchorage for intrusion of the posterior teeth. Elastic chain was applied from the MI heads and looped around a rectangular archwire (0.019 × 0.025 inch). A third MI was inserted between the maxillary central incisors, adjacent to the midline frenum, with the MI angled apically by 10° (Fig. 39.2F–H).

The larger helix of a Ulysses extrusion auxiliary spring (American Orthodontics) (Fig. 39.2I) was applied over the head of the MI. The spring was activated (i.e. stretched out with the smaller loop of the spring about 5 mm incisal to the main archwire). The archwire was then inserted through the lumen of the smaller helix of the auxiliary, thereby compressing the spring between the wire and the MI. The archwire was subsequently tied into the brackets with the spring force to extrude the anterior teeth. Light-cured adhesive was placed over the head of the MI to reduce any tissue irritation. Simultaneous intrusion of the maxillary posterior teeth and extrusion of the anterior teeth was performed, which closed the open bite and improved the smile line in 6 months (Fig. 39.2B,J–L).

Treatment Results

Final results, 1 year after completion of treatment, demonstrated favorable stability.

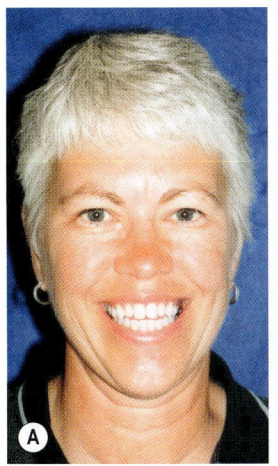
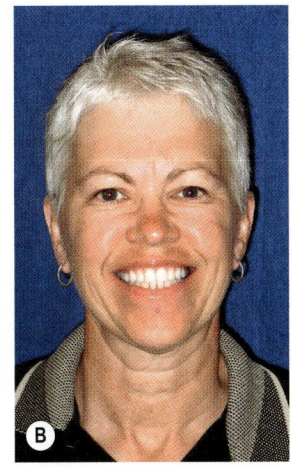

Fig. 39.2 Case 2: increasing incisor display for anterior open bite and poor smile. (A,C–E) Pretreatment. (F–H) Aarhus miniscrew implants (MIs) were inserted between maxillary posterior teeth for intrusion with direct anchorage using elastic chains around a rectangular archwire. A third MI was placed in the anterior region and a Ulysses spring was stretched from the MI to the archwire to extrude the anterior teeth, close the open bite and improve the incisor display and smile line. (I) The Ulysses extrusion auxiliary spring. (B,J–L) Post-treatment.

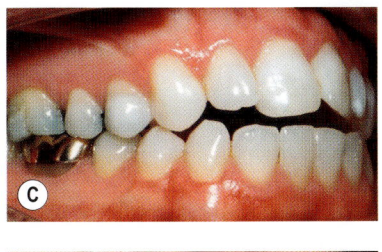
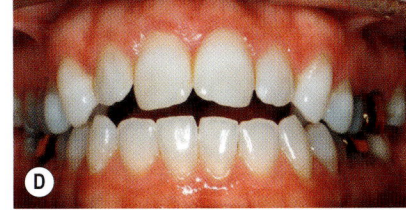
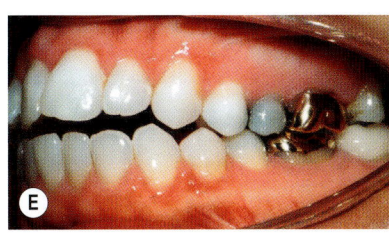
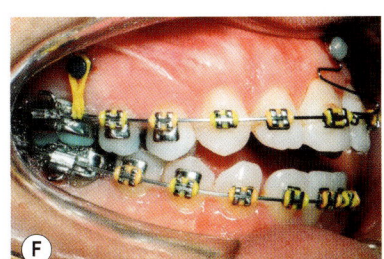
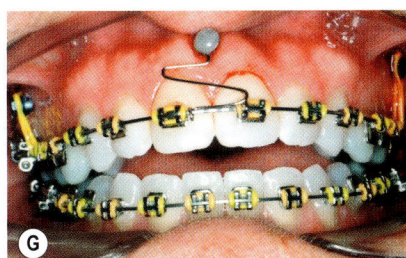
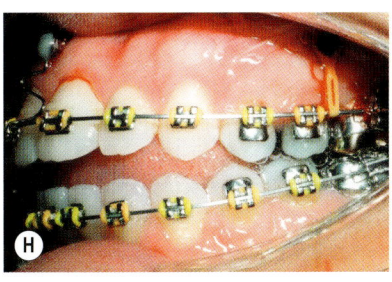
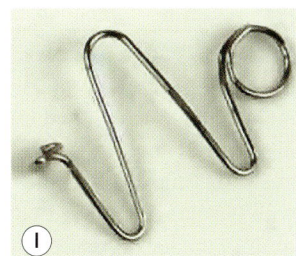
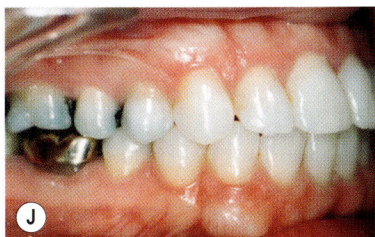
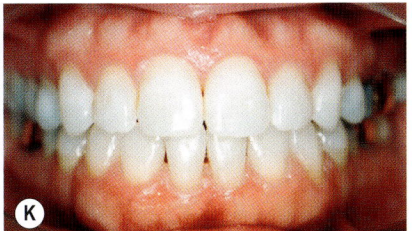
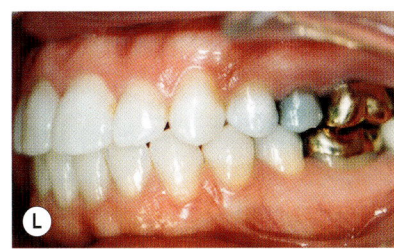

TREATMENT OF DEEP OVERBITE

Altering the smile line in deep bite requires careful diagnosis to ascertain if intrusion of anterior teeth is appropriate, as well as to determine the correct dental arch to address. A knee-jerk reaction to intrude maxillary incisors (e.g. intrusion arch or J-hook headgear) for a patient with a deep bite, but with long upper lip and minimal incisor display, would certainly be inappropriate. In some instances, intrusion of hypererupted mandibular anterior teeth may, in fact, be indicated. A number of examples are given of methods to deal with this problem.

Fig. 39.3A shows a 13-year-old boy with a deep overbite and a favorable smile line for whom maxillary anterior intrusion was contraindicated. A MI was inserted between the mandibular incisors to provide direct anchorage for intrusion of the mandibular anterior teeth. A Monkey Hook (American Orthodontics) was attached to the head of the MI and elastic thread was tied from the hook to the archwire (Fig. 39.3A). Total treatment required 26 months, but the MI was removed after 8 months of intrusion.

Indirect anchorage from MIs may also be employed for intrusion of anterior teeth. MIs, inserted between the mandibular laterals and canines,

were used to maintain leeway space to avoid extraction or unstable inter-canine expansion while resolving crowding for a 13-year-old girl with mixed dentition. Sectional square wire segments were bonded into the heads of the MIs and into auxiliary tubes on the first molars to support sequential retraction of the mandibular teeth into the residual leeway space (Fig. 39.3B). This same anchorage system then supported Class II elastics to reduce unwanted flaring of mandibular incisors or extrusion of mandibular molars. The MIs were also employed to intrude the hypererupted mandibular incisors (using elastic thread from the support wires to the base archwire).

Occasionally, simple retraction (with or without intrusion) is the key to an improved smile line. Figure 39.3C shows a 14-year-old boy with a moderate bimaxillary protrusion, some lip incompetence and mildly excessive gingival display. MIs were inserted in all four posterior quadrants (between the second premolars and first molars). Direct anchorage was employed for en masse retraction of both dental arches using elastic chain for 9 months (Fig. 39.3C). Improvement in the smile line, gingival display and facial profile were achieved in 18 months.

If, however, a gummy smile is the chief complaint, then mechanics specifically designed to intrude are compulsory (Fig. 39.3D–F).[6,7]

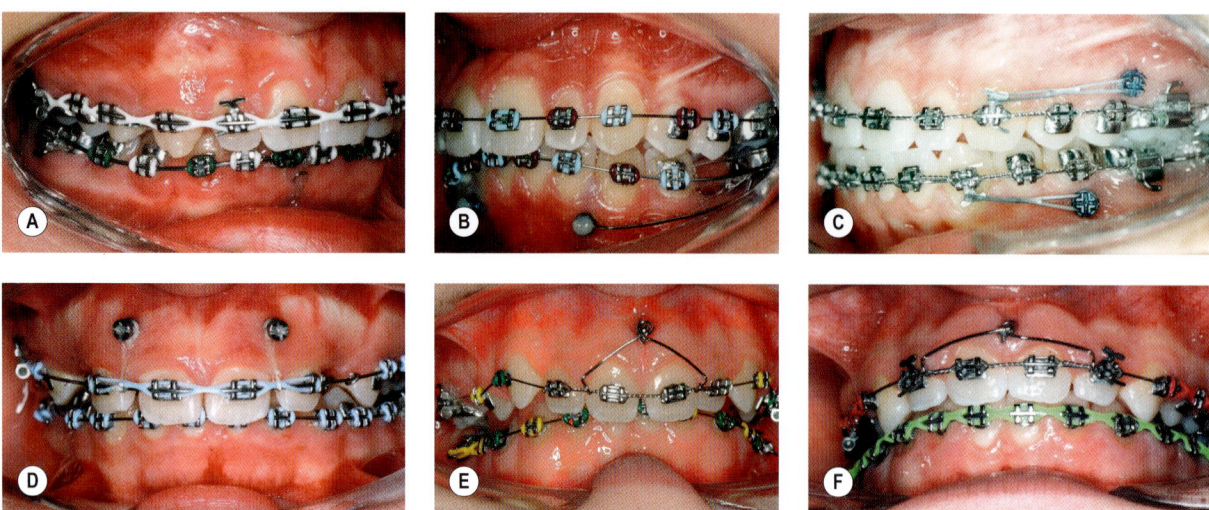

Fig. 39.3 Improving smile line for deep overbite. (A) Direct anchorage from a miniscrew implant (MI) inserted between the lower incisors for intrusion of the mandibular incisors. (B) Indirect anchorage from MIs inserted between the mandibular lateral incisors and the canines to maintain leeway space and to support sequential retraction of lower teeth into the residual leeway space. The same anchorage supported Class II elastics to reduce unwanted flaring of lower incisors and extrusion of lower molars, as well as to provide indirect anchorage to intrude the hypererupted lower incisors. (C) Direct MI anchorage in all four quadrants for bimaxillary en masse retraction to improve smile line, gingival display and facial profile. (D) Direct MI anchorage for the intrusion of maxillary anterior teeth to reduce an asymmetric gummy smile; impacted canines were exposed and erupted at the same time. (E,F) A "TAD Bite-Opening Spring" auxiliary placed on a MI to intrude the maxillary central incisors to improve the patient's smile line.

Fig. 39.3D shows a 13-year-old girl with a gummy smile, moderate overbite and also palatally impacted canines. Two MIs were inserted between the maxillary central and lateral incisors and used as direct anchorage for intrusion of the maxillary anterior teeth using elastic thread. Simultaneously, the impacted canines were surgically exposed and Monkey Hooks with elastic chains were used to pull the crowns distally, away from the roots of the lateral incisors, thereby, tipping the teeth occlusally. Only then were they moved laterally into the arch form as the smile line was improved. The patient was later referred to a periodontist to further improve her dental display.

Another option for a gummy smile as the chief complaint is to use a specific auxiliary designed to produce intrusive forces (Fig. 39.3E,F). A 13-year-old girl with concerns about her prominent canines and gum tissue display was treated with a TAD Bite Opening Spring[7] (American Orthodontics) placed over the head of a MI that had been inserted between the roots of the maxillary incisors (Fig. 39.3E). An SS ligature was inserted through the head in the neck of the MI to secure the auxiliary. The arms of this auxiliary were lifted incisally and hooked over the archwire to produce an intrusive force on the anterior teeth, supported by the MI. Improvement in the occlusal plane and smile line were achieved without a J-hook headgear and the MI removed at the halfway point of a 2-year treatment (Fig. 39.3F).

GUMMY SMILE CAUSED BY MAXILLARY ALVEOLAR EXCESS

Gummy smiles are a common complaint of patients, and their correction may be as simple as the use of a J-hook headgear. However, predictability is problematic because of issues of patient cooperation. The option of incorporating MI anchorage can improve treatment predictability through avoiding compliance issues and by reducing the side effects of reciprocal anchorage mechanisms.

Some adults with Class II, division 2 malocclusion respond favorably to mandibular anterior repositioning, and the potential for a positive response is best predicted by the difference between centric occlusion and centric relation.[9] Since in adults there is no mandibular growth to support

Class II correction, an en masse retraction of the maxillary dentition is required.

CASE 3: DEEP OVERBITE AND CONSIDERABLE GINGIVAL DISPLAY

A 24-year-old woman presented with a complaint of considerable gingival display. She had a Class II, division 2 with a deep overbite (Fig. 39.4A) and upon smiling, the right side risorius muscle contracted more, lifting the right corner of the mouth, warranting myofunctional therapy during orthodontics.[8]

Treatment Progress

MIs were inserted between the maxillary lateral incisors and canines to provide direct anchorage support for their intrusion. This area is easily accessible and the root prominences are often readily identifiable on the labial alveolus, simplifying the insertion process. Since the canine is at the corner of the arch form, the insertion angle of the MIs must be oriented distally to account for the rotation of the ovoid root.

A maxillary midline frenectomy was performed at the time of MI insertion to release tension on the upper lip, thereby reducing retention of food debris in the buccal vestibule and permitting improved oral hygiene (Fig. 39.4B). Elastic forces were applied from the MIs directly to the maxillary archwire to intrude the anterior teeth.

As this patient was likely to respond well to en masse retraction of the maxillary dentition, a Transpalatal Arch Plus Hooks (TPA-PH) device (see Chapter 37) and two additional MIs were inserted into the palatal alveolus between the roots of the second premolars and first molars (Fig. 39.4C). Elastic chains (replaced monthly) were stretched from the hooks on the TPA-PH to the MIs to produce a distalizing force of about 200 g per side, transmitted throughout the dental arch using a full-size rectangular archwire to reduce attendant dental tipping. The TPA-PH device comes in various designs that are suitable for specific patient facial patterns, bone structures and locations of the sinus (see Chapter 37). In this case, bonded anterior bite plates[10] were added to the construction of the TPA-PH to assist in correcting the overbite.

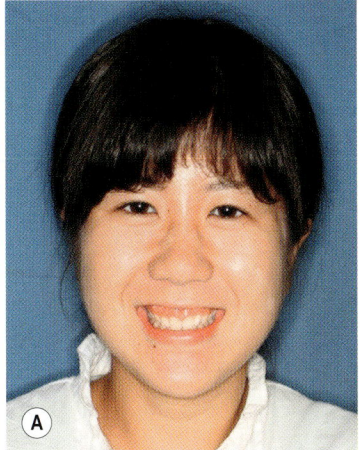

Fig. 39.4 Case 3: deep overbite and considerable gingival display. (A) Pretreatment. (B) Maxillary midline frenectomy and insertion of miniscrew implants. (C) Transpalatal Arch Plus Hooks device in place. (D) Post-treatment.

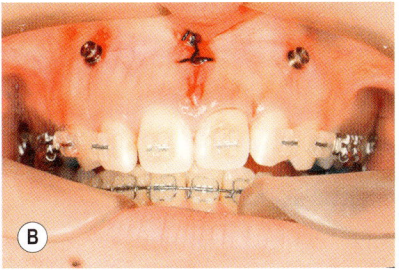
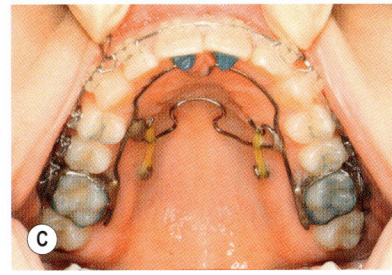
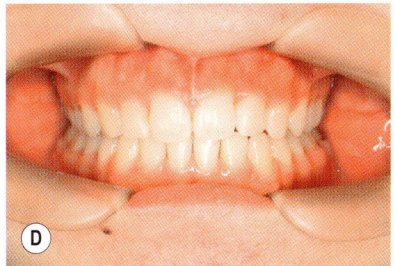

En masse maxillary retraction and intrusion of the anterior teeth was continued with the combination of TPA-PH device, anterior bite planes and Class II elastics until the centric occlusion/centric relation was deemed to be coincident. Completion of treatment required 11 months (Fig. 39.4D). Myofunctional therapy also improved the asymmetrical nature of her smile. The anterior bite plates were left in place to reduce relapse of the overbite.[10]

Treatment Results

Cephalometric superimposition demonstrated some flaring and 2 mm of intrusion of the maxillary and mandibular incisors, improved overbite and overjet, and some distalization without alteration of the mandibular plane.

IMPROVING A DEVIATED SMILE LINE

Patient perceptions of their unattractive teeth may cause them to adopt asymmetric or unnatural smiles. Both myofunctional therapy and orthodontic treatment can assist in this problem.

CASE 4: A HABITUAL ASYMMETRIC SMILE

A 15-year-old female with Class III malocclusion, featuring substantial crowding of the anterior teeth (including an impacted maxillary left canine), had assumed a habitual asymmetric smile that had warranted myofunctional therapy during her orthodontic care (Fig. 39.5A,D).[8] The original treatment plan included the extraction of maxillary second molars with an intention to open space to direct the eruption of the impacted canine.

Treatment Progress

During initial leveling and alignment, several issues become apparent: (1) an anterior open bite, (2) substantial midline deviation, (3) ankylosis

of the impacted canine and (4) canted occlusal plane (Fig. 39.5B,D). The maxillary left canine and the third molars were removed instead of the originally planned second molars. Consequently, the maxillary left posterior segment had to be moved mesially using MI anchorage and associated auxiliaries.

Asymmetric extraction exacerbated the midline deviation. Extraction of a corresponding premolar on the right side was avoided by intra-arch mechanics supported with MIs (Fig. 39.5E). MIs were inserted in the palatal alveolus between the roots of the premolars and connected with elastic chains to a TPA-PH device (with finger springs) to protract the upper left posterior dentition and simultaneously retract the right dentition.

A short propeller arm auxiliary (American Orthodontics) was connected to a MI placed in the buccal alveolus between the roots of the maxillary left premolars, and the sliding hook was fastened with SS ties to the first premolar bracket (Fig. 39.5F).[11,12] The coil spring was compressed between the MI and the premolar to protract the posterior teeth into the extraction site of the ankylosed canine. Elastic chain was also connected from an extended hook on the first molar band to the same MI anchor for additional protraction force.

After the left space was closed, a Ulysses extrusion auxiliary spring was compressed between a MI inserted between the roots of the lateral incisor and the first premolar and the anterior brackets to close the anterior left open bite (Fig. 39.5G). In the mandibular arch, minor en masse retraction of the dentition to resolve crowding was accomplished using direct anchorage from MIs inserted between the roots of the mandibular first molars and second premolars.

Treatment Results

After 36 months of treatment, significant improvement in dental and smile esthetics was achieved (Fig. 39.5C,H). Assessments of the pre- and post-treatment cephalometric radiographs showed a mild extrusion of the maxillary left posterior dentition. Although substantial improvement in the original malocclusion and the unintended iatrogenic effects that occurred

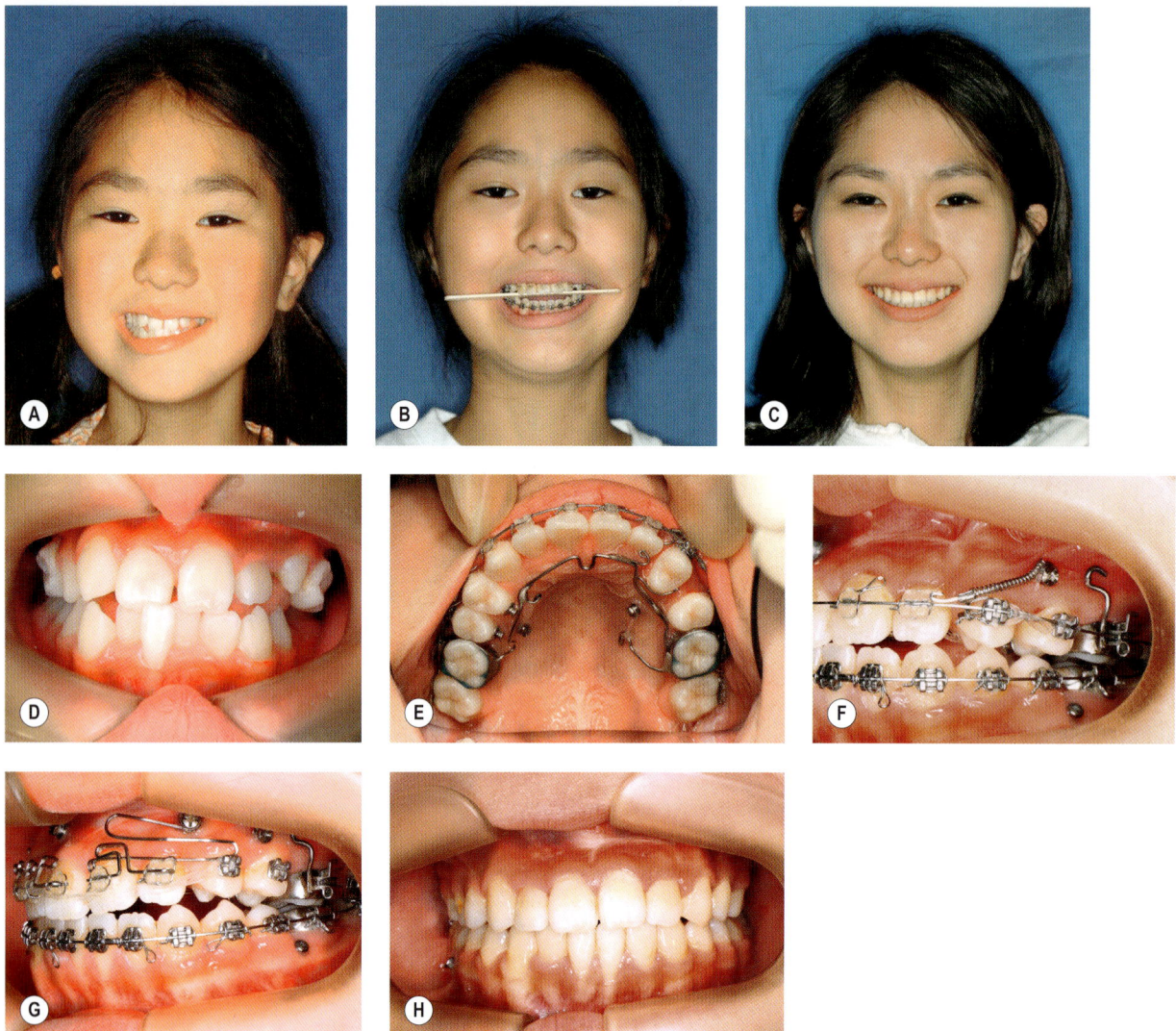

Fig. 39.5 Case 4: a habitual asymmetric smile. (A,D) Pretreatment. (B) En face during treatment indicating the canted occlusal plane. (E) The maxilla following asymmetric extraction of the ankylosed canine and insertion of miniscrew implants and the Transpalatal Arch Plus Hooks device. (F) Application of the short "propeller arm" auxiliary. (G) Application of a Ulysses extrusion auxiliary spring. (C,H) Post-treatment.

during initial leveling were accomplished during 36 months of treatment, some compromises resulted, but the overall esthetic improvement in the patient's deviated smile was significant.

DISCUSSION

Recently, orthodontists have placed great emphasis on soft tissue and smile esthetics rather than concentrating purely on tooth alignment and occlusion. This may be because the appearance of their smile is a major concern for patients, even though they may also benefit from an improvement in their bite.[13,14] Combined surgical–orthodontic options provide substantial improvements but are not always acceptable to patients. The addition of MI anchorage into the orthodontic armamentarium has improved the predictability of traditional orthodontic biomechanics and has permitted the simulation of some orthognathic effects without surgery. These types of improvement, specifically on patient smile lines, have been demonstrated in this chapter.

REFERENCES

1. Sarver DM. The importance of incisor positioning in esthetic smile: the smile arc. Am J Orthod 2001;120:98–111.

2. Paik CH, Woo YJ, Boyd RL. Non-surgical treatment of an adult skeletal Class III patient with insufficient incisor display. J Clin Orthod 2005;39:515–21.

3. Liou EJW, Lin JCY. The Lin/Liou Orthodontic Mini Anchor System (LOMAS). In: Cope JB, editor. Ortho TADs: clinical guide and atlas. Dallas, TX: Under Dog Media; 2007. p. 213–30.

4. Kokich VG. Altering vertical dimension in the perio-restorative patient: the orthodontic possibilities. In: Cohen M, editor. Interdisciplinary treatment planning, principle, design, implementation. Hanover Park, IL: Quintessence; 2008. p. 49–80.

5. Spear F, Kinzer G. Approaches to vertical dimension. In: Cohen M, editor. Interdisciplinary treatment planning, principle, design, implementation. Hanover Park, IL: Quintessence; 2008. p. 249–82.

6. Lin JCY, Yeh CL, Liou EJW, et al. Treatment of skeletal origin gummy smiles with miniscrew anchorage. J Clin Orthod 2008;42:285–96.

7. Lin JCY, Liou EJW, Bowman SJ. Simultaneous reduction in vertical dimension and gummy smile using miniscrew anchorage. J Clin Orthod 2010;44:1–14.

8. Winchell B. Orofacial myofunctional therapy for adult patients. Int J Orofacial Myol 1989;15:14–18.

9. Dawson P. Evaluation, diagnosis and treatment of occlusal problems. 2nd ed. St. Louis, MO: Mosby; 1989.

10. Carano A, Mannarini C, Bowman SJ. Deep bites: correction and retention with permanent bite planes. Ortho Prod 2006;42–5.

11. Ludwig B, Baumgaertel S, Bowman SJ. Mini-implants in orthodontics: innovative anchorage concepts. London: Quintessence; 2008.

12. Bowman SJ. Thinking outside the box with mini-screws. In: McNamara J Jr, editor. Microimplants as temporary orthodontic anchorage [Craniofacial Growth Series], vol. 45. Ann Arbor, MI: University of Michigan; 2008. p. 327–90.

13. Bowman SJ. The social six redux: is that really all there is? Ortho Tribune 2007;2:11–15.

14. Burrow SJ. Biomechanics and paradigm shift in orthodontic treatment planning. J Clin Orthod 2009;43:635–44.

Lingual orthodontics and the use of miniscrew implants for the management of Class II malocclusion in adults

Kee-Joon Lee and Young-Chel Park

40

INTRODUCTION

Classically, orthodontic treatment in adults was considered inappropriate where there was inadequate space to move teeth into, where movement of teeth against occlusal apposition or into occlusal trauma was needed, where anchorage was inadequate or where the periodontal health, function or esthetics of the teeth would not be improved. Nevertheless, ideal occlusion with proper interdigitation is still a treatment goal regardless of a patient's age. There are a number of specific issues that need to be taken into consideration before initiation of orthodontic treatment in adults.

The adult will present with a history that may include tooth wear, caries and previous prosthesis use. Preventive measures, including space maintenance around peg-shaped or fused incisors, are often impossible in adults, particularly when mesial migration of the posterior teeth has already taken up the interdental space adjacent to the target tooth. Even regaining a minor space around a small tooth may demand overall restructuring of the dentition, including molar distalization. Consequently, making a provisional cast is essential to assess the specific type and amount of tooth movement possible at each area and if a radical change in the molar relation may be indicated.

Adults will also present with variations in alveolar bone thickness. Reduced alveolar bone height is a significant risk factor in orthodontic treatment in adults as this will alter the center of resistance (CR) of teeth. Consequently, a force-driven appliance should be selected that can deliver a precision force system, for example extension of a lever arm. The posterior segment may also have some alveolar bone loss, which would suggest that reciprocal anchorage within the arch may not be suitable and bone-borne temporary anchorage devices may better serve the purpose.

As bone formation capacity diminishes with age, treatment for the relief of crowding in adults should avoid modalities such as incisor flaring or transversal expansion that are regarded as tooth movement against the thin labial/buccal cortical plate, as these may cause irreversible gingival recession or bony dehiscences. The third approach, molar distalization, takes place within the alveolar housing and is, therefore, considered a safer way to regain the space in the arch than the other types of tooth movement (Table 40.1).

Temporomandibular joint disorders are also prevalent in young adults, with clicking, crepitus and limitation of mouth opening as major symptoms. Idiopathic condylar resorption, which mainly occurs in young females in their late teens and early twenties, is considered a major pathological sequence that eventually alters the facial morphology into a Class II profile with mandibular retrusion and open bite. Although condylar change is prevalent in many Class II patients with retrusive mandibles, it is not clear whether the Class II morphology is a cause or a result of the morphological change. There are no clear guidelines for detection or prevention of the pathology. Orthodontists are advised to avoid the use of intermaxillary elastics in these patients in order to minimize or eliminate possible loading of the joint. Once again, this indicates that the anchorage for either incisors or molars should be established within the arch, necessitating the use of MIs.

BIOMECHANICAL CONSIDERATIONS

Class II malocclusion has been shown to be more common than Class III malocclusion in many ethnic groups.[1] Class II means not only a Class II denture relation but also a Class II skeletal/facial pattern, represented by a convex profile, retrusive mandible and protrusive upper lips. Treatment plans should be tailored to the individual patient's needs but the following issues should be taken into account.

ESTHETICS OF APPLIANCE

Esthetic issues during treatment are significant for the majority of adults, who prefer lingual or clear appliances over the more highly visible labial (buccal) appliances.[2] Although removable clear plastic appliances provide esthetics and comfort, as they can be removed for eating and cleaning, the type of tooth movement that can be induced is significantly limited. In contrast, lingual fixed appliances can overcome these technical limitations, although they do have difficulties for speech and maintenance of oral hygiene. So-called lingual treatment does not necessarily mean that all of the attachments must be located on the lingual sides of the teeth. Patients are mainly concerned about the exposure of the attachments during normal function, such as speech, mastication and smiling. Therefore, esthetics of the maxillary anterior teeth is usually the major concern. Labial/buccal attachments may be included if these are in areas other than the maxillary anterior region, and some clear attachments, such as clear plastic buttons, can also be used. Awareness of this flexibility will expand the scope of lingual orthodontics that can be offered.

CONTINUOUS OR SEGMENTAL APPROACHES

In most adults with tight occlusions and possibly some degree of alveolar bone loss, precision tooth movement without round tripping is an absolute requirement, since a jiggling type of movement can be detrimental. Careful assessment of the required tooth movement followed by use of the continuous or the segmented approach, depending on the purpose, is advised. If movement of a specific teeth segment is not desired, additional temporary

Table 40.1 Effect of tooth movements on esthetics, function and safety

	Anterior flaring	Transverse expansion	Distalization
Esthetics	Poor	Not much	N/S
Function	Not much	Risky (tipping)	N/S
Safety	Risky	Very risky (tipping, adults)	high

N/S, Not significant.

anchorage devices such as MIs can be used to move the target segment that has to be moved.

EXTRUSIVE OR INTRUSIVE MECHANICS

Class II intermaxillary elastics tend to extrude both maxillary incisors and mandibular molars, contributing to a posteroinferior rotation of the mandible and an increase in the vertical dimension. Even without intermaxillary elastics, vertical bowing of a continuous arch often causes extrusion of the posterior teeth, which, in turn, leads to opening of the mandibular plane and worsens the Class II profile. Therefore, extrusion of a tooth/teeth segment is contraindicated in most Class II patients. Careful application of intrusive mechanics is recommended. The use of MIs inserted in the interdental alveolar region is, therefore, justified in that they create intrusive force vectors.[3]

MINISCREW IMPLANTS

The monocortical type of MIs is versatile, economic and less invasive than other types of bone-borne anchorage devices, such as miniplates, onplants and dental implants.

From a biomechanical standpoint, the force applied using MIs as anchors can be characterized as a constant single line of force, moderate in amount and intrusive. This makes MIs very advantageous anchorage modalities in treating adults with Class II malocclusion.

As lingual appliances are normally attached on the lingual sides of the teeth, both lingual and palatal alveolar areas may be readily used for MI insertion to allow direct application of forces from the MIs to the archwires. MIs can be effective for both incisor and molar correction in Class II patients.

The main insertion sites for MIs in the maxilla are the buccal and palatal interdental alveolar areas (Fig. 40.1A,B).[4] It is recommended that longer MIs are used on the palatal side than on the buccal side, for example, 7 mm on the buccal and at least 8–9 mm on the palatal side (Fig. 40.1B). To avoid damage to adjacent roots, sufficient inter-radicular space and bone thickness needs to be secured. In the maxilla, inter-radicular areas between the second premolars and first molars, and between the first and second molars, are regarded as safe insertion sites (Fig. 40.1C). Placement on the lingual side avoids any risk of damage to the major nerves and vessels that run along the palatal side. Extension of a lever arm is easier on the maxillary palatal side than on the labial side and will allow control of the type of tooth movement using the line of force. The midpalate is a reliable insertion site, particularly for lingual appliances. Variable molar and/or incisor control is feasible using midpalatal MIs. However, midpalatal MIs will create a vertical force vector, which leads to intrusive movement of the target segment.

There are fewer suitable sites for MIs in the mandible because of the presence of the tongue although both buccal and lingual alveolar inter-radicular areas are available for insertion. Buccal bone thickness and inter-radicular space in the premolar and molar region are sufficient to maintain the MI in place, but the retromolar area has thick soft tissue covering dense cortical bone and this can cause difficulties in MI maintenance (Fig. 40.1D). The retromolar area is regarded as a stable MI insertion site during mandibular teeth distalization and uprighting.

PRACTICAL GUIDELINES FOR CLASS II LINGUAL ORTHODONTICS

TREATMENT GOALS

Treatment goals should be visualized prior to treatment, in particular from the occlusal view.

Tooth Movements

The amount and direction of tooth movement and the arch length discrepancy should be quantified in each quadrant, with the midline as the reference line. This allows the amount of either symmetric or asymmetric tooth movement at each side to be assessed, particularly when the initial occlusal relationship is asymmetric. The clinician must also determine whether a specific tooth/teeth segment has to be moved or not by defining the amount of required movement, sagittal, vertical and transverse, in each quadrant using imaging.

The type of tooth movement in anterior and posterior segments should also be defined before treatment: tipping, translation, root movement or intrusive/extrusive. For example, in the anterior segment, flared incisors may need to be uprighted via controlled tipping, whereas transition from a Class II to Class I molar relationship may be accomplished mainly through posterior translation of the maxillary molars or anterior translation of the mandibular molars.

Incisor Relations

In skeletal Class II patients, the common approach for anteroposterior dental compensation in the incisor region includes labial flaring of the mandibular incisors and/or lingual inclination of the maxillary incisors.[5] This reflects the adaptation of the dentoalveolar complex within the soft tissue envelope during growth. In contrast, the decompensation indicated before orthognathic surgery often includes a tipping (uprighting) movement of the incisors toward an ideal position within the basal bones: lingual tipping of mandibular incisors and labial tipping of maxillary incisors. However, in order to attempt a successful camouflage treatment with an ideal occlusion and desirable esthetics in spite of the underlying skeletal discrepancy, it is crucial to move not only the crown but also the root of the tooth, implying the need for translational movement instead of tipping. The required type of tooth movement is often translation of the maxillary incisors and uprighting of the mandibular incisors. Hence, removable appliances are not readily indicated for camouflage treatment as they cannot move the roots of the teeth. Fixed appliances that can deliver a precision force system are better indicated for most patients requiring camouflage treatment.

There are two ways to control incisor movement: by changing the moment-to-force ratio applied to a bracket or by changing the line of force by extending lever arms from the main archwire.

Translation of maxillary incisors with a line of force at the palatal side of the arch can be easy. The palatal vault is normally deeper than the labial/buccal vestibule and, therefore, the clinician can extend longer lever arms than on the labial side. Long lever arms may induce translation or root movement depending on the position of the line of force relative to the CR of the tooth. Incisors with reduced alveolar bone height need longer lever arms since the CR is lowered in relation to the alveolar bone height.

MOLAR DISTALIZATION IN CLASS II MALOCCLUSION

Precise anteroposterior control of the molars is often indicated in Class II camouflage treatment. Assuming that the initial molar relation tends to be Class II, treatment objectives with regard to molar control can be twofold; mesial movement of molars into a full cusp Class II position or distalization into complete Class I position. The former is mainly indicated where extractions are used, the latter with no extractions.

Molar correction can be by single tooth movement (Fig. 40.2A,B) or segmental movement (Fig. 40.2C,D). Single tooth control needs precision appliance construction when it comes to translation or root movement. In

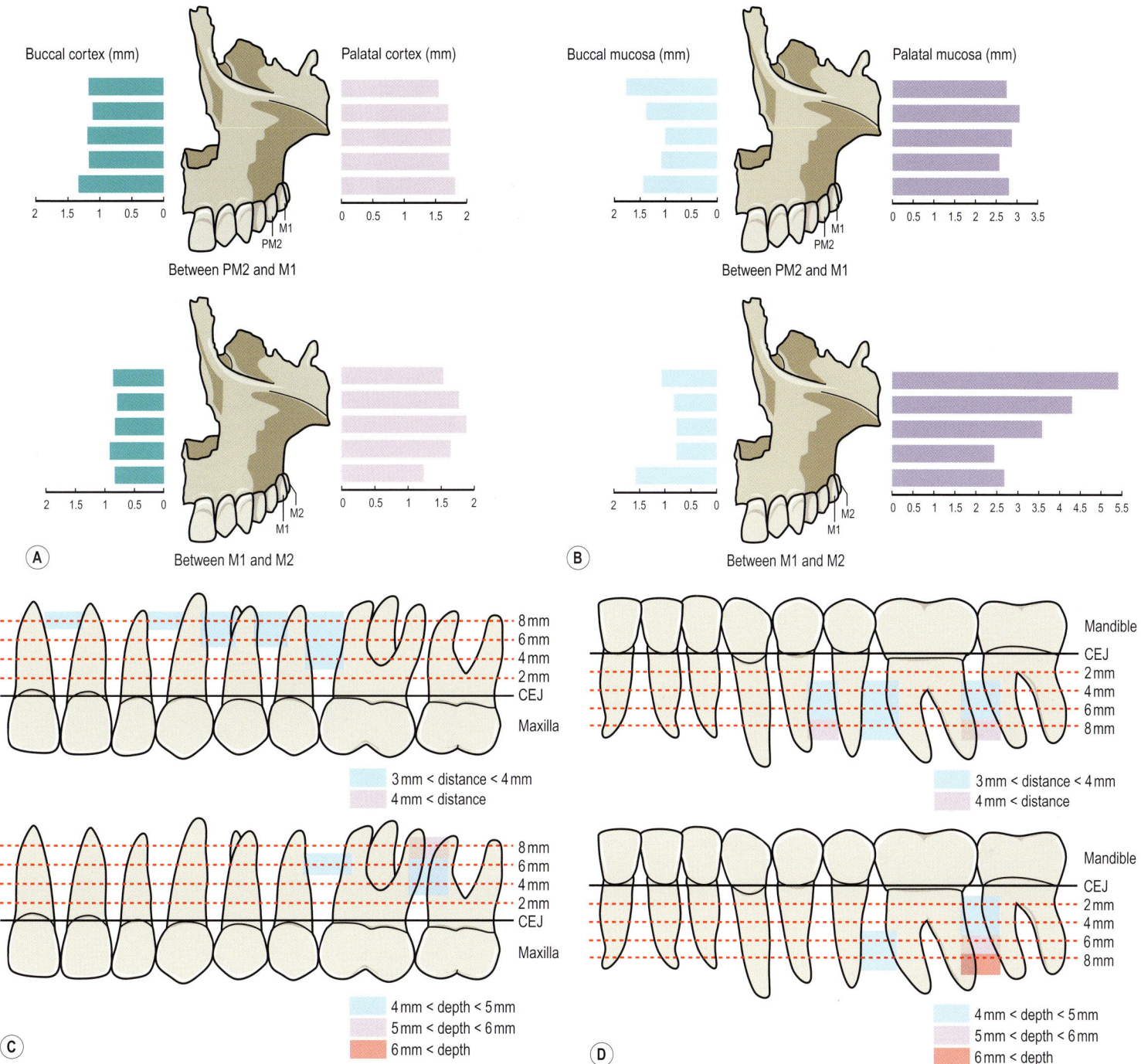

Fig. 40.1 Insertion sites. (A,B) Maxillary buccal and palatal alveolar area cortical bone thickness (A) and soft tissue thickness (B). (C,D) Available inter-radicular bone in the maxilla (C) and mandible (D). CEJ, cementoenamel junction. (With permission from Lee et al., 2009.[4])

contrast, segmental control of molars can be easy in terms of appliance fabrication when it is combined with inter-radicular MIs. Anteroposteriorly, a long segment can be more resistant to tipping than a single tooth, which enables distal translation without additional apparatus such as lever arms.

Segmental distalization using MIs as anchorage is limited by the possible contact between the roots and MIs; the maximum amount of movement is 2–3 mm, which is sufficient to correct end-to-end Class II molars. For more distalization, removal of MIs and reinsertion at nearby interradicular sites is recommended. Angulation of the insertion path is recommended to secure more clearance between the MI and the roots of the teeth. Simultaneous segmental or total arch distalization can be possible using continuous archwires, which may reduce the total chair-time by eliminating the need for additional appliances.

THE LEVER ARM DESIGN

In a two-dimensional model, lever arms can be extended as an extension wire up to or beyond the CR of the target segment (Fig. 40.3A).[6] Three-dimensional finite element analysis has shown that long lever arms extended toward the palatal vault may show elastic deformation to the distal side according to the force direction, which, in turn, may tip the central incisors lingually (Fig. 40.3B).[7] In order to secure precision tooth movement, it is advised that the two lever arms extending from each side

Fig. 40.2 Molar correction. (A,B) Clinical (A) and schematic (B) representation of single molar distalization using midpalatal miniscrew implants (MIs). (C,D) Clinical (C) and schematic (D) representation of segmental distalization using buccal alveolar MIs.

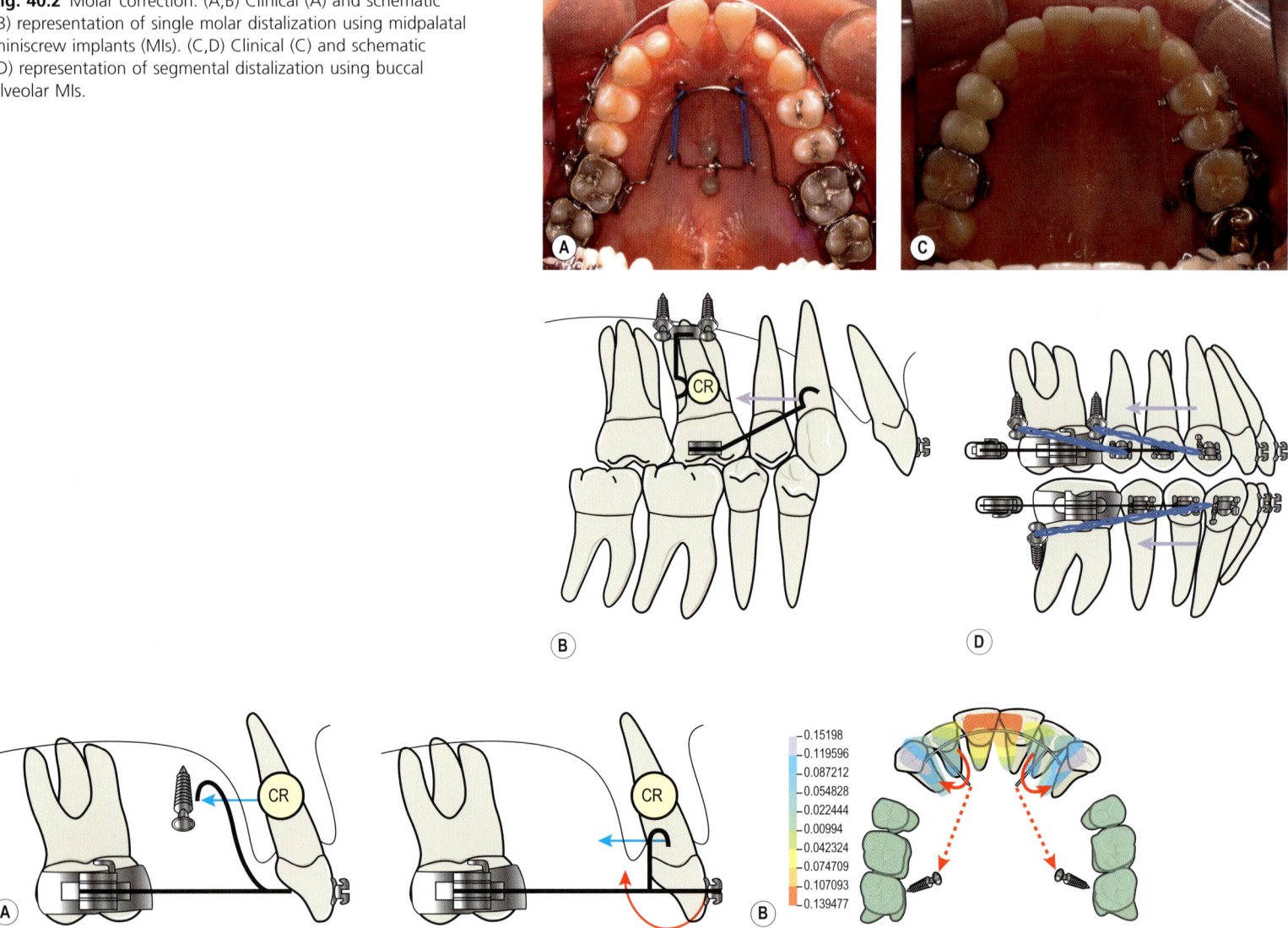

Fig. 40.3 Lever arm design. (A) Two-dimensional model. (B) Occlusal view with application of forces from the miniscrew implants to hooks attached to the lingual archwire.

are reinforced with rigid connecting wires. The lever arms along the floor of anterior maxilla should be as long as 20 mm.

FINISHING STAGE

Following segmental correction, continuous archwires are normally used to stabilize the entire arch. Up-and-down vertical elastics can be used short term for occlusal seating. However, the use of either Class II or Class III elastics for a relatively long period of time for incomplete anteroposterior correction is not recommended because of their extrusive nature.

CLINICAL APPLICATIONS

Some clinical examples of treatment of adults with Class II malocclusion using lingual appliances and MIs are presented and discussed below.

CASE 1: PROTRUSION OF MAXILLARY AND MANDIBULAR INCISORS

A 29-year-old woman presented with protrusion of the maxillary and mandibular incisors (Fig. 40.4A,C–E). There was prominent labial displacement of the maxillary right central incisor and a mild Class II molar relation on both sides. There was a 3.0 mm arch length discrepancy in both the maxillary and mandibular arches. Her facial profile was convex, possibly because of protrusive lips and retrusive chin. Initial cephalometric analysis revealed moderate Class II pattern (Table 40.2). Considering the severity of the protrusion, extraction of the first premolars was indicated. However, the maxillary and mandibular left second premolars had received root canal treatment. Consequently, second premolar extraction was considered as more appropriate in order to save the sounder teeth. To be able to retract the eight teeth encompassing the incisors, canines and first premolars as a unit, firm anchorage preparation was crucial. For this reason, insertion of the MIs was planned on both the maxillary and mandibular lingual sides.

To relieve the anterior crowding while ensuring maximum retraction at the same time, the canines and the first premolars were first retracted on round SS wire (0.016 inch) from the MIs (diameter, 1.8 mm; length, 7 mm; tapered body; Orlus 18107, Ortholution, Seoul, Korea) with elastic chains (Fig. 40.4F,G). The MIs were inserted on the palatal slope between the maxillary molars. Following partial retraction of the premolars and canines, brackets were bonded on the incisors for full-arch alignment. Retraction of premolars and canines in the mandibular arch was initially accomplished with reciprocal elastic chains engaged on the second molars.

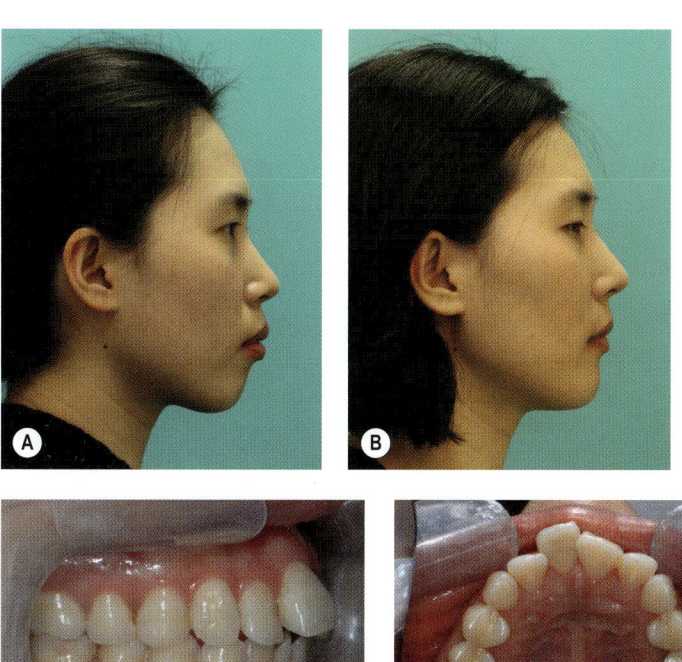

Fig. 40.4 Case 1: protrusion of maxillary and mandibular incisors. (A,C–E) Pretreatment. (F,G) The two arches during retraction of the premolars and canines. (H,I) The two arches during retraction of the upper and lower anterior segments immediately after insertion of a splinted H-lever arm. (B,J–L) Post-treatment.

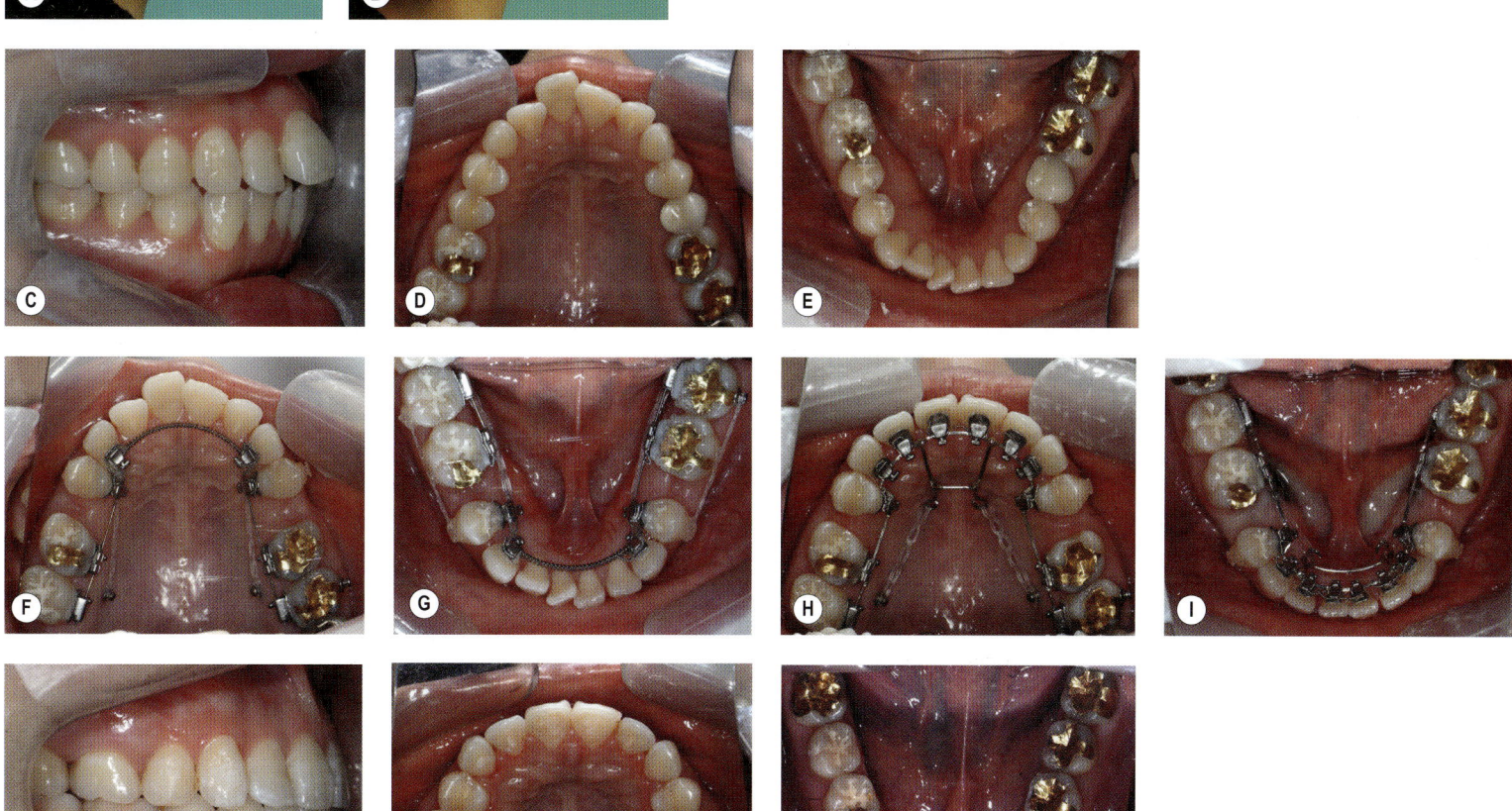

Table 40.2 Case 1: cephalometric measurements

Variables	Before treatment	After treatment
SNA (°)	86.59	84.79
SNB (°)	79.65	78.69
ANB (°)	6.94	6.09
Wits appraisal (mm)	0.04	−2.63
Sum (°)	396.40	396.23
SN-GoMe (°)	36.40	36.23
U1 to SN (°)	115.43	99.21
IMPA (°)	103.86	92.63
Upper lip to E-line (mm)	3.73	−2.05
Lower lip to E-line (mm)	5.82	−0.73

IMPA, incisor mandibular plane angle.

After full alignment, both upper and lower anterior segments were retracted with a splinted H-lever arm, which was fabricated with 0.8 mm round SS wire, soldered on the main SS archwire (Fig. 40.4H,I). In the mandibular arch, the MIs were inserted on the lingual alveolar bone mesial to the first molars.

Following anterior retraction and detailing, the appliances were removed (Fig. 40.4B,J–L). The maxillary and mandibular incisors had been moved 8.5 mm and 5.5 mm, respectively. Lateral facial profile was improved through a significant lip profile change.

Discussion

For this patient, significant displacement of the roots and crowns of the incisors was indicated in both arches for improvement of the profile. Hence, the incorporation of the rigid lever arm on the main continuous archwire aimed was intended to achieve this desired tooth movement.

Extraction of the second instead of the first premolar was another limiting factor. In order to secure maximum anchorage for the retraction of both the anterior teeth and the premolars, as well as to produce an appropriate line of force passing through the CR of the incisors, the MIs were placed on the lingual alveolar slope in both arches. Subsequently, tooth movement was translation of the maxillary incisors and a combination of translation and lingual tipping of the mandibular incisors.

CASE 2: ANTERIOR OPEN BITE AND PROTRUSION

A 20-year-old woman presented with a chief complaint of anterior open bite and protrusion (Fig. 40.5A,C–E). In the past, she had suffered from problems with her temporomandibular joint, which had subsided some years ago. Associated with this, flattening of the condylar head was noted in the initial panoramic radiograph. Cephalometric and model analysis revealed a severe Class II skeletal pattern, incisor dental compensation (flared mandibular incisors and uprighted maxillary incisors) and a negative overbite of 2 mm with hyperactivity of the mentalis muscle at reposed lip position (Table 40.3). Her major concern was to improve the lateral profile with invisible braces. However, in spite of the severe skeletal pattern, she did not want invasive orthognathic surgery procedures. Therefore, orthodontic camouflage treatment was chosen, aiming to induce a significant profile change without mandibular advancement. The limitations of this approach were explained to the patient and informed consent was gained. Considering the compensated incisor relation, maximum

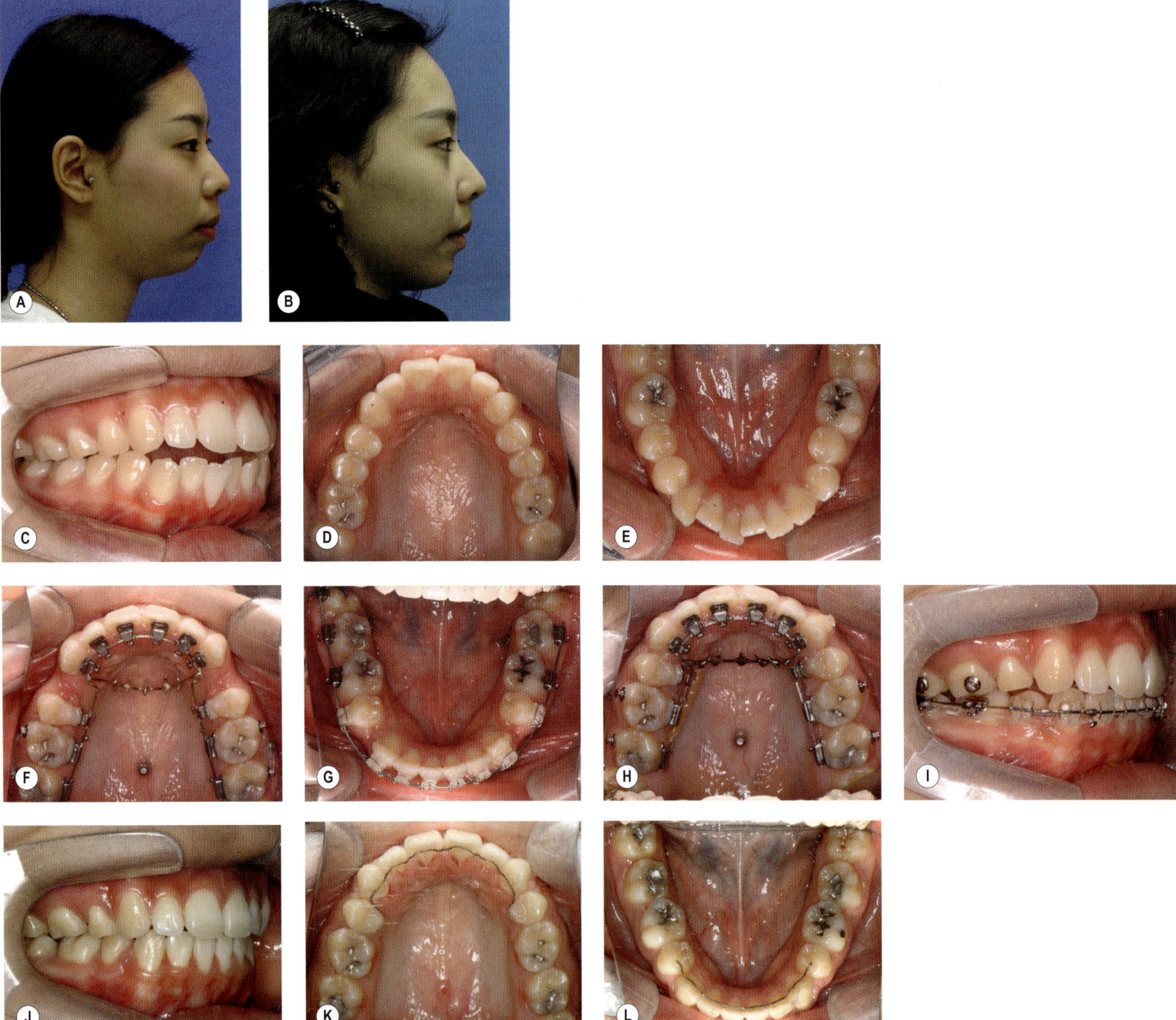

Fig. 40.5 Case 2: anterior open bite and protrusion. (A,C–E) Pretreatment. (F,G) Premolars have been extracted, a lingual appliance placed in the maxillary arch and conventional buccal fixed appliances in the mandibular arch. (H) Four months later. (I) Completion of segmental retraction. (B,J–L) Post-treatment.

Table 40.3 Case 2: cephalometric measurements		
Variables	Before treatment	After treatment
SNA (°)	87.14	85.31
SNB (°)	76.96	77.42
ANB (°)	10.18	7.89
Wits appraisal (mm)	1.95	3.88
Sum (°)	401.59	400.42
SN-GoMe (°)	41.59	540.42
U1 to SN (°)	104.44	97.91
IMPA (°)	115.15	96.45
Upper lip to E-line (mm)	4.42	1.49
Lower lip to E-line (mm)	7.63	1.64

IMPA, incisor mandibular plane angle.

Table 40.4 Case 3: cephalometric measurements		
Variables	Before treatment	After treatment
SNA (°)	76.68	76.00
SNB (°)	71.45	71.4
ANB (°)	5.24	4.60
Wits appraisal (mm)	2.73	0.48
Sum (°)	397.58	396.95
SN-GoMe (°)	37.58	36.95
U1 to SN (°)	107.19	98.76
IMPA (°)	106.43	112.55
Upper lip to E-line (mm)	1.63	1.31
Lower lip to E-line (mm)	2.41	1.26

IMPA, incisor mandibular plane angle.

translation of maxillary incisors was planned, together with controlled tipping of the mandibular incisors.

To achieve maximum translation of the maxillary incisors, a high line of force application was needed, which was provided using a cross-arch lever arm soldered from the main archwire positioned at the deepest palatal arch to a MI (diameter, 1.8 mm; length, 7 mm; tapered body; Orlus 18107) inserted in the midpalatal area (Fig. 40.5F,G).

Vertical bowing was noted during retraction, and so the main archwire was segmented distal to the canines. A high line of force was constantly provided for the root movement of incisor segment (Fig. 40.5H).

After further segmental retraction of 8 months, flattening of the occlusal plane was observed (Fig. 40.5I). Further space closure was performed on the segmented arch.

After 18 months of active treatment, space closure and detailing were complete (Fig. 40.5B,J–L). Proper incisor and molar relationship was attained through pure translation of the maxillary incisors. Her lateral profile was improved mainly by retraction of the upper and lower lips and the relief of soft tissue tension, particularly in the mentalis muscle.

At 1 year following active treatment, the temporomandibular joint did not show any drastic change and the occlusion remained stable. Incisor relation, midline and molar relation were maintained during the short-term retention phase.

Discussion

In order to overcome the underlying severe Class II skeletal pattern, extrusion of the teeth was strictly contraindicated in this patient. The midpalatal MI position in combination with the long lever arm from the incisor brackets was, therefore, selected in order to produce the highest line of force for the intrusive translation of the maxillary incisors. The resulting movement was consequently lingual translation of the maxillary incisors and lingual tipping (uprighting) of the mandibular incisors. The labial appliances on the mandibular arch were tolerated well by the patient.

CASE 3: MAXILLARY ANTERIOR PROTRUSION

A 37-year-old woman presented with a chief complaint of maxillary anterior protrusion (Fig. 40.6A,C-E). Initial cephalometric and model analysis showed severe Class II skeletal pattern with end-to-end Class II molars on both sides (Table 40.4). Both the maxillary and the mandibu-

lar incisors were proclined and in particular, root shortening of the upper incisors and alveolar bone loss in the anterior area were severe. The patient refused to receive orthognathic surgery, asking for a less invasive orthodontic treatment. Considering her maxillary incisors, distalization of the upper arch by 3.5 mm on both sides was better indicated than the extraction of premolars. In order to avoid round tripping of incisors, the use of tooth- (or/and tissue-) borne intraoral distalizers, such as the Distal Jet or the Pendulum, were contraindicated. Instead, a simultaneous distalization of both molar and incisor segments, i.e. total arch, was planned.

To reduce the friction during alignment, 2D lingual brackets were selectively bonded on the anterior teeth. After leveling and alignment, the anterior 2D brackets were removed, and the total maxillary arch was retracted using a modified lever arm, which was composed of a mesh pad bonded on the anterior segment to avoid any jiggling movement by the bracket-wire play and a conventional main archwire inserted into the brackets of the posterior teeth (Figure 40.6F,G). The MIs were initially inserted on the palatal slope between the molars.

In order to induce a sufficient amount of distalization, alternative lingual and buccal MIs were used. After significant distalization was achieved, conventional lingual brackets were bonded for finishing (Figure 40.6H,I).

After 27 months of treatment, all appliances were removed (Figure 40.6J-L). The maxillary incisors were retracted 6.0 mm, the maxillary molars were distalized 3.5 mm, the mandibular incisors were flared 2.0 mm, and the patient's profile was improved (Figure 40.6B).

Discussion

With the limitation of the camouflage treatment understood beforehand, the patient was satisfied with the result of treatment.

CONCLUSIONS

Based on both esthetic factors during treatment and treatment effects, lingual appliances may be a very strong option for adults. The greatest strength of the utilization of MIs in lingual orthodontic treatment is the fact that they can induce arbitrary segmental movement depending on the insertion sites. This versatility enables the orthodontist to attempt lingual treatment even in very challenging cases.

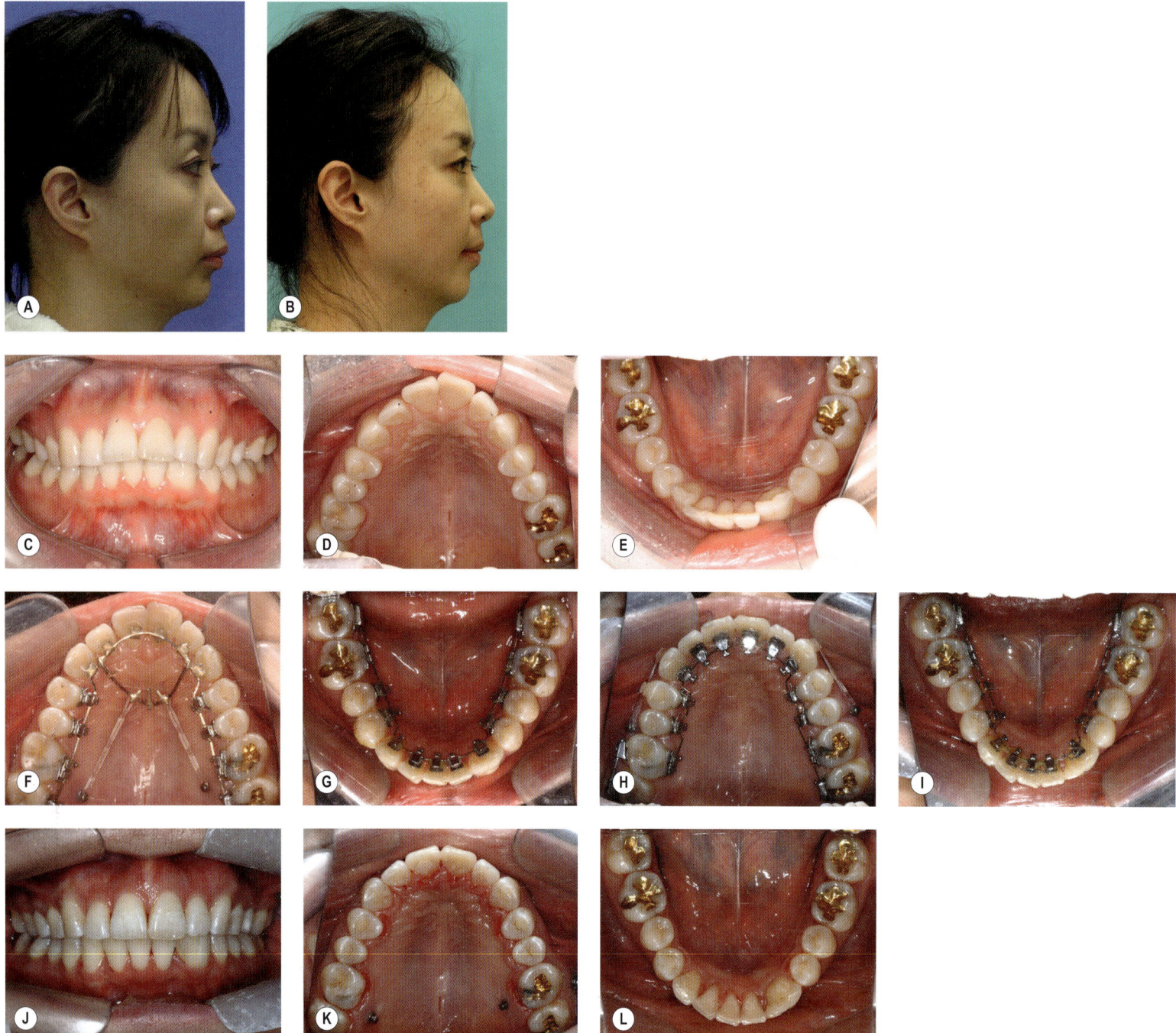

Fig. 40.6 Case 3: maxillary anterior protrusion. Pre- (A) and post-treatment (B) extraoral photographs. (C-E) Pre-treatment intraoral photographs. (F,G) After placement of a modified lever arm, insertion of the MIs and application of elastic chains for the retraction of the maxillary arch. (H,I) After insertion of buccal MIs and placement of conventional lingual brackets for finishing. (J-L) Post-treatment intraoral photographs.

REFERENCES

1. Tod MA, Taverne AA. Prevalence of malocclusion traits in an Australian adult population. Aust Orthod J 1997;15:16–22.
2. Hohoff A, Wiechmann D, Fillion D, et al. Evaluation of the parameters underlying the decision by adult patients to opt for lingual therapy: an international comparison. J Orofac Orthop 2003;64:135–44.
3. Lee KJ, Park YC, Hwang CJ, et al. Displacement pattern of the maxillary arch depending on miniscrew position in sliding mechanics. Am J Orthod Dentofacial Orthop 2011;140:224–32.
4. Lee KJ, Joo E, Kim KD, et al. Computed tomographic analysis of tooth-bearing alveolar bone for orthodontic miniscrew placement. Am J Orthod Dentofacial Orthop 2009;135:486–94.
5. Kinzinger G, Frye L, Diedrich P. Class II treatment in adults: comparing camouflage orthodontics, dentofacial orthopedics and orthognathic surgery. A cephalometric study to evaluate various therapeutic effects. J Orofac Orthop 2009;70:63–91.
6. Park YC, Choy K, Lee JS, et al. Lever-arm mechanics in lingual orthodontics. J Clin Orthod 2000;34:601–5.
7. Kim KH, Lee KJ, Cha JY, et al. Finite element analysis of effectiveness of lever arm in lingual sliding mechanics. Korean J Orthod 2011;41:324–36.

Skeletal anchorage in lingual orthodontic treatment with sliding mechanics

41

Kyoto Takemoto and Moschos A. Papadopoulos

INTRODUCTION

Treatment of Class II malocclusion usually involves maxillary molar distalization and subsequent retraction of the anterior teeth. This can be performed either without friction (using loop mechanics) or with friction (using sliding mechanics). Table 41.1 compares these approaches as it is important for the clinician to understand the advantages and disadvantages in order to choose an appropriate mechanism for a patient's treatment.

Miniscrew implants (MIs) can provide greater anchorage in the mandibular arch than in the maxilla, while posterior anchorage needs to be reinforced in lingual orthodontics, particularly in the maxillary arch.[1-3] Various methods of maximum, moderate and minimum anchorage (e.g. MIs, transpalatal arches, headgears, Class II elastics) can support loop and sliding mechanics in the maxillary dental arch.

This chapter focuses on the management of Class II malocclusion with lingual orthodontics and application of sliding mechanics combined with MIs to reinforce posterior anchorage during en masse retraction of the maxillary teeth.

Table 41.1 Advantages and disadvantages of loop and sliding mechanics

	Loop mechanics	Sliding mechanics
Wire friction	+	−
Anti-tipping bend	+	+/−
Control of retraction force	+	+/−
Unilateral extraction cases	+	+/−
Bite opening control	+	−
Discomfort	+/−	+
Wire bending	−	+

+, achievable with these mechanics; −, difficult to achieve with these mechanics.

CLINICAL APPLICATION

For en masse retraction of the maxillary teeth in lingual orthodontic treatment of Class II malocclusion, strong retraction forces may cause a tip-forward of the posterior teeth, and consequently lateral occlusal function may be impaired. The use of MIs for anchorage reinforcement can help to avoid these undesirable countermovements of the posterior teeth during anterior teeth retraction or during closure of extraction sites.

MIs can be positioned either inter-radicularly on the palatal side in the alveolar bone between the roots of the teeth or in the midpalatal suture.

INTER-RADICULAR SITES

The most common site is inter-radicularly on the palatal side, usually between the second premolars and the first molars on both sides of the maxillary arch (Fig. 41.1A,B), since these regions provide the best bone quality and quantity. For MIs in this position, power chains or closed coil springs are placed between the MIs and the hooks attached between the canines and second premolars on the upper archwire, and the maxillary anterior teeth are retracted en masse with sliding mechanics.

The wire is usually furnished with a gable-bend to maintain the torque of the maxillary anterior teeth. This procedure may induce lingual tipping of the maxillary anterior teeth and deep bite, particularly when the retraction force is strong. However, the maxillary posterior teeth may intrude and, consequently, posterior disocclusion tends to occur (Fig. 41.1B). Therefore, this procedure is indicated for the treatment of patients with open bite, particularly when the maxillary anterior teeth are proclined. It is not suitable for patients with deep bite, such as those with Class II, division 2 malocclusion.

Midpalatal Suture Sites

The MI is inserted in the midpalatal suture at the level between the second premolars and first molars (Fig. 41.1C,D). For MIs in this position, a

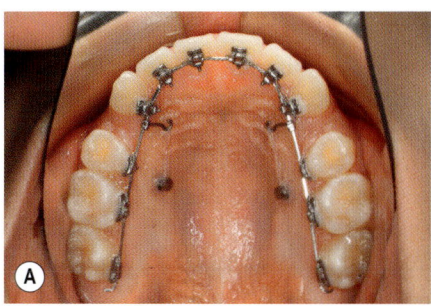

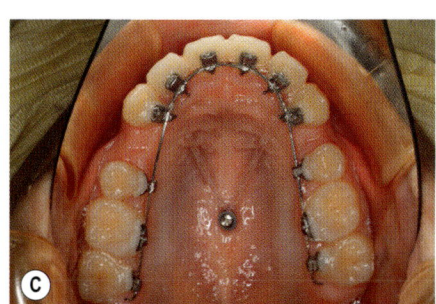

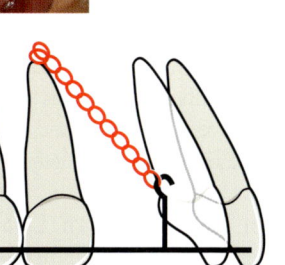

Fig. 41.1 En masse retraction of the maxillary anterior teeth. (A,B) Clinical view (A) and schematic (B) of inter-radically placed miniscrew implants (MIs). (C,D) Clinical view (C) and schematic (D) of MI inserted in the midpalatal suture.

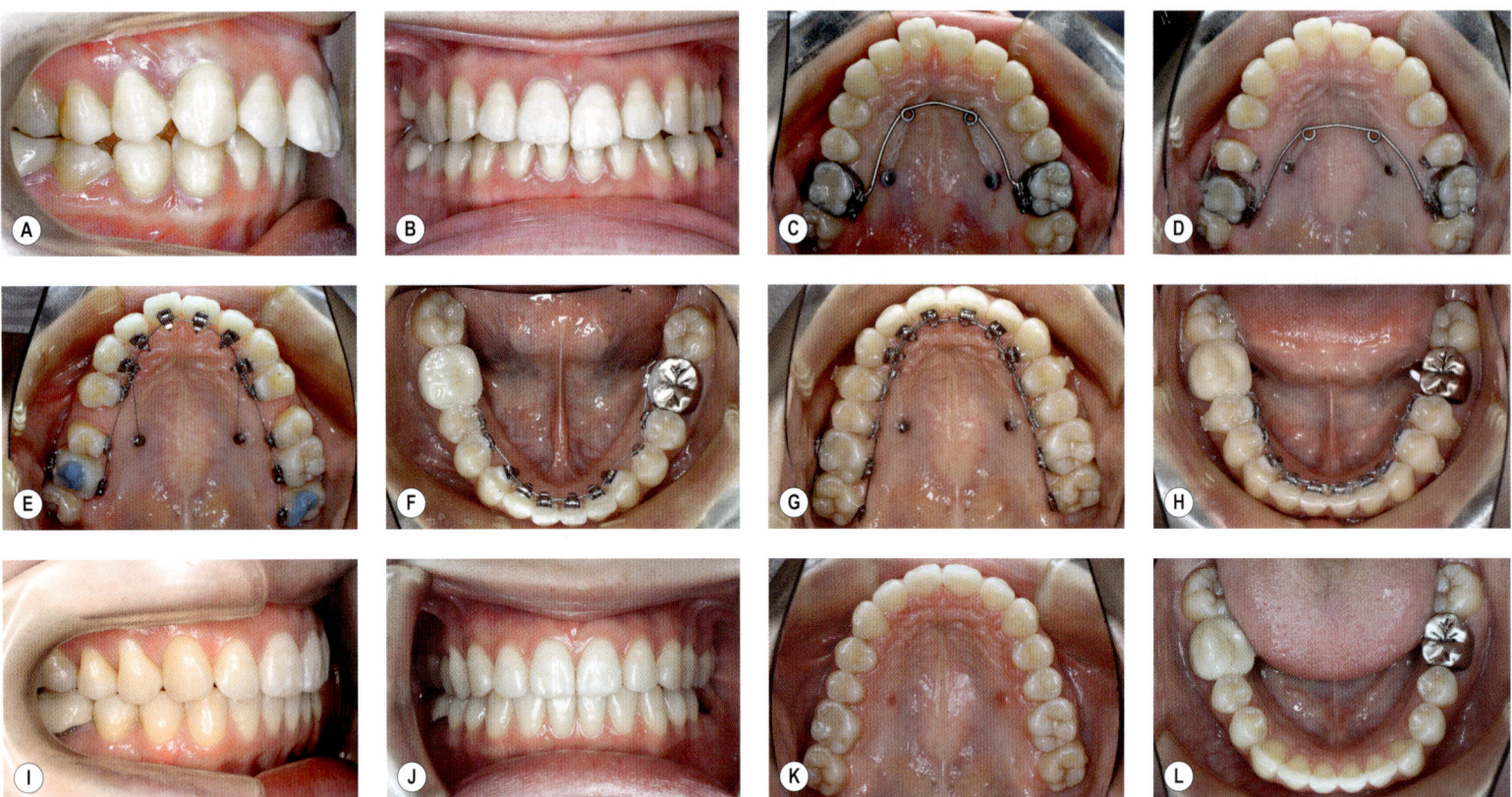

Fig. 41.2 Case 1: non-extraction treatment for protrusion of maxillary anterior teeth. (A,B) Pretreatment. (C) Insertion of a lingual arch and two inter-radicularly placed microscrew implants. (D) Nine months later at end of maxillary molar distalization. (E,F) Removal of the lingual arch and insertion of lingual fixed appliances at 10 months after initiation of treatment. (G,H) Start of the finishing stage at 2 years after initiation of treatment. (I–L) Post-treatment.

closed coil spring or a power chain is placed between the MIs and the hooks attached between maxillary lateral incisors and canines, and the maxillary anterior teeth are retracted en masse with sliding mechanics.

The MI should be inserted more mesially if a stronger intrusive force is desired and more distally if a stronger distalization force is desired. This procedure allows retraction without deepening the bite, since the posterior teeth maintain stability as simultaneous intrusive and retraction forces can be applied. However, because of the application of these additional intrusive forces, it may take additional time for the retraction of the maxillary anterior teeth. Therefore, this procedure is mainly indicated for patients presenting with a normal to deep bite, but not for patients with an open bite.

CASE EXAMPLES

CASE 1: NON-EXTRACTION TREATMENT OF PROTRUSION OF MAXILLARY ANTERIOR TEETH

A 21-year-old woman presented with protrusion of her maxillary anterior teeth. She had a Class II, division 1 malocclusion and Class II molar and canine relationship on both sides, plus Class I skeletal relationships of the maxilla and mandible (Fig. 41.2A,B).

Initially, a maxillary lingual arch was bonded on the maxillary first molars and two MIs were inserted inter-radicularly between the maxillary second premolars and first molars (Fig. 41.2C). Maxillary molar distalization was initiated by applying elastic chains between the MIs and the lingual arch as shown in Fig. 41.2C. Molar distalization was completed in 9 months (Fig. 41.2D).

The lingual arch was removed and lingual appliances (STb Light Lingual System, Ormco, Orange, CA, USA) were bonded on both dental arches (Fig. 41.2E,F). Using this lingual system and the straight wire

Table 41.2 Case 1: wire sequence followed during treatment

Date	Maxillary arch	Mandibular arch
Nov 2008	0.012 inch Ni-Ti	0.012 inch Ni-Ti
Jan 2009	0.016 × 0.016 inch Ni-Ti	
March 2009	0.0175 × .0.0175 inch TMA	
May 2009	0.016 × 0.016 inch SS	0.016 × 0.016 inch Ni-Ti
June 2009	0.018 × 0.018 inch SS	
Nov 2009	0.0175 × 0175 inch TMA	
Nov 2010		0.0175 × 0.0175 inch TMA

approach, the maxillary and mandibular dental arches were leveled and aligned, while the anterior teeth and first premolars were retracted. Anterior teeth retraction was initiated by applying open coil springs between the brackets of the canines and first premolars, while the MIs were connected through wire ligatures to the canine brackets to support anchorage. Elastic chains were applied between the MIs and hooks attached on the maxillary archwire between the brackets of the canines and the first premolars (Fig. 41.2G). Two years after treatment start, short Class II elastics were used and the finishing stage of treatment was initiated (Fig. 41.2G,H). The wire sequence used during treatment is presented in Table 41.2.

After a total treatment time of 3 years, the fixed appliances and MIs were removed (Fig. 41.2I–L). The final result was a well-functioning occlusion presenting Class I canine and molar relationships, ideal torque of the anterior teeth, as well as ideal overjet and overbite.

CASE 2: EXTRACTION TREATMENT OF PROTRUSION OF MAXILLARY ANTERIOR TEETH

A 21-year-old woman presented with maxillary anterior teeth protrusion. She had Class I molar relationships on both sides, severe proclination of

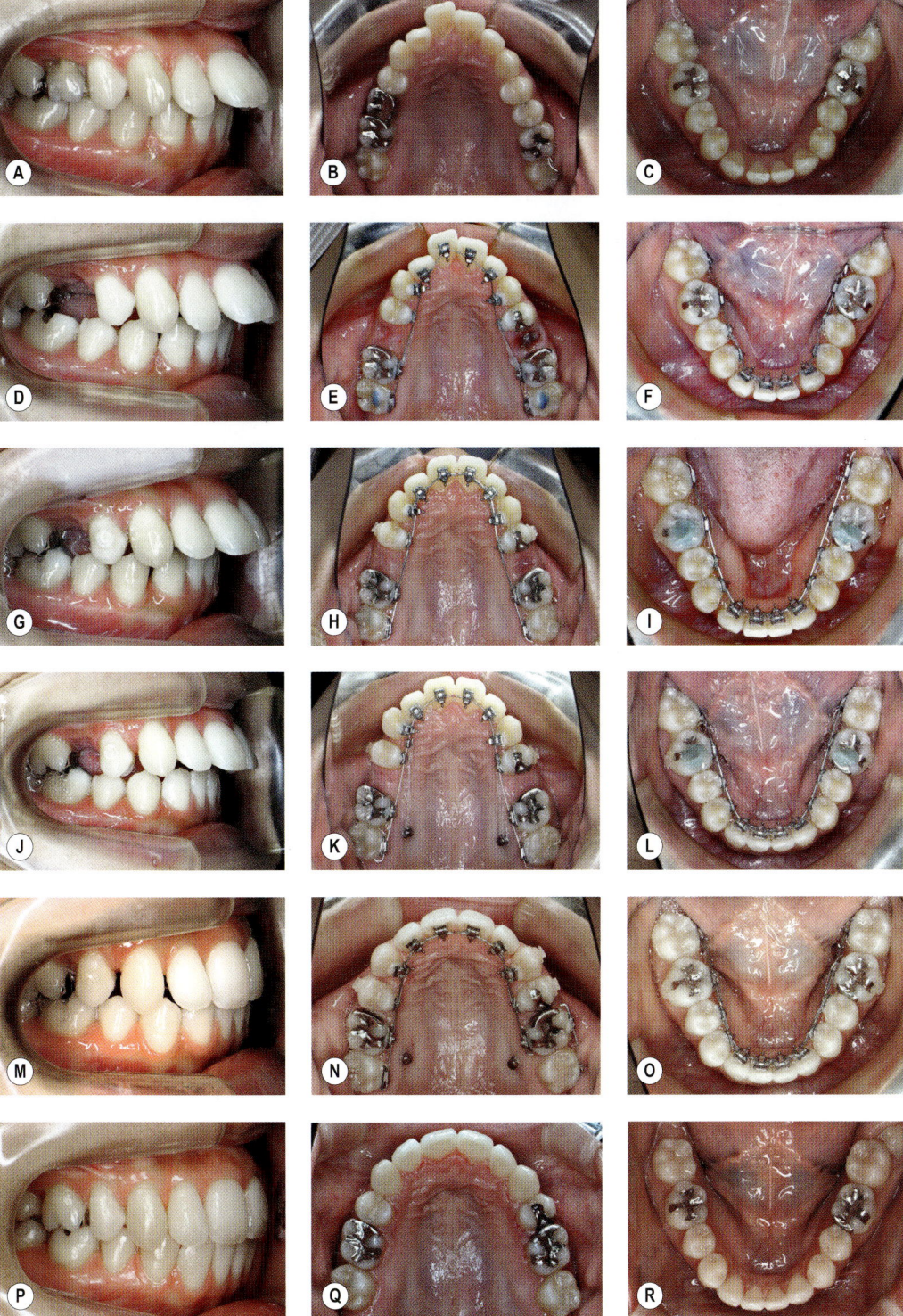

Fig. 41.3 Case 2: extraction treatment for protrusion of maxillary anterior teeth. (A–C) Pretreatment. (D–F) After extraction of teeth and insertion of fixed lingual appliances. (G–I) Leveling stage at 2 months after initiation of treatment. (J–L) Insertion of two miniscrew implants between the first and second maxillary molars at 3 months after initiation of treatment. (M–O) Retraction of the maxillary first premolars and anterior teeth at 9 months after treatment start. (P–R) Post-treatment.

the maxillary anterior teeth and a large overjet (Fig. 41.3A,B). The overjet was partially attributed to the missing mandibular lateral incisors. In addition, the maxillary right second primary molar was present but the corresponding second premolar was missing. The mandibular lateral incisors and the maxillary right second premolar were congenitally missing. She had Class II skeletal relationships of the maxilla and mandible with a slight dolichofacial tendency.

Before initiating treatment, the maxillary right primary second molar and the left second premolar were extracted. Lingual appliances (STb Light Lingual System) were bonded on both dental arches (Fig. 41.3D–F) for leveling and alignment, which was undertaken using the straight wire approach (Fig. 41.3G–I).

Three months after initiation of treatment, two MIs were inserted inter-radicularly between the first and second maxillary molars to support the retraction of the maxillary anterior teeth (Fig. 41.3J–L). Elastic chains were applied between the MIs and hooks attached on the archwire between the brackets of the canines and first premolars.

Nine months after treatment start, the retraction of the maxillary first premolars and the anterior teeth was completed (Fig. 41.3M–O). Since lingual tipping of the maxillary anterior teeth and posterior disocclusion had occurred, the maxillary dental arch was leveled again, and final extraction space closure and finishing was carried out. The wire sequence used during treatment is presented in Table 41.3.

Table 41.3 Case 2: wire sequence followed during treatment

Date	Maxillary arch	Mandibular arch
Apr 2008	0.012 inch Ni-Ti	0.012 inch Ni-Ti
June 2008	0.016 × 0.016 inch Ni-Ti	0.016 × 016 inch Ni-Ti
July 2008	0.016 inch SS	
Aug 2008		0.0175 × 0.0175 inch TMA
Dec 2008	0.016 × 0.016 inch Ni-Ti	
Jan 2009	0.0175 × 0.0175 inch TMA	
Apr 2009	0.016 × 0.022 inch SS	
Aug 2009		0.018 × 0.01 inch TMA
Oct 2009	0.018 × 0.01 inch β-Ti	

The total treatment time was 2.5 years. After completion of treatment, the fixed lingual appliances and MIs were removed (Fig. 41.3P–R). The final result revealed a good and stable occlusion with Class I canine and molar relationships, normal overbite and overjet, and ideal torque of the anterior teeth.

REFERENCES

1. Geron S. Anchorage considerations in lingual orthodontics. Semin Orthod 2006;12: 167–77.
2. Papadopoulos MA, Papageorgiou SN, Zogakis IP. Clinical effectiveness of orthodontic miniscrew implants: a meta-analysis. J Dent Res 2011;90:969–76.
3. Scuzzo G, Takemoto K. Invisible orthodontics. Current concepts and solutions in lingual orthodontics. Berlin: Quintessence; 2003.

42

Lever arm and miniscrew implant system for distalization of maxillary molars and anterior teeth retraction

Seung-Min Lim and Ryoon-Ki Hong

INTRODUCTION

This chapter will discuss the lever arm and miniscrew implant (MI) system for the treatment of Class II malocclusion through distal movement of maxillary molars and anterior teeth retraction.

DISTALIZATION OF MAXILLARY MOLARS

An ideal force system for distal movement of the maxillary molars in three dimensions should have distinct effects in different planes:

- sagittal plane: produce a bodily distal movement of molars without undesired effects of the reciprocal force on the anterior teeth
- vertical plane: exert intrusion forces simultaneously to distalization without changing the mandibular plane angle (i.e. avoid unintended molar extrusion)
- transverse plane: provide rotational control of the molars.

THE LEVER ARM AND MINISCREW IMPLANT SYSTEM

The lever arm and MI system fulfills these needs. Lingual lever arms can be easily fabricated and positioned in the maxillary arch to fit the available width and depth of the palate. Their use facilitates alteration of the point of force application and consequently of the moment-to-force ratio in a much easier way than using calibrated springs, since springs cannot be adjusted independently to produce differential forces and moments.

For bodily translation of a tooth, two forces are applied at some distance from the center of resistance (CR) of the tooth. One force at the level of the crown and another at the root apex creates a resultant force through the CR and, thus, causes no rotational movement.

The lever arm and MI system allows adjustment of the distalizing force through a buccal and a palatal force system, thus varying the overall line of force, as shown in Fig. 42.1.[1] If the expansion of a posterior tooth is needed during distalization, it can be obtained simultaneously using a transpalatal arch (TPA). To prevent hanging down of the palatal cusp of the maxillary first molars during expansion, buccal root torque should be applied when using the TPA or an adequate intrusive force should be

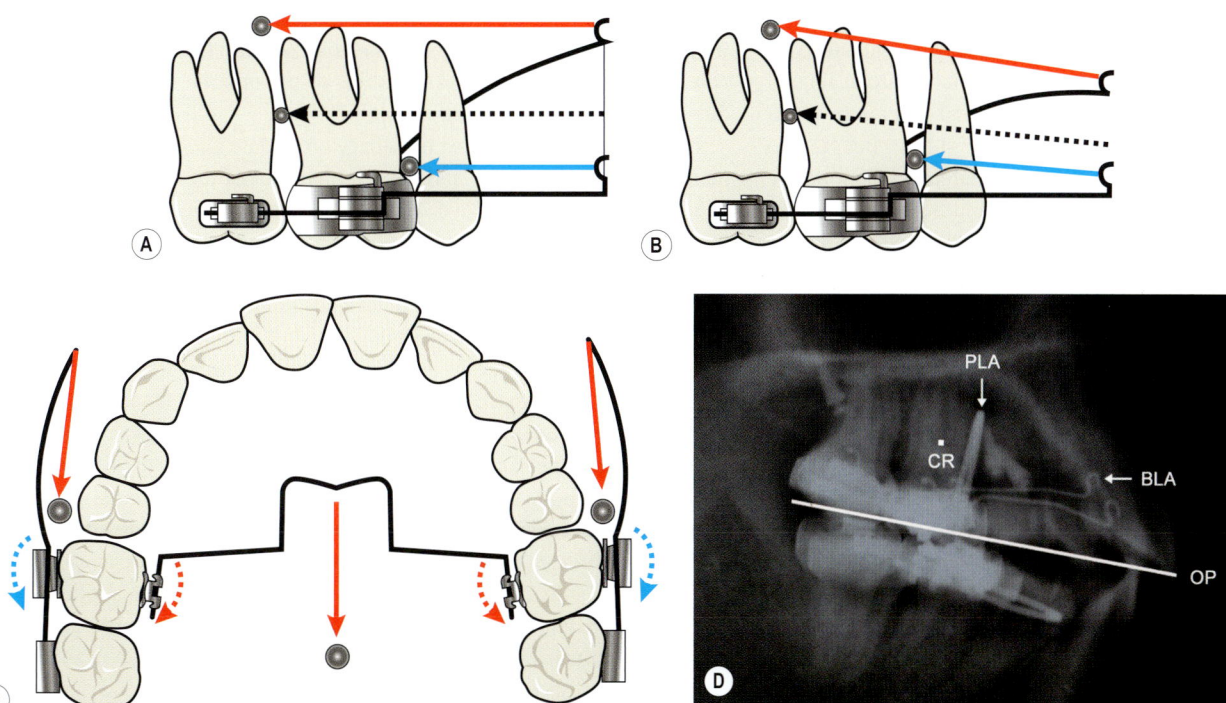

Fig. 42.1 The lever arm and miniscrew implant (MI) system. (A) The line of action of the resultant distalizing force passes through the center of resistance (CR) of the maxillary molars, producing a bodily movement parallel to the occlusal plane. (B) The line of action of the resultant force passes through the CR of the maxillary molars in a superior direction, producing bodily distal movement along with intrusion. (C) Buccal and palatal forces together facilitate rotation control of the maxillary molars. (D) Determination of the length of the lever arm and of the position of the MIs using lateral cephalometric radiography. OP, occlusal plane; BLA, buccal lever arm; PLA, palatal lever arm.

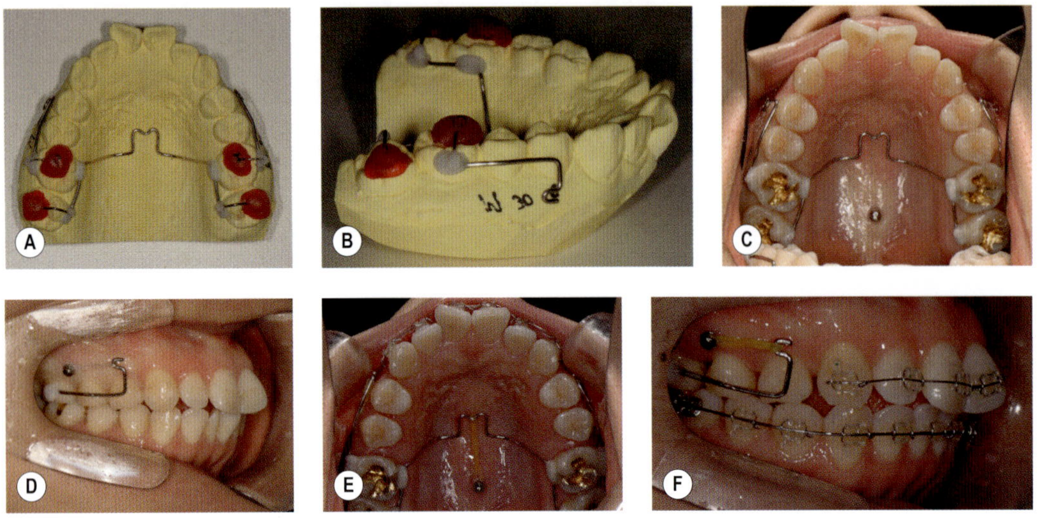

Fig. 42.2 Indirect bonding method. (A,B) Occlusal (A) and lateral (B) views of the transfer trays and lever arms on the cast. (C,D) Intraoral occlusal (C) and lateral (D) views of the lever arm and miniscrew implant (MI) system immediately after bonding, insertion of one palatal and two buccal miniscrew implants and application of distalizing forces with elastic chains. (E,F) Intraoral occlusal (E) and lateral (F) views of the same patient after distalization of the maxillary molars.

utilized by altering the height between the midpalatal MI and the TPA. The lever arm and MI system comprises three MIs (one inserted in the palate and two inserted buccally between the roots of the maxillary first molars and second premolars on both sides), two buccally positioned lever arms, a TPA functioning as a palatal lever arm, bands on first maxillary molars (and occasionally brackets on second maxillary molars) (Fig. 42.1A–C). Forces are applied using elastic chains.

Appliance Construction

The maxillary first molars are banded with double combination tubes (0.022 inch) welded on the buccal side and Burstone lingual brackets (0.032 × 0.032 inch) on the palatal side. The maxillary second molars are bonded with 0.022 inch tubes. A TPA fabricated from either TMA (0.032 × 0.032 inch) or SS wire (0.9 mm) is used as the palatal lever arm. When SS wire is used, the portion engaged in the Burstone lingual brackets is ground with a green stone bur. The buccal lever arm is SS wire (0.019 × 0.025 inch). The positions of the MI and the buccal and palatal lever arms are determined by evaluating the lateral cephalometric radiograph (Fig. 42.1D) and the maxillary cast. Figure 42.2 shows the indirect bonding method for the buccal and palatal lever arms. If there is no need for expansion of the maxillary molars, or if both first and second molars need to be intruded, the TPA can be bonded on both the first and the second molars.

The length of the lever arm is set to place the applied force in the desired position with regard to the CR of the molars, which is assessed by thoroughly evaluating a lateral cephalometric radiograph (Fig. 42.1D). If the height of alveolar bone is low, the CR of the tooth moves toward the root apex; therefore, alveolar bone height should be carefully determined. The occlusal plane and facial pattern should be evaluated to decide the type of tooth movement needed, for example whether the tooth should be just distalized parallel to the occlusal plane or with simultaneous intrusion.

Position for Miniscrew Implants

The depth of the palatal vault should also be taken into consideration. If it is extremely shallow, bodily movement of maxillary molars is accomplished by inserting a MI in the midpalatal suture. However, in most patients, the head of the MI is positioned vertically on the root apex level. Therefore, the vertical position of the buccal MIs should be set so the

resultant force passes through the CR of the maxillary molars. If the palatal vault is deep, the MIs are implanted more occlusally, while if it is shallow, the MIs are implanted more gingivally.

CLINICAL APPLICATION

CASE 1: SEVERE ANTERIOR CROWDING AND MAXILLARY PROTRUSION

A 27-year-old Korean woman presented with the chief complaint of severe anterior crowding and maxillary protrusion. She had a convex profile and Class II molar relationships (Fig. 42.3A,B). There was an arch length discrepancy of 18.5 mm and 12 mm in the maxillary and mandibular dental arches, respectively. Bilateral maxillary posterior dental constriction and slight anterior open bite were also present. Cephalometric analysis revealed Class II skeletal relationships of the maxilla and mandible and a dolichofacial growth pattern (Table 42.1).

Prior to treatment, the first maxillary premolars and second molars, right mandibular first premolar and the retained root of the left first molar were extracted (Fig. 42.3D). Two MIs (length, 6 mm) were inserted between the maxillary first molars and second premolars bilaterally and both maxillary canines were retracted with elastic chains (Fig. 42.3C,D). An additional MI was inserted in the palate and, after 3 months, distalization of the maxillary molars was initiated.

Because of the anterior open bite tendency and the hyperdivergent growth pattern, the extrusion of maxillary molars that usually takes place during distalization could lead to a clockwise rotation of the mandible and opening of the bite. Consequently, the vertical levels of the MI heads and lever arms on both sides were adjusted to produce an intrusive force in addition to the distalization force (Fig. 42.3E,F). Using elastic chain modules, a force of approximately 150 g was applied on each lever arm on the buccal side and a force of approximately 300 g was applied on the TPA on the palate (i.e. in total a force of approximately 300 g on each maxillary molar). In addition, a 0.9 mm SS expanded TPA was used to correct bilateral posterior maxillary dental constriction.

After 9 months of treatment, the lever arms and the TPA were removed and two additional MIs were inserted on the palate between the roots of the second premolars and first molars (Fig. 42.3G,H). Elastic chains and power hooks were utilized to retract the anterior teeth and treatment was continued for an additional 12 months.

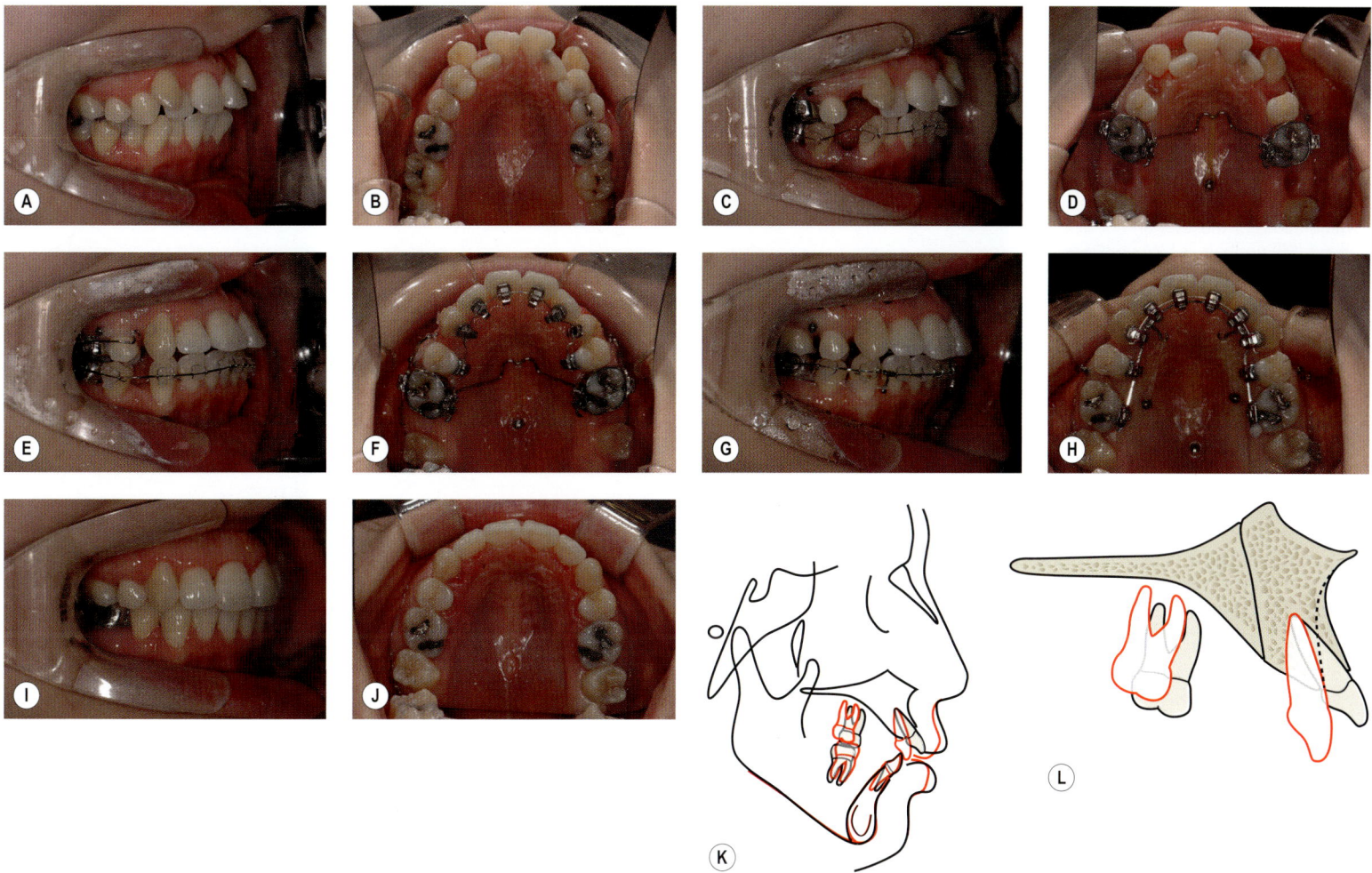

Fig. 42.3 Case 1: distalization of maxillary molars for severe anterior crowding and maxillary protrusion. (A,B) Pretreatment. (C,D) Placement of buccal fixed appliances on the lower arch, and insertion of the palatal lever arm and of one palatal and two buccal miniscrew implants (MIs) on the maxilla. The buccal MIs facilitate canine retraction, while the palatal MI effects distalization of maxillary molars. (E,F) Insertion of the buccal lever arms on the maxillary arch. Adjustment of the vertical level of all MI heads and lever arms to apply an intrusive force simultaneous to distalization. (G,H) Insertion of two additional MIs on the palate between the roots of the second premolars and first molars to facilitate anterior teeth retraction. (I,J) Post-treatment. (K,L) Superimposition of the cephalometric tracings before (black) and after (red) treatment; overall superimposition on the SN line (K) and maxillary superimposition (L).

Table 42.1 Case 1: cephalometric measurements		
Measurement	**Pretreatment**	**Post-treatment**
Skeletal		
SNA (°)	81	80
SNB (°)	73	73
ANB (°)	8	7
FMA (°)	29.5	29.5
NPo-FH (°)	73.5	73.5
Dental		
U1to FH (°)	124	105
FMIA (°)	55	55.5
Overbite (mm)	−1	2
Overjet (mm)	8	2.5
Soft tissues		
Upper lip to E-line (mm)	1.5	−2
Lower lip to E-line (mm)	3	−0.5

FMA, Frankfort-mandibular plane angle; FMIA, Frankfort-mandibular incisor angle.

The fixed appliances were removed 24 months after initiation of treatment. Ideal Class I molar and canine relationships, overbite and overjet were achieved (Fig. 42.3I,J). On the cephalometric superimposition before and after treatment, a 3.0 mm bodily distalization and 1.5 mm intrusion of the maxillary molars were evident, while the mandibular plane angle did not change (Fig. 42.3K,L).

ANTERIOR TEETH RETRACTION

Temporary anchorage devices seem to be effective for intraoral anchorage reinforcement for en masse retraction of the anterior teeth. However, torque control is still a significant issue to be taken into consideration.

The design of a force system for retraction of the anterior teeth is based on knowledge of the CR of the unit (the six anterior teeth) to be moved. Based on retraction with sliding mechanics, the CR of the six anterior teeth has been determined as 77% of the total root length away from the apex, which is approximately 11–12 mm apical to the incisal edge of the incisors (6.5–7.5 mm apical to labial brackets position).[2,3]

Factors such as wire size, the bracket slot size and the interplay between bracket slot and archwire are some of the variables affecting the biomechanical behavior of tooth movement. A three-dimensional finite element analysis of sliding mechanics showed that a lever arm placed

Fig. 42.4 Analysis of anterior teeth retraction. (A,B) Effects of bracket positioning and point of force application on tooth movement when bonding on the labial (A) or the lingual (B) surface of the maxillary central incisor. When using lingual appliances, the resultant force produces a larger moment, which tips the incisor more lingual than when using conventional labial appliances. (C–E) Line of action of the retraction forces with varying configurations of the lever arm or miniscrew implant (MI) position. (C) When the resultant force vector passes through the CR of the incisors; the anterior teeth will be retracted bodily and intruded (left), retracted bodily (middle) or retracted bodily and extruded (right). (D) With simultaneous lingual crown torque of the anterior teeth where the resultant force vector passes below the CR of the incisor, the anterior teeth will be retracted and intruded (left), retracted (middle) or retracted and extruded (right). (E) With simultaneous lingual root torque of the anterior teeth where the resultant force vector passes above the CR of the incisors, the anterior teeth will be retracted and intruded (left), retracted (middle) or retracted and extruded (right). CR, center of resistance; F_R, retraction force; F_I, intrusion force; F_{R+I}, resultant force; LA, lever arm; M_1 and M_2, moments.

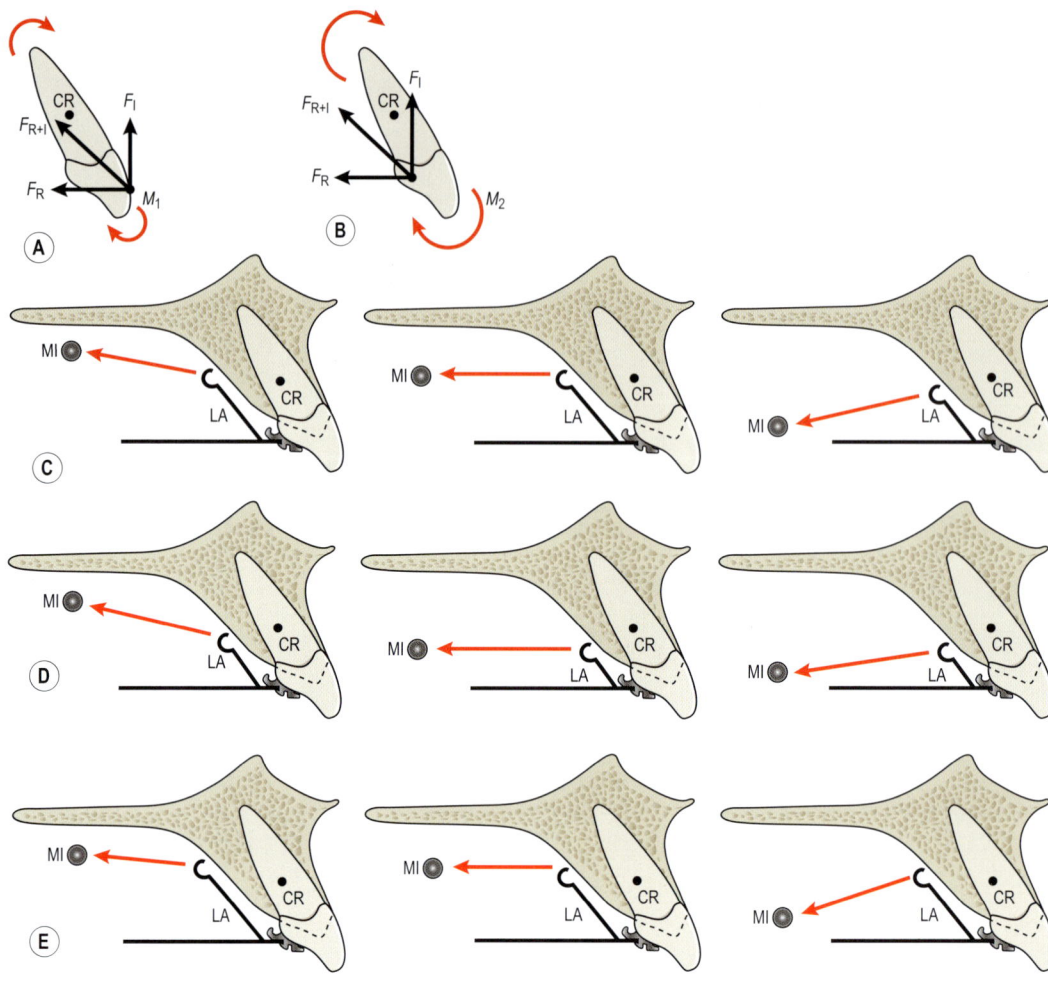

mesial to the canine at a height of 5.5 mm apical to the bracket position produced bodily movement for anterior teeth retraction.[4] As the position of the lever arm on the archwire was moved from the incisor to the premolars, the length of the lever arm had to be increased in order to produce parallel translation: the length should be 4.99 mm apical to the bracket position when the lever arm was located between the lateral incisors and the canines and 8.22 mm when located between the canines and the first premolars.[5] If the interplay between the bracket slot and archwire is increased, the height of the lever arm is also increased in order to produce bodily movement, and vice versa. Therefore, the lever arm should be placed mesial to the canines in order to attain better control of the anterior teeth with sliding mechanics.

Several other variables affecting the biomechanical behavior of tooth movement must be taken into consideration in clinical lingual orthodontics, for example anatomic parameters, such as the length and the shape of teeth roots, the width of the periodontal ligament, the palatal alveolar bone height, the angle of crown inclination and the physical properties of periodontal tissue.

In lingual orthodontics, torque control of anterior teeth during retraction is more challenging than using labial fixed appliances because of the specific position of the brackets on the lingual surfaces of the teeth (Fig. 42.4A,B). Anterior torque control is achieved either by directly applying a moment and a force to a lingual bracket or by using lever arm mechanics to obtain the desired line of action of the force with respect to the CR of the tooth (Fig. 42.4C–E).[6–8] The desired tooth movement is attained by adjusting the length of the lever arm and the point of force application. Using lingual appliances allows the lever arm system to be ideally located because appropriate space is almost always available within the width and depth dimensions of the palate. Therefore, in combination with a lever arm, MIs can be used not only for anchorage reinforcement but also for anterior torque control in lingual orthodontics.

THE LEVER ARM AND MINISCREW IMPLANT SYSTEM

To design the optimal lever arm and MI system for obtaining the desired force system during retraction with respect to the CR of the anterior segment, the point of force application and the line of action of the retraction force are planned using lateral cephalometric radiographs.

Figure 42.4C–E illustrates the overall reaction that can be expected with retraction forces in various configurations. Force parallel to the occlusal plane and applied through the CR of the anterior teeth will bodily retract the anterior segment, alone or with simultaneous intrusion or extrusion (Fig. 42.4C).

If the length of the lever arm is adjusted so that the line of action of the retraction force is located below the CR of the anterior teeth, there will be lingual crown torque of the anterior segment (Fig. 42.4D), while if the line of action of the retraction force is located above the CR, there will be lingual root torque of the anterior segment (Fig. 42.4E).

Appliance Construction

Because the interplay between the bracket slot and archwire is a very important factor, affecting the height of the lever arm, clinicians must be aware of the real slot size and shape of the lingual brackets (Table 42.2).[9]

In lingual orthodontics during anterior teeth retraction with sliding mechanics using brackets with horizontal slots, there is a tendency of the archwire to come out of the lingual bracket slot. Consequently, there is a bigger chance of losing control of anterior segment torque if the bracket slot walls are divergent. In such a case, a longer lever arm should be used and additional anterior torque should be applied to the archwire.

Fujita lingual brackets are provided with horizontal and vertical slots (Fig. 42.5). The size of the main horizontal slot is 0.018 × 0.025 inch and of the vertical slot is 0.019 × 0.019 inch. An SS archwire (0.016 × 0.022 inch) is inserted into the horizontal slot as the main archwire, while

Table 42.2 Bracket slot size, shape and difference between slot top and slot base

Bracket-type prescription	Mean slot size (%)		Slot shape	Difference from slot top to base
	Slot base	Slot top		
Ormco 7th generation	13.95	17.23	D	3.28
STB	−0.92	2.58	D	3.5
Fujita	6.08	4.33	C	−1.75
Stealth	7.61	7.63	P	0.2
In-Ovation L	3.94	5.2	D	1.26

D, divergent; C, convergent; P, parallel.

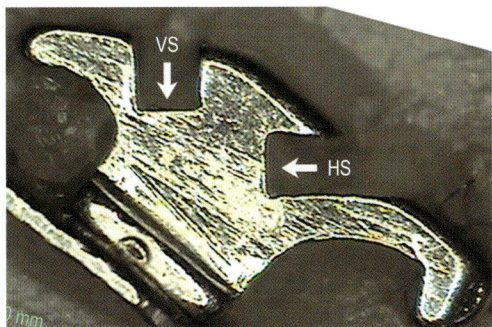

Fig. 42.5 Anterior Fujita bracket. VS, vertical slot; HS, horizontal slot.

an SS segmented archwire (0.018 × 0.018 inch or 0.019 × 0.019 inch) is inserted into the vertical slot. This segmented archwire can be used for additional anterior torque control and can prevent unintentional anterior torque loss, thus allowing shorter lever arms to be used during anterior teeth retraction.[10]

When the lever arm is located between the lateral incisor and the canine, its length in the vertical is 2–3 mm shorter than its actual length because of the inclination of the palatal vault. Therefore, a crimpable hook 7 mm in length is recommended to be used as lever arm for controlled tipping during anterior teeth retraction and one of 10 mm in length for bodily movement. Alternatively, a 7 mm crimpable hook fabricated from SS segmented archwire (0.019 × 0.019 inch) can be applied for additional lingual root torque. However, when a lever arm of more than 10 mm in length is needed for bodily movement, for example with low bone level or requiring lingual root movement, soldering of a 0.9 mm SS wire is recommended to prevent deformation.

CLINICAL APPLICATION

CASE 2: LIP PROTRUSION AND ANTERIOR CROWDING

A 33-year-old Korean woman presented with the chief complaint of lip protrusion and anterior crowding. She had a convex profile and Class I malocclusion (Fig. 42.6A,B). Cephalometric analysis revealed Class II skeletal relationships of the maxilla and mandible (Table 42.3).

Initially, all four first premolars were extracted and the brackets were bonded indirectly. After 5 months of treatment, both maxillary and mandibular teeth were leveled and aligned (Fig. 42.6C,D). During space closure, bodily movements of maxillary anterior teeth without anchorage loss were required. Two 9 mm MIs were inserted between the maxillary first molars and second premolars. A 7 mm crimpable hook (SS wire, 0.016 × 0.022 inch) was used as lever arm and positioned distal to the canines. An SS wire (0.019 × 0.019 inch) was also placed into the vertical

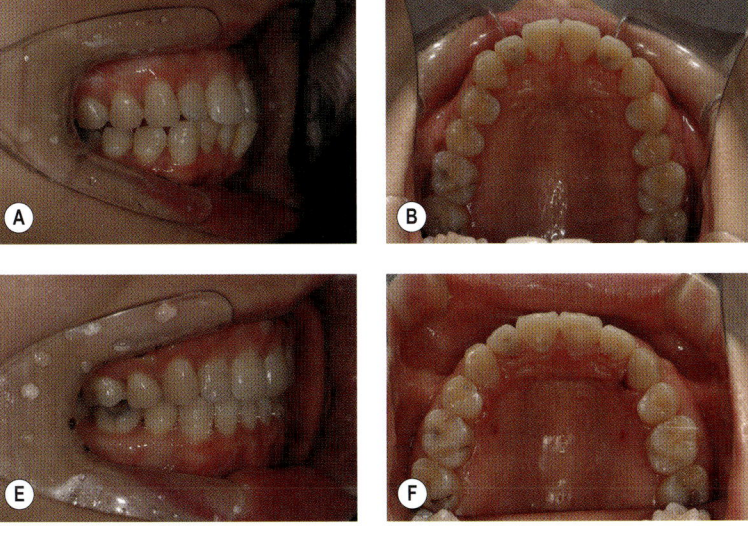

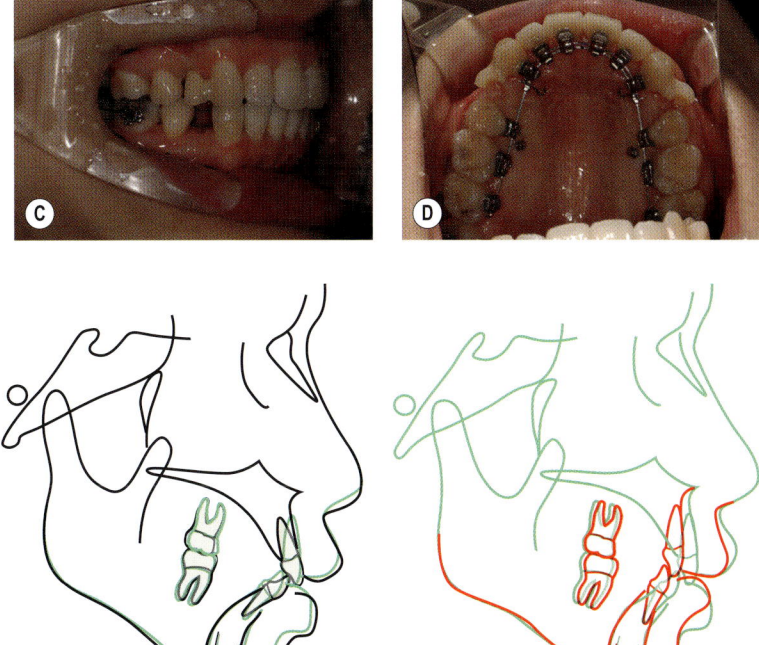

Fig. 42.6 Case 2: anterior teeth retraction for lip protrusion and anterior crowding. (A,B) Pretreatment. (C) Bonding of lingual appliances on both dental arches. (D) Insertion of the lever arm and miniscrew implant system for anterior teeth retraction on the maxilla. (E,F) Post-treatment. (G,H) Superimposition of cephalometric tracings before treatment (black) and before retraction (green) (G), and before retraction (green) and after treatment (red) (H).

Table 42.3 Case 3: cephalometric measurements

Measurement	Pretreatment	Before retraction	Post-treatment
Skeletal			
SNA (°)	86	86	85
SNB (°)	78	78	78
ANB (°)	8	8	7
FMA (°)	32	31.5	31.5
NPo-FH (°)	87	86.5	86.5
Dental			
U1 to FH (°)	107	95	93
FMIA (°)	45	56	69
Overbite (mm)	3	4.5	3.5
Overjet (mm)	4.5	5	3.5
Soft tissues			
Upper lip to E-line (mm)	5.5	4.5	0.5
Lower lip to E-line (mm)	6.5	5	1

FMA, Frankfort-mandibular plane angle; FMIA, Frankfort-mandibular incisor angle.

slot, with 10° of additional lingual root torque. According to the evaluation of the lateral cephalometric radiograph, the upper ending of the lever arm was constructed 12 mm away from the incisal edge. After 3 further months, 6 mm MIs were inserted between the mandibular first molars and second premolars for anchorage reinforcement and treatment was continued for an additional 10 months. After a total of 18 months, treatment was completed.

After treatment, the convex profile was favorably improved, and crowding was corrected (Fig. 42.6E,F). Superimpositions of the cephalometric tracing before and after treatment showed that bodily movement of the maxillary incisors occurred without evidence of loss of anchorage of the posterior teeth (i.e. maxillary molars did not move mesially during retraction; Fig. 42.6G,H). In addition, no downward or backward rotation of the mandible was evident, and lip protrusion was improved.

REFERENCES

1. Lim SM, Hong RK. Distal movement of maxillary molars using a lever-arm and miniscrew implant system. Angle Orthod 2008;78:167–75.
2. Sia SS, Koga Y, Yoshida N. Determining the center of resistance of maxillary anterior teeth subjected to retraction forces in sliding mechanics: an in vivo study. Angle Orthod 2007;77:999–1003.
3. Sia SS, Shibazaki T, Koga Y, et al. Experimental determination of optimal force system required for control of anterior tooth movement in sliding mechanics. Am J Orthod Dentofacial Orthop 2009;135:36–41.
4. Tominaga JY, Tanaka M, Koga Y, et al. Optimal loading conditions for controlled movement of anterior teeth in sliding mechanics. Angle Orthod 2009;79:102–7.
5. Kim TS, Suh JS, Lee MK. Optimum conditions for parallel translation of maxillary anterior teeth under retraction force determined with the finite element method. Am J Orthod Dentofacial Orthop 2010;137:639–47.
6. Bantleon HP. Modified lingual lever arm technique: biomechanical considerations. In: Nanda R, editor. Biomechanics in clinical orthodontics. Philadelphia, PA: Saunders; 1997. p. 229–45.
7. Park YC, Choy KC, Lee JS, et al. Lever-arm mechanics in lingual orthodontics. J Clin Orthod 2000;34:601–5.
8. Hong RK, Heo JM, Ha YK. Lever-arm and miniscrew implant system for anterior torque control during retraction in lingual orthodontic treatment. Angle Orthod 2005;75:129–41.
9. Lim SM, Hong RK. An evaluation of slot size in lingual orthodontic brackets. Kor J Lingual Orthod 2012;1:19–23.
10. Lim SM, Hong RK. The tandem archwire technique in lingual orthodontics. J Clin Orthod 2013;47:232–40.

Molar and group distalization for the correction of Class II malocclusion using bone anchorage

Nazan Kucukkeles, Mustafa B. Ates and Nejat Erverdi

43

INTRODUCTION

Distalization using skeletal anchorage devices allows group movement of buccal segments without any side effects on the other teeth of the dental arch or the need for extended treatment in stages to complete the Class II correction (see Chapter 2).

This chapter describes (1) the initial use of a tooth-based anchorage that was converted to one using miniscrew implants (MIs) to support the tooth anchorage, (2) use of palatal implants, (3) use of zygomatic miniplate anchorage, and (4) use of MIs for maxillary molar distalization.

MOLAR DISTALIZATION WITH MINISCREW IMPLANTS SUPPORTING THE TOOTH-ANCHORING SYSTEM

Using MIs in the dental arch to support a tooth-anchored system can avoid some of the unwanted side effects seen when using tooth anchoring alone,

such as loss of anchorage of the anterior teeth in terms of maxillary incisor proclination and increase of overjet.

CASE 1: MAXILLARY MOLAR DISTALIZATION WITH THE KELES SLIDER AND MINISCREW IMPLANTS

A 15-year-old girl presented with the chief complaint of crowding of her upper anterior teeth. She had a symmetrical face, incompetent lips, an asymmetrical smiling line and a convex profile. She presented a Class II, division 1 malocclusion with Class I skeletal relationships in conjunction with a normal to high-angle vertical growth pattern. The lower incisors were proclined. The amount of crowding was 3.05 mm and 2.55 mm in the maxillary and mandibular arches, respectively (Fig. 43.1A,B). The treatment plan included a Keles Slider to distalize the upper posterior segments to correct the Class II dental relationships and fixed appliances to align the arches.

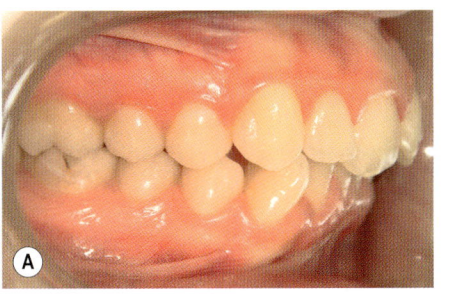
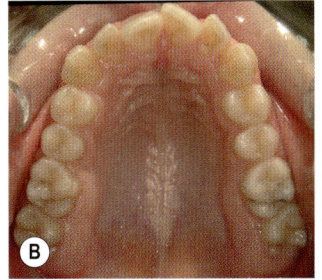
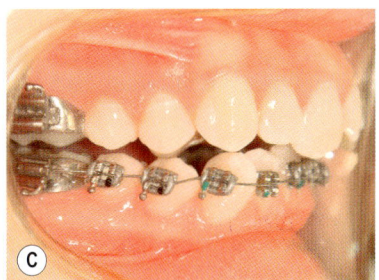
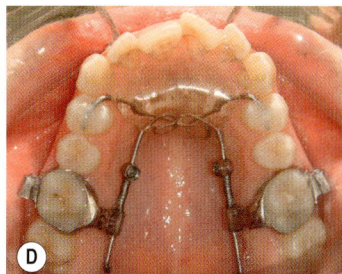
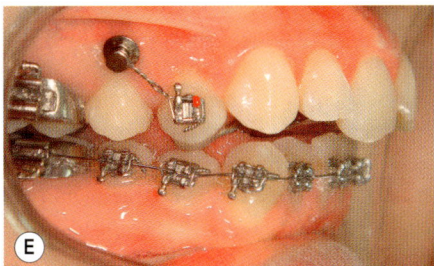
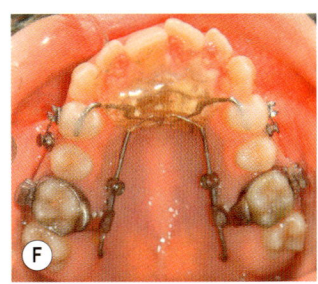
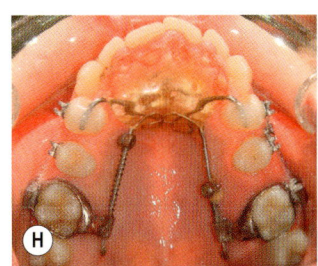
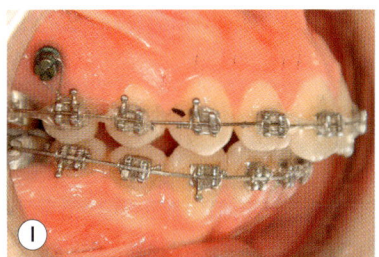
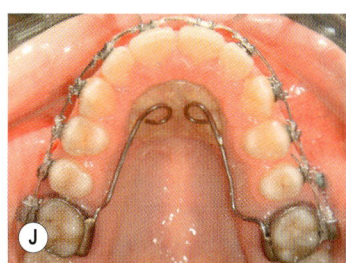
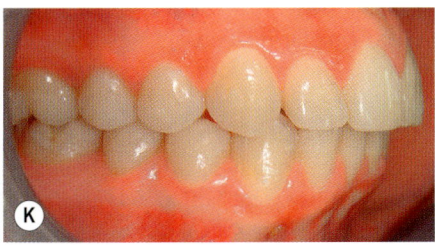
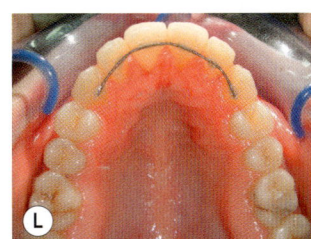

Fig. 43.1 Case 1: maxillary molar distalization with the Keles Slider and miniscrew implants (MIs). (A,B) Pretreatment. (C,D) Keles Slider cemented and bonding of the mandibular arch. (E,F) Insertion of MIs. (G,H) Molar distalization completed. (I,J) Premolars and canines have been distalized. (K,L) Post-treatment.

Treatment Progress

The Keles Slider was cemented to the first premolars and first molars. A Roth multibracket system with a slot (0.018 × 0.025 inch) was bonded on the lower arch and leveling was started with Ni-Ti archwire (0.014 inch) (Fig. 43.1C,D). Over the next 3 months, spaces developed between the premolars and first molars on both sides, but there was little improvement in molar relationship and little molar distalization. Activation of the appliances was discontinued, and two MIs (diameter, 1.6 mm; length, 8.0 mm) were placed between the premolars and ligated with the first premolars to control anchorage loss (Fig. 43.1E,F). Activation of the Keles Slider was restarted and maintained for 6 months until a super-Class I molar relationship was achieved on both sides (Fig. 43.1G,H).

The Keles Slider was then removed and a Nance appliance was placed to maintain molar position (Fig. 43.1I,J). In addition, the initial MIs were removed and two new MIs were placed mesial to the upper first molars. Using these MIs as anchorage, both premolars and canines were distalized using elastic chains on SS archwire (0.016 inch) (Fig. 43.1I,J). Anchorage of posterior teeth was then reinforced by ligating the canines with the MIs during retraction of anterior teeth with a TMA archwire (0.016 × 0.022 inch) with closing loops. Total treatment time was 28 months (Fig. 43.1K,L).

Treatment Results

Placement of MIs in the maxillary buccal inter-radicular space between the second premolars and the first molars at an oblique angle proved useful for moving the maxillary teeth distally en masse in this patient. Mesial movement of anchor teeth did not occur during distalization, and after molar movement, the premolars and canines were also distalized and the incisors retracted successfully. This protocol allowed effective non-compliance maxillary molar distalization without side effects.

Use of sandblasted MIs (diameter, 1.8 mm; length, 14.0 mm) in the anterior palatal region avoided mesial movement of the first premolars when they were used as anchor teeth during molar distalization through buccal mechanics.[1] Average distal movement of the first molars in this study was 3.9 mm and there was no anchorage loss. However, there was 8.8° of tipping as well as some distopalatal rotation with the buccal force application.

If distal tipping occurs alongside molar distalization, some of the space attained by distalization can be lost during molar uprighting when full fixed therapy is initiated.[2,3] Consequently, this should also be considered when using molar anchorage during fixed appliance treatment.[1]

MOLAR DISTALIZATION WITH PALATAL IMPLANTS

While it has been shown that dental implants placed in alveolar bone can withstand the forces required for orthodontic movements,[1,4–6] many patients seeking orthodontic treatment have complete dentitions and, therefore, no available alveolar bone sites for implant placement. Consequently, several studies have looked at alternative sites, such as the hard palate, the mandibular retromolar area, the inferior border of the zygomatic buttress, the symphysis region and the labial or buccal inter-radicular bone areas.[7]

Several criteria should be considered when selecting an implant site:

- whether the site can support the planned biomechanics required for indirect or direct anchorage
- if implant placement can be achieved without causing any root, nerve or artery injury
- if a bone site is available that presents adequate depth and thickness

- if an area rich in cortical bone is available, as this improves the primary stability of the implant.

Palatal bone is widely used as a site for orthodontic implants because of its favorable cortical bone thickness.[8] The midpalatal suture area seems particularly suitable as it has both thin soft tissue and thick cortical bone[9] and so will allow maximum retention (good quality and quantity of bone) with least risk of soft tissue inflammation. There are also no anatomical structures, such as nerves, blood vessels or roots, that can be damaged during implant placement.[10] The palatal area within 1 mm of the midpalatal suture presents the thickest bone in the whole palate, with thickness tending to decrease toward lateral and posterior.[11] The best area seems to be at the level of the first and second premolars. The soft tissue of the median palate in this area is, on average, 0.45–3.06 mm thick. This, with the intrinsic characteristics of the palatal mucosa, guarantees biomechanical stability for the placement of implants and MIs.[10]

There are some studies reporting results following the use of osseointegrated palatal implants or onplants as direct or indirect anchorage modalities during molar distalization.[8,12–13] When maxillary molars are distalized using palatal implants as anchorage, two side effects are commonly observed, depending on the location of the line of action of the force. First, when the force vector from the sagittal aspect does not pass through the center of resistance of the maxillary molars, the molar crowns tip mesially or distally. Second, depending on the location of the distalizing force (buccal side for mesial-out, lingual side for distal-out) from the occlusal aspect, the molar crown will rotate mesial-out or distal-in. Preventing this rotational tendency is usually more difficult because of anatomical constraints. A rigid TPA may help to prevent it.[14]

A 17-year-old patient presented with the chief complaint of crowding of her upper teeth. She had a symmetrical face and a balanced profile. She had a Class II molar and canine relationship and severe crowding of the maxillary anterior teeth (Fig. 43.2A,B). Both upper canines were buccally positioned, the left canine totally out of the arch, while the left lateral incisor was in full crossbite. The upper dental midline was in line with the face, but there was a 1.5 mm midline deviation of the mandibular arch to the left. Overbite was 1.0 mm and overjet 1.5 mm. She had skeletal Class I relationships and an average vertical growth pattern. The treatment plan included maxillary molar distalization using palatal implants.

Treatment Progress

A stepped screw titanium implant (diameter, 4.5 mm; length, 3.8 mm) (Frialit-2 Implant System, Synchro Screw Implants, Friadent, Mannheim, Germany) was placed in the anterior palatal region (paramedian to the suture) for anchorage reinforcement. After waiting 3 months for osseointegration of the implant, molar distalization was initiated using mini-expansion screws that were anchored on the palatal implant (Fig. 43.2C,D). The patient was instructed and trained to open the screws twice a week (0.25 mm each turn) and was reviewed every 4 weeks to monitor progress. Once a super-Class I molar relationship was achieved, the device was kept in place for at least 3 months for retention to prevent relapse and to allow maxillary premolars to drift distally (Fig. 43.2E–G). The distalizing screws were then removed and a 1.2 mm SS transpalatal arch was adjusted and inserted into the abutment slot to maintain molar position (Fig. 43.2G) during the subsequent orthodontic treatment (Fig. 43.2H,I).

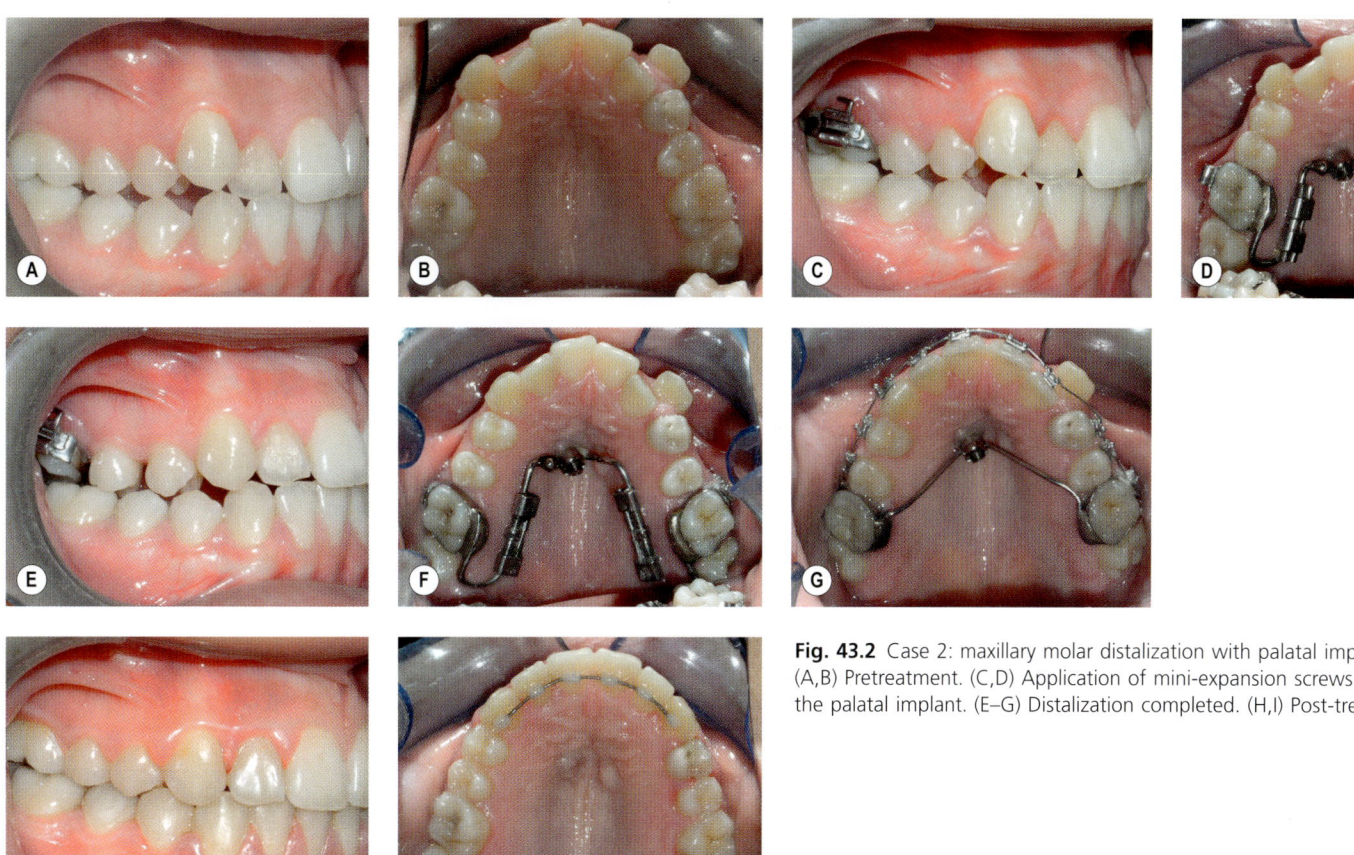

Fig. 43.2 Case 2: maxillary molar distalization with palatal implants. (A,B) Pretreatment. (C,D) Application of mini-expansion screws in conjunction with the palatal implant. (E–G) Distalization completed. (H,I) Post-treatment.

Treatment Results

Molar distalization took 6 months and overall treatment time was 20 months. Maxillary first molars moved 4.5 mm distally. Maxillary second bicuspids followed the first molars through distal drifting. Distal tipping of the maxillary molars and retrusion of incisors also occurred.

The amount of maxillary molar distalization was similar to that reported elsewhere: 6.4 mm in 7 months,[8] 6 mm in 7.8 months,[12] 3.4–4.5 mm in 6 months[5] and 5.9 mm in 5 months.[13] Although bodily molar distalization had been expected, cephalometric radiographs revealed that the molars also tipped during treatment.

Distal molar tipping ranging from 4.0° to 15.7° has been reported in many studies using intraoral distalization mechanics without skeletal anchorage.[15,16] However, it is also seen in studies using skeletal anchorage[5] even when attempts were made to avoid it, for example using coil springs or elastic chains along the archwire and an orthodontic titanium miniplate system (Skeletal Anchorage System).[6] Although some studies have used a distalization device soldered directly to a steel cap[17] or a specially designed cap with a rectangular slot to overcome tipping (Oric Cap, Basel, Switzerland), no data are available on the type of molar movement that occurs.

In the patient described here, the maxillary molars and premolars were rotated slightly in the distobuccal direction because the force vectors were applied on the palatal side.[18] Although this was not expected from such a rigid system, it can be attributed to bending of the arms of the device under the high forces delivered by activation of the expansion screws.[19]

Retroclination of the incisors was also observed, probably because of the pull of the transeptal fibers as the distalization forces acted on the maxillary arch. This effect was opposite to the effects of other intraoral molar distalization systems, which result in proclination of the maxillary incisors.[2,20,21] However, increases in the overjet (of 1.3 to 4.7 mm) have been noted in studies with conventional intraoral distalization systems,[2,15,22] which is not unexpected as the devices included the incisor segment as anchorage.

MOLAR DISTALIZATION WITH ZYGOMATIC ANCHORAGE

The maxilla is made up of thin cortical bone in its buccal and labial aspects. Bone thickness is not more than 2 mm, except in the three buttress areas: (1) the posterior buttress close to the tuber area, (2) the zygomatic buttress and (3) the nasal buttress close to the nasal area. All these areas have a thick and solid bony structure, which makes implant placement possible. The location of the posterior buttress prevents easy access and the nasal buttress area is not suitable because of its close location to the infraorbital foramen and nasal cavity. However, the inferior border of the zygomatico-maxillary buttress is suitable as direct access is easy and it is away from critical anatomical structures. Because it is close to the maxillary molars, the zygomatic buttress can be used for their anchorage either directly or indirectly.

Zygomatic miniplates are easily placed and removed under local anesthesia. They can be used in various clinical situations, such as arch expansion, retraction and distalization, as well as for the treatment of open bite, without the need for patient cooperation in wearing an appliance. However, although they provide new treatment possibilities, careful case selection is needed.

CASE 3: MAXILLARY MOLAR DISTALIZATION WITH ZYGOMATIC MINIPLATES

A 15-year-old girl was referred with the chief complaint of protrusion of the upper incisors. She had a symmetrical face, high smiling line, competent lips and a convex profile (Fig. 43.3A,B). Clinical examination revealed a unilateral Class II canine and molar relationship on the right side and Class I on the left. The maxillary arch was constricted, while both arches

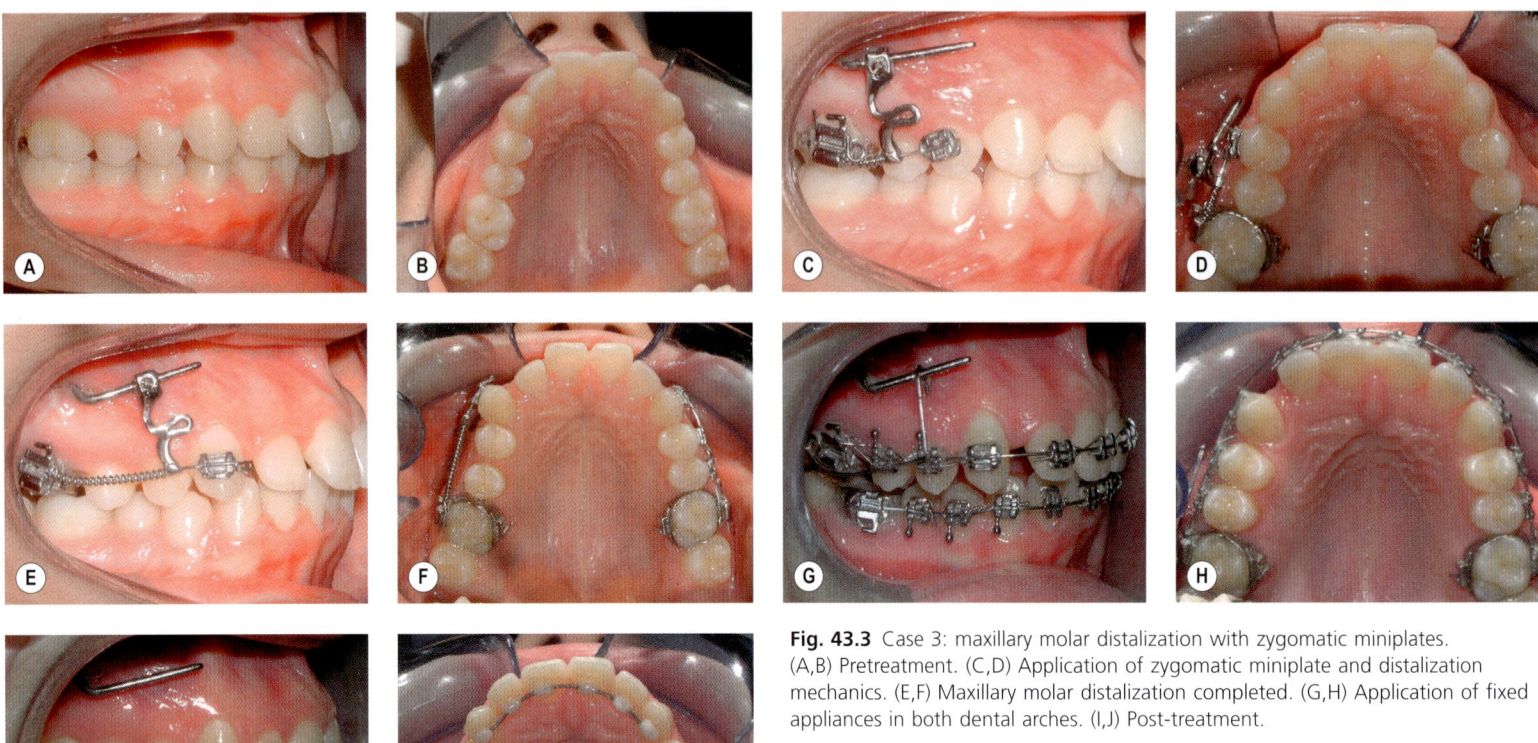

Fig. 43.3 Case 3: maxillary molar distalization with zygomatic miniplates. (A,B) Pretreatment. (C,D) Application of zygomatic miniplate and distalization mechanics. (E,F) Maxillary molar distalization completed. (G,H) Application of fixed appliances in both dental arches. (I,J) Post-treatment.

showed slight crowding of the anterior teeth. The treatment objectives included correction of the unilateral Class II molar and canine relationship and improvement of smile esthetics by eliminating the posterior gummy smile and dark buccal corridors. The treatment plan involved distalization of the right maxillary molars using zygomatic anchorage, followed by fixed appliance therapy.

Treatment Progress

A zygomatic miniplate (Multi Purpose Implant MPI 1000, Tasarim, Istanbul, Turkey) with a 0.9 mm bar thickness was used as anchorage for maxillary molar distalization. The upper part of the miniplate was adapted to the curve of the zygomatic buttress area, 5 mm mesial to the line passing from the mesial edge of the first molar tube. The round bar was extended downwards to the level of the first molar tube and then bent towards mesial along the sulcus depth, 3 mm away from the vestibular mucosa to maintain hygiene in this area (Fig. 43.3C,D). An SS round wire (diameter 1 mm) was soldered on to the lower surface of the custom fabricated metal sliding lock (Dentaurum, Ispringen, Germany), extending towards the archwire to transfer the point of force application to the level of the archwire. A horizontal U-bend was made in the wire to adjust the force vector. A segmental round tube was soldered to the lower edge of this wire at the same level as the main archwire in order to facilitate compression of an open coil spring. The metal sliding lock was engaged on the mesial extension of the zygomatic implant. An SS archwire (0.016 inch) was engaged passing through the segmental tube, a segmental Ni-Ti open coil spring was placed on the archwire after the segmental tube, and the archwire was engaged in the main tube of the molar band. A metal sliding lock was moved in a distal direction so that sufficient activation of the open coil spring was obtained and it was then fixed in position.

The patient was seen every 4 weeks to monitor progress, while the system was reactivated every 2 months by shifting the sliding lock towards distal or by placing a longer open coil spring. Distalization was completed in approximately 4 months (Fig. 43.3E,F).

After completion of distalization, the second premolars had also moved distally, partially under the influence of the transeptal fibers. Orthodontic treatment was continued using fixed appliances for the final alignment of the arches and detailing of the occlusion, during which time molar position was maintained using wire ligation between the implant and the molar tubes (Fig. 43.3G,H).

Treatment Results

At the end of treatment, a Class I canine and molar relationship was achieved on both sides; the maxillary arch was slightly expanded and smile esthetics were improved (Fig. 43.3I,J). Zygomatic miniplates were easily removed under local anesthesia.

MOLAR DISTALIZATION WITH MINISCREW IMPLANTS

Recently, MIs have gained wide acceptance for use as stationary anchorage modalities. They have several clinical advantages: minimal anatomical placement limitations, lower cost and simpler placement with less traumatic surgery. In patients who had MI insertion, 50% did not feel pain at any time after placement, and most reported minimal discomfort from swelling and few speech or chewing difficulties. However, use of MIs does have several disadvantages and risks: damage can occur to anatomical structures such as dental roots, nerves and blood vessels; a MI can break during placement or removal; and failure can occur, mainly through

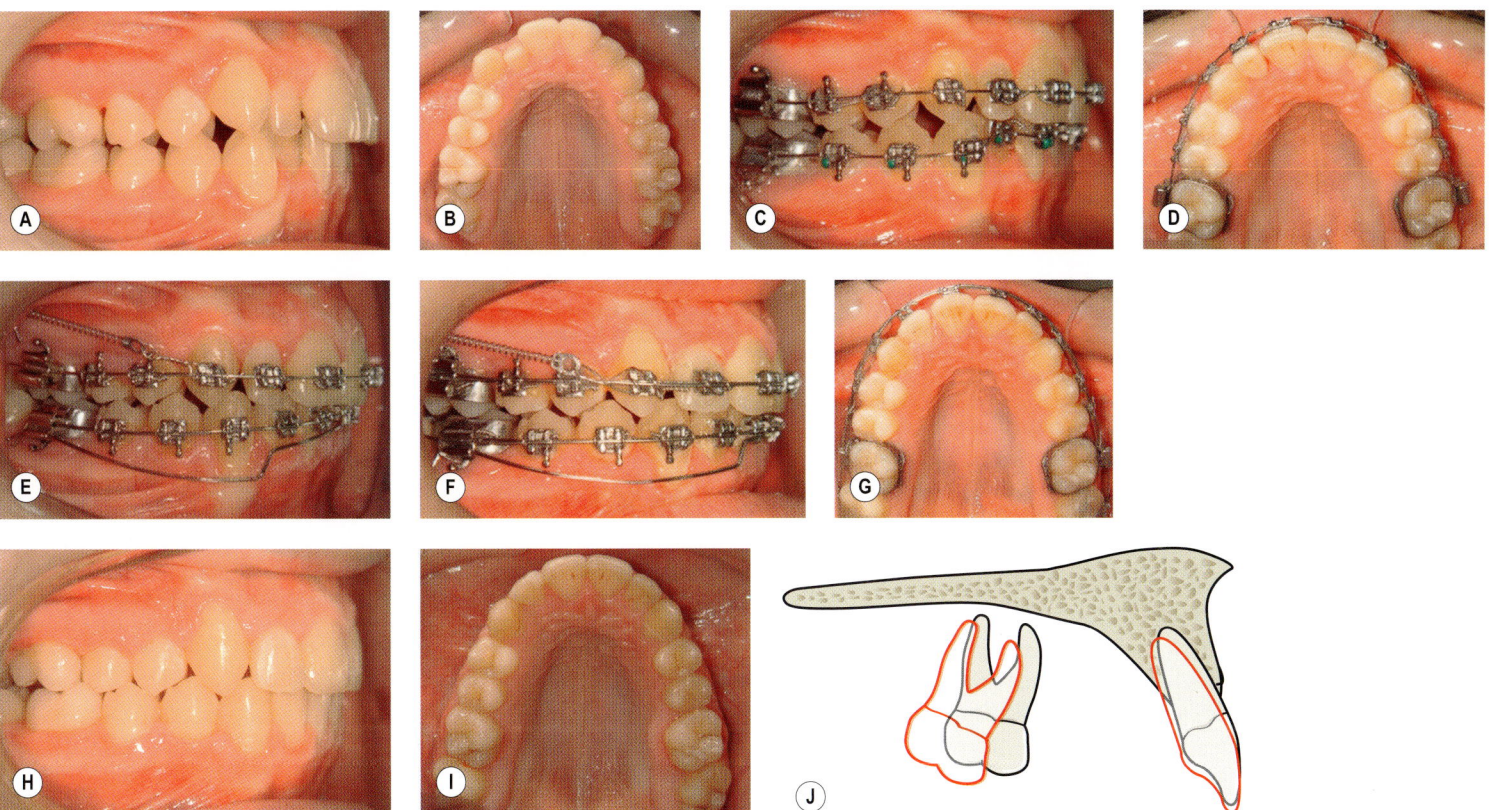

Fig. 43.4 Case 4: unilateral maxillary molar distalization with miniscrew implants (MIs). (A,B) Pretreatment. (C,D) Fixed orthodontic appliances inserted. (E) Application of the MI. (F,G) Molar distalization completed. (H,I) Post-treatment. (J) Cephalometric superimposition of the maxilla before (black) and after (red) treatment shows the distalization effect.

peri-implant inflammation. Success rates with MIs are reported between 80 and 95%.[23]

Various anatomical sites have been proposed for MI insertion. Placement into the basal bone below the roots of the teeth prevents root damage but limits the amount of vertical force vectors that can be applied.[24,25] Implanting MIs into alveolar bone between the roots of the posterior teeth increases the horizontal component of the applied force.[26] The inter-radicular spaces between the roots of the second premolars and those of the first molars in the maxillary arch and between the roots of the first molars and those of the second molars in the mandibular arch are generally now accepted as the best sites for MI placement on the buccal side of the jaws.[27]

In the maxilla, the greatest amount of bone mesiodistally is on the palatal side between the second premolars and the first molars, while the least amount of bone is in the tuberosity. In addition, the greatest bone thickness in the buccopalatal dimension is between the first and second molars, whereas the least is again in the tuberosity.[28]

Skeletal anchorage can be obtained directly, where force is transmitted directly to the implant, or indirectly, where the skeletal anchorage device is connected to the anchor teeth and forces are applied to these teeth and to a tooth or group of teeth that have to be moved.[14]

CASE 4: UNILATERAL MAXILLARY MOLAR DISTALIZATION WITH MINISCREW IMPLANTS

A 16-year-old boy presented with the chief complaint of crowding of his upper anterior teeth. He had a symmetrical face, normal smiling line and a convex profile (Fig. 43.4A,B). He had a Class II, subdivision malocclusion and Class I skeletal relationships with an average vertical growth pattern. The lower incisors were proclined and there was a 3.75 mm arch length discrepancy in the maxillary arch and 1.2 mm in the mandibular

arch. The treatment plan included use of a MI to support distalization of the upper right posterior segment and correction of the Class II dental relationship plus fixed appliances to correct crowding of the maxillary and mandibular dental arches and create some space for the peg-shaped right lateral incisor to enable it to be restored to a normal shape.

Treatment Progress

A Roth multibracket system with a slot (as used in Case 1) was bonded first on the maxillary arch and after 2 months to the mandibular teeth. Leveling was started with Ni-Ti archwires (0.014 inch) (Fig. 43.4C,D). Following insertion of SS wire (0.016 inch), a MI (diameter, 1.6 mm; length, 7 mm) was placed between the maxillary first and second molars in order to distalize the upper right posterior segment and correct Class II malocclusion. The MI was positioned 8 mm above the sulcus between the roots. The MI was then tied to the right canine and a distalization force of 150 g was provided using a closed coil spring. In order to correct the occlusal cant of the mandibular arch, an asymmetric intrusion arch was tied to the main Ni-Ti archwire (0.016 × 0.016 inch) at the left lateral incisor (Fig. 43.4E). At every appointment, both the closed coil spring tied to the maxillary right canine and the intrusion utility arch were activated. After 6 months, the occlusal cant was corrected and the intrusion arch was removed and replaced by SS archwire. Because of the existence of Bolton excess on the anterior region of the mandibular arch, interproximal stripping of the incisors (approximately 1.5 mm) was undertaken. After distalization of the maxillary right posterior segment, a diastema was created between the upper right lateral incisor and canine. Since the right lateral incisor was peg shaped, a composite restoration was performed to recreate the normal shape (Fig. 43.4F,G). Total treatment time was 18 months.

Treatment Results

After completion of treatment, a Class I canine and molar relationship was achieved on both sides, and the smile esthetics were improved (Fig. 43.4H,I). The right maxillary molar moved distally approximately 4 mm against the MI and slightly extruded during leveling. However, this was not a bodily movement since the molar also exhibited 6° of tipping (Fig. 43.4J). Maxillary incisor position was almost stable. The MI was also stable during distalization as well as during the subsequent treatment, without any complications, and it was removed easily during debonding. No root resorption was observed in the post-treatment panoramic radiograph.

Placement of MIs in the maxillary buccal inter-radicular spaces between the first and the second molars at an oblique angle proved very useful for moving a group of teeth distally in this patient. Molar distal movement was achieved without active patient compliance and with no undesirable side effects such as incisor proclination, clockwise mandibular rotation or root resorption.

The procedure reported for this patient was slower than other published distalization methods. However, the overall treatment time was similar or even shorter because all the posterior teeth were retracted simultaneously with MI-aided mechanics. The anterior teeth were retracted with conventional methods after distalization of the posterior segment, while maintaining the corrected position of the right segment by means of the MI.

CONCLUSIONS

Use of skeletal anchorage to provide an anchor for distalization forces allows tooth movements to occur without any reciprocal unwanted effects on other teeth of the dental arch. Use of MIs for skeletal anchorage has become popular as they are available in many sizes, facilitating their application in various areas; they provide stable anchorage for the application of orthodontic forces; and are easy to insert. However, the location for insertion, as for all anchorage devices, is very important when designing the treatment plan for distalization, and planning must consider the vertical components of the force vectors among other issues.

REFERENCES

1. Gelgor IE, Buyukyilmaz T, Karaman IE, et al. Intraosseous screw-supported upper molar distalization. Angle Orthod 2004;74:836–48.
2. Ghosh J, Nanda RS. Evaluation of intraoral maxillary molar distalization technique. Am J Orthod Dentofacial Orthop 1996;10:639–46.
3. Bolla E, Muratore F, Carano A, et al. Evaluation of maxillary molar distalization with the distal jet: A comparison with other contemporary methods. Angle Orthod 2002;72:481–94.
4. Karaman AI, Basçiftçi FA, Polat O. Unilateral distal molar movement with an implant-supported distal jet appliance. Angle Orthod 2001;72:167–74.
5. Oncag G, Seckin O, Dincer B, et al. Osseointegrated implants with pendulum springs for maxillary molar distalization: A cephalometric study. Am J Orthod Dentofacial Orthop 2007;131:16–26.
6. Sugawara J, Kanzaki R, Takahashi I. Distal movement of maxillary molars in non-growing patients with the skeletal anchorage system. Am J Orthod Dentofacial Orthop 2006;129:723–33.
7. Erverdi N, Keleş A, Nanda R. Orthodontic anchorage and skeletal implants. In: Nanda R, editor. Biomechanics and esthetic strategies in clinical orthodontics. Missouri: Elsevier, Saunders; 2005. p. 278–94.
8. Kircelli BH, Pektas ZO, Kircelli C. Maxillary molar distalization with a bone-anchored pendulum appliance. Angle Orthod 2006;76:650–9.
9. Asscherickx K, Vannet BV, Bottenberg P, et al. Clinical observations and success rates of palatal implants. Am J Orthod Dentofacial Orthop 2010;137:114–22.
10. Gracco A, Lombardo L, Cozzani M, et al. Quantitative cone-beam computed tomography evaluation of palatal bone thickness for orthodontic miniscrew placement. Am J Orthod Dentofacial Orthop 2008;134:361–9.
11. Martinelli FL, Luiz RR, Faria M, et al. Anatomic variability in alveolar sites for skeletal anchorage. Am J Orthod Dentofacial Orthop 2010;138:252.e1–e9.
12. Escobar SA, Tellez PA, Moncada CA, et al. Distalization of maxillary molars with the bone-supported pendulum: A clinical study. Am J Orthod Dentofacial Orthop 2007;131:545–9.
13. Oberti G, Villegas C, Ealo M, et al. Maxillary molar distalization with the dual-force distalizer supported by mini-implants: A clinical study. Am J Orthod Dentofacial Orthop 2009;135:282.e1–e5.
14. Uribe FA, Nanda R. Skeletal anchorage based on biomechanics. In: Nanda R, Uribe FA, editors. Temporary anchorage devices in orthodontics. Missouri: Elsevier, Mosby; 2009. p. 145–63.
15. Keles A, Sayinsu K. A new approach in maxillary molar distalization: Intraoral bodily molar distalizer. Am J Orthod Dentofacial Orthop 2000;117:39–48.
16. Kucukkeles N, Doganay A. Molar distalization with bimetric molar distalization arches. J Marmara Univ Dent Fac 1994;2:399–403.
17. Giancotti A, Muzzi M, Greco M, et al. Palatal implant-supported distalizing devices: Clinical application of the Strauman Orthosystem. World J Orthod 2002;3:135–9.
18. Kucukkeles N, Cakirer B, Mowafi M. Cephalometric evaluation of molar distalization by hyrax screw used in conjunction with a lip bumper. World J Orthod 2006;7:261–8.
19. Zimring J, Isaacson R. Forces produced by rapid maxillary expansion. Angle Orthod 1965;35:178–86.
20. Byloff FK, Darendeliler MA, Clar E, et al. Distal molar movement using the pendulum appliance. Part 2: The effects of maxillary molar root uprighting bends. Angle Orthod 1997;67:261–70.
21. Scuzzo G, Pisani F, Takemoto K. Maxillary molar distalization with a modified pendulum appliance. J Clin Orthod 1999;33:645–50.
22. Joseph AA, Butchart CJ. An evaluation of the pendulum distalizing appliance. Semin Orthod 2000;6:129–35.
23. Yamada K, Kuroda S, Deguchi T, et al. Distal movement of maxillary molars using miniscrew anchorage in the buccal interradicular region. Angle Orthod 2009;79:78–84.
24. Kanomi R. Mini implant for orthodontic anchorage. J Clin Orthod 1997;31:763–7.
25. Costa A, Raffainl M, Melsen B. Miniscrews as orthodontic anchorage: A preliminary report. Int J Adult Orthod Orthognath Surg 1998;13:201–9.
26. Park HS. The skeletal cortical anchorage using titanium microscrew implants. Korean J Orthod 1999;26:699–706.
27. Park HS. An anatomical study using CT images for the implantation of micro-implants. Korean J Orthod 2002;32:435–41.
28. Poggio PM, Incorvati C, Velo S, et al. 'Safe Zones': A guide for miniscrew positioning in the maxillary and mandibular arch. Angle Orthod 2006;76:191–7.

Treatment of Class II open bite malocclusion supported by skeletal anchorage

44

Kazuo Tanne, Junji Ohtani, Hiroko Sunagawa, Masato Kaku and Tadashi Fujita

INTRODUCTION

Class II open bite morphologically is characterized by large molar height and subsequent mandibular displacement backward and downward. The large mandibular plane angle in Class II open bite is regarded as the most difficult malocclusion for orthodontic treatment because of the associated nasopharyngeal respiratory disorders that may have induced it. Nasopharyngeal disorders may lead to Class II open bite by the following sequence.[2,3]

- Nasopharyngeal airway obstruction
- Habitual mouth opening and breathing
- Reduction in masticatory muscle activity, masseter muscle in particular, with abnormal swallowing and tongue thrusting
- Prominent vertical growth of posterior dentoalveolar structures with large molar height
- Backward and downward displacement of the mandible
- Onset of Class II open bite with small and/or distally located mandible.

Based on this, it could be reasonably assumed that open bite can be corrected efficiently by molar intrusion and the resultant forward and upward rotation of the mandible (in other words, mandibular autorotation). An edgewise technique with extraction of teeth does enable correction of open bite through alignment of teeth, movement of the molar teeth into the extraction site and extrusion of the anterior teeth. However, this anterior teeth extrusion can lead to substantial root resorption. The multiloop edgewise archwire (MEAW) technique[1] was developed for distalizing and intruding molars for the treatment of open bite (Fig. 44.1) and for treatment of mandibular prognathism and maxillary protrusion.

However, the MEAW technique and the vertical elastics create repetitive intrusion and extrusion forces on the anterior teeth experience, and a certain amount of anterior teeth extrusion is almost always produced, which could lead to relapse of open bite and root resorption of the anterior teeth. Consequently, approaches using miniscrew implants (MIs) and miniplates may be an opportune way to obtain the desired results without unwanted side effects.

TREATMENT OF CLASS II OPEN BITE WITH MINISCREW IMPLANT-SUPPORTED TREATMENT

It has been shown that molar intrusion is superior to incisor extrusion for open bite treatment in terms of lower incidences of relapse and root resorption.[4] The treatment biomechanics when using MI anchorage may be similar to that when using the MEAW technique; however, the efficiency of molar intrusion is substantially higher with MI anchorage than with the MEAW technique.

Successful use of MIs and miniplates as anchorage is dependent upon the clinician's knowledge of the many factors that may affect their primary stability, both host factors (e.g. age, comorbidities, oral hygiene, bone quality) and technical factors (e.g. length, diameter of the MI, insertion technique, torque). Section II discusses in detail the factors for successful use of MIs and miniplates as temporary anchorage devices for orthodontic treatment. The twisting torque used during MI insertion has been shown to be one key determinant for successful implantation. The optimal twisting torque for MI insertion in humans is 5–15 Ncm for the maxilla and 6–17 Ncm for the mandible and clinicians are recommended to maintain MI insertion torques within these optimal ranges. Our group has recently developed an electrical driver (approved by the Japanese Ministry of Health) that facilitates control of rotation direction, speed and twisting torque (Fig. 44.2). This electrical hand driver is rechargeable, very light and easy to use.

CASE EXAMPLES

The cases described below illustrate treatment approaches based on MIs (Cases 1 and 2) and a miniplate (Case 3).

CASE 1: AN ADULT WITH OPEN BITE

A 23-year-old woman presented with open bite with a Class II molar relationship and large overjet and overbite (7.2 mm and −3.6 mm, respectively; Fig. 44.3A,B). Tooth–jaw discrepancy was prominent, and

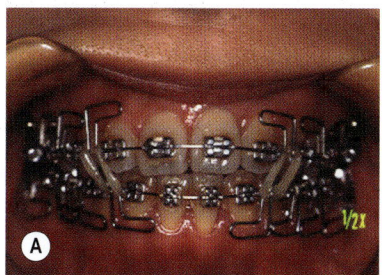
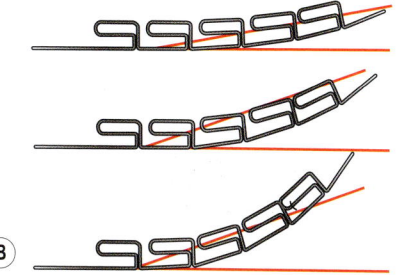
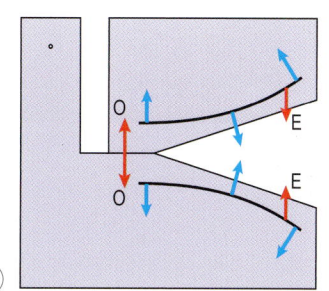
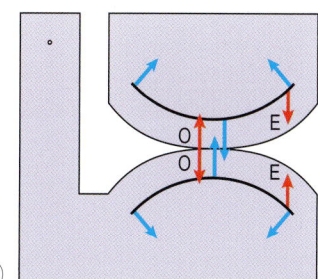

Fig. 44.1 (A-D) Biomechanics of the MEAW technique for the correction of open bite.

so the maxillary first premolars and mandibular second premolars were extracted.

After initial leveling with fixed appliances, four MIs were placed interradicularly in the maxilla, two on the buccal side and two on the palatal side (Fig. 44.3C,D). Elastics were used for the intrusion of the maxillary first and second molars and second premolars. The mandibular molars were fixed with a lingual arch because the curve of Spee was straight, indicating that molars were not extruded.

After 8 months of treatment, the overbite was corrected from −3.6 to 2.0 mm. At the end of active treatment after 29 months, overjet and overbite were improved from 7.2 to 2.5 mm and from −3.6 to 2.5 mm, respectively, and a well-functioning occlusion was established (Fig. 44.3E,F). On the superimposition of the cephalometric tracings before and after treatment, maxillary molar intrusion and subsequent counterclockwise rotation of the mandible were observed (Fig. 44.3G). These changes constitute the principal mechanism for an upward and forward displacement

of the mandible, directly leading to the correction of the Class II open bite. In addition, both maxillary and mandibular incisors experienced a prominent lingual tipping movement, which contributed to the correction of lip protrusion.

CASE 2: A 19-YEAR-OLD WOMAN WITH OPEN BITE AND IMPAIRED MASTICATORY FUNCTION

A 19.5-year-old woman with open bite tendency complained that she had impaired masticatory function from the reduced occlusal contacts. Four premolars had been extracted previously. Her facial profile was convex, with mentalis muscle overactivity. She had Class II molar relationships with 5.5 mm overjet and 0.5 mm overbite (Fig. 44.4A). Functional examination showed that the patient had pain on the temporomandibular joints (TMJ) during chewing and mouth opening. She had skeletal Class II relationships of the jaws (ANB angle, 9.8°) with severe mandibular deficiency (ANB angle, 66.7°) and a steep mandibular plane angle (37.1°) (Table 44.1). On TMJ radiographs taken by the Schüller method, the condyles occupied a relatively posterior position on the glenoid fossa (Fig. 44.4E), implying an anterior displacement of the articular disk. Her diagnosis was as a skeletal Class II open bite with TMJ problems. The initial treatment plan, involving surgery, was refused by the patient.

Treatment commenced with bonding of fixed appliances in both arches; a self-drilling titanium alloy MI (diameter, 1.6 mm; length, 6 mm; Dual-Top Auto Screw) was inserted into the midpalatal region at the level of the maxillary first molars in order to intrude the maxillary posterior teeth (Fig. 44.4B,C). A transpalatal arch was also placed in order to maintain the transversal dimension of the maxillary molars. The molars were intruded using elastic chains attached between the MI and the lingual sheaths of the first molar bands. Class II elastics were never used during treatment to avoid extrusion of mandibular posterior teeth. After 1 year of treatment, intrusion of the maxillary molars was completed. Overjet was changed from 5.5 to 2.0 mm and overbite from 0.5 to 2.5 mm; the teeth were well aligned in a good intercuspal position and the TMJ pain had disappeared. After a 3-year retention period, the occlusion was stable with no symptoms of TMJ problems (Fig. 44.4D). Radiography revealed that

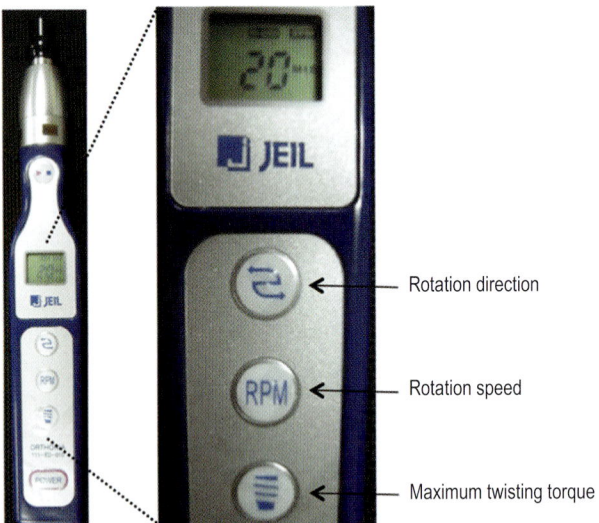

Fig. 44.2 The electronic torque controllable hand driver.

Rotation direction
Rotation speed
Maximum twisting torque

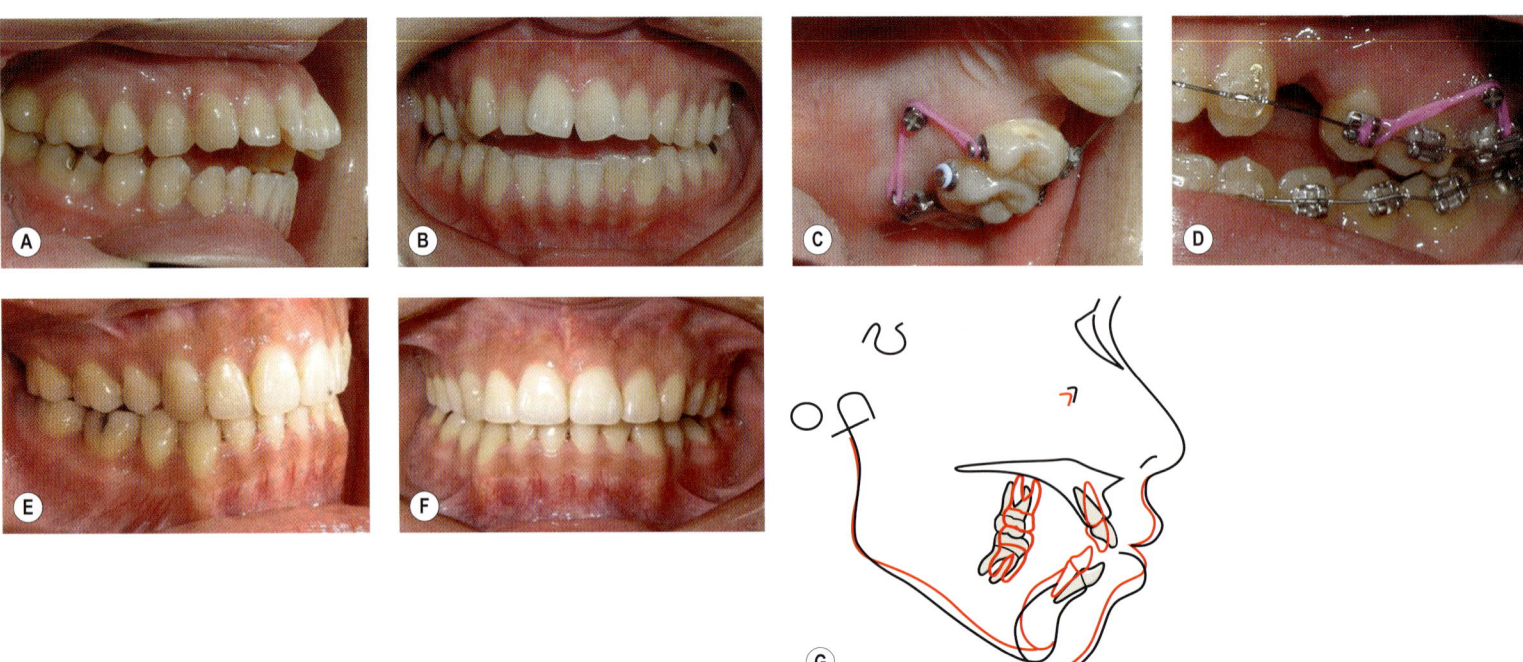

Fig. 44.3 Orthodontic treatment of Case 1. (A,B) Pre-treatment intraoral photographs. (C,D) Intrusion of the maxillary molars using MIs. (E,F) Post-treatment intraoral photographs. (G) Superimposition of the cephalometric tracings on the anterior cranial base (SN) before (black line) and after (red line) treatment.

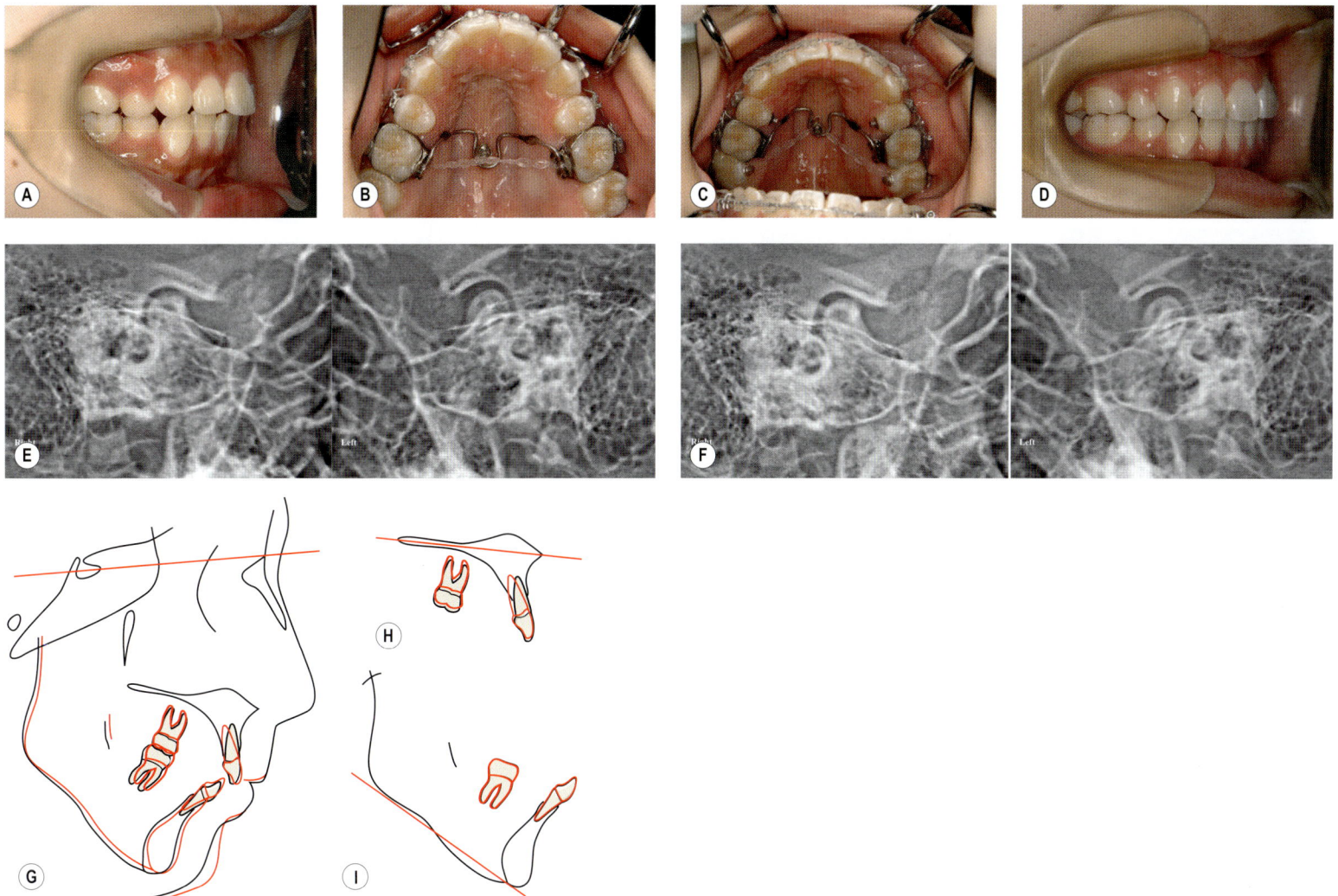

Fig. 44.4 Orthodontic treatment of Case 2. (A) Pretreatment intraoral photograph. (E) Pretreatment TMJ radiograph of the right and left condyle. (B,C) Progress intraoral photographs during intrusion of maxillary molars using an MI. (D) Post-treatment intraoral photographs. (F) Post-treatment TMJ radiograph of the right and left condyle. (G-I) Superimpositions of the cephalometric tracings on the anterior cranial base (G), on the maxilla (H), and on the mandible (I) before (black line) and after (red line) treatment.

Table 44.1 Case 2: cephalometric measurements

Measurements	Pre-retreatment	Post-treatment
SNA (°)	76.5	76.5
SNB (°)	66.7	67.8
ANB (°)	9.8	8.6
FMA (°)	37.1	35.1
FMIA (°)	41.2	44.3
IMPA (°)	101.6	100.6
U1-FH (°)	111.8	106.3
Z-angle (°)	56.0	62.7
Overjet (mm)	5.5	2.0
Overbite (mm)	0.5	2.5

IMPA, incisor mandibular plane angle; FMA, Frankfort-mandibular plane angle; FMIA, Frankfort-mandibular incisor angle.

after treatment both condyles were shifted significantly to an anterior position, occupying a more central position in the glenoid fossa (Fig. 44.4F). The facial profile was slightly changed, with a more relaxed mentalis muscle.

Superimposition of the lateral cephalometric tracings before and after treatment revealed that the maxillary molars were intruded by 2 mm, the mandible rotated in a counterclockwise direction (Fig. 44.4G–I), while the maxillary incisors experienced a lingual root torque. The ANB angle changed from 9.8 to 8.6°, the mandibular plane angle from 37.1 to 35.1° and the Z-angle from 56.0 to 62.7°, indicating an improvement of the lateral soft tissue profile (Table 44.1).

CASE 3: AN ADULT WITH SEVERE OPEN BITE AND DIFFICULTY IN LIP CLOSURE

A 32-year-old woman with severe open bite complained of difficulty in lip closure, which was caused by the severe maxillary protrusion and the open bite. Although orthognathic surgery was proposed, she requested a conservative non-surgical treatment plan. She had a convex lateral soft tissue profile with mentalis muscle overactivity caused by habitual mouth opening and breathing. She had bilateral Class II molar relationships and a severe open bite, with an overjet and overbite of 5.0 mm and −4.0 mm, respectively (Fig. 44.5A,B). Cephalometric analysis revealed skeletal Class II relationships of the jaws (ANB angle, 11.0°) and a skeletal open bite with a large mandibular plane angle (39.3°).

The treatment plan included molar intrusion and retraction of the anterior teeth after the extraction of maxillary second premolars with use of a miniplate placed on the zygomatic bone to provide skeletal anchorage (Fig. 44.5C).

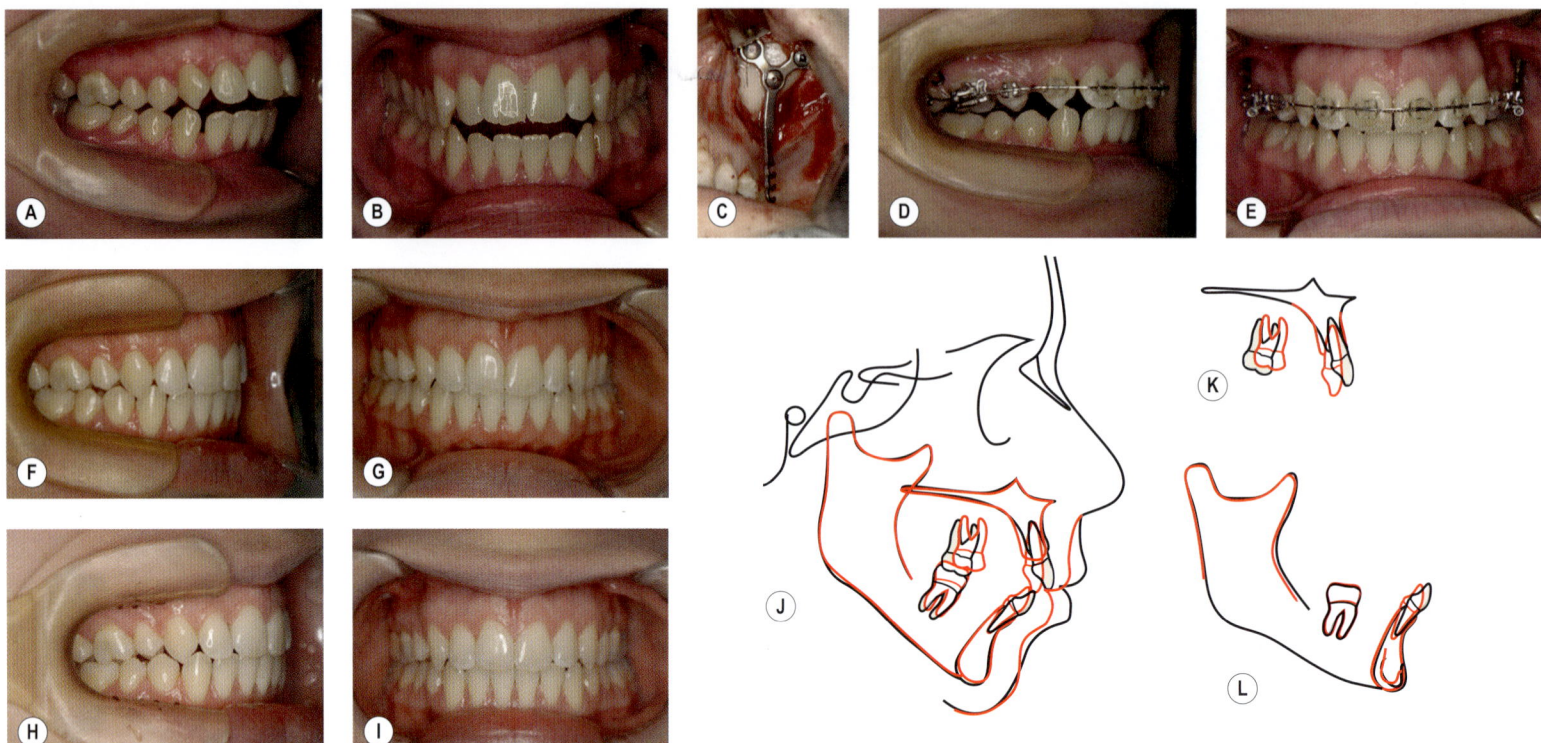

Fig. 44.5 Orthodontic treatment of Case 3. (A,B) Pre-treatment intraoral photographs. (C) Intraoral photograph depicting the positioning of the zygomatic miniplate. (D,E) Progress intraoral photographs during intrusion of the molars with miniplates. (F,G) Post-treatment intraoral photographs. (H,I) Post-retention intraoral photographs. (J-L) Superimpositions of the cephalometric tracings on the anterior cranial base (J), on the maxilla (K), and on the mandible (L) before (black line) and after treatment (red line).

After insertion of fixed appliances and leveling of both dental arches, intrusion of the first and second molars was initiated using elastic chains connected to the miniplate. Seven months later, the open bite was corrected (Fig. 44.5D,E). After 2 years of treatment, an acceptable occlusion was achieved and retention was initiated with lingual bonded retainers on both dental arches and removable retainers for night wear (Fig. 44.5F,G). The occlusion was stable even after 2 years in retention (Fig. 44.5H,I).

The overall facial balance was improved. Superimposition of the cephalometric tracings before and after treatment showed that the maxillary molars were intruded by 4.0 mm and a counterclockwise rotation of the mandible had occurred (Fig. 44.5J–L). The ANB angle changed from 11.0 to 5.2° and the mandibular plane angle from 39.3 to 37.0°.

CONCLUSIONS

The treatment outcomes described here indicate that MIs are more reliable and efficient for the treatment of open bite than the MEAW approach, in terms of quick molar intrusion and distalization with less dependence on patient cooperation. Skeletal anchorage with miniplates on the zygomatic bone (Case 3) provided more extensive and efficient tooth movements than MIs in terms of molar intrusion, molar distalization and retraction of anterior teeth, all of which are essential for the treatment of Class II open bite.

These findings suggest that some patients with skeletal open bite, which would ideally have been treated by surgical correction, may be treated solely orthodontically. However, more extensive studies are required to examine the nature of relapse of molar intrusion and the long-term stability of the results.

REFERENCES

1. Kim YH. Anterior open bite and its treatment with MEAW. Angle Orthod 1987;57: 290–321.
2. Tanne K. Association between nasopharyngeal disease and orthodontic treatment. Part 1: the onset of malocclusion resulted from nasorespiratory disturbances. J Orthod Pract 2000;16:11–20.
3. Shikata N, Ueda HM, Kato M, et al. Association between nasal respiratory obstruction and vertical mandibular position. J Oral Rehabil 2004;31:957–62.
4. Chang YI, Moon SC. Cephalometric evaluation of the anterior open bite treatment. Am J Orthod Dentofacial Orthop 1999;115:29–37.

INTRODUCTION

Molar and canine Class II relationships can result from skeletal discrepancies of a hypoplastic mandible relative to a normal maxilla, a hyperplastic maxilla relative to a normal mandible or a combination of hyperplastic maxilla to hypoplastic mandible to varying degrees. In bimaxillary skeletal harmony, dental Class II patterns can still occur if the maxillary posterior molars drift mesially as a result of early loss or exfoliation of primary teeth.

If there is minimal anticipated growth, such as in older adolescents and adults, and the skeletal discrepancy is determined to be within the boundaries of dental camouflage, the malocclusion is usually corrected using conventional orthodontic biomechanics, which rely on dentoalveolar compensation and on extractions of permanent teeth. However, many individuals and parents are extremely resistant to removal of permanent teeth and are adamant in treating their problems without extractions.

The use of skeletal anchorage, such as miniscrew implants (MIs) or miniplates, avoids issues of patient compliance, provides a consistent intraoral anchor unit and allows the desired tooth movements without any untoward movement of peripheral teeth.

This chapter describes the clinical applications of the C-type orthodontic bone anchors (OBAs), such as the C-implant and C-tube miniplate, including immediate relocation procedures for these in the correction of Class II malocclusions without extracting permanent teeth.

The treatment philosophy follows the fundamental principles of biocreative therapy (C-therapy). Biocreative therapy is a novel treatment philosophy advocated and clinically applied by K. R. Chung in Korea since 2001. The objectives are simplified and patient-friendly orthodontic biomechanics using OBAs plus reduced time for orthodontic adjustment at each visit. The treatment protocol dictates that conventional fixed orthodontic appliances are placed only on teeth that need to be moved. Biocreative therapy uses C-type OBAs, which include C-implants, C-tube

miniplates and/or C-palatal miniplates,[1] in a manner quite distinct from the systems that use MIs, focusing on them as the core construct of the dental movement protocol and supplemented by orthodontic brackets and wires.[2-4] The C-type OBAs can endure multidirectional heavy orthodontic and orthopedic forces with better stability, which is essential to moving multiple teeth at the same time and may reduce the total treatment time. Higher resistance to heavy forces also effectively reduces the total number of C-type OBAs needed to achieve the orthodontic tooth movement.

This chapter will discuss two types of C-type OBAs applied for the non-extraction correction of Class II malocclusion: the C-implant and the C-tube miniplate.

C-TYPE ORTHODONTIC BONE ANCHORS

There are many different force application options for OBAs in the oral cavity. For example, molar distalization can be achieved either by placing OBAs in the anterior region and pushing the posterior dentition distally (pushing mechanics), or by placing them in the posterior region in such a way that a sliding jig can pull against them to move molars distally (pulling mechanics). They can also be placed in the maxillary posterior region in conjunction with Class III elastics to the mandibular anterior dentition to distalize both maxillary and mandibular posterior dentitions (Fig. 45.1). If an OBA is placed in the palatal region and rigidly fixed to the lingual premolar region to establish stationary anchorage, the posterior molar dentition can also be pushed distally. OBAs can be used to move the maxillary posterior dentition distally without losing anchorage when they are positioned in the maxillary buccal region. The most commonly recommended site for placement when distalizing the posterior dentition is between the maxillary first molars and maxillary second premolars. Consequently, the OBA will need to be relocated once sufficient space has been created since it can obstruct distal movement of premolars.

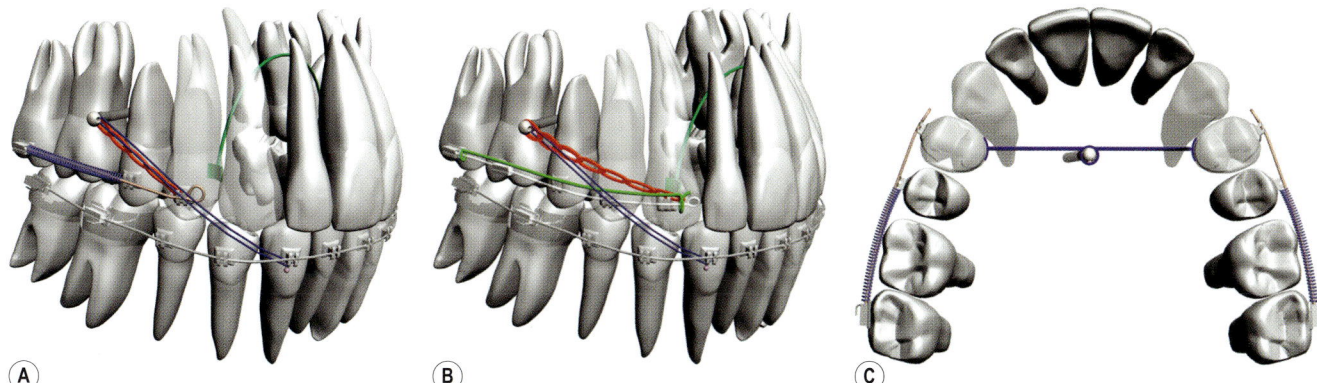

(A) (B) (C)

Fig. 45.1 The C-implant used for different force application options. (A) Use as direct anchorage in a pulling mechanism. A power chain from the C-implant to the maxillary first premolar (red) distalizes the entire maxillary posterior segment, while the open coil (blue tube) between the second molar and second premolar creates room for the first molar. The transpalatal arch (green) bonded to the first premolar prevents buccal flaring of the teeth during distalization. The C-implant concurrently serves as direct anchorage to support Class III elastics (blue lines) to distalize mandibular posterior segments. (B) Use in direct anchorage for individual tooth distalization of second molars using open coil spring pushing directly against installed C-implants. (C) Use as indirect anchorage with a transpalatal arch. The open coil spring between the second molar and second premolar will push the two teeth apart. When the C-implant is anchored to the transpalatal arch bonded to the lingual surfaces of the first premolars, it will hold these teeth in position and there will be no mesial movement of these teeth. The net space gained will be complete distalization of the second molar.

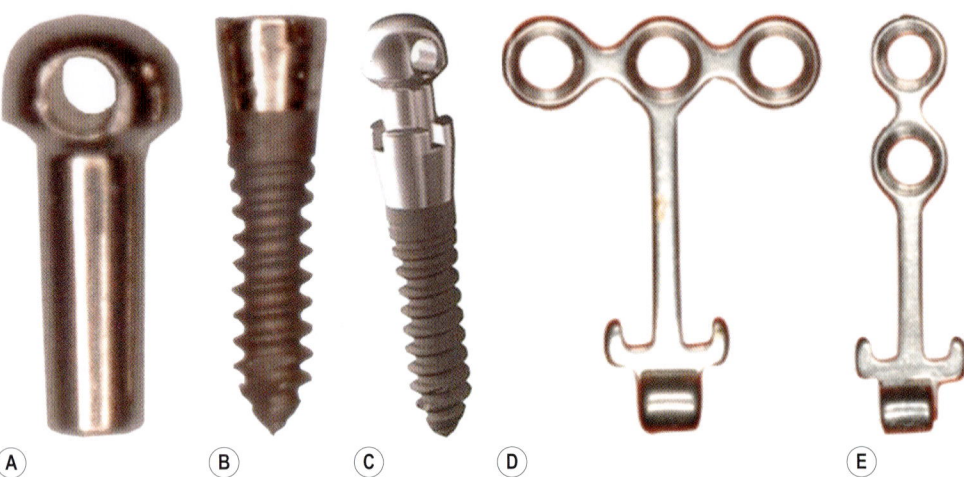

Fig. 45.2 C-type orthodontic bone anchors. (A–C) The two separate parts of the C-implant (A,B) and as one piece (C). (D,E) The C-tube miniplate.

Relocation to the distal in the molar region allows the force vector to be changed from a push to a pull system.

THE C-IMPLANT

The C-implant is made of titanium grade V alloy (C-implant Co., Seoul, Korea) and has a screw base (diameter, 1.8 mm; lengths, 6.5, 7.5 or 8.5 mm) and head attachment (lengths, 1, 2 or 3 mm) (Fig. 45.2A–C). Choice of screw base is determined by bone thickness and of head attachment by gingival thickness. The screw base is inserted into the bone first and then the head attachment is placed, thereby avoiding any torque fracture of the implant neck during insertion and removal. The sandblasted, large-grit and acid-etched surface induces only partial osseointegration and enables easily removal. The C-implant is relatively small in size and can be easily inserted into the inter-radicular areas of the maxilla and mandible, making it very versatile in a variety of clinical applications.

In complex orthodontic situations, many different directions of force vector may be needed at once and sequentially. Frequently, this may require the insertion of OBAs in many sites, or removal from a site once the OBA is in danger of becoming a physical obstruction to additional tooth movement.[5] Buccal OBAs may need to be replaced after distal movement of a posterior part is accomplished or palatal implants can be used for large amounts of distal movement of teeth.[6] How easy it is to take out an OBA and reinsert it at a different location depends on the degree of osseointegration that occurs, and whether this osseointegration is sustained under functional loading.

Recommended Protocol for Immediate Relocation of C-implant

After applying local anesthesia, an explorer can be located in the hole on the head component to pull it with a counterclockwise rotational force to separate the head attachment from the screw base. The screw base is then removed with a counterclockwise rotational force using a manual screwdriver provided with the C-implant system. The C-implant is relocated either by drilling a pilot hole 1.5 mm in diameter at 1000 rpm to a depth sufficient just to perforate compact bone or by manually inserting a self-drilling MI of 1.5 mm in diameter to create a pilot hole.

The concavity of the removed C-implant body should be snugly fitted into the screwdriver before being inserted by rotating the screwdriver clockwise with mild pressure. The angle of the C-implant body is directed parallel to the occlusal plane. Irrigation should be avoided in order to maximize contact between the C-implant and the patient's own blood for better adaptation. The head is then attached and tapped gently to fix it in place. Orthodontic force is immediately applied afterwards.

THE C-TUBE MINIPLATE

The C-tube miniplate is made of commercially pure titanium (Jin Biomed, Bucheon, Korea) (Fig. 45.2D,E) with its free end rolled to form a tube-shaped head with a 0.036 inch lumen to be exposed through the oral mucosa in order to engage orthodontic archwires. The anchor part is usually I-shaped and has two to three holes for the insertion of the corresponding miniplate anchoring screws. The anchoring screws are self-drilling and self-tapping MIs (diameter, 1.5 mm; length, 4-5 mm). The C-tube miniplates are recommended when there is insufficient inter-radicular space for C-implant placement or when much heavier forces are expected to be used in order to control en masse teeth movements.

SEVERE MAXILLARY CROWDING AND MINIMAL MANDIBULAR CROWDING

Two cases illustrate the use of C-implants for direct and indirect anchorage.

CASE 1: C-IMPLANT USED FOR DIRECT AND INDIRECT ANCHORAGE

A 15-year-old girl presented with a chief complaint of crowding of the maxillary anterior teeth (Fig. 45.3). She had an end-on Class II molar and a Class III canine relationship with 2 mm skeletal open bite. The maxillary anterior segment showed severe dental crowding while there was minimal crowding in the mandibular arch. A non-extraction treatment plan was suggested using dramatic distal and intrusive movements of the maxillary posterior dentition.

C-implants were placed in the inter-radicular space between the maxillary second premolars and first molars. The C-implant head attachment incorporated a 0.8 mm diameter hole, which was used as an orthodontic wire slot. The second molars were first distalized by placing an open Ni-Ti coil spring between the second molar and the second premolar on SS wire (0.018 × 0.025 inch), with the premolars ligated by SS wire to the C-implant head for indirect anchorage to prevent mesial migration of the anterior dentition (Fig. 45.3A). The first molars were engaged and distalized in the same manner, while the second molars were held in position

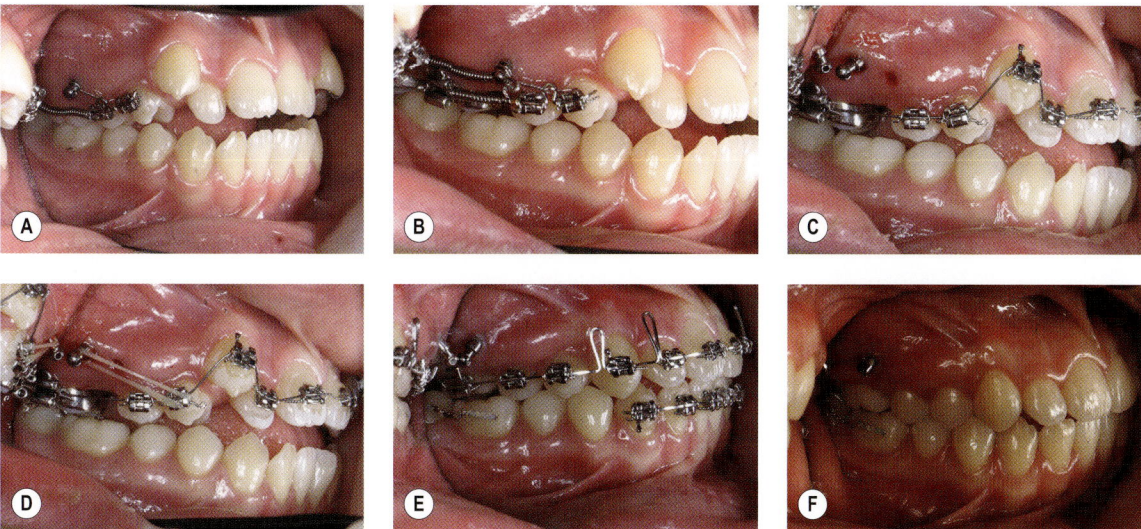

Fig. 45.3 Case 1: C-implant used for direct and indirect anchorage. (A) C-implant inserted between the maxillary first molar and second premolar for indirect anchorage. (B) Distalization of molars using the C-implant as both direct and indirect anchorage. (C) Relocation of the C-implant more distally in the same surgical site. (D) Retraction of premolars using the C-implant as direct anchorage with orthodontic elastic bands. (E) Before debonding. (F) After a further year of retention with the C-implant.

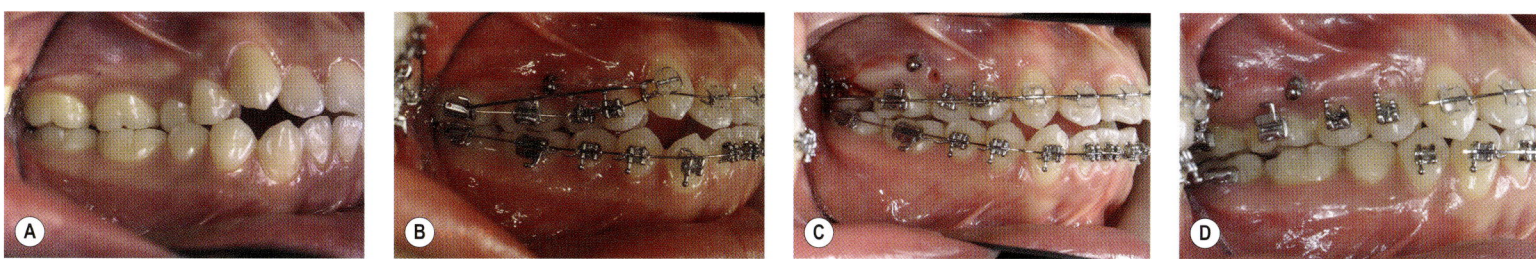

Fig. 45.4 Case 2: C-implant used as direct anchorage with auxiliary distalization appliances. (A) Dental Class II end-on molar relationship. (B) Distal movement of molars using a sliding jig. (C) Relocation of the C-implant. (D) Detailing and finishing of the occlusion after 17 months of C-implant relocation.

with an auxiliary wire and open Ni-Ti coil springs between the second molar and the hole of the C-implant head (Fig. 45.3B). Once molar distalization had been achieved, the C-implants were carefully removed and immediately repositioned superodistally but still in the region mesial to the roots of the first molars (Fig. 45.3C). The maxillary premolar segments were pulled distally against the newly repositioned C-implants with direct anchorage by connecting them with elastics to the premolar brackets (Fig. 45.3D). As the premolar segments moved distally, crowding of the anterior dentition resolved. Mandibular bands or brackets were unnecessary until the final stage of the treatment since all the required anchorage was obtained by maxillary OBAs. The initially placed C-implants were reused successfully without failure for 18 months in this immediate relocation procedure (Fig. 45.3E). Since the maxillary canines were extremely high at the start of treatment, C-implants were retained in position and connected to the canine brackets (replaced with ceramic brackets for esthetic reasons) with SS ligatures for an additional year after removal of orthodontic appliances (Fig. 45.3F).

CASE 2: C-IMPLANT USED AS DIRECT ANCHORAGE WITH AUXILIARY DISTALIZATION APPLIANCES

Instead of Ni-Ti push-coil springs as in Case 1, a sliding SS wire jig (0.018 × 0.025 inch) was used against the C-implant to distalize the maxillary posterior dentition to a Class I molar relationship (Fig. 45.4A,B). During this approach, the C-implant was repositioned superodistally to further retract the premolars and anterior teeth (Fig. 45.4C). The C-implant was continuously used for an additional 17 months by using an immediate

relocation procedure (Fig. 45.4D). It should be noted that a transpalatal arch between maxillary premolars is often critical in preventing an unwanted buccal divergence of maxillary premolars during molar distalization when OBAs are used as indirect anchors.

MINIMAL MAXILLARY CROWDING AND SEVERE MANDIBULAR CROWDING

Three cases illustrate the use of C-implants and C-tube miniplates.

CASE 3: RELOCATION OF C-IMPLANT WITHIN THE MANDIBLE

A 32-year-old man with a history of orthodontic treatment 15 years previously presented with relapse and expressed concerns about anterior teeth crowding and the loss of the left mandibular first molar (Fig. 45.5). The treatment plan included protraction of the left mandibular second molar against a unilateral C-implant (Fig. 45.5A).

Initially, the C-implant was placed immediately distal to the mandibular left second premolar. A lever arm was positioned on the second molar buccal tube and engaged to the C-implant with an elastic chain to have the line of protraction force passing closely to the center of resistance of the second molar. A lingual attachment was also bonded on the lingual surface of the second molar crown and connected to the C-implant with elastic chains to prevent rotation of the tooth during mesialization. The C-implant was angulated parallel to the long axis of the tooth and raised to the

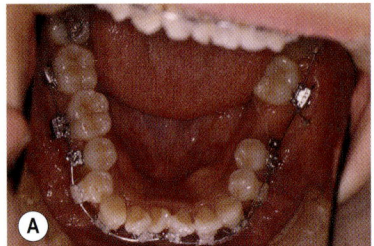 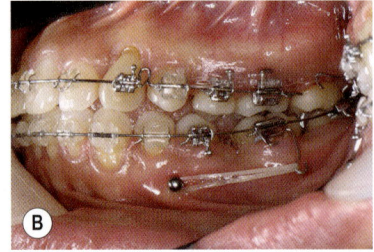 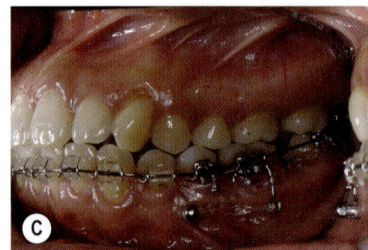

Fig. 45.5 Case 3: relocation of C-implant within the mandible. (A) Initial phase of space closure. The C-implant inserted distal to the second premolar. (B) C-implant relocated between the premolars. (C) All spaces closed and progressing to the finishing stage 14 months after relocation of the C-implant.

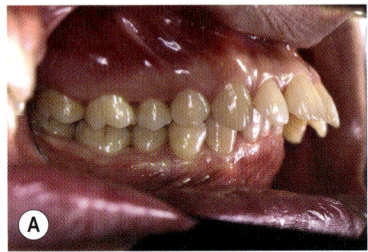 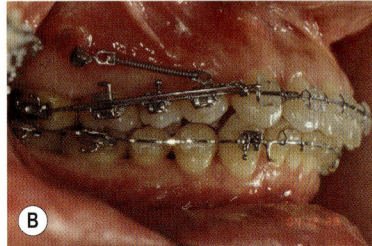 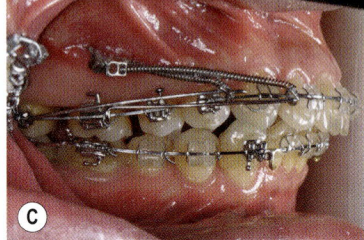 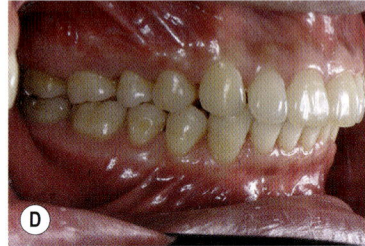

Fig. 45.6 Case 4: C-tube miniplates used as direct anchorage with auxiliary distalization appliances. (A) Pretreatment. (B) Distal movement of molars using C-tube miniplates as direct anchorage and a sliding jig. (C) Multiple sliding jigs simultaneously engaged against the C-tube miniplate using multiple Ni-Ti closed coils. A transpalatal arch between the maxillary second premolars was installed to prevent unwanted buccal divergence of the midsegment of the maxillary dentition. (D) Debonding after 27 months of distalization.

occlusal surface to prevent gingival impingement of the power chains. After extensive mesialization of the second molar to the point where it was starting to impinge on the C-implant, the C-implant was removed and immediately repositioned between the first and second premolar (Fig. 45.5B). The lever arm was repositioned flush distal to the second molar tube and engaged to the C-implant with a longer elastic chain. Final space closure was achieved and detailing of the occlusion and root parallelism was followed (Fig. 45.5C). The C-implant was maintained successfully for 14 months during mesialization of the second and third molars after immediate relocation.

CASE 4: C-TUBE MINIPLATES USED AS DIRECT ANCHORAGE WITH AUXILIARY DISTALIZATION APPLIANCES

A 30-year-old man presented with a chief complaint of mandibular anterior incisor crowding (Fig. 45.6A). A skeletal and dental Class II malocclusion was confirmed and a non-extraction treatment plan was suggested with the intention to distalize the entire maxillary dentition as well as the mandibular posterior teeth to relieve the mandibular anterior crowding.

Two C-tube miniplates were used in the maxillary posterior areas since large force loads were anticipated in order to distalize the maxillary dentition en masse. Initially, a single sliding jig was used to distalize the maxillary second molars (Fig. 45.6B). Soon after, multiple sliding jigs were simultaneously engaged against the C-tube miniplates using multiple Ni-Ti closed coils (Fig. 45.6C). A transpalatal arch between the maxillary second premolars was immediately installed to prevent an unwanted buccal divergence of the midsegment of the maxillary dentition. Full fixed orthodontic appliances were placed on both dental arches from the start of treatment, since the maxillary dentition required full distalization and the mandibular dentition required a significant amount of leveling for molar uprighting and curve of Spee correction. The full maxillary arch was distalized until Class I molar and canine relationships were established, with a total of 27 months of treatment time (Fig. 45.6D).

CASE 5: RELOCATION OF C-IMPLANT FROM BUCCAL MAXILLARY BONE TO PALATE

A 28-year-old woman presented with a chief concern of maxillary protrusion. She had Class I molar and Class II canine relationships with crowding of the maxillary and mandibular anterior teeth. Non-extraction correction of crowding was planned by distalizing the maxillary and mandibular posterior teeth.

Initially, a C-implant was placed on each side between the maxillary first molars and second premolars, and Class III elastics were used against the C-implants to the mandibular canines (direct anchorage) to effectively upright and distalize the mesially tipped posterior segment (Figs 45.1B and 45.7A,B). The C-implants were also ligated with SS wire to the premolar region (indirect anchorage) to distalize the maxillary posterior molar teeth (Fig. 45.7B). After sufficient molar distalization, the buccal C-implants were removed. One of the removed C-implants was immediately relocated to the median palatal suture area (Fig. 45.7C,D) and a transpalatal arch of SS wire (diameter, 0.8 mm) was engaged to the palatal C-implant to fix the molars in position in order to use them as anchorage to retract the maxillary premolars. A solid Class I molar and canine relationship with well-intercuspated occlusion and with an ideal overbite and overjet was achieved (Fig. 45.7E,F). No orthodontic appliances were used for the maxillary anterior teeth until the final stage of treatment, minimizing the total time of wearing braces on the front teeth (in line with the principles of biocreative therapy, which discourages unnecessary and extended use of orthodontic appliances). The C-implant was maintained well for an additional 8 months of treatment from the time of its relocation to the palate.

DISCUSSION

The design of the C-implant enables good bone–implant contact and stability and having the two components avoids issues of fracture of the neck region of the implant during placement and removal.[2] The screw base has

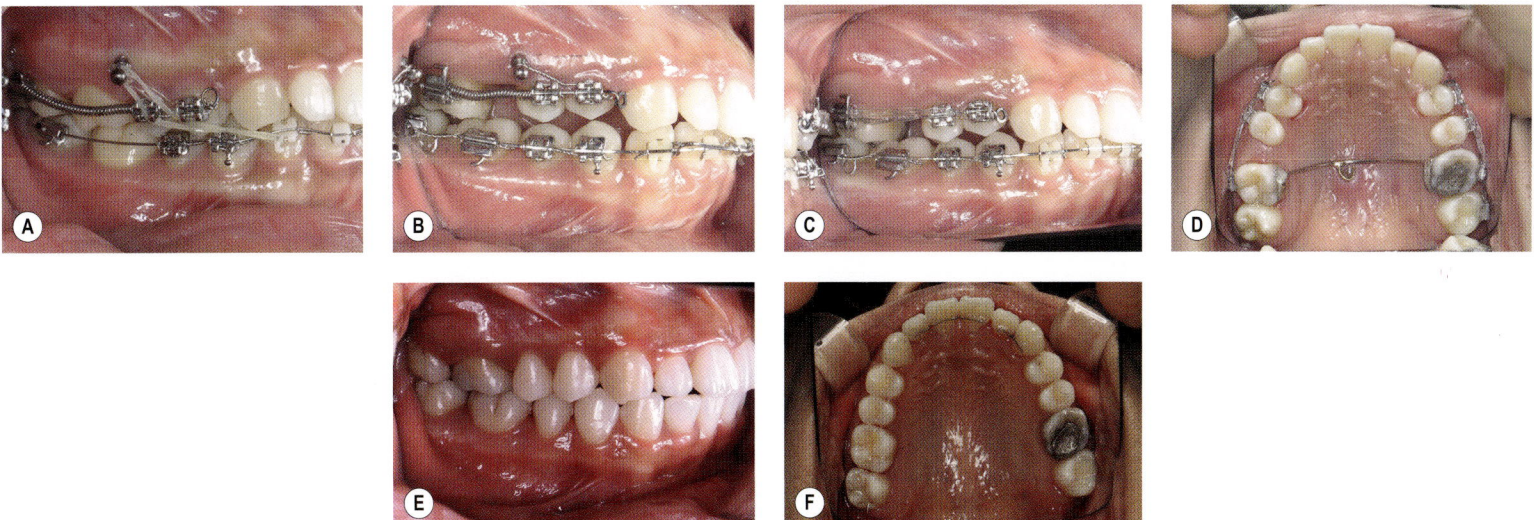

Fig. 45.7 Case 5: relocation of C-implant from buccal maxillary bone to palate. (A) Mandibular molar distalization using Class III elastics from a buccally positioned C-implant to the mandibular canines on each side. (B) Maxillary molar distalization using the C-implant as indirect anchorage. (C,D) Relocation of C-implant to the palate to be used as indirect anchorage via a transpalatal arch bonded to the molars. (E,F) Completion of orthodontic treatment 8 months after C-implant relocation.

a blunt pitch and dull apex, effectively reducing the risk of root damage compared with many other self-drilling and self-tapping MI systems. The dual components also give greater flexibility, since there is the option to select different sizes of head attachment to avoid gingival inflammation. The lumen in the head attachment can accommodate orthodontic wires for supplemental auxiliary biomechanics if necessary.

Animal experiments have indicated that the removal torque of a repositioned C-implant is not significantly different from that of the C-implant being removed from its initial position.[7] Partial osseointegration was observed at the surface of the repositioned C-implant, which implies that it could be used as a source of skeletal anchorage even when relocated.

Relocation of the OBAs in most cases appears to occur without adverse effects of bone remodeling.

It is imperative that the C-implants are handled with care and isolated from other contamination sources during repositioning. A contaminated C-implant body can be autoclaved and reused, but only for the same patient. If existing C-implants have failed because of root contact, or insertion is not feasible, orthodontic miniplates can be used.[8] For example, a C-tube miniplate can be used where the inter-radicular alveolar bone is narrow, the maxillary sinus is enlarged, the roots of the teeth are curved or the alveolar bone shows severe resorption.

REFERENCES

1. Chung KR. C-palatal plate. In: Chung KR, editor. Textbook of speedy orthodontics. Seoul: Jeesung; 2001. p. 99–113.
2. Chung KR, Kim SH, Kook YA. C-orthodontic micro implant as a unique skeletal anchorage. J Clin Orthod 2004;38:478–86.
3. Chung KR, Nelson G, Kim SH, et al. Severe bidentoalveolar protrusion treated with orthodontic microimplant-dependent en-masse retraction. Am J Orthod Dentofacial Orthop 2007;132:105–15.
4. Chung KR, Kim YS, Linton JL, Lee YJ. The miniplate with the tube for skeletal anchorage. J Clin Orthod 2002;36:407–12.
5. Sung SJ, Jang GW, Chun YS, et al. Effective en-masse retraction design with orthodontic mini-implant anchorage: a finite element analysis. Am J Orthod Dentofacial Orthop 2010;137:648–57.
6. Chung KR, Choo H, Kim SH, et al. Timely relocation of mini-implants for uninterrupted full-arch distalization. Am J Orthod Dentofacial Orthop 2010;138:839–49.
7. Go TS, Jee YJ, Kim SH, et al. The comparison of removal torque values and SEM findings of orthodontic C-implant before and after recycling procedure. J Korean Assoc Hosp Dent 2006;2:88–95.
8. Lee JH, Choo H, Kim SH, et al. Replacing a failed mini-implant with a mini-plate to prevent interruptions during orthodontic treatment with temporary skeletal anchorage device (TSAD). Am J Orthod Dentofacial Orthop 2011;139:849–57.

46

Correction of Class II malocclusion with the bone-anchored Forsus Fatigue Resistant Device

Narayan H. Gandedkar

INTRODUCTION

Fixed functional appliances have been in routine use for treatment of skeletal Class II jaw relationships arising from a mandibular deficiency but do have undesired dentoalveolar effects because of the use of teeth for anchorage. The use of temporary anchorage devices such as miniscrew implants (MIs) and miniplates can allow treatment to proceed successfully with none of these untoward effects.

This chapter discusses the use of bone anchorage in treating patients with Class II, division 1 malocclusion of skeletal origin arising from mandibular deficiencies and the use of three-dimensional imaging for orthodontic diagnosis and treatment planning. Cone beam CT (CBCT) allows quantitative evaluation of hard tissues with accuracy and ease, and at comparatively low effective radiation doses.[1] The chapter attempts to answer the following questions with regard to the use of MIs and miniplates in treating Class II, division 1 malocclusion:

- Is the approach beneficial for Class II, division 1 malocclusion arising from mandibular deficiency?
- What are the potential benefits, merits, problems of the approach?
- Does three-dimensional evaluation of condylar growth and the maxillary restraining effect of fixed functional appliances provide useful information on changes in the maxillomandibular complex?

MINISCREW IMPLANTS AS ANCHORING UNITS FOR FIXED FUNCTIONAL APPLIANCES

The application of MIs with the Forsus Fatigue Resistant Device (FRD) is presented in detail with the following case report.

CASE 1: USE OF MINISCREW IMPLANTS AS ANCHORAGE FOR ADVANCEMENT OF THE MANDIBLE

A 14-year-old boy in the acceleration phase of the pubertal growth spurt presented with a chief complaint of protruding maxillary front teeth and small mandible (Fig. 46.1A,D). His medical history was unremarkable, and temporomandibular joint function was normal. He had a severe convex facial pattern and lip trap, mild crowding in the maxillary anterior region and severe crowding of the mandibular anterior teeth plus proclination (Fig. 46.1D). Overjet was 14 mm and overbite 100%, with a full complement of teeth. Based on the boy's profile and growth status, it was decided to extract the maxillary and mandibular first premolars to correct the inclination and alleviate crowding of the maxillary and mandibular dental arches, and subsequently to anchor a fixed functional appliance on the lower archwire to advance the mandible. However, such anchoring would cause inadvertent proclination of the mandibular anterior teeth and so it was decided to level and align the teeth (Fig. 46.1E.F) and then place the MIs in the inter-radicular area between the mandibular canine and first premolar bilaterally for anchoring the appliance (Fig. 46.1G).

Treatment for 11 months with the fixed functional appliance had no untoward effects linked to use of MIs (Fig. 46.1H). Treatment was continued with fixed appliances (Fig. 46.1I). A Class I molar relation with pleasing profile was achieved at the end of treatment (Fig. 46.1B,J) and the patient showed excellent retention 1 year after treatment with no relapse (Fig. 46.1C,K,L).

Discussion

The MI insertion site between the mandibular canines and the first premolars is known to be suitable because there is no risk of damage to roots or neurovascular structures. Several factors have a significant role in the success of MIs as anchoring units for fixed functional appliances, including the patient's age and growth status plus the type of appliance and the duration of treatment.

Ideally, treatment should occur when the patient is in an acceleration phase of the pubertal growth spurt, with 65–85% residual pubertal growth remaining. This typically corresponds to 14.2 ± 4 years for boys and 12.3 ± 3 years for girls.[2]

The type of functional appliance has a decisive role in the success of applying functional appliances for the correction of Class II malocclusion. If a removable functional appliance is used for advancement of the mandible, two separate phases of treatment have to be carried out and there must be optimum patient compliance. There is also some evidence of intermittent condylar displacement with removable functional appliances, leading to varying degrees of glenoid fossa remodeling.[3] In contrast, fixed functional appliances show a remarkably significant change in the glenoid fossa–condyle complex.[4]

Fixed functional appliances have clear advantages over removable ones, with the correction achieved being a combination of skeletal and dental changes. However, with fixed functional appliances anchored on the dentition, most of the dental correction comes from proclination of the mandibular anterior teeth. This suggests that the use of MI/miniplate anchorage for fixed functional appliances would be highly advantageous in that it would produce all the expected changes apart from the unwanted proclination of the mandibular anterior teeth.

Treatment duration with fixed functional appliances is also of importance. Use of the Forsus Nitinol Flat Spring (less rigid than the Forsus FRD) over a functional period of 4 months gave a mix of skeletal and dental effects, with the dental effects contributing to 66% of the changes.[5] By comparison, using the Forsus FRD with MI anchorage needed a longer functional phase (in Case 1, 11 months) but created no mandibular anterior dentition effects (Fig. 46.1L).

MINIPLATES AS ANCHORING UNITS FOR FIXED FUNCTIONAL APPLIANCES

Miniplates seem to provide better primary and secondary stability than MIs. The advantage of these plates is that they are located away from the dentition and do not interfere with tooth movements. However, placement of miniplates is far more invasive than placement of MIs, and infections can occur. One orthodontic miniplate system that has been widely used is the titanium Skeletal Anchorage System.[6] Other designs are the Ortho-Anchor System[7] and the Zygoma Anchorage System.[8] These systems have been shown to provide excellent anchorage for Class II functional

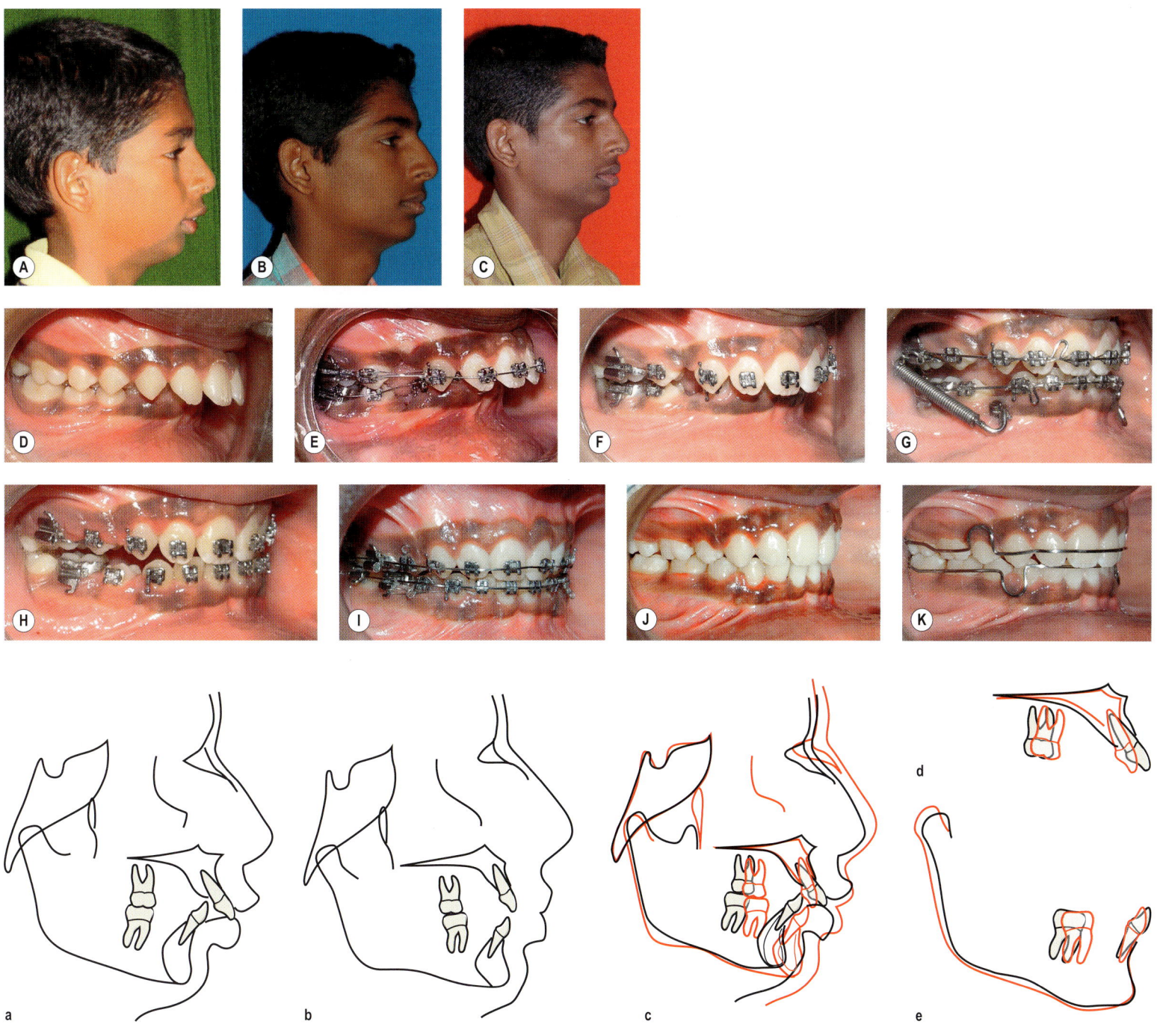

Fig. 46.1 Case 1: use of miniscrew implants as anchorage for advancement of the mandible. (A,D) Pretreatment. (E) Fixed appliances bonded and initial arch wire placed. (F) Prefunctional view. (G) Forsus FRD anchored on miniscrew implants. (H) After functional treatment. (I) Before continuation of treatment with fixed appliances. (B,J) Post-treatment. (C,K) One year after completion of treatment (with Hawley's retainers). (L) Superimposition of the cephalometric tracing before (a) and after (b) treatment on the anterior cranial base (c), the maxilla (d) and the mandible (e).

treatment but their use in Class II, division 1 malocclusion has not been thoroughly evaluated.

Almost any type of skeletal miniplate can be used as an anchor unit but the triangular design with its three parts is versatile and can be used in many indications. The first part, the retentive plate, has three holes at three corners of a triangular plate, which can resist the force applied in a comprehensive fashion through its tripod design (see Fig. 13.1). The second part is an extension arm and the third is the anchor, which is essentially a fourth hole extending from the retentive plate. The extension arm's length (8, 10, 12 or 14 mm) depends on the mandibular height at the canine and premolar region, and the skeletal plate is placed so that the anchor part of

the plate lies immediately at the mucogingival junction level. The fixation screws are 8 or 10 mm in length, with a 1.2 mm head dimension.

CLINICAL PROCEDURE

The miniplate is inserted in the area between the mandibular first premolar and incisors (see Chapter 13 for the insertion technique). Although the miniplate can be loaded immediately, a period of 5–7 days before loading is recommended to allow the soft tissues to heal.

The distance from the distal aspect of the maxillary first molar headgear tube to the hole of the anchor plate is measured with the Forsus FRD

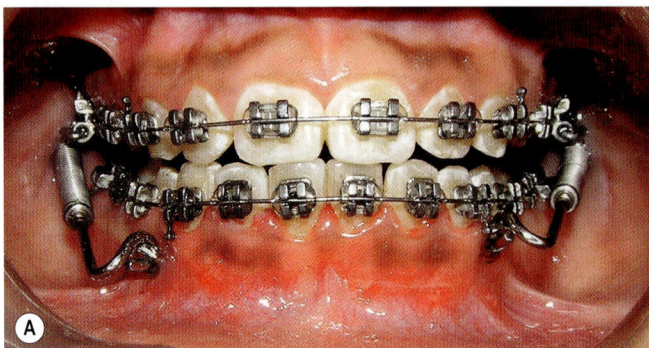 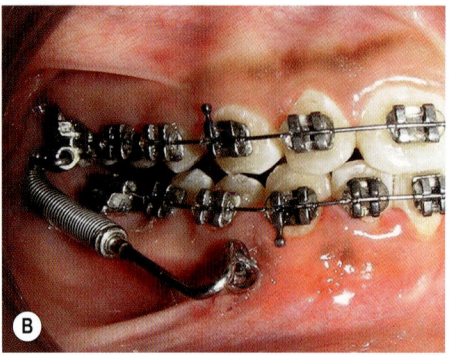 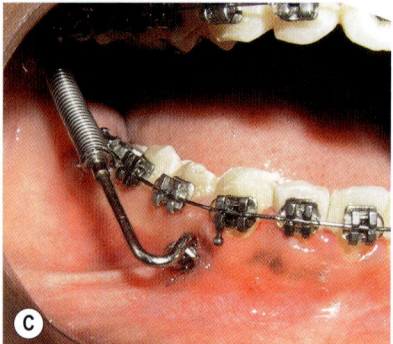

Fig. 46.2 Anchorage of the Forsus Fatigue Resistant Device to the hook of miniplates. (A,B) Attachment of the device. (C) Assessing mouth opening to ensure that the device does not roll into occlusion while functioning.

measuring jig (usually 29–32 mm). The push rod hook of the Forsus FRD is crimped on to the hook of the anchor part of the miniplate (Fig. 46.2A,B), and the patient is asked to open and close the mouth several times to check whether the appliance is injuring the soft tissues or the push rod is rotating into the bite (Fig. 46.2C). Once the push rod is correctly fitted, the patient is asked not to open the mouth too wide and is given regular instructions plus advice with special emphasis on oral hygiene maintenance, particularly around the miniplate extensions.

ASSESSMENT OF THE USE OF BONE ANCHORAGE FOR FIXED FUNCTIONAL APPLIANCES

The benefits of using bone anchorage for the application of a fixed functional appliance in treating Class II, division 1 malocclusion include:

- does not require teeth leveling and alignment before initiating mandibular advancement and so the fixed functional appliances are incorporated into the treatment plan at its initiation, thus allowing maximum benefit from growth potential in growing patients
- linking the device directly to the miniplates or MI avoids the need for bypass wires or heavy rectangular wire
- labial flaring of the mandibular anterior teeth is avoided, which eliminates root resorption of the mandibular anterior teeth and alveolar bone dehiscence
- rapid flaring of the mandibular anterior teeth is avoided
- no requirement to use brackets, thus avoiding additional bracket inventory, negative crown torque on the mandibular anterior teeth and the frequent debonding of canine brackets.

There are also disadvantages, which should not be underestimated:

- placement and removal of MIs and miniplates is an invasive procedure with all the attendant issues
- a potential for damage to adjacent roots or other neighboring structures, such as the neurovascular bundle, during placement, particularly if the clinician is inexperienced
- migration of MIs is always possible, particularly if dimensions are smaller; MIs of 1.4 mm diameter and 14.0 mm length and miniplates with a triangular configuration are recommended
- soft tissue injury can occur, particularly in individuals with a shallow mandibular vestibular depth; vestibuloplasty can increase vestibular height if required.

BIOMECHANICAL ASPECTS OF BONE ANCHORAGE FOR THE FORSUS FATIGUE RESISTANT DEVICE

The impact of fixed functional appliances can be considered for the maxilla and mandible separately.

Effects on the maxilla and maxillary teeth include:

- primarily, the maxillary first molar is affected as it is hooked on the headgear tube of the maxillary first molar band (Fig. 46.3A–C)
- there is a clockwise rotation of the maxilla with restraining effect of the maxillary complex (Fig. 46.3E).

Effects on the mandible and on mandibular teeth include:

- clinically, cephalometrically and tomographically, no effect is evident on the mandibular teeth in terms of labial flaring, anterior teeth intrusion, anterior teeth root resorption
- MIs and miniplates are placed closer to the center of resistance of the mandibular arch to allow derived force to be most effective in advancing or anterior repositioning of the mandible (Fig. 46.3D).

EVALUATION OF CONDYLAR GROWTH AND THE EFFECT ON THE MAXILLARY COMPLEX OF THE FIXED FUNCTIONAL APPLIANCES

A prospective CBCT study assessed the effect of the Forsus FRD on the maxilla and mandible in six growing individuals (four girls, two boys; mean age, 13 ± 0.6 years) with skeletal Class II jaw relationships (SNA angle, 84 ± 2°; SNB angle, 76 ± 2°), and Class II, division 1 malocclusion, as well as an overjet of more than 7 mm with minimal or no crowding of the maxillary and mandibular dental arch. The exclusion criteria included the presence of any primary teeth, absence of maxillary posterior permanent teeth, prosthetic restorations on the maxillary posterior teeth, periodontal disease and previous orthodontic treatment. Figure 46.4 illustrates the treatment of a typical patient. All the teeth were bonded with slot brackets (0.022 inch) and the maxillary first molars were banded with triple tube buccal attachments incorporating a headgear tube. Initially, Ni-Ti archwires (0.014 inch) were placed in the maxillary and mandibular dental arch, and an SS transpalatal arch (0.032 inch) was placed on the maxillary first molars. Two miniplates with a triangular design were placed bilaterally in the anterior part of the mandible and were loaded 5–7 days after insertion (Fig. 46.4B). The functional phase lasted 11.0 ± 0.8 months. All patients were subjected to CBCT imaging before treatment, immediately after completion of the advancement of the mandible and 1 year after treatment (Table 46.1). The images were converted into a DICOM (digital imaging and communications in medicine) format and evaluated using InVivo 5.1 software (Anatomage, San Jose, CA, USA). The images were superimposed using the software by selecting certain stable skeletal structural landmarks of the anterior cranial base (Fig. 46.4C,D).

Data analysis shows that the treatment outcome was significant, with overall reduction of overjet of 0.67 mm on average. The greatest effect was on the mandible, with a significant increase of total mandibular length (GoGn) and in the sagittal positioning of the mandible, with an increase in

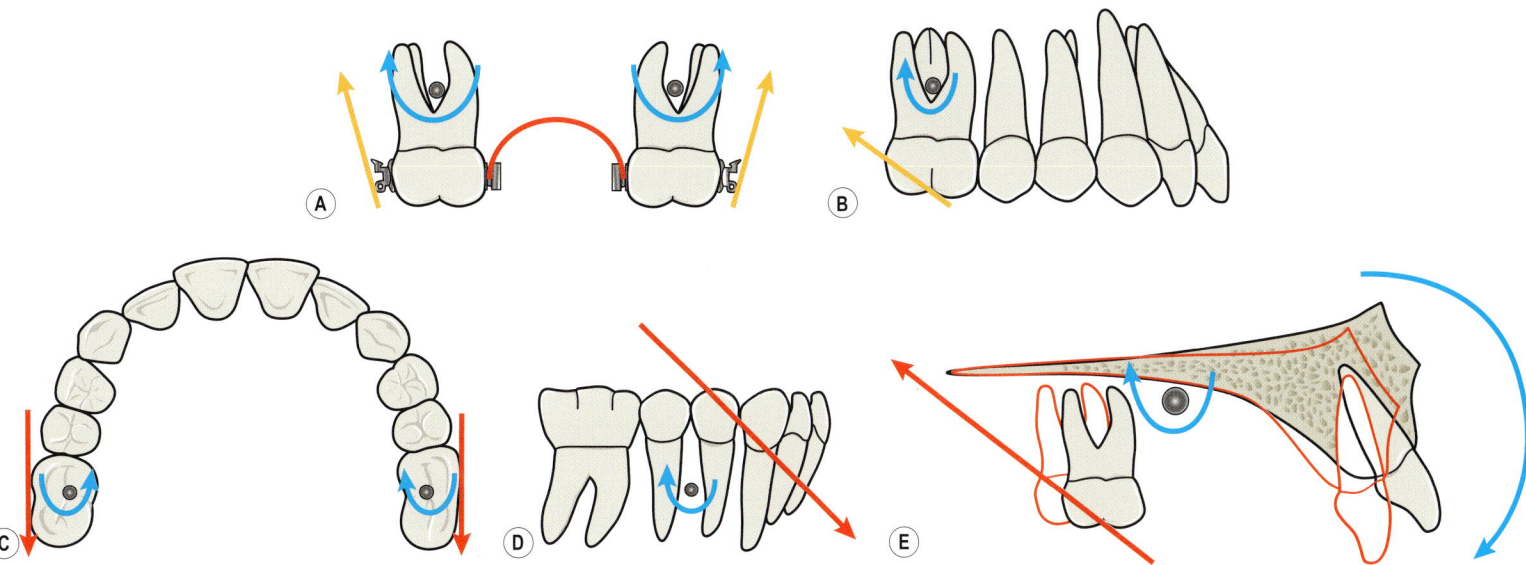

Fig. 46.3 The effects on the maxillary posterior teeth of the Forsus Fatigue Resistant Device with miniplates. (A–C) The first molar is affected in all three dimensions with buccal tipping (A) distal tipping (B) and distopalatal rotation (C). A transpalatal arch is essential to counter these untoward effects. (D,E) The appliance anchored on the miniplate is placed close to the center of resistance of the upper (D) and lower (E) dentition.

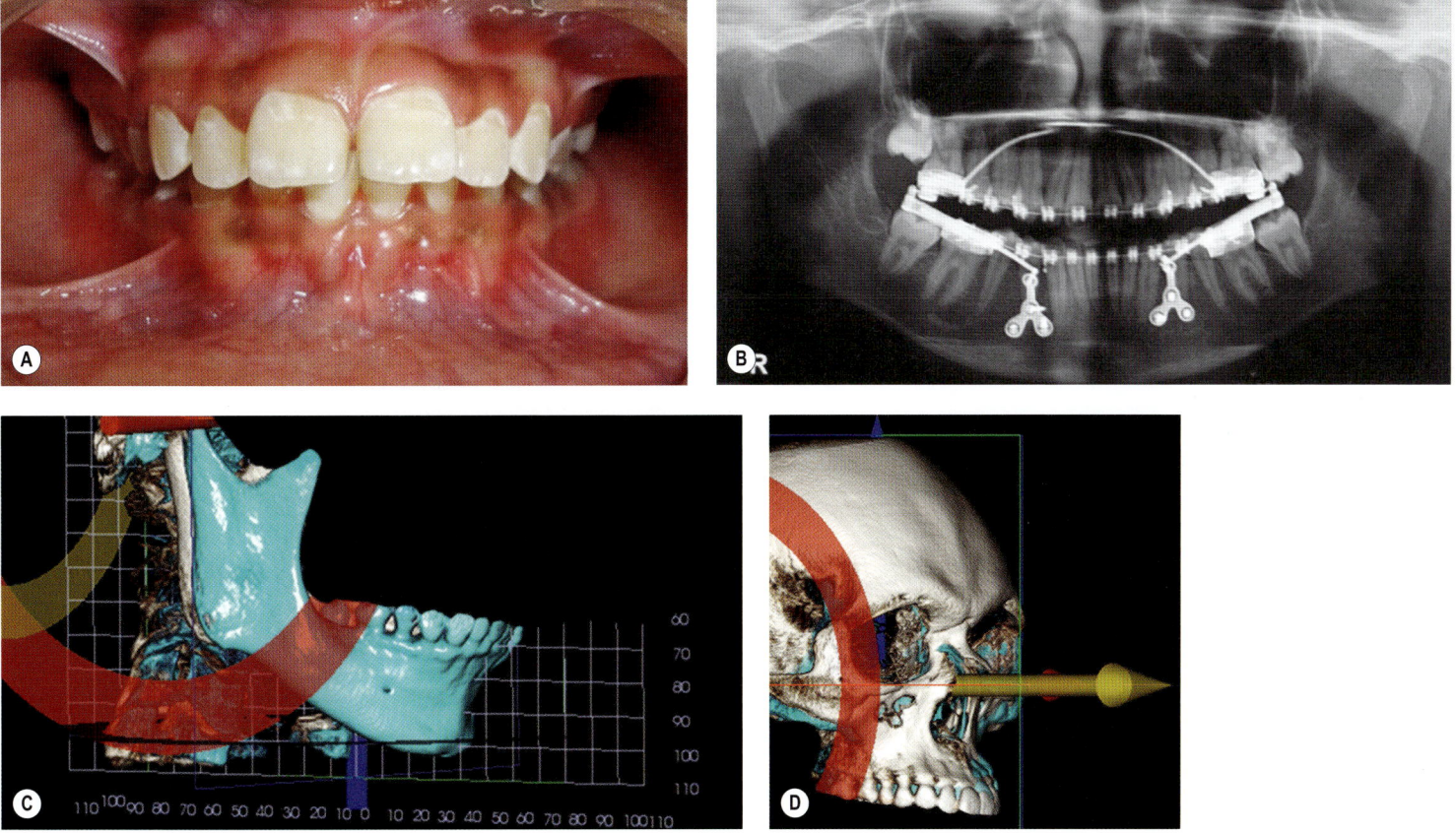

Fig. 46.4 Treatment of a typical patient in the study of the Forsus Fatigue Resistant Device. (A) Pretreatment. (B) Panoramic radiograph taken immediately after insertion of the miniplate, showing sufficient clearance from the mental foramen. (C,D) Use of InVivo software to assess changes in the mandible, where there was a forward and downward movement (C), and the maxilla, where there was an overall restraining effect along with backward and downward movement (D).

bony chin position. There was little change in the inclination of the anterior mandibular teeth, which contrasts with the significant proclination and intrusion of mandibular incisors seen with tooth-borne fixed functional appliances. This supports the fact that anchorage via the miniplate rather than via the anterior teeth completely eliminates unwanted tooth movements.

The maxilla showed mild clockwise rotation with a restraining effect on the entire maxillary complex; the main influence of the appliance was on the maxillary molars, followed by the anterior teeth. The maxillary molars, and particularly the first molars, showed an intrusive and distal tipping effect despite the presence of a transpalatal arch, with mild retrusion and extrusion of the maxillary anterior teeth.

The lack of a control group is an inherent defect of this study. However, the data presented here are part of an ongoing study with a larger sample and an appropriate control group; this study will be published when completed.

Table 46.1 Cone beam CT evaluation

Variables	T1	T2	T3
Anteroposterior			
ANB (°)	8 ± 1	2 ± 1	2 ± 1
A-B (mm)	14 ± 3	4 ± 1	3 ± 1
Wits appraisal (mm)	6 ± 2.5	2 ± 0.5	2 ± 0.5
NA-Pog (mm)	10 ± 2.5	3.5 ± 1	3 ± 1
Vertical			
SN-GoGn (°)	23 ± 4	27 ± 2	27 ± 2
FH-GoMe (°)	21 ± 2	24 ± 2	24 ± 1
MM plane (°)	18 ± 3	20 ± 1	20 ± 1
Y-axis (°)	86 ± 2	90 ± 2	90 ± 1
Maxilla			
SNA (°)	86 ± 2	82 ± 2	82 ± 1
A-N (mm)	3 ± 1	1 ± 1	1 ± 1
A-Ptm (mm)	52 ± 1.5	51 ± 1	51 ± 1
S-Ptm (mm)	21 ± 1	21 ± 1	21 ± 1
Mandible			
SNB (°)	76 ± 2	81 ± 2	81 ± 1
Go-Pg (mm)	70 ± 2	75.5 ± 2	76 ± 1.5
Dental			
U1-SN (°)	114 ± 4	102 ± 3	102 ± 2
U1-NA (°) [mm]	26 ± 3 [8 ± 4]	18 ± 2 [2 ± 1]	18 ± 2 [2 ± 1]
L1-MP(°)	96 ± 2	96 ± 2	96 ± 2
L1-NB (°) [mm]	24 ± 2 [3 ± 1]	22 ± 2 [2 ± 1]	22 ± 2 [2 ± 1]
U1-L1 (°)	124 ± 2	128 ± 2	128 ± 2
Overjet (mm)	7 ± 1.5	1.8 ± 0.5	1.2 ± 0.5
Overbite (mm)	7 ± 1.2	1.0 ± 0.8	1.2 ± 1.0
Temperomandibular joint			
Gl-Cpr (mm)	4.5 ± 1.2	6.8 ± 1.3	6.7 ± 1.2
Gl-Cdis (mm)	5.2 ± 0.8	7.3 ± 0.7	7.1 ± 0.4
Gl-Cmed (mm)	4.2 ± 0.7	6.1 ± 0.5	6.4 ± 0.2

T1, pretreatment; T2, post-functional treatment; T3, 1-year follow-up; IMPA, incisor mandibular plane angle; Gl, inside innermost concavity of glenoid fossa of temporal bone; Cpr, center of head of condyle; Cdis, head of the condyle distal aspect; Cmed, head of the condyle medial aspect.

The study results also show that use of the Forsus FRD with a miniplate anchorage allowed the growing mandible to express its full growth potential without any labial flaring of the anterior teeth.

Post-treatment stability needs to be ensured through stable cuspal interdigitation of the maxillary and mandibular dentition; minor relapse of overjet and overbite has been documented 1-year after treatment, caused by relapse in mandibular incisor inclination.[9] In our study, no relapse was noted in the 1-year retention period, because the prefunctional incisor inclination was maintained by the fixed functional appliance being anchored directly on the bone.

The functional phase in our study was 11 months, which is longer than many other studies with fixed functional appliances (approximately 6 months on average); this might explain the excellent orthopedic response and stability. Moreover, there is histological evidence to suggest that additional growth occurs with longer treatment times, perhaps through mineralization and adaptation of muscle attachments.[10–12]

REFERENCES

1. Kau CH, English JD, Muller-Delgardo MG, et al. Retrospective cone-beam computed tomography evaluation of temporary anchorage devices. Am J Orthod Dentofacial Orthop 2010;137:166.
2. Rajagopal R, Kansal S. A comparison of modified MP3 stages and the cervical vertebrae as growth indicators. J Clin Orthod 2002;36:398–406.
3. Baume L, Derichsweiler H. Is the condylar growth centre responsive to orthodontic therapy? An experimental study in *Macaca mulata*. Oral Surg Oral Med Oral Path 1961;14:347–62.
4. Ruf S, Pancherz H. Temporomandibular joint remodeling in adolescents and young adults during Herbst treatment: a prospective longitudinal magnetic resonance imaging and cephalometric radiographic investigation. Am J Orthod Dentofacial Orthop 1999;115:607–18.
5. Heinig N, Göz G. Clinical application and effects of the Forsus spring. A study of a new Herbst hybrid. J Orofac Orthop 2001;62:436–50.
6. Umemori M, Sugawara J, Mitani H, et al. Skeletal anchorage system for open-bite correction. Am J Orthod Dentofacial Orthop 1999;115:166–74.
7. Chung KR, Kim YS, Linton JL, et al. The miniplate with tube for skeletal anchorage. J Clin Orthod 2002;36:407–12.
8. De Clerck H, Geerinckx V, Siciliano S. The Zygoma Anchorage System. J Clin Orthod 2002;36:455–9.
9. Pancherz H. The Herbst appliance: its biologic effects and clinical use. Am J Orthod 1985;87:1–20.
10. Buschang PH, Santos-Pinto A. Condylar growth and glenoid fossa displacement during childhood and adolescence. Am J Orthod Dentofacial Orthop 1998;113:437–42.
11. Voudouris JC, Woodside DG, Altuna G, et al. Condyle-fossa modifications and muscle interactions during Herbst treatment. Part 2. Results and conclusions. Am J Orthod Dentofacial Orthop 2003;124:13–29.
12. Auf der Maur HJ. Electromyographic recordings of the lateral pterygoid muscle activity in activator treatment of Class II, Division 1 malocclusion cases. Eur J Orthod 1980;2:161–71.

The Twin Force Bite Corrector and skeletal anchorage for Class II correction

47

Aditya Chhibber, Ravindra Nanda and Flavio Uribe

INTRODUCTION

Fixed functional appliances may be broadly classified as rigid, flexible and semirigid appliances.[1] The major difference between functional appliances and fixed functional appliances is probably that the mandible is forcefully postured in an anterior position with the latter, with the help of interarch anchorage using the maxillary denture base as the anchor unit. As discussed in many chapters in this book, the use of temporary anchorage devices such as miniscrew implants (MIs) to provide the anchorage for fixed functional appliances avoids the unwanted effects of using teeth as the only anchorage. This chapter describes the use of the Twin Force Bite Corrector (TFBC), which is a hybrid type of fixed functional appliance,[2] together with direct and indirect anchorage supplied by MIs.

THE TWIN FORCE BITE CORRECTOR

The TFBC is a fixed push type appliance clamped bilaterally to SS archwires in both the maxillary and mandibular dental arches (upper, 0.019×0.025 inch; lower, 0.021×0.025 inch) (see Fig. 2.7C). Each unit is made of two 15 mm telescopic parallel cylinders containing a Ni-Ti coil that is activated as the patient occludes. A plunger is incorporated within each cylinder on opposite ends. Hex nuts at the free end of each plunger attach the appliance mesial to the maxillary molars and distal to the mandibular canines on the archwires. At full compression, a force of approximately 210 g is delivered on each side by the compression of the coil spring. This force is synergistic to that applied indirectly by the muscles of mastication to the denture bases through the anterior positioning of the mandible. A unique feature of the appliance is that, since the point of force application is closer to the center of resistance (CR) of the maxillary dentition, less clockwise moment is generated with the appliance (Fig. 47.1A) than with other fixed functional appliances, where the point of force application on the maxillary arch is distal to the maxillary molars (Fig. 47.1B). In addition, since the appliance is clamped on to the archwire, the intrusive component of the spring force is dissipated along the entire arch,

redistributing the intrusive force along the entire denture base. The appliance is placed on the two archwires for a period of 3 months. A transpalatal arch is placed to counteract the buccal forces exerted by the appliance on the maxillary dentition.

Class II correction using the TFBC appliance occurs through a combination of skeletal and dental effects.[3] Retention of the correction of any type of malocclusion is a challenge in orthodontics and relapse is a common problem reported in the literature.[4] Therefore, assessment of outcomes must consider both short- and long-term effects with an appliance to determine which therapies may be considered stable. Examination of patient groups at the end of treatment with the TFBC appliance and after at least 2 years of retention shows that the occlusal plane clockwise canting and intrusion of maxillary molars that occurred with the TFBC appliance is not stable and reverts back, leading to flattening of the functional occlusal plane. Flaring of the mandibular incisors could possibly limit the amount of anterior displacement of the mandible during the Class II correction phase and, therefore, limit the amount of skeletal correction. A mechanism capable of minimizing the dental effects in the anterior region could capitalize on the significant skeletal change, observed as orthopedic mandibular lengthening, and improve outcomes in the long term. The use of skeletal anchorage could provide such a mechanism, and temporary anchorage devices such as MIs and miniplates have been shown to avoid the unwanted effects of reactive forces on dental anchor units, limiting mandibular incisor flaring and possibly maximizing mandibular advancement (see Chapter 46).

THE TWIN FORCE BITE CORRECTOR WITH TEMPORARY ANCHORAGE DEVICES

DIRECT ANCHORAGE

Various possible combinations of miniplates and MIs could be implemented for direct anchorage with the TFBC. Since the magnitude of force indirectly exerted to the appliance by the musculature is high, a single MI at each end would be unlikely to tolerate this load. Therefore, two MIs

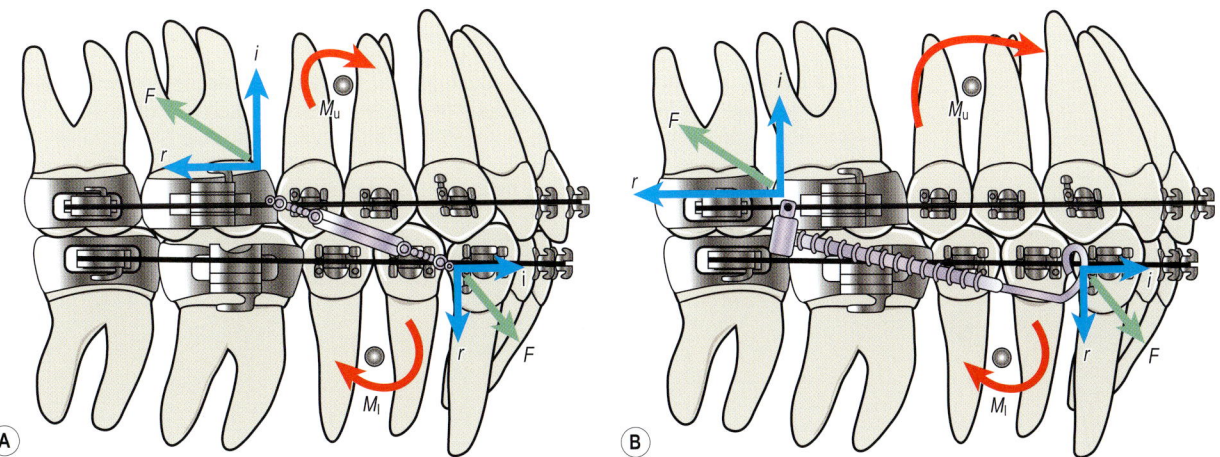

Fig. 47.1 Biomechanics of the Twin Force Bite Corrector (A) and a conventional fixed functional appliance (B). *F*, total force; *i*, vertical (intrusive) component; *r*, horizontal component; M_u, moment created on the upper arch; M_l, moment created on the lower arch.

splinted together, resembling a miniplate, may be placed between the maxillary first and second molars and distal to the mandibular canines with the head of the TFBC appliance stabilized to a wire segment (Fig. 47.2A). However, analysis of the force system indicates that there will be a greater vertical component of the force and so the moment generated on the maxillary dentition would be less as the point of force application would be very close to the CR of the maxillary dentition. The stability of the MIs may

also be compromised through jiggling forces generated by the appliance spring and the muscles when the patient forcefully bites in a forward posture.

Excessive vertical forces could be reduced by using a miniplate on the maxillary zygomatic buttress splinted to the two MIs with a rigid wire in the mandibular arch (Fig. 47.2B). The advantage is that the forces would be more horizontal on both the maxilla and mandible and that the miniplate

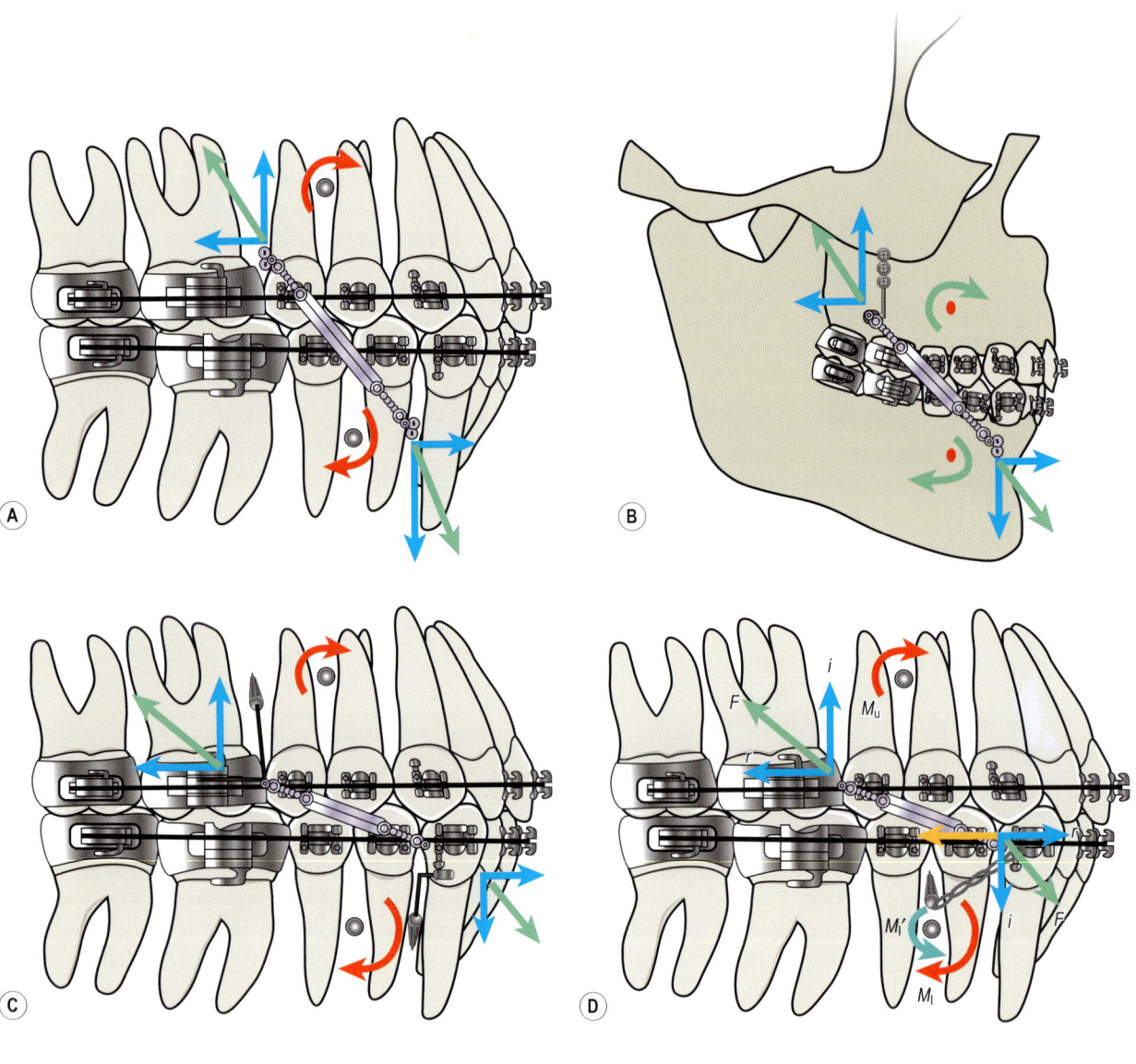

Fig. 47.2 Biomechanics with the Twin Force Bite Corrector. (A) Anchored with miniscrew implants (MIs). (B) Anchored with miniplates. (C) Tooth-borne appliance anchored indirectly from MIs. (D) Tooth-borne appliance with a ligature tie for indirect anchorage to the MI. (E) Tooth-borne appliance with an elastic chain for indirect anchorage to the MI. F, total force; i, vertical (intrusive) component; r, horizontal component; M_u, moment created on the upper arch; M_l, moment created on the lower arch; M_l', moment created on the lower arch from ligation; r', retractive force applied on the lower arch equal to r of the TFBC when the anterior segments move forward; a, horizontal/retractive component of elastic force; b, vertical component of elastic force; M_e, moment in lower arch from elastic force.

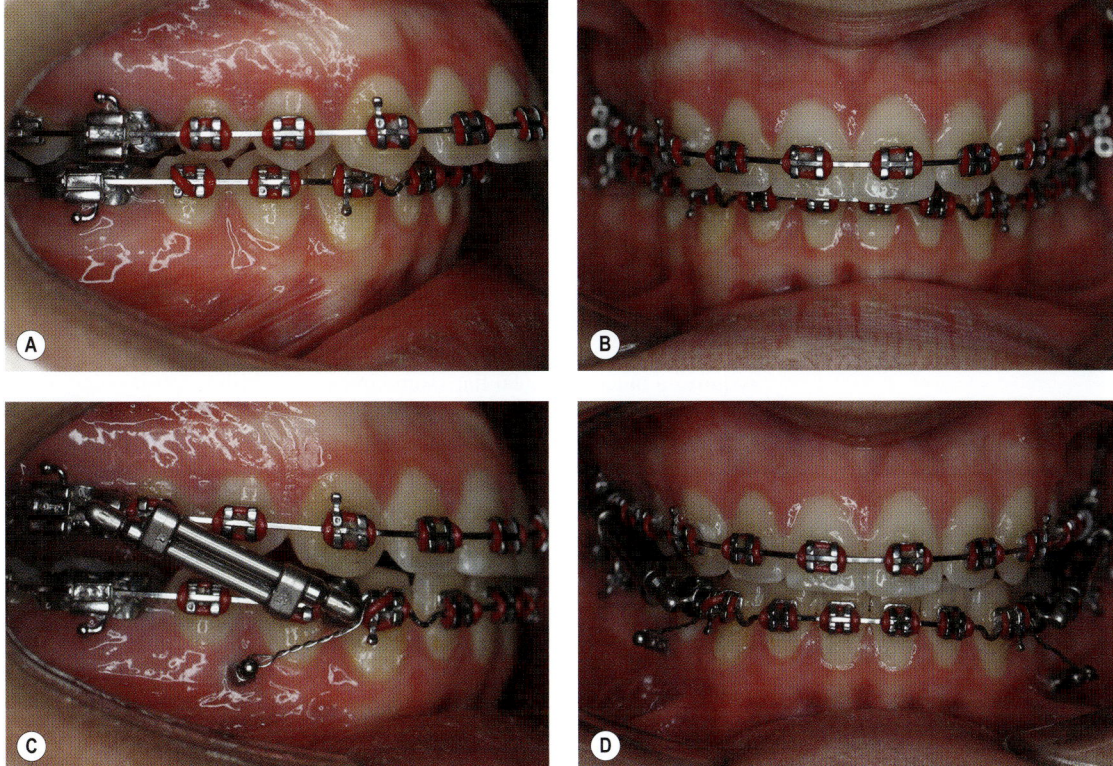

Fig. 47.3 Case example of Twin Force Bite Corrector with miniscrew implant anchorage. (A,B) Leveled and aligned arches just prior to appliance fitting. (C,D) Placement of the appliance with indirect anchorage using a miniscrew implant between the premolars in the mandible.

would be better suited to bear the high forces exerted by the TFBC appliance. However, a very large moment would be generated in the maxilla as the point of force application would be further away from the CR.

INDIRECT ANCHORAGE

To overcome the issues of direct anchorage, MIs can be placed mesial to the maxillary first molar with an archwire connecting the first molar and the MI to provide indirect anchorage against the distal movement of the maxillary molar (Fig. 47.2C). However, based on the magnitude of distal movement of the maxillary molar observed with the TFBC, this approach seems unnecessary. Furthermore, our long-term results support the fact that the maxillary molar will revert back to its original position with the natural mesial drift of the dentition. In order to prevent the undesired flaring of the mandibular incisors, a MI can be placed distal to the canine with an arm extending from the MI to an auxiliary tube bonded on the canine.

The most practical way to implement indirect anchorage is by utilizing a single MI on each side in the mandibular arch to prevent mandibular incisor flaring. The MI would be placed between the roots of the mandibular first molar and second premolar or between the two premolars. The TFBC appliance is then placed mesial to the maxillary molar and distal to the mandibular canine and the MI can either be ligated to the canine bracket (Fig. 47.2D) or an active force can be applied from the MI to the canine by placing a coil spring or elastic chain (Fig. 47.2E). The vertical component of force increases drastically with an elastic chain, which may generate an unfavorable open bite tendency. Against this, based on the vertical positioning of the MI, there may be a mild favorable (if mandibular incisor flaring is to be avoided) counterclockwise moment generated in the

mandibular dental arch. Overall, a passive ligature seems to have a more favorable effect in preventing incisor flaring with minimal side effects, as shown in the case example in Fig. 47.3.

CONCLUSIONS

The TFBC is a very versatile appliance for the correction of the Class II malocclusion. Short- and long-term results appear to be favorable and stable; however, true orthopedic effects seem to be minimal if any. Skeletal anchorage could, in theory, provide an avenue to increase the orthopedic effect, reflected in enhanced mandibular growth. Although this is an appealing approach, the preliminary clinical research results do not show promising evidence supporting the use of MIs in tandem with fixed functional appliances. It could be argued that dentoalveolar effects are at the heart of the correction of this type of malocclusion and, therefore, should not be prevented. True skeletal changes of significant magnitude would probably require an extended period of appliance wear.

REFERENCES

1. Papadopoulos MA. Classification of the non-compliance appliances used for Class II correction. In: Papadopoulos MA, editor. Orthodontic treatment of the Class II non-compliant patient: current principles and techniques. Edinburgh: Elsevier-Mosby; 2006. p. 9–17.
2. Rothenberg J, Campbell ES, Nanda R. Class II correction with the Twin Force Bite Corrector. J Clin Orthod 2004;38:232–40.
3. Campbell E. A prospective clinical analysis of a push-type fixed intermaxillary Class II correction appliance, Master Thesis. Farmington: University of Connecticut; 2003.
4. Proffit WR. Retention. In: Proffit WR, Fields HW Jr, Sarver DM, editors. Contemporary orthodontics. 4th ed. St. Louis, MO: Elsevier; 2007. p. 617–34.

48 Success rates, risk factors and complications of miniplates used for orthodontic anchorage

Marie A. Cornelis and Catherine Nyssen-Behets

INTRODUCTION

Miniscrew implants (MIs) and miniplates have been developed specifically for orthodontic purposes and can be inserted in multiple locations close to the dental arch. Their primary stability allows immediate loading, or early loading within 4 weeks of placement. Their surface is generally smooth, in contrast to dental implants, to avoid levels of osseointegration that would hinder their removal with a screwdriver.

Ideally, such temporary skeletal anchorage devices should not require invasive surgery for placement and removal, should be simple to connect to the orthodontic appliance and be able to withstand orthodontic forces. They are also expected to be inexpensive, early loadable, biocompatible and to provide superior clinical results to traditional anchorage systems.[1]

MIs are of smaller size than miniplates and are frequently placed by orthodontists themselves, but have a high risk of failure when placed in unattached gingiva and a high risk of root injury when placed in keratinized mucosa.[2,3] While root impingement is less likely with the smaller MIs, the risk of failure and fracture during placement increases as the MI's diameter decreases.[4,5] Unscrewing moments must be avoided during force application, and MIs inserted between roots might need to be repositioned during treatment to complete tooth movements.

Orthodontic miniplates are surgical osteosynthesis plates modified to allow a connection to orthodontic appliances.[6–8] Miniplates work as an onplant screwed on the bone surface, while the fixation screws act as an implant. Both plates and fixation screws are affected by a certain amount of osseointegration if they are made of titanium, but this is usually limited because the surfaces are smooth.

Miniplates have some advantages over MIs. The fixation screws are typically shorter than MIs and placed at a safe distance from the roots, while the connection to the orthodontic appliances is still located in attached gingiva close to the dental arch. The roots can, therefore, slide past the device and en masse distalization of an entire dental arch, for example, can occur without any root–screw impingements.[9] Miniplates can also sustain torquing moments and have higher success rates.[10,11] Consequently, they may provide more secure anchorage when higher forces are needed and may allow orthopedic forces.[18] Their disadvantage is that placement requires flap elevation, an invasive approach, and so is usually carried out by an oral surgeon or periodontist.

A number of miniplate systems have been developed, such as the Skeletal Anchorage System (Chapters 13 and 46), the C-tube system (KLS Martin, Umkirch, Germany; Chapter 45), the Bone Anchor system (Surgi-Tec, Belgium), the Dentsply-Sankin system (Tokyo, Japan) etc. Miniplates are usually made of titanium grade II, while their stabilizing screws are made of either commercially pure titanium or titanium grade V (Ti-Al6-V4), which has superior strength. The screws are self-tapping or self-drilling and usually measure between 4 and 7 mm in length.

The recommended locations in the maxilla are the zygomatic buttress and the piriform rim (in between, the bone covering the sinus is very thin), while in the mandible, the alveolar bone apical to the roots is suitable, apart from the mental foramen area. Miniplates are usually placed under local anesthesia with or without intravenous sedation. Placement surgery requires a mucoperiosteal flap, sometimes pilot drilling, positioning of the screws to fix the plate, and sutures (see Chapter 13). Orthodontic force is usually applied after soft tissue healing, at 1–4 weeks after placement. Removal surgery is recommended immediately after completion of orthodontic treatment, and again requires an incision before removal of the plates and screws, and stitches.

Miniplates are indicated particularly for intrusion of maxillary and/or mandibular molars in non-surgical treatment of open bite.[12,13] Beside intrusion, which is the most documented application, miniplates have also been used for distalization of the anterior teeth after premolar extractions,[14,15] and for maxillary[9,16] and/or mandibular[17] molar distalization in non-extraction treatment. Finally, a promising indication for miniplates is orthopedic protraction of the maxilla.[18] Use of miniplates in these multiple applications tends to reduce the need for extractions and orthognathic surgery.

The specific issues of success rates, risk factors and complications are addressed below.

SUCCESS RATES

Case series report success rates varying from 85 to 98% (Table 48.1). A meta-analysis of temporary anchorage devices estimated the failure rate of miniplates at 7.3% and concluded that miniplates and palatal implants, when grouped together, showed a 1.9-fold lower failure rate than MIs.[11] Success rates are usually higher in the maxilla than in the mandible,[8,23] and in adults than in growing patients.[23] Definition of success generally implies achievement of orthodontic objectives with the initial miniplate, some miniplates being successfully used throughout treatment even though slightly mobile.[8,22,23] Although the vast majority of failures can be linked to increased mobility, failure can also be caused by anchor

Table 48.1 Success rates reported in miniplate case series

Study	No. patients	No. miniplates	Success rate (%)
Retrospective			
Miyawaki et al., 2003[4]	7	17	96.4
Choi et al., 2005[8]	17	68	92.6
Kuroda et al., 2007[19]	22	38	86.8
Chen et al., 2007[20]	25	44	95.5
Chen et al., 2008[21]	194	171	95.3
Prospective			
Cheng et al., 2004[3]	N/A	48	85.4
Mommaerts et al., 2005[22]	18	35	91.4
Cornelis et al., 2008[23]	97	200	92.5
Eroglu et al., 2010[24]	37	74	98.6

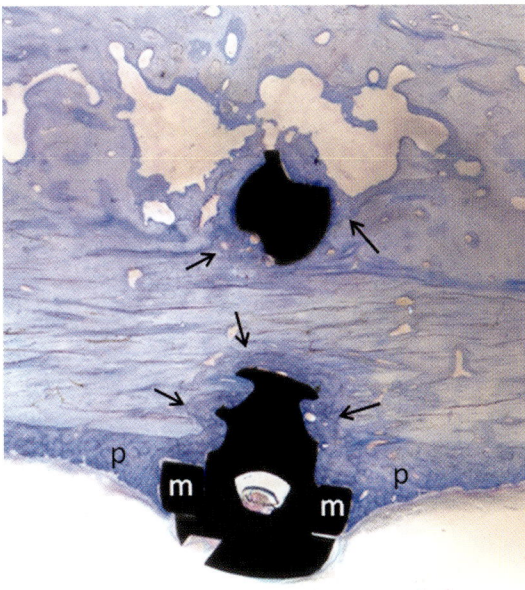

Fig. 48.1 Undecalcified longitudinal section through a dog mandible supporting a two-screw miniplate. The miniplate was loaded 2 weeks after placement, and loading was maintained for 27 weeks. The miniplate (m) is visible around the inferior screw and is in contact with abundant periosteal new bone (p). Remodeled bone is present at the surface of both screws, as attested by cementing lines (arrows). (Methylene blue staining; bar = 1 mm.)

breakage, cheek ulceration or poor location, all requiring miniplate removal and replacement.

The issue of success rate raises the question of optimal time before loading. Whereas for MIs it is stated that immediate loading is as successful as loading after a few weeks of healing,[25,26] healing times for miniplates vary between 1 and 4 weeks. However, various healing times have not been compared under experimental conditions. Although optimal healing time is not clearly defined, it has been shown that mobility occurs in general 5 weeks after miniplate placement in dogs,[27,28] which is consistent with MI failure. This might represent the critical stage of transition between primary stability obtained by tight fitting of the screws in cortical bone and secondary stability generated by remodeling (Fig. 48.1).[29] If correct, this observation would suggest that loading should be planned either earlier or later than this transition period, but not close to it.

The effect of magnitude of load on bone healing around miniplates is another important question raised by the issue of success rate. No comparative data are available at present with regard to the selection of appropriate forces and so it is impossible to know what the lower and upper thresholds might be that would trigger a positive balance, which if exceeded might possibly compromise the ease of removal of the plate, to a negative one, perhaps decreasing stability. This is an important area for future research as applications of miniplates have already broadened to include such indications as single tooth or whole arch intrusion, and orthopedic correction of skeletal problems.

The effect of loading on dental implants has been studied in detail; remodeling around implants generates a compliant layer of bone preventing microdamage accumulation and allowing long-term success of endosseous implants.[30] Microcalli have been observed under orthodontic load, and attributed to microrepair.[31] However, as the bone–implant contact is not affected by the orthodontic load of dental implants, strain levels are probably lower than the adapted window magnitudes.[32] With regard to miniplates, loading in the range of orthodontic forces appeared to have no effect on stability under experimental conditions in dogs, since the success rate was not significantly different in loaded versus unloaded plates, and loading did not affect bone-to-screw contact or bone density.[27,28]

RISK FACTORS

According to the literature, some possible risk factors can be advanced, including the insertion location, lack of primary stability of the screws, screw-to-root contact, soft tissue inflammation patient's age and occlusal interferences.

INSERTION LOCATION

An increased failure rate in the mandible compared with the maxilla has been shown in many studies, both clinical [3,8,21,23,33] and experimental.[28,34] The higher failure rate in the mandible could be attributed to the smaller amount of attached gingiva or it might be that maxillary trabecular bone responds better to miniplate placement than compact mandibular bone, since ensuring a better transition between primary and secondary stability. This would suggest that successful anchorage depends not only on bone density but also on specific features of the receptor site.[27]

LACK OF PRIMARY STABILITY OF THE SCREWS

Although no specific data are available for miniplates, it is evident that lack of primary stability of the screws fixing the plates is a major factor for failure. It is known from dental implants that excessive surgical trauma impedes the ability to establish the necessary intimate bone–implant contact.[35] For example, when the initially drilled hole had to be redrilled on a slightly different axis during miniplate placement, woven bone could be observed in dogs as a repair process,[27] which might argue in favor of a drill-free technique. Screw-to-bone contact with self-drilling screws has been shown to be superior to that of self-tapping screws when used for osteosynthesis after orthognathic surgery or fracture.[36]

From MI reports, it is clear that primary stability depends on the thickness and quality of the cortical bone. Although this issue has not been clearly established for orthodontic miniplates, miniplates placed in hyperdivergent patients were reported to be more at risk, possibly because cortical bone is usually thinner in these patients.[4]

SCREW-TO-ROOT CONTACT

For MIs, root proximity seems to be a major risk factor, either because there is less bone surrounding the screw or because of the transmission of occlusal forces to the screws; however, for miniplates, root proximity and contact of the anchoring screws seem to have minimal effects on stability.[37]

SOFT TISSUE INFLAMMATION

Failures are associated with inflammation of the soft tissues.[4,8,20,24] Good oral hygiene, with mouth rinses during the first week after placement and careful brushing of the exposed parts of the miniplate and surrounding mucosa throughout treatment, is, therefore, critical for miniplate success.[4,8,20,24,38] Indeed, crevices around miniplates have been shown to be supportive of anaerobic growth of bacteria likely to stimulate soft tissue inflammation.[39] Although antibiotic coverage appears to be the preferred protocol after placement surgery, high success rates even without antibiotics suggest that antibiotic prophylaxis might not be so important.[38] Clinical trials should be conducted to confirm this hypothesis. Concentration on surgical asepsis would probably further reduce the risk of introducing pathogens at the surgical site.

Sof tissue perforation through the non-keratinized mucosa is a risk factor, possibly impeding tight closure of the tissues around the miniplate in this more mobile mucosa and thus stimulating inflammation through

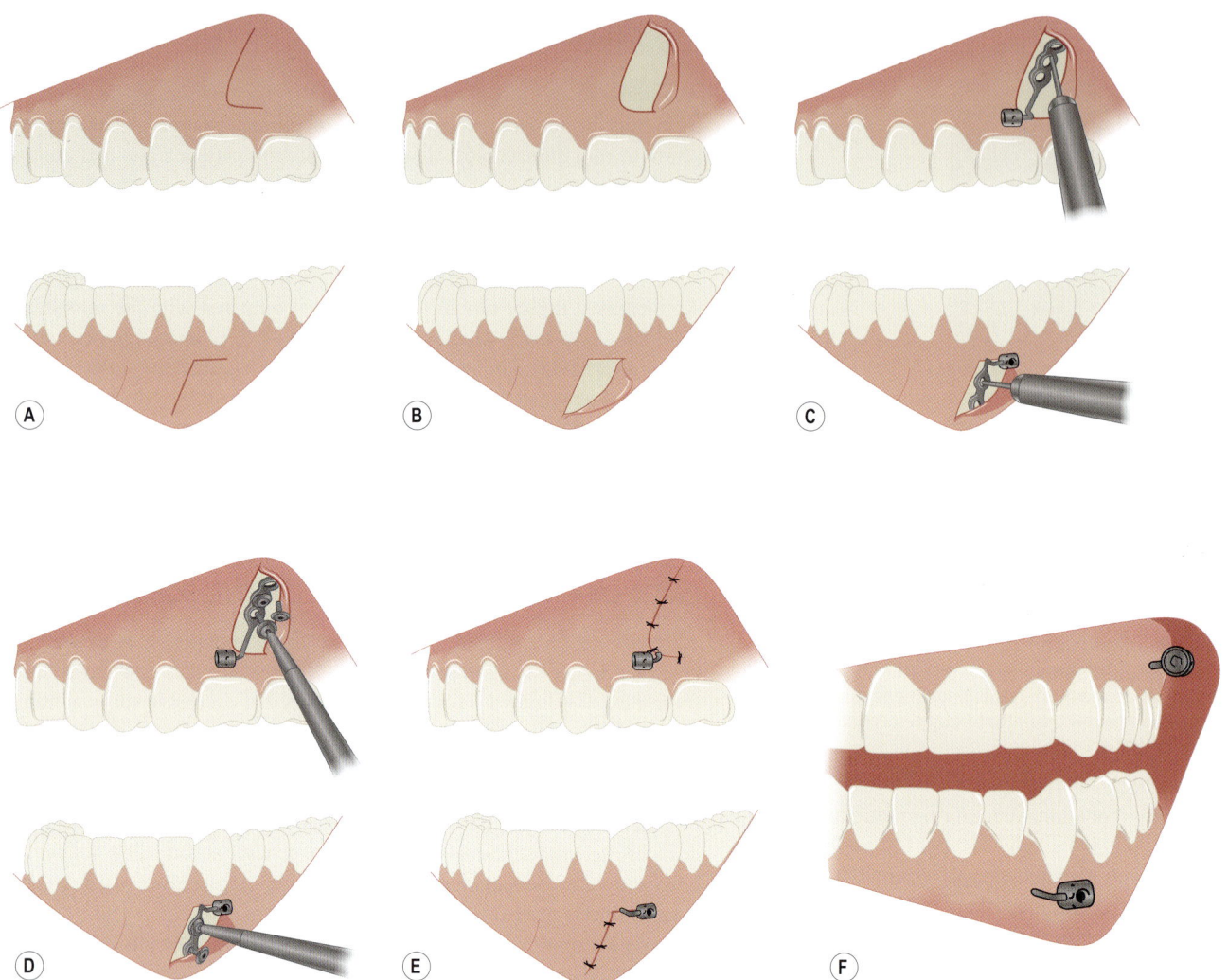

Fig. 48.2 Placement surgery in the maxilla and mandible. (A) L-shaped incisions with the horizontal part of the incision being 1 mm into the attached gingiva. (B) Mucoperiosteal flap. (C) Drilling of the middle hole (for the three-hole plate) or of the hole located closest to the attachment unit (for the two-hole plate). (D) Insertion of the screws. (E) Closure with resorbable sutures. (F) Bollard miniplates with the attachment units facing anterior in the posterior maxilla and posterior in the anterior mandible. (With permission from Cornelis et al., 2008.[38])

exposure to the oral cavity.[3] Soft tissue perforation is, therefore, recommended to occur at either the mucogingival junction or immediately within the keratinized mucosa in order to allow for good soft tissue healing (Fig. 48.2).[23]

Combining miniplate placement with extractions in the same area should also be avoided since the inflammation around the extraction socket may interfere with bone and soft tissue healing.[38]

PATIENT'S AGE

Miniplate placement in children and adolescents has not been documented extensively. However, one study revealed that the majority (73%) of the failures occurred in growing patients.[23] It may be that during placement of the miniplates, perforating the soft tissues at the mucogingival junction is more difficult in younger patients where the alveolar height tends to be shallow, the width of attached gingiva decreased and the access restricted.

OCCLUSAL INTERFERENCES

The presence of occlusal interferences has been reported to be critical for miniplates success.[20] However, this is seldom a problem in clinical conditions as the part of the miniplate exposed to the oral cavity is generally away from the teeth, since mucosal perforation is recommended to

occur at the mucogingival junction or immediately within the attached gingiva.

COMPLICATIONS

Complications can be divided into postoperative complications, soft tissue complications, damage to teeth and adjacent structures, miniplate mobility, practical complications and complications during miniplate removal.

POSTOPERATIVE COMPLICATIONS

Swelling

The most frequent problem reported by patients is postsurgical swelling, lasting on average 5 days after miniplate placement and after removal (Fig. 48.3A).[38] Swelling is sometimes accompanied by hematoma (Fig. 48.3B). After surgery, anti-inflammatory agents and/or painkillers are usually recommended to patients. It is probable that more aggressive management of postoperative edema, including the use of ice packs 1–2 hours postoperatively, the addition of preoperative anti-inflammatory agents or corticosteroids delivered intravenously, could prevent or at least reduce this complication.

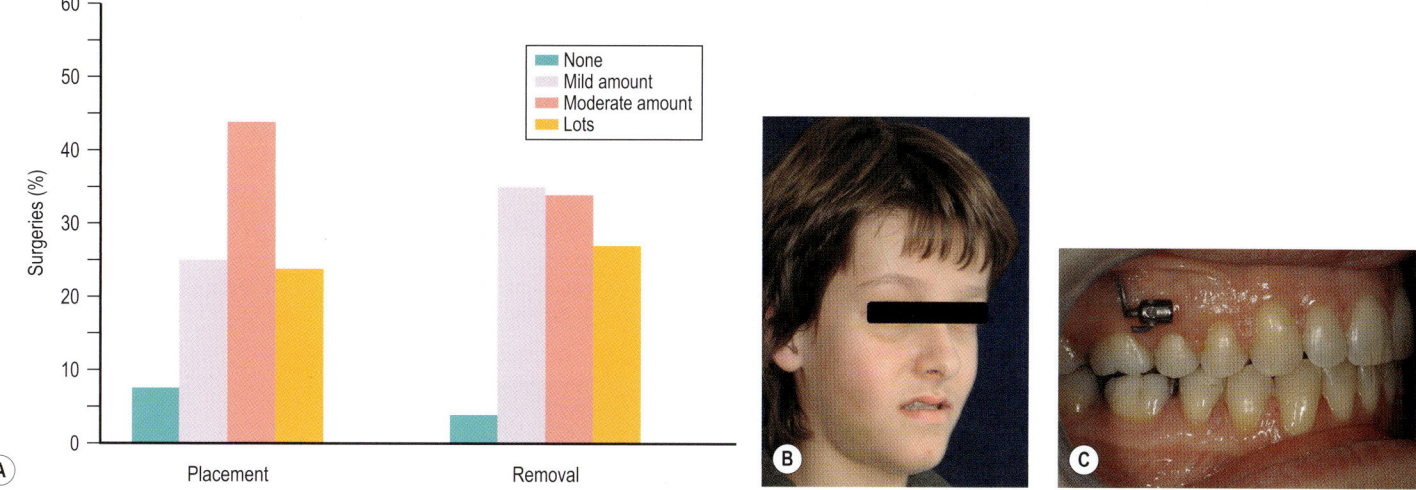

Fig. 48.3 Postoperative complications. (A) Frequency of swelling reported by patients for placement and removal surgery. (B) Cheek and infraorbital hematomas on the right side of the face 1 week after placement of four miniplates. (C) Gingival dehiscence of the lower part of the miniplate. (A with permission from Cornelis et al., 2008.[38])

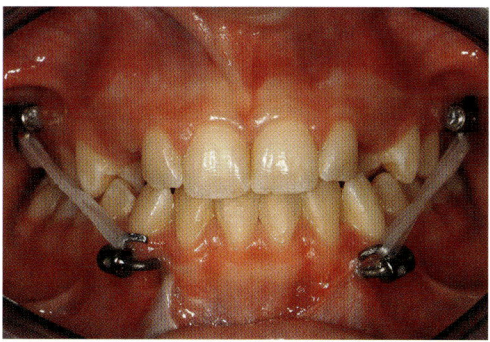

Fig. 48.4 Four miniplates placed in a growing child to achieve maxillary protraction with interanchor elastics. The mandibular miniplates were placed between the lateral incisors and canines to reduce the risk of cheek irritation.

Pain

Although the placement of miniplates requires surgery to raise a mucoperiosteal flap and retract the tissues, the procedure appears to be associated with minimal perioperative pain. Four out of five patients report that the surgical experience is better than expected, with little or no pain, while their discomfort is less or equivalent to extractions.[23]

SOFT TISSUE COMPLICATIONS

Cheek Irritation

Cheek irritation is experienced initially by more than one-third of the patients but reduces over time.[23] In the mandible, locating the miniplates between the lateral incisor and canine generates less cheek irritation than between the canine and first premolar, probably because the miniplate head is then more prominent in the region of the orbicularis oris musculature (Fig. 48.4).

Gingival Dehiscence

Poor adaptation of the miniplate to the bone at the exit point into the oral cavity can generate gingival dehiscence with consequent exposure of part of the miniplate (Fig. 48.3C).[22,38] Importantly, the connection bar must be slightly bent at the lower limit of the plate to ensure tight contact with the bone surface where the bar emerges through the mucosa and good soft tissue healing (see Fig. 22.2C).

DAMAGE TO TEETH AND ADJACENT STRUCTURES

Root Damage

Root damage was probably underestimated initially but has been reported since 2005 for MIs[40] and, more recently, for miniplates.[37] Surprisingly, although the risk should theoretically be less for miniplates than for MIs, a cone beam CT evaluation of miniplates in the posterior maxilla showed that 1 out of 10 anchoring screws penetrated the dental roots, even when very short (4 mm) and self-drilling fixation screws were used.[37] However, this happened with a relatively short plate (C-tube), forcing the anchoring screws closer to the roots. Although the authors concluded that root contact did not interfere with miniplate stability, this raises the question of cementum repair after root impingement.[37] While experimental studies describe cementum repair and healing of the periodontal structure a few weeks after MI removal when the damage is limited to cementum or dentin, abnormal healing responses are observed when pulpal invasion occurs.[40–42] The finding that MI placement less than 1 mm from the root surface can cause root resorption is also of considerable concern.[42]

Sinus Perforation

Miniplate anchoring screws have been shown to penetrate the maxillary sinus, but no harmful consequences were reported.[37]

MINIPLATE MOBILITY

Miniplate mobility is the most frequent reason for failure. Histologically, screws without the bone-to-screw contact needed for stability are surrounded with a large radiotransparent space, with bone resorption and absence of osteoblastic activity, and are exclusively in contact with dense fibrous tissue.[27] However, although miniplates can become mobile, some are still sufficiently firm to provide the necessary anchorage to achieve the treatment objectives (Fig. 48.5).[23]

PRACTICAL COMPLICATIONS

Anchor Breakage

Breakage is a complication that occurs in less than 2% of miniplates. It seems to be associated with repeated bending, causing in order to change the force vector (Fig. 48.6).[23]

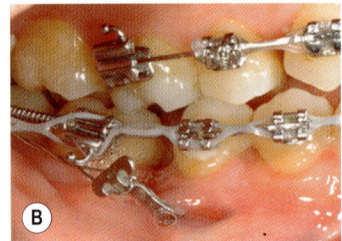

Fig. 48.5 Miniplate used for uprighting and mesializing a mandibular molar. Although the miniplate was clearly mobile and the gingival conditions were far from ideal, planned molar movement was achieved with the initial inserted miniplate. (A) Initiation of molar mesialization. (B) Miniplate displaced to the distal but still used. (C) Final position of the molar, a few months after miniplate removal. (Courtesy of Drs. Diane Pham and Fabienne Pernet.)

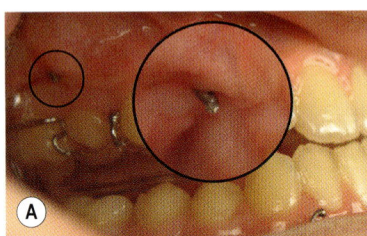
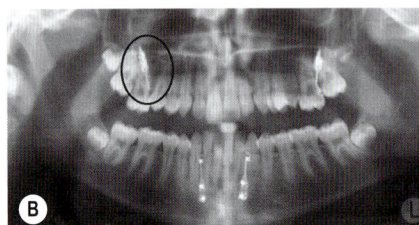
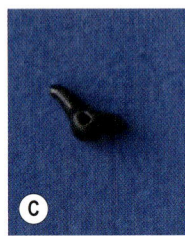

Fig. 48.6 Fracture of an upper right miniplate in a child having four miniplates placed for maxillary protraction. (A) Intraoral view of fracture. (B) Panoramic radiograph showing the upper right miniplate fractured. (C) Fractured button of the miniplate.

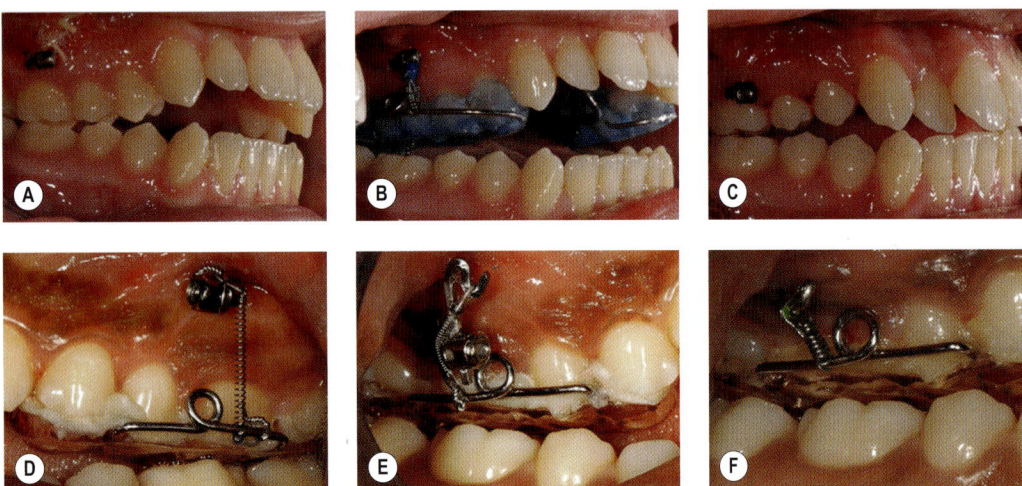

Fig. 48.7 Miniplates with tooth movement during molar intrusion in two open bite patients. (A–C) Progress of open bite closure in one patient. (A) After miniplate placement, with sutures still present. (B) Intrusion with a bonded acrylic plate. (C) Occlusion at the end of the molar intrusion phase. Overcorrection could not be achieved because of the proximity of the miniplates to the intruded molars. (D–F) Alteration of the shape of a miniplate interfering with movement. (D) Miniplate placed correctly at the left side. (E) Miniplate placed too low on the right side; a connecting wire had to be inserted into the miniplate button in order to increase the distance between the acrylic plate and the miniplate. (F) In order to proceed with the intrusion, a flap was later reopened, the lower screw was removed, the button was cut away and the plate was bent upwards, in order to make a hook. (A–C courtesy of Dr. Alexander Johner.)

Interference with Tooth Movement

During molar intrusion, a miniplate may interfere with the tooth in its new position; consequently the miniplate needs to be repositioned to allow the completion of intrusion (Fig. 48.7A–C).[23] Alternatively, a less traumatic solution would be to open a flap, cut away the part of the miniplate interfering with movement and bend the remaining part in order to make a hook (Fig. 48.7D–F).

COMPLICATIONS AT REMOVAL

Bone Overgrowth

The main difficulty encountered during removal surgery is bone overgrowth over the plates, although this varies considerably from patient to patient (Fig. 48.8). Bone covering 25% or more of the plate has been reported for more than 1 in 10 patients, but it did not seem to be correlated with the location of the plate (maxilla or mandible, anterior or posterior) or with the age of the patient.[38] As long as titanium is used for miniplate fabrication, even if uncoated and polished, some degree of bone-to-screw contact does occur, which increases with time and in some cases even extends from the screws to the plate.[27] Therefore, it is recommended that plates are removed as soon as they are no longer needed.

CONCLUSIONS

The most important clinical conclusions can be summarized as follows.

- Before surgery, patients should be informed about postoperative swelling. They might be reassured about pain, which is usually milder than expected.

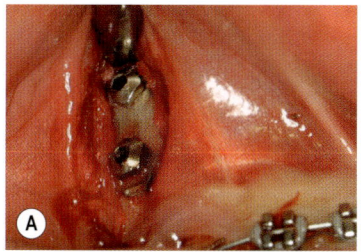 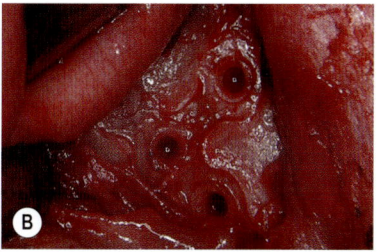

Fig. 48.8 Bone overgrowth. (A) Miniplate covered by bone overgrowth after flap opening, before miniplate removal. (B) Imprint of miniplate appearing in bone after miniplate removal, clearly demonstrating the bone overgrowth.

- Surgery should respect strict guidelines and avoid excessive trauma. In particular, redrilling, which is associated with bone-remodeling healing reactions, has to be avoided in order to optimize primary stability.

- When possible, the maxilla should be preferred as receptor site over the mandible, since the number of failures is higher in the mandible.

- Placement in children is more subject to failures than in adults, which needs to be clarified to the parents during consultation.

- Oral hygiene is of major importance to avoid inflammation of the soft tissues. Even though the need for patient compliance is reduced compared with other anchorage devices, it remains essential in terms of plaque control.

- It is recommended that miniplates are removed as soon as they are no longer necessary, since osseointegration of the screws increases with time which may in some cases impede miniplate removal.

REFERENCES

1. Cope JB. Temporary anchorage devices in orthodontics: a paradigm shift. Semin Orthod 2005;11:3–9.
2. Poggio PM, Incorvati C, Velo S, et al. "Safe zones": a guide for miniscrew positioning in the maxillary and mandibular arch. Angle Orthod 2006;76:191–7.
3. Cheng SJ, Tseng IY, Lee JJ, Kok SH. A prospective study of the risk factors associated with failure of mini-implants used for orthodontic anchorage. Int J Oral Maxillofac Implants 2004;19:100–6.
4. Miyawaki S, Koyama I, Inoue M, et al. Factors associated with the stability of titanium screws placed in the posterior region for orthodontic anchorage. Am J Orthod Dentofacial Orthop 2003;124:373–8.
5. Buchter A, Wiechmann D, Koerdt S, et al. Load-related implant reaction of mini-implants used for orthodontic anchorage. Clin Oral Implants Res 2005;16:473–9.
6. De Clerck H, Geerinckx V, Siciliano S. The Zygoma Anchorage System. J Clin Orthod 2002;36:455–9.
7. Chung KR, Kim YS, Linton JL, et al. The miniplate with tube for skeletal anchorage. J Clin Orthod 2002;36:407–12.
8. Choi BH, Zhu SJ, Kim YH. A clinical evaluation of titanium miniplates as anchors for orthodontic treatment. Am J Orthod Dentofacial Orthop 2005;128:382–4.
9. De Clerck HJ, Cornelis MA. Biomechanics of skeletal anchorage. Part 2: Class II nonextraction treatment. J Clin Orthod 2006;40:290–8, quiz 307.
10. Chen YJ, Chang HH, Lin HY, et al. Stability of miniplates and miniscrews used for orthodontic anchorage: experience with 492 temporary anchorage devices. Clin Oral Implants Res 2008;19:1188–96.
11. Schatzle M, Mannchen R, Zwahlen M, et al. Survival and failure rates of orthodontic temporary anchorage devices: a systematic review. Clin Oral Implants Res 2009;20:1351–9.
12. Sherwood KH, Burch JG, Thompson WJ. Closing anterior open bites by intruding molars with titanium miniplate anchorage. Am J Orthod Dentofacial Orthop 2002;122:593–600.
13. Sugawara J, Baik UB, Umemori M, et al. Treatment and post-treatment dentoalveolar changes following intrusion of mandibular molars with application of a skeletal anchorage system (SAS) for open bite correction. Int J Adult Orthodon Orthognath Surg 2002;17:243–53.
14. Erverdi N, Acar A. Zygomatic anchorage for en masse retraction in the treatment of severe Class II, division 1. Angle Orthod 2005;75:483–90.
15. Iino S, Sakoda S, Miyawaki S. An adult bimaxillary protrusion treated with corticotomy-facilitated orthodontics and titanium miniplates. Angle Orthod 2006;76:1074–82.
16. Cornelis MA, De Clerck HJ. Maxillary molar distalization with miniplates assessed on digital models: a prospective clinical trial. Am J Orthod Dentofacial Orthop 2007;132:373–7.
17. Sugawara J, Daimaruya T, Umemori M, et al. Distal movement of mandibular molars in adult patients with the skeletal anchorage system. Am J Orthod Dentofacial Orthop 2004;125:130–8.
18. Kircelli BH, Pektas ZO, Uckan S. Orthopedic protraction with skeletal anchorage in a patient with maxillary hypoplasia and hypodontia. Angle Orthod 2006;76:156–63.
19. Kuroda S, Sugawara Y, Deguchi T, et al. Clinical use of miniscrew implants as orthodontic anchorage: success rates and postoperative discomfort. Am J Orthod Dentofacial Orthop 2007;131:9–15.
20. Chen CH, Hsieh CH, Tseng YC, et al. The use of miniplate osteosynthesis for skeletal anchorage. Plast Reconstr Surg 2007;120:232–5.
21. Chen YJ, Chang HH, Lin HY, et al. Stability of miniplates and miniscrews used for orthodontic anchorage: experience with 492 temporary anchorage devices. Clin Oral Implants Res 2008;19:1188–96.
22. Mommaerts MY, Michiels ML, De Pauw GA. A 2-year outcome audit of a versatile orthodontic bone anchor. J Orthod 2005;32:175–81.
23. Cornelis MA, Scheffler NR, Nyssen-Behets C, et al. Patients' and orthodontists' perceptions of miniplates used for temporary skeletal anchorage: a prospective study. Am J Orthod Dentofacial Orthop 2008;133:18–24.
24. Eroglu T, Kaya B, Cetinsahin A, et al. Success of zygomatic plate-screw anchorage system. J Oral Maxillofac Surg 2010;68:602–5.
25. van de Vannet B, Sabzevar MM, Wehrbein H, et al. Osseointegration of miniscrews: a histomorphometric evaluation. Eur J Orthod 2007;29:437–42.
26. Freire JN, Silva NR, Gil JN, Magini RS, et al. Histomorphologic and histomorphometric evaluation of immediately and early loaded mini-implants for orthodontic anchorage. Am J Orthod Dentofacial Orthop 2007;131:704.
27. Cornelis MA, Vandergugten S, Mahy P, et al. Orthodontic loading of titanium miniplates in dogs: microradiographic and histological evaluation. Clin Oral Implants Res 2008;19:1054–62.
28. Cornelis MA, Mahy P, Devogelaer JP, et al. Does orthodontic loading influence bone mineral density around titanium miniplates? An experimental study in dogs. Orthod Craniofac Res 2010;13:21–7.
29. Schenk RK, Buser D. Osseointegration: a reality. Periodontol 2000 1998;17:22–35.
30. Huja SS, Katona TR, Burr DB, et al. Microdamage adjacent to endosseous implants. Bone 1999;25:217–22.
31. Trisi P, Rebaudi A. Progressive bone adaptation of titanium implants during and after orthodontic load in humans. Int J Periodontics Restorative Dent 2002;22:31–43.
32. Cattaneo PM, Dalstra M, Melsen B. Analysis of stress and strain around orthodontically loaded implants: an animal study. Int J Oral Maxillofac Implants 2007;22:213–25.
33. Chen CH, Chang CS, Hsieh CH, et al. The use of microimplants in orthodontic anchorage. J Oral Maxillofac Surg 2006;64:1209–13.
34. Owens SE, Buschang PH, Cope JB, et al. Experimental evaluation of tooth movement in the beagle dog with the mini-screw implant for orthodontic anchorage. Am J Orthod Dentofacial Orthop 2007;132:639–46.
35. Esposito M, Thomsen P, Ericson LE, et al. Histopathologic observations on early oral implant failures. Int J Oral Maxillofac Implants 1999;14:798–810.
36. Heidemann W, Terheyden H, Gerlach KL. Analysis of the osseous/metal interface of drill free screws and self-tapping screws. J Craniomaxillofac Surg 2001;29:69–74.
37. Kim GT, Kim SH, Choi YS, et al. Cone-beam computed tomography evaluation of orthodontic miniplate anchoring screws in the posterior maxilla. Am J Orthod Dentofacial Orthop 2009;136:628, discussion 628–9.
38. Cornelis MA, Scheffler NR, Mahy P, et al. Modified miniplates for temporary skeletal anchorage in orthodontics: placement and removal surgeries. J Oral Maxillofac Surg 2008;66:1439–45.
39. Sato R, Sato T, Takahashi I, et al. Profiling of bacterial flora in crevices around titanium orthodontic anchor plates. Clin Oral Implants Res 2007;18:21–6.
40. Asscherickx K, Vannet BV, Wehrbein H, et al. Root repair after injury from miniscrew. Clin Oral Implants Res 2005;16:575–8.
41. Brisceno CE, Rossouw PE, Carrillo R, et al. Healing of the roots and surrounding structures after intentional damage with miniscrew implants. Am J Orthod Dentofacial Orthop 2009;135:292–301.
42. Kim H, Kim TW. Histologic evaluation of root-surface healing after root contact or approximation during placement of mini-implants. Am J Orthod Dentofacial Orthop 2011;139:752–60.

49 Success rates and risk factors of miniscrew implants used as temporary anchorage devices for orthodontic purposes

Moschos A. Papadopoulos, Spyridon N. Papageorgiou and Ioannis P. Zogakis

INTRODUCTION

Miniscrew implants (MIs) are widely used as supporting anchorage auxiliaries in orthodontics. They are usually manufactured from pure titanium or titanium alloy (Ti6-Al4-V) with a diameter of 1–2 mm and length of 8–20 mm. Their value lies in their ability to remain relatively stationary in bone and to increase anchorage capacity without adverse effects or anchorage loss. MIs seem to be more effective in supporting anchorage when they are used in the mandible between the second premolar and the first molar; when two MIs are inserted instead of one; when the MIs are directly connected; when they are used in adults; and when treatment lasts more than 12 months.

COMPLICATIONS OF MINISCREW USE

Complications can occur at various stages;

1. during insertion
   - lack of initial stability if placed in inadequate cortical bone thickness
   - injury of adjacent structures (periodontal ligament, tooth root, nerves, blood vessels or sinus perforation)
2. during orthodontic treatment
   - inflammation and infection of surrounding tissues
   - loss of MI stability attributable to inflammation or bone remodeling
3. during MI removal
   - fracture.

ASSESSMENT OF SUCCESS RATES AND RISK FACTORS

Factors possibly associated with the success or survival of orthodontic MIs have been assessed in several clinical studies[1-7] and partially in published systematic reviews.[8-10] However, these reviews only included a limited number of studies, assessed only a few factors qualitatively and included other methods of anchorage reinforcement such as miniplates. Cohort studies can provide reliable evidence under controlled experimental conditions, and they usually include larger samples. Nevertheless, prospective studies tend to have higher reporting quality and more complete data than retrospective ones, although both present medium or high risk of bias.

Failure is considered to mean the need for MI removal or its inability to act as the required stationary anchor. Based on three retrospective cohort studies that investigated MI failures by month of treatment, it seems that, on average, the first 2 months after insertion are crucial, with 58% of all failures occurring in this period and with 20% of the overall failures taking place between months 2 and 3 (Fig. 49.1).[4,5,11] At this point change in treatment plan may be difficult or even impossible.

This chapter presents a meta-analysis of the existing knowledge from published controlled and uncontrolled clinical trials regarding the success/failure rates of MIs used for orthodontic anchorage purposes in order to identify associated risk factors.[12] An unrestricted electronic search for published and unpublished studies in any language was followed by study selection, data extraction and risk of bias evaluation in duplicate by two investigators. Random-effects meta-analyses were performed implementing failure rates in percentages, relative risks and the corresponding 95% confidence intervals (CIs). Additional analyses included subgroup analyses, meta-regression and stratification by jaw.

Following proper selection according to specific inclusion and exclusion criteria, a total of 52 studies were identified: 5 randomized controlled trials (RCTs), 8 prospective controlled trials, 27 prospective cohort studies and 12 studies with unclear design that were considered through detailed reading to be prospective cohort studies (Table 49.1). Reporting quality varied among studies, and risk of bias analysis indicated that most of the studies were of medium quality.

The 52 studies included a total of 4987 MIs, which were placed in 2281 patients in order to reinforce orthodontic anchorage. The reported percentage of failure rates in these original studies ranged between 0.0% and

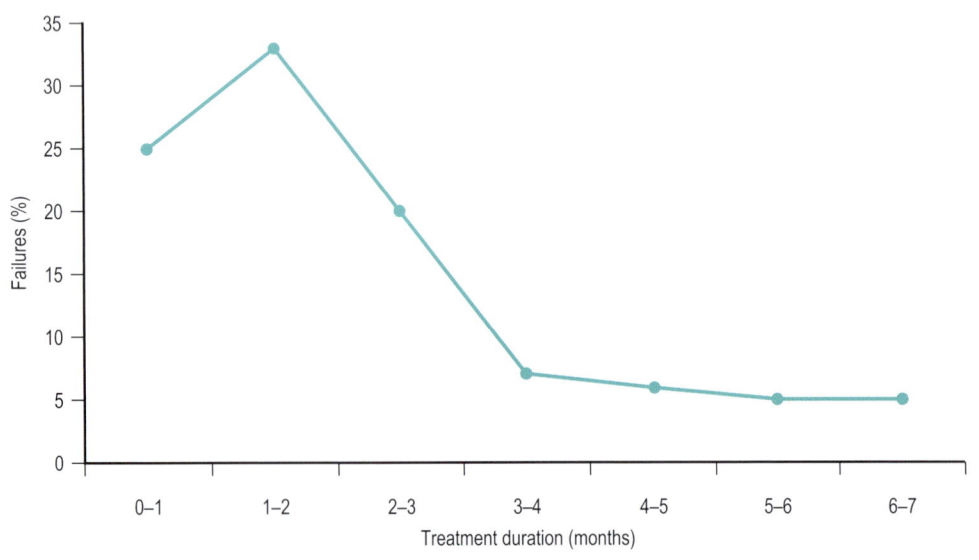

Fig. 49.1 Distribution of the percentages of miniscrew implant failures over treatment duration according to the data derived from three retrospective cohort studies.[4,5,11]

Table 49.1 Characteristics of the trials included in the meta-analysis

Source	Setting	Total No. MIs	MIs per patient (per jaw)	Brand[a]	Diameter (mm)	Length (mm)	Success criteria	Failure rate (%)	Action
RCT (randomized anchorage type per patient									
Basha et al. (2010)[13]	U	14	2 (2)	SS	1.3	8	Stability	28.6	New
Liu et al. (2009)[14]	NR	68	2 (2)	Ningbo Cibei	1.2	8	Stability	11.8	New
Upadhyah et al. (2008)[15]	U	72	4 (2)	Modified Ti fixation screws	1.3	8	Stability	6.9	New
RCT (risk factors per patient)									
Aboul-Ela (2011)[16]	U	26	2 (2)	AbsoAnchor	1.3	8	Stability	7.7	Repositioned
Lehnen et al. (2011)[17]	NR	60	2 (2)	Tomas-pin	1.6	8	NR	11.7	Excluded
PCCT (randomized anchorage type per patient)									
Hedayati et al. (2007)[18]	U	27	3 (1/2)	Orthognathic screws	2	9/11	Stability	18.5	Repositioned
Maddalone et al. (2010)[19]	NR	25	NR	3M Unitek	1.8	8	Stability	8.0	NR
Park et al. (2008)[20]	U	46	2/4 (2)	AbsoAnchor/ Osteomed/ Leibinger	1.2	6/8	Tx completion	13	New
Shi et al. (2008)[21]	U	28	2 (2)	Miniscrew Anchorage System	1.5	8	NR	10.7	New
Upadhyah et al. (2008)[22]	U	30	2 (2)	Modified Ti fixation screws	1.3	8	Stability	10.0	New
Wilmes et al. (2009)[23]	NR	10	1 (1)	Dual-Top	2	10	NR	0.0	NR
PCCT (risk factors per patient)									
Apel et al. (2009)[24]	U	76	2/4 (2)	Tomas-pin	1.6	8	Stability/Infection	10.5	Excluded
Garfinkle et al. (2008)[25]	U/Private	82	4/8 (4)	Osteomed	1.6	6	Stability/Tx completion	19.5 (Only loaded MIs included)∧	NR
PCS									
Upadhyay et al. (2009)[26]	U	46	2 (2)	Ti mini-implants	1.3	8	NR	4.3	New
Blaya et al. (2010)[27]	U/Private	30	1 (1)	Sin Implant System	1.2	10	Stability	0.0	NR
Brandão & Mucha (2008)[28]	U	40	4 (2)	Ortoimplante Básicos	1.5	9	Stability	0.0	NR
Cheng et al. (2004)[29]	U	92	NR	Leibinger/ Mondeal	2	5–15	Stability/ Infection/Tx completion	8.7 (Only MI data are reported from the various anchorage-reinforcement methods)	NR
Gelgör et al. (2004)[30]	U	25	1 (1)	IMF Stryker, Leibinger, Germany)	1.8	14	Stability	0.0	NR
Herman et al. (2006)[31]	NR	49	1/2 (1/2)	Ortho Implant, Sendax MDI	1.8	6/8/10	Stability	40.8	New/Excluded
Justens & de Bruyn (2008)[32]	U	50	NR	Dual-Top	1.8/2	8/10	Stability/Tx completion	34.0 (Including failed miniscrews which did not need to be replaced to complete treatment)	New
Kim et al. (2010)[33]	U	50	2 (2)	C-Implant	1.8	8.5	Stability	4.0	New
Liou et al. (2004)[34]	NR	32	2 (2)	Leibinger	2	17	Stability	0.0	NR
Luzi et al. (2007)[35]	U	140	NR	Aarhus Mini-Implants	1.5/2	9.6/11.6	Stability/Tx completion	15.7 (Including failed miniscrews which did not need to be replaced to complete treatment)***	Excluded
Miyazawa et al. (2010)[36]	U	44	NR	Dual-Top	1.6	8	Tx completion	9.1	NR
Motoyoshi et al. (2006)[37]	U	124	1–4 (1/2)	ISA orthodontic implants	1.6	8	Stability	14.5	NR
Motoyoshi et al. (2007)[38]	U	169	1–4 (1/2)	ISA orthodontic implants	1.6	8	Stability/Tx completion	14.8	NR
Motoyoshi et al. (2007)[39]	U	87	NR	ISA orthodontic implants	1.6	8	Stability/Tx completion	12.6	NR

Continued

Table 49.1 Characteristics of the trials included in the meta-analysis—cont'd

Source	Setting	Total No. MIs	MIs per patient (per jaw)	Brand[a]	Diameter (mm)	Length (mm)	Success criteria	Failure rate (%)	Action
Motoyoshi et al. (2009)[40]	U	209	1–4 (1/2)	ISA orthodontic implants	1.6	8	Stability/Tx completion	11.5	NR
Motoyoshi et al. (2010)[41]	U	148	NR	ISA orthodontic implants	1.6	8	Stability	9.5	Excluded
Oh et al. (2011)[42]	U	78	NR	AbsoAnchor/ Osteomed	1.2/NR	NR	NR	10.3 (4 MIs omitted as intentionally moved to another location)‡	New
Park et al. (2006)[2]	U	227	NR	Stryker Leibinger/ Osteomed/ KLS-Martin	1.2/2	4–15	Stability/Tx completion	8.4	New
Polat-Ozsoy et al. (2009)[43]	U	22	2 (2)	AbsoAnchor	1.2	6	Stability/Infection	13.6 (One MI was replaced due to root proximity and was also classified as failure)§	New
Suzuki et al. (2011)[44]	U	280	NR	Sistema Nacional de Implantes/ ACR Mini-Implant	1.5	6/8	NR	6.8	NR
Thiruvenkatachari et al. (2006)[45]	U	18	1/2 (1)	Titanium microimplant	1.3	8	Stability	0.0	NR
Türköz et al. (2010)[46]	U	112	1/2 (1/2)	AbsoAnchor	1.4	7	Stability	22.3	NR
Viwattanatipa et al. (2009)[47]	U	97	2 (2)	Osteomed	1.2	8–12	Mobility/ Dislodgement/ Infection	33.0	NR
Wang et al. (2009)[48]	U	298	2 (2)	Micro-planting nail	1.6	11	Stability/Tx completion	22.8	Excluded
Wiechmann et al. (2007)[49]	NR	133		AbsoAnchor/ Dual-Top	1.2/1.6	5–10	Stability/Tx completion/ Infection	23.3	NR
Wu et al. (2009)[7]	U	414	NR	AbsoAnchor/ LOMAS/A1	1.1–1.7/2	7–13	Stability/Tx completion	10.1	NR
Alves et al. (2011)[50]	U	41	2/3 (2/3)	INP	1.4/2	6/8	NR	14.6	New (in an adjacent location)†
PCS, unclear design[b]									
Baek et al. (2008)[11]	NR	109	1/2 (1/2)	THOplant	2	5	Stability/ Infection/Tx completion	24.8 (Reinstalled MI failures not considered)	New
Bayat & Bauss (2010)[51]	Private	110	1–4 (1/2)	LOMAS	2	7/9/11	Stability/Infection	18.2	NR
Berens et al. (2006)[52]	Private	239	1–3 (1/2)	AbsoAnchor/ Dual-Top	1.4/1.8/2	NR	Stability	15.1	Rescrewed/ Excluded
Chaddad et al. (2008)[53]	NR	32	2/4 (2)	C-Implant/ Dual-Top	1.4–2	6–10	Stability/ Infection/Tx completion	12.5	NR
El-Beialy et al. (2009)[54]	U	40	NR	AbsoAnchor	1.2	8	Stability	17.5	Excluded
Freudenthaler et al. (2001)[55]	NR	15	NR	Leibinger	2	13	Stability/Soft tissue problem	6.7	Excluded/New
Gelgor et al. (2007)[56]	NR	40	1 (1)	IMF	1.8	14	Stability	0.0	NR
Fritz et al. (2004)[57]	U	36	NR	Dual-Top	1.4/1.6/2	6/8/10	Stability	30.6	NR
Kim et al. (2010)[58]	U	197	1 (1)	KLS-Martin/ Orthoplant	1.5/2	5	Stability	9.2	New
Kuroda et al. (2007)[59]	U	216	NR	AbsoAnchor/ Gebrüder Martin	1.3/1.5	6–12	Tx completion	16.2	NR
Lee et al. (2010)[6]	NR	260	2 (2)	C-Implant	1.8	8.5	NR	8.5	NR
Wang et al. (2009)[60]	U	77	NR	MIA system/SDIA system	1.2/2	7/8	NR	7.8	NR

[a]3M Unitek A1, Bio-ray, Syntec Scientific Co, Chang Hua, Taiwan; Aarhus Mini-Implants, Medicon, Germany; AbsoAnchor, Dentos, Daegu, Korea; ACR Mini-Implant, BioMaterials Korea, Guro-gu, Seoul, Korea; C-Implant, Implantium, Seoul, Korea; Dual-Top, Jeil Medical, Seoul, Korea; Gebrüder Martin, Tuttlingen, Germany; IMF, Stryker Leibinger, Germany; INP, São Paulo, Brazil; ISA orthodontic implants, BIODENT, Tokyo, Japan; Jeil Medical, Seoul, Korea; KLS-Martin, Jacksonville, FL, USA; Leibinger, Freiburg, Germany; LOMAS, Mondeal Medical Systems; MIA system, Dentos, Daegu, Korea; Micro-planting nail, North Medical, Ningbo Chi, China; Miniscrew Anchorage System, Titanium Biological Products, Xi'an Bang, China; Mondeal, Tuttlingen, Germany; Ningbo Cibei, Ningbo City, China; Ortho Implant, IMTEC, Ardmore, OK, USA; Ortoimplante Básicos, Conexão, Arujá São Paulo, Brazil; Osteomed, Addison, TX, USA; SDIA system, Zhejiang Cixi Oral Biomaterials, Cixi City, China; Sendax MDI, Irvine, CA, USA; Sin Implant System, São Paulo, Brazil; Sistema Nacional de Implantes, São Paulo, Brazil; SS, Surgical Steel; Stryker Leibinger, Freiburg, Germany; THOplant, Biomaterials Korea, Seoul, South Korea; Tomas-pin, Dentaurum, Ispringen, Germany

[b]Unclear design, judged to be prospective cohort study.

NR, not reported; PCCT, prospective controlled clinical trial; PCS, prospective cohort study; RCT, randomized controlled trial; Tx, treatment; U, university.

Reference	Weight	Risk ratio random, 95% CI
11	19.4%	2.10 (1.10–3.98)
58	11.7%	1.43 (0.57–3.62)
6	12.4%	1.28 (0.52–3.12)
37	3.3%	0.67 (0.10–4.53)
40	8.1%	0.52 (0.16–1.67)
39	3.2%	0.69 (0.10–4.89)
2	13.1%	1.72 (0.73–4.07)
47	13.6%	0.56 (0.24–1.30)
7	15.2%	0.85 (0.39–1.84)
Total (95% CI)	**100.0%**	**1.11 (0.77–1.60)**

Total events

Heterogeneity: Tau^2 = 0.07; Chi^2 = 10.37, df = 8 (p = 0.24); I^2 = 23%
Test for overall effect: Z = 0.57 (p = 0.57)

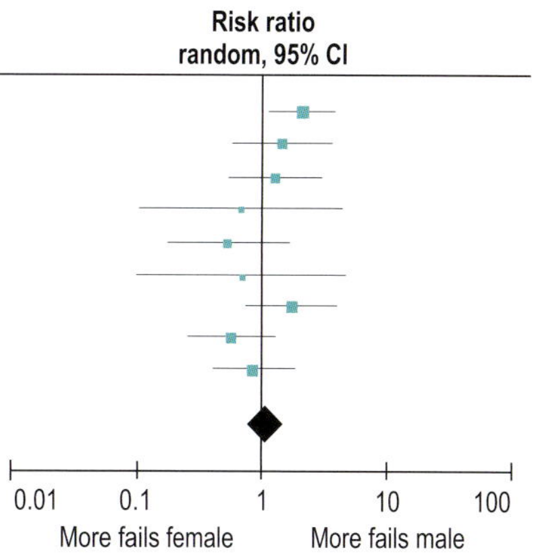

More fails female — More fails male

 A

Reference	Weight	Risk ratio random, 95% CI
11	20.6%	0.86 (0.41–1.66)
58	18.6%	2.13 (0.89–5.10)
6	19.5%	2.84 (1.28–6.27)
39	19.3%	0.32 (0.14–0.72)
7	22.0%	1.55 (0.87–2.77)
Total (95% CI)	**100.0%**	**1.20 (0.59–2.44)**

Total events

Heterogeneity: Tau^2 = 0.51; Chi^2 = 18.40, df = 4 (p = 0.001); I^2 = 78%
Test for overall effect: Z = 0.50 (p = 0.62)

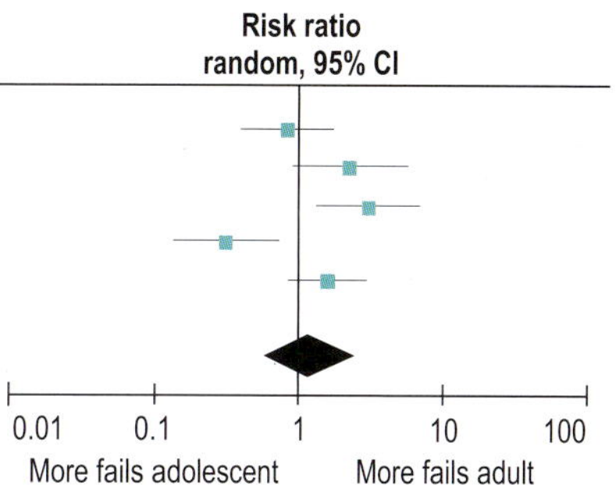

More fails adolescent — More fails adult

B

Reference	Weight	Risk ratio random, 95% CI
11	24.9%	1.04 (0.62–1.75)
6	10.8%	1.06 (0.48–2.37)
37	9.5%	1.00 (0.43–2.35)
40	11.8%	0.71 (0.33–1.52)
38	12.5%	0.72 (0.34–1.50)
39	5.7%	0.78 (0.26–2.36)
2	4.8%	0.20 (0.06–0.67)
47	20.0%	0.79 (0.44–1.41)
Total (95% CI)	**100.0%**	**0.81 (0.62–1.06)**

Total events

Heterogeneity: Tau^2 = 0.00; Chi^2 = 7.17, df = 7 (p = 0.41); I^2 = 2%
Test for overall effect: Z = 1.51 (p = 0.13)

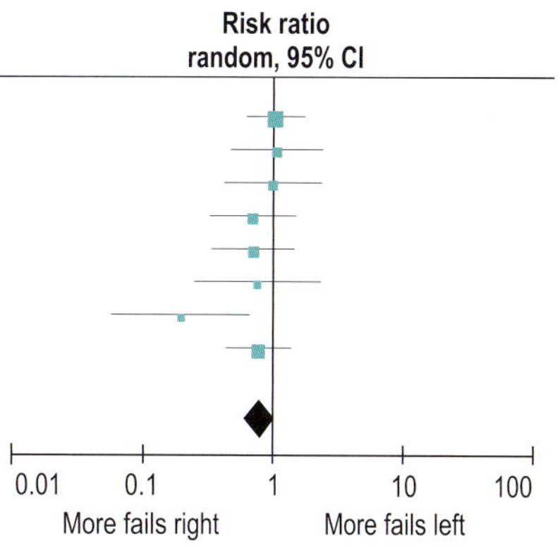

More fails right — More fails left

C

Fig. 49.2 Non-significant findings as risk ratios (Mantel–Haenszel method) of the meta-analyses of miniscrew implant failures supported by numerous studies regarding gender (nine studies; A), age (five studies; B) and side of insertion (eight studies; C). CI, confidence interval.

40.8%. Using the random-effects model, the meta-analysis of all trials yielded an overall failure rate of 13.5% (95% CI, 11.5–15.8), in other words a success rate of 86.5%. Meta-analysis of "large" trials with ≥100 MIs each (including a total of 3385 MIs), yielded an overall failure rate of 14.0% (95% CI, 11.5–17.0). This failure rate is close to another meta-analysis of uncontrolled studies (16.4%),[8] as well as to previous work of the authors on prospective controlled studies (13.3%).[61]

This translates to 14 failed implants per 100 inserted, which is a relatively low rate. In addition, although more than one MI was placed in each patient, it was a rare event for a patient to experience multiple MI failures. Most of the "failed patients" (80.5%) experienced only one loss of MI. Only 12.2% of the patients with MI failure experienced loss of two MIs, 4.9% experienced loss of three MIs, and 2.4% experienced loss of four MIs. However, MI failures can be successfully handled in most cases by reinstalling the MI in the same or adjacent areas without penalty, replacing it with another anchorage-reinforcing device or continuing treatment without it, when a new MI is no longer needed.

RISK FACTORS ASSOCIATED WITH FAILURES

A total of 30 original studies including 4008 MIs in 1827 patients reported two or more MI failure rates in relation to various characteristics and they were compared through subgroup analyses. In many of the comparisons however, a limited number of studies contributed and therefore no reassuring conclusions could be drawn. The non-significant findings (Fig. 49.2), as well as the major significant findings (Fig. 49.3) supported by adequate studies, are also expressed as risk ratios. The observed MI failure rates can be considered in six categories:

- patient related
- clinician related
- characteristics and properties of MIs
- insertion procedure
- type of MI utilization during orthodontic treatment
- treatment outcome related.

Fig. 49.3 Significant findings as risk ratios (Mantel–Haenszel method) of the meta-analyses of miniscrew implant failures regarding jaw (17 studies; A), cortical bone thickness (CBT) (2 studies; B), insertion torque (IT) (2 studies; C) and root contact (4 studies; D). CBT, cortical bone thickness; CI, confidence interval; IT, insertion torque.

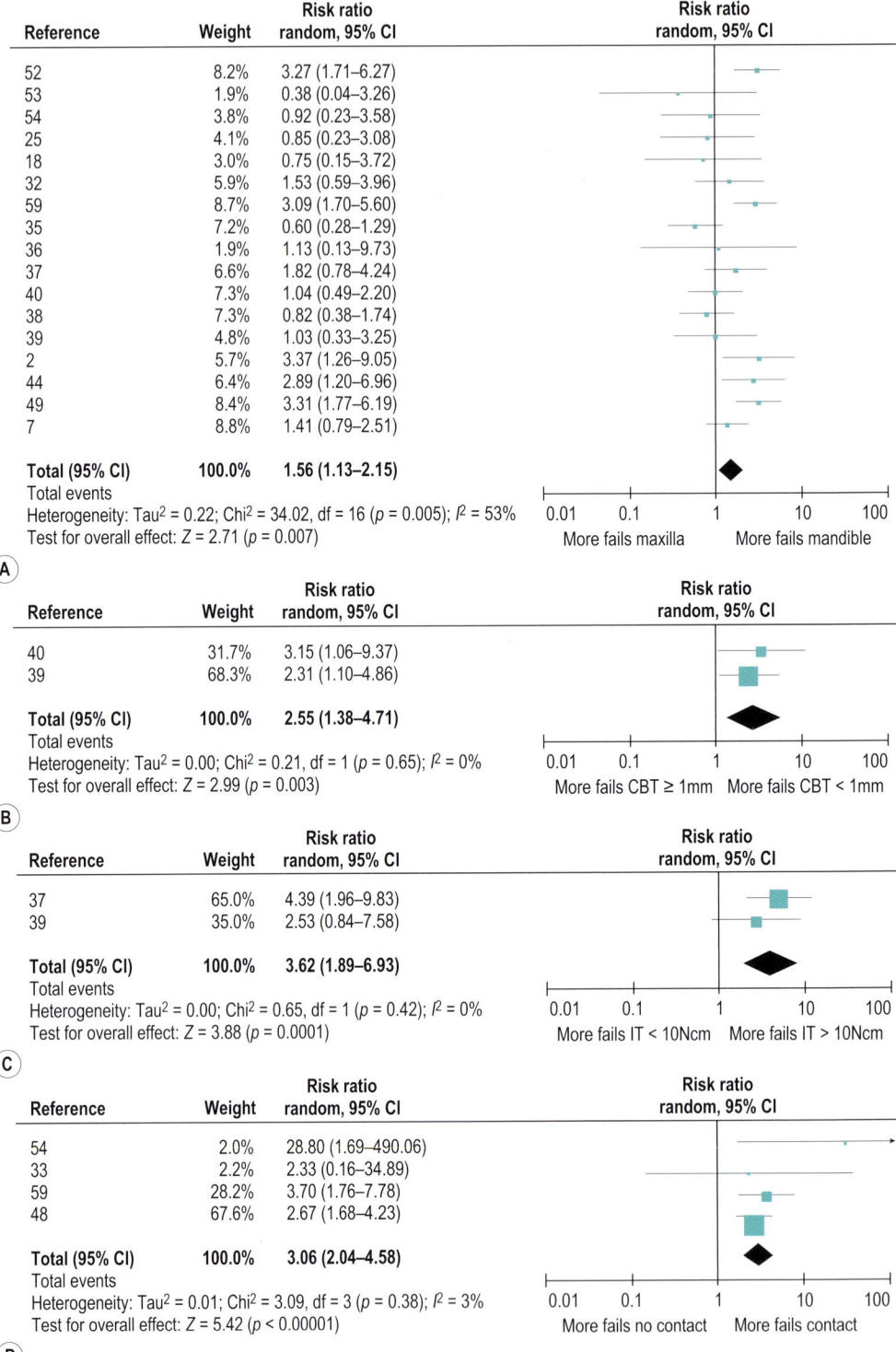

PATIENT-RELATED FACTORS

Patient-related factors that may possibly affect the failures of MIs are outlined in Table 49.2. Within the analysis, there were a sufficient number of studies to provide data on gender and age, while the other factors need additional evidence to support any association.

Gender

Non-significant differences in MI failures related to the patient's gender were observed in the prospective studies included in our analysis,[2,6,7,11,37–40,47,58] which agrees with the results of large retrospective studies[1,3–5,62–64] and a systematic review.[10] Interestingly, most of the studies

had significantly more females. A retrospective study found that males had twice the risk of MI failure compared with females.[65] This may be related to lower cortical bone thickness under the attached gingiva mesial to the maxillary first molar in women.

Age

No evidence for the association of age with MI failure was found in the meta-analysis or in large retrospective studies.[1,3–5,62–64] There is some evidence of a higher risk of failure (multivariate odds ratio, 4.22; $p = 0.016$) in younger patients (<20 years) than older patients (>30 years);[66] however, this retrospective study included miniplates and MIs. A possible

Table 49.2 Summary estimates of miniscrew implant failure rates with patient-related factors

Factor	Studies	Heterogeneity (p value)	Event rate	95% CI	Between subgroups p value
Gender					
Male	9	0.006	13.4	8.4–20.7	0.907
Female	9	<0.001	12.9	8.9–18.5	
Smoking					
Non-smokers	1	1.000	9.6	4.6–18.8	**0.002****
Smokers	1	1.000	35.1	21.6–51.5	
Subgroup smokers					
Light (<10 per day)	1	1.000	11.1	2.8–35.2	**0.007****
Heavy (>10 per day)	1	1.000	57.9	35.6–77.4	
Age					
Adult (>20 years)	5	0.136	15.5	11.2–21.0	0.575
Adolescent (<20 years)	5	<0.001	12.6	6.4–23.3	
Malocclusion					
Class I	2	<0.001	23.4	4.8–65.1	0.191
Class II	2	0.034	17.3	5.1–45.1	
Class III	1	1.000	2.9	0.4–18.1	
Skeletal sagittal: ANB (°)					
<0	1	1.000	11.8	5.4–23.8	**0.002****
0–4	1	1.000	52.2	32.5–71.2	
>4	1	1.000	25.7	14.0–42.5	
Skeletal vertical: FMA (°)					
Low (20)	2	0.117	16.6	8.9–28.3	0.836
Middle (30)	2	0.016	18.3	7.2–39.1	
High (40)	2	0.032	9.3	1.0–51.0	
Skeletal vertical: Sn-GoGn (°)					
Low (28)	1	1.000	10.0	3.3–26.8	0.456
Middle (38)	1	1.000	10.1	6.1–16.4	
High (48)	1	1.000	2.9	0.4–18.1	
Plaque index (%)					
<20	1	1.000	37.9	22.4–56.4	0.187
20–40	1	1.000	44.4	17.7–74.9	
>40	1	1.000	8.3	1.2–41.3	
Gingival index (%)					
<20	1	1.000	36.4	23.6–51.4	**0.037***
20–40	1	1.000	92.9	42.3–99.6	
Oral hygiene					
Good	2	0.872	7.5	5.0–11.1	0.376
Bad	2	0.979	9.8	6.3–14.8	

CI, confidence interval; FMA, FMA, Frankfort-mandibular plane angle.
*$p < 0.05$; **$p < 0.01$.

explanation is a variation in cortical bone thickness of the mandible mesial to the first molars with age.[38]

Smoking

Higher MI failure rates were observed in smokers (35.1%) than in non-smokers (9.6%), as well as in heavy smokers (>10 cigarettes per day; 57.9%) compared with light smokers (<10 cigarettes per day; 11.1%). Lower bone–implant contact and lower peri-implant bone density have been reported in smokers, with marginal bone loss, gap and fibrous tissue around implants.[67] Both wound healing and bone healing are known to be impaired in smokers. Modification of the MI surface could possibly improve outcome in such patients.

Type of Malocclusion

No association was identified with the patient's type of malocclusion according to Angle's classification, which is in agreement with other retrospective studies.[1,5,62,66]

Sagittal Skeletal Relationships

Sagittal skeletal relationships seem to affect MI failures. More specifically, patients with an ANB angle between 0 and 4° (i.e. skeletal Class I skeletal relationships) presented higher MI failure rates (52.2%) than patients with an angle greater than 4° (i.e. skeletal Class III skeletal relationships; 25.7%) or less than 0° (i.e. skeletal Class II skeletal relationships; 11.8%).

Vertical Skeletal Relationships

No linkage between MI failure and vertical skeletal relationships was found for Frankfort–mandibular plane angle or the Sn–mandibular length angle. However, patients with high mandibular plane angle did have four times the failure rate compared with patients with average or low mandibular plane angle in a retrospective study.[3] Data from a retrospective cohort study indicate that dental relationships are important, with higher MI failure rates associated with patients with open bite.[1]

A recent retrospective study included a comprehensive investigation of various skeletal cephalometric variables and their association with MI failures using multiple logistic regression analysis.[5] No significant association was observed for articular angle, mandibular plane to palatal plane angle, mandibular plane angle, gonial angle and lower gonial angle. In contrast, patients with a low Frankfort–mandibular plane angle (<20°) were likely to present approximately a five times higher success rate compared with patients with a high angle (≥30°). In addition, patients with an average upper gonial angle (44–50°) had fewer MI failures (almost double the success rate) than those with an angle below this range.

Crowding

Crowding of teeth (maxillary and mandibular arch length discrepancies of less than 6 mm) was not identified by retrospective studies as a significant risk factor for MI failures.[3,5] Although case reports have described successful treatment of patients with crowding using MI anchorage,[68,69] evidence on influencing factors is scarce.

Physical and Dental Statuses

Health and dental status have been reported in a few studies but none associated them with MI failures. Osteoporosis, uncontrolled diabetes, radiotherapy, reduced mouth opening and various drugs (e.g. bisphosphonates) have been indicated as risk factors for osseointegrated dental implants[2] due to lower bone quality, poor wound healing or proneness to gingival inflammation. However, whether these risk factors may also compromise the outcome of MI-assisted orthodontic therapy remains to be investigated.

Oral Hygiene

Two of the studies in the meta-analysis assessed oral hygiene at MI insertion subjectively,[2,59] but the pooled MI failures did not differ significantly. The one study that reported plaque and gingival indexes at the time of insertion found significantly higher failure rates in patients with increased gingival indexes: indexes between 20 and 40% with a failure rate of 92.9% compared with 36.4% in patients with an index less than 20%.[32] There appears to be no differences between patients verbally instructed to avoid irritating/traumatizing the MI head and those who were not.

The basis for these factors in terms of MI stability and maintenance lies in the crucial role for inflammation control.[3,29,59,63] Prophylactic oral anti-inflammatory drugs have been prescribed for 5 days after the surgical procedure, and the use of single tufted brushes, 0.2% chlorhexidine mouth rinses or dental floss dipped in 2% chlorhexidine have been proposed as useful aids.

Periodontal and Temporomandibular Joint Problems

Periodontal and temporomandibular problems do not seem to affect MI success.[3] Controlled periodontitis and peri-implant inflammation alone seem also not to be predictive of MI failure. MIs have been used successfully in patients with symptoms of temporomandibular disorder.

CLINICIAN-RELATED FACTORS

The number of clinicians who insert the MIs, the clinician's expertise and the operator's learning curve are all potential risk factors (Table 49.3). However, there is little strong evidence evaluating these factors.

Number of Clinicians

The number of clinicians who insert the MIs seems not to be associated with MI failures.[6]

Expertise

Clinician expertise is significantly associated with fewer failures: MI failure rates were 29.2% for postgraduate students and 1.9% for faculty members.

Table 49.3 Summary estimates of miniscrew implant failure rates with clinician-related factors

Factor	Studies	Heterogeneity (p value)	Event rate	95% CI	Between subgroups p value
No. clinicians					
One	1	1.000	8.6	5.3–13.8	0.896
Two	1	1.000	8.1	3.9–16.1	
Clinician					
Professor	1	1.000	1.9	0.3–12.0	0.005**
Postgraduate student	1	1.000	29.2	14.6–49.8	
Learning curve (per 18 MI insertions)					
1st	1	1.000	25.0	13.6–41.5	0.009**
2nd	1	1.000	8.8	4.0–18.3	
3rd	1	1.000	2.1	0.3–13.6	
4th	1	1.000	4.3	1.1–15.8	

MI, miniscrew implant; CI, confidence interval.
**$p < 0.01$.

Operator's Learning Curve

Learning curve of insertion technique is a significant factor, as for every additional group of 18 MIs inserted, the failure rate decreased: a failure rate of 25% was observed for the first 18 MIs, 8.8% for the second ones, 2.1% for the third ones and 4.3% for the fourth ones.[49] A retrospective study also reported lower failure rates after the first 40 MIs.[64] This can be attributed, at least partially, to the lower risk of root contact during predrilling among experienced operators compared to inexperienced ones.

A retrospective analysis of MIs and miniplates indicated that the risk for failure was three times higher when they were placed by an orthodontist than when placed by an oral surgeon.[62]

MINISCREW-RELATED FACTORS

Table 49.4 summarizes the MI-related factors of significance. Thread length, diameter and design were assessed by many studies but the diversity of data collected, and its variation, suggests that additional studies are needed to reach definite conclusions.

Brand

Data concerning failures of MIs of different brands could be pooled from three studies included in the meta-analysis[2,7,49] and indicated no significant differences, which is in agreement with the results of other retrospective studies.[1] However, future studies would benefit from more emphasis on the individual characteristics of each specific MI rather than the manufacturer.

Thread Diameter

Seven studies evaluated the association between MI thread diameter and MI failure rates and showed a non-significant effect.[2,7,50,53,59,60] This is in agreement with some retrospective data,[64] while other data indicate that MIs of increased diameter have a lower risk of failure.[65] One retrospective study reported higher failure rates for MIs with diameters of 1 mm or less,[3] which is smaller than the diameter of MIs used in the included studies.

The actual effect of MI diameter on outcome might be distorted by a small number of implants being used in many different ways and by possible uncontrolled confounding factors. When deciding on the diameter of a MI, it seems important to take into consideration the tipping moment at the bone rim.[70] The clinician must also bear in mind that increasing the MI diameter also raises the risk of root damage during placement, particularly when the MIs are inserted inter-radicularly.[38] MI diameter is closely related to where they can be safely inserted: MIs up to 1.3 mm in diameter can be inserted in several "safe zones" but should be avoided in areas of thick cortical bone; MIs up to 1.5 mm in diameter can be used inter-radicularly; MIs of 2 mm in diameter can only be considered for placement in the posterior inter-radicular spaces of the maxilla between the first molar and the second premolar on the palatal side and between the canine and the first premolar on the palate (median or paramedian).[71] MI diameter appears to be one of the main factors negatively influencing strain development in vitro, but in vivo a significant influence on stability is only seen at high applied forces (2.5 N).[72]

Thread Length

Seven studies showed a non-significant association of thread length with MI failures.[7,18,44,47,50,53,60] A negative correlation between MI thread length and MI failure was reported by two retrospective analyses as a significant effect,[73,74] and another study showed a non-significant trend approaching significance.[66] A possible explanation for these contradictory results might be that MI length may significantly influence MI displacement only when high forces (2.5 N) are applied.[72] There may also be an interaction between diameter and length, whereby a decrease in diameter requires an increase in length for the same stability.

Head Length

No association was found between the length of the MI head and failure rates in the one study that examined this parameter.[55] However, in vitro/in silico studies do indicate that the length of the exposed head is one of the main factors influencing increased strain. This is not surprising as an increased moment of force would increase bending moment at the neck.

Thread Shape

The thread shape was not investigated in any of the prospective cohort studies included in the analysis, but in vitro studies indicate better mechanical stability for dual-threaded MIs than for cylindrical or tapered ones,[75] as well as better mechanical properties for cylindrical MIs compared with conical ones (see Chapter 6). Thread shape, depth and pitch have been reported to influence load both at pitch and at break but this may only be a minor influence on developed strain in cortical bone (shape, 2%; depth, 1%).[76]

Thread Design: Self-drilling or Non-self-drilling

Lower MI failure rates were observed for self-drilling MIs (7.7%) compared with non-self-drilling MIs (17.3%) in pooled data from three studies,[44,46,50] but this was not significant. Although animal studies support these lower failure rates of self-drilling MIs, retrospective analyses have varied in results, with one reporting more than two times more failures for self-drilling MIs compared with non-self-drilling[62] and another detecting no significant differences after adjusting for possible confounders.[64]

A possible explanation for the lower failure rates observed with self-drilling MIs might be that drill-free insertion tends to increase primary stability or it may be that the pilot drilling of the bone needed for non-self-drilling MIs may cause overheating and consequently bone damage.[9]

The temperature of manually inserted self-drilling MIs may affect bone response around the implant: cold MIs (0.7°C) produced a significant increase in cortical bone necrosis when compared with ones at room temperature (22.0°C).[77]

Thread Surface

The preparation of the surface of the MI thread does not appear to alter MI success since no significant differences were found between machined MIs compared to sandblasted and acid-etched MIs in the one study that examined this parameter.[53] A number of studies have indicated that sandblasting and acid etching increase bone–MI contact and consequently osseointegration and removal torques (see Chapter 6).

Other modifications, such as the incorporation of microgrooves on the thread surface, might also be worth investigation.

INSERTION-RELATED FACTORS

A number of factors related to the insertion of MIs are discussed that could possibly affect success (Table 49.5) and these are subdivided into the data for the maxilla and mandible in Table 49.6.

Table 49.4 Summary estimates of miniscrew implant failure rates with miniscrew-related factors

Factor	Studies	Heterogeneity (p value)	Event rate	95% CI	Between subgroups p value
Product					
AbsoAnchor	3	<0.001	16.8	6.4–37.4	0.223
Aarhus	1	1.000	13.0	6.3–24.8	
Osteomed	1	1.000	15.8	5.2–39.2	
LOMAS	2	0.416	5.9	3.3–10.3	
A1	1	1.000	20.0	7.7–42.8	
Microsrew, Mondeal	1	1.000	5.3	0.7–29.4	
C-Implant	1	1.000	8.5	5.6–12.5	
KLS-Martin	1	1.000	20.0	2.7–69.1	
Diameter (mm)					
1.1	1	Meta-regression			0.387
1.2	3				
1.3	2				
1.4	3				
1.5	2				
1.6	1				
1.7	1				
1.8	1				
2	6				
Diameter category (mm)					
1.1–1.3	4	0.042	10.9	7.7–15.3	0.729
1.4–1.6	5	0.796	12.7	8.1–19.3	
1.7+	6	0.013	14.3	7.4–25.8	
Thread length (mm)					
6	3	Meta-regression			0.183
7	2				
8	6				
8.5	1				
9	1				
10	3				
11	2				
12	2				
13	1				
14	1				
15	1				
Thread length category (mm)					
5–8	11	0.101	12.3	8.3–17.9	0.281
8.5–12	9	<0.001	20.1	10.8–34.3	
13–15	3	0.561	7.8	1.9–26.7	
Head length (mm)					
4.5	1	1.000	8.3	1.2–41.3	0.806
2.5	1	1.000	12.5	0.7–73.4	
Thread design					
Self-drilling	3	0.824	7.7	4.8–12.0	0.210
Not-self-drilling	3	<0.001	17.3	5.1–44.9	
Thread surface					
Machined	1	1.000	17.6	5.8–42.7	0.366
Sandblasted & acid-etched	1	1.000	6.7	0.9–35.2	

CI, confidence interval.

Table 49.5 Summary estimates of miniscrew implant failure rates with insertion-related factors

Factor	Studies	Heterogeneity (p value)	Event rate	95% CI	Between subgroups p value
Cortical notching					
No	3	0.734	6.8	4.1–11.1	0.154
Yes	3	<0.001	13.7	5.9–28.4	
Flap					
No	1	1.000	51.3	36.0–66.4	0.037*
Yes	1	1.000	4.5	0.3–44.8	
Insertion torque (Ncm)					
<10	2	0.925	8.8	5.3–14.2	0.004**
>10	2	0.172	29.9	15.5–49.7	
Insertion angle (°)					
10–20	1	1.000	9.0	4.1–18.5	0.113
30–40	1	1.000	4.8	2.0–10.9	
90	1	1.000	14.8	7.6–26.9	
Screw head exposed					
No	2	<0.001	21.2	1.3–84.8	0.696
Yes	2	0.849	12.8	8.3–19.1	
Cortical bone thickness (mm)					
≥1	2	0.892	8.3	5.3–12.8	0.003**
<1	2	0.592	21.3	13.7–31.7	
Jaw					
Maxilla	17	0.014	12.0	9.6–14.9	0.012*
Mandible	17	<0.001	19.3	14.3–25.6	
Side					
Left	8	<0.001	13.2	7.9–21.3	0.382
Right	8	<0.001	17.4	11.9–24.6	
Region					
Posterior	2	<0.001	16.1	4.7–42.6	0.771
Anterior	2	0.680	22.0	2.9–72.6	
Soft tissue					
Keratinized	3	0.459	12.5	7.0–21.5	0.450
Non-keratinized	3	<0.001	21.6	5.5–56.7	
Site					
Inter-radicular	5	0.268	10.9	8.3–14.0	0.412
Palate	5	0.108	15.6	6.6–32.7	
Palate subgroup					
Midpalatal	4	0.113	16.8	6.6–36.7	0.135
Para-palatal	1	1.000	7.5	4.4–12.5	
Inter-radicular subgroup					
Teeth: P2M1	1	1.000	23.3	15.0–34.3	0.553
Teeth: M1M2	1	1.000	28.6	16.1–45.4	
Root contact					
Yes	4	0.102	29.9	21.0–40.7	<0.001***
No	4	0.122	7.8	3.9–15.0	

CI, confidence interval; P2M1, between the second premolar and the first molar; M1M2, between the first and second molar.
*$p < 0.05$; **$p < 0.01$; ***$p < 0.001$.

Notching of the Cortical Bone

Three prospective studies[7,44,46] examined notching of cortical bone prior to MI insertion and found no significant association. Another retrospective study also showed no difference when MIs were inserted with a reduction handpiece or a normal handpiece or whether cooling was used for notching of the cortical bone.[65]

Use of Flap Surgery

Insertion of MIs following flap surgery was associated with lower MI failure rates.[31] More specifically, higher MI failure rates were observed in flapless insertion of the MIs (51.3%) compared with flap deflection (4.5%). Other studies found no difference between MI insertion without flap or incision and insertion by making a

Table 49.6 Summary estimates of miniscrew implant failure rates with insertion-related factors, stratified by jaw

Factor	Studies	Heterogeneity (p value)	Event rate	95% CI	Between subgroups p value
Maxilla					
Side					
Left	4	0.035	15.8	7.4–30.7	0.307
Right	4	0.035	20.1	12.6–30.4	
Region					
Posterior	2	0.459	23.7	9.7–47.4	**0.006****
Anterior	1	1.000	4.2	1.7–9.6	
Soft tissue					
Keratinized	1	1.000	8.8	2.9–24.0	0.635
Non-keratinized	1	1.000	6.4	2.9–13.5	
Cortical bone thickness (mm)					
≥1	1	1.000	3.0	0.4–18.6	**0.031***
<1	1	1.000	26.1	12.2–47.2	
Site 1					
Alveolar process	4	0.069	12.0	7.0–19.9	0.924
Palate	4	0.027	11.1	2.3–39.8	
Site 2					
Midpalatal	2	0.017	6.6	0.2–73.3	0.948
Inter-radicular	2	0.538	7.4	4.5–11.8	
Inter-radicular subgroup 1					
Buccal	2	0.802	9.7	4.4–20.0	0.107
Palatal	2	0.381	21.1	11.5–35.4	
Inter-radicular subgroup 1					
Teeth: P1P2	1	1.000	6.3	0.4–53.9	0.357
Teeth: P2M1	2	0.187	18.7	9.3–34.0	
Teeth: M1M2	1	1.000	28.6	16.1–45.4	
Mandible					
Side					
Left	3	0.516	15.9	9.0–26.5	0.935
Right	3	0.899	15.4	8.7–25.7	
Region					
Posterior	3	<0.001	18.8	7.4–40.3	0.679
Anterior	3	0.837	23.7	11.4–42.9	
Site 1					
Symphysis	1	1.000	23.5	9.1–48.6	0.271
Retromolar	1	1.000	20.0	5.0–54.1	
Inter-radicular	1	1.000	9.7	4.7–19.0	
Inter-radicular subgroup 1					
Buccal	2	0.905	9.1	3.0–24.7	**<0.001*****
Lingual	1	1.000	73.3	46.7–89.6	
Inter-radicular subgroup 2					
Teeth: P1P2	1	1.000	5.6	0.3–50.5	0.565
Teeth: P2M1	1	1.000	16.7	1.0–80.6	

CI, confidence interval; SG, Subgroup; P1P2, between the first and second premolar; P2M1, between the second premolar and the first molar; M1M2, between the first and second molar.
*$p < 0.05$; **$p < 0.01$; ***$p < 0.001$.

cross-shaped incision and reflecting a flap.[3-5] However, the latter was associated with higher patient discomfort and is not preferred by patients.[3] Although flapless insertion is simple enough and can be easily done by the orthodontist, sometimes flap deflection is still needed in order to achieve the precise location and the prescribed angle during MI insertion.[31]

Dimension of Pilot Hole

Pilot hole diameter was not assessed by any prospective studies included in our analysis. However, one study found that the larger the diameter of the pilot hole in relation to the diameter of the MI the lower the primary stability of the MI, but the smaller the pilot hole in relation to the MI diameter, the more likely was implant fracture.[78] It was suggested that MIs of 2.0 mm in diameter inserted into dense compact bone should have a pilot hole of 1.3 mm.

Insertion Torque

Insertion torque was positively associated with MI failure rates in pooled data from two studies.[37,39] More specifically, higher MI failure rates were observed when insertion torque exceeded 10 Ncm (29.9%), compared with 8.8% with smaller torque values. As high levels of stress could cause necrosis and local ischemia of the surrounding bone, specific values of insertion torque have been proposed.[37–39]

Angle of Insertion

The angle of MI insertion was not associated with MI failure in our analysis. A cohort study identified the angle of MI insertion as a secondary risk factor, with higher angles associated with less oral trauma,[79] which can be attributed to the reduced retention of obliquely inserted MIs. Other studies have supported an insertion angle of 60–70° in order to increase insertion torque and primary stability.[80] In some locations, the insertion angle is predetermined (e.g. at the infrazygomatic crest where a steeper angle is required) but, in general, placing MIs at an obtuse angle may lower the risk of root damage and increase contact with cortical bone.

Exposure of Miniscrew Implant Head

Whether the head of the MIs was exposed to the oral environment does not seem to affect failure rates.

Cortical Bone Thickness

Cortical bone thickness seems to be important for the success of MIs, with a cortex zone of 1 mm being the limit. Data from the meta-analysis indicate that higher failure rates (2.5 times more failures) were observed at insertion sites with a cortical bone thickness less than 1 mm (21.3%; 8.3% for ≥1 mm). One numerical analysis indicated that higher cortical bone thickness was associated with less deflection of the MI,[81] while another indicated that a cortical bone thickness of less than 2 mm led to increased stresses that could possibly cause resorption of the cancellous bone.[82] Since the risk of overheating is higher when drilling sites of dense cortex, continuous saline irrigation must be used to avoid necrosis.

Jaw of Placement

There are significant differences between the maxilla and the mandible for MI failure rates in pooled data from 17 studies.[2,7,18,25,32,35–37,39,40,44,49,52–54,59] More specifically, in our investigation higher overall MI failure rates were observed in the mandible (19.3%) than the maxilla (12.0%). This is in agreement with some retrospective studies (two times more failures for mandibular MIs),[65,66] while other retrospective studies and animal studies report non-significant differences.[1,4,64] The higher MI failure rates observed for the MIs inserted in the mandible can be attributed to higher bone density, which can lead to higher insertion torque value and bone overheating during insertion; less cortical bone at the upper part of the MI in the mandible; and/or a narrower vestibule, which makes thorough cleaning harder.

Overall failure comparisons between the two jaws are of no great clinical significance to the orthodontist. The reported failure rates were also stratified separately by the jaw of insertion (Table 49.6) in order to facilitate clinical decision making.

PLACEMENT IN THE MAXILLA

No significant difference was observed in the MI failure rate with the side of insertion, type of soft tissue (keratinized or non-keratinized) or the site of insertion (alveolar process or palate; midpalatal or inter-radicular; buccal or palatal; between the first and second premolars, the second premolars and first molars and the first and second molars). However, significantly higher failure rates were observed for MIs inserted in the posterior region of the maxilla (23.7%) compared with the anterior region (4.2%), as well as for a cortical bone thickness of less than 1 mm (26.1%) compared with 1 mm or more (3.0%).

PLACEMENT IN THE MANDIBLE

No significant difference was observed in the MI failure rate with the side of insertion, the region of insertion (anterior or posterior) or the site of insertion (symphysis, retromolar or inter-radicular; between the first and second premolars or between the second premolars and first molars). The only exception was the higher failure rates observed for inter-radicular MIs inserted lingually (73.3%) compared with buccally (9.1%). Some studies have shown differentials in failures rates: slightly more failures in the posterior region of the mandible;[29] higher failure rates for placement between the mandibular second premolars and first molars compared with between first and second premolars;[4] highest failure rates (30.9%) between the mandibular first and second molars and lowest between the mandibular first and second premolars (11.0%);[4] higher failure rates for buccal placement in the molar area than in the premolar area;[4] and higher failure rates in the right side of the mandible between the first and second molars compared with all other sites of both jaws.[1] By comparison, one retrospective study found no significant associations of MI failure with the site (buccal, lingual or crest) or the inter-radicular area of insertion after adjusting for possible confounding factors.[66]

Side of Placement

No differences were observed in MI failure rate according to side of placement in the eight studies examining this (when pooling data from both jaws).[2,6,11,37–40,47] This agrees with the findings of other studies,[1,4,5,65] although, where studies have found differences, these have been explained by various factors such as unilateral preference for mastication, unequal level of oral hygiene among left- and right-handed patients or random statistical error.

Region of Placement

Region of MI placement (posterior or anterior) was not associated with MI failures when pooling the data from MIs inserted in both the maxilla and mandible,[2,32] which is in agreement with the findings of retrospective studies.[62,65]

Soft Tissues

Keratinized gingiva is regarded by many clinicians as presenting a lower risk of developing hypertrophic tissues and inflammation, with the oral mucosa having the highest risk around MIs. However, the current meta-analysis found no significant differences in MI failure rates when the MIs were placed in areas covered by keratinized (attached) gingiva or in areas of oral mucosa, which is in agreement with one retrospective study.[64] Other studies have found lower failure rates for MIs placed in attached gingiva of the maxilla than in all other keratinized or non-keratinized tissues.[1,29,65] Full coverage of the MIs with oral mucosa has been proposed for MIs

Table 49.7 Summary estimates of miniscrew implant failure rates with treatment-related factors

Factor	Studies	Heterogeneity (p value)	Event rate	95% CI	Between subgroups p value
Two MIs splinted					
Yes	1	1.000	4.1	1.7–9.4	0.003**
No	1	1.000	17.6	10.5–27.9	
Loading time					
Early (up to 2 weeks)	3	0.125	26.8	16.4–40.6	0.304
Delayed (after 2 weeks)	3	0.073	15.6	5.6–36.7	
Tooth movement					
Intrusion	1	1.000	11.1	4.2–26.1	0.826
Distalization	1	1.000	7.3	2.8–17.8	
Mesialization	1	1.000	10.0	1.4–46.7	
En masse retraction	1	1.000	11.3	5.7–20.9	
Combination	1	1.000	4.0	0.6–23.5	
Treatment duration					
<6 months	1	1.000	27.3	9.0–58.6	0.046*
>6 months	1	1.000	8.1	4.9–12.9	

MI, miniscrew implant; CI, confidence interval.
$*p < 0.05$; $**p < 0.01$.

placed in non-keratinized tissues, with wires or attachments passing through the mucosa.[2]

Root Contact

Root contact was associated with more MI failures in all four studies included in the meta-analysis, yielding a significant association.[33,54,59,48] More specifically, root contact during insertion increased failure rates to 29.9%, from 7.8% for no root contact ($p < 0.001$). The rate and pattern of root contact have been reported to be associated with surgery site and operator experience.[83] Root contact produces increased stresses and inflammation, which could affect MI stability.[82] There is evidence that damaged root is finally repaired after MI removal with a narrow zone of mineralized tissue.[84] Successful restoration of the damaged roots has been reported using surgical treatment and mineral trioxide aggregate.[85]

TREATMENT-RELATED FACTORS

Treatment-related factors are discussed below and summarized in Table 49.7.

Use of Splinted Miniscrew Implants

The use of two splinted MIs reduced failure rates (4.1%) compared with a single MI (17.6%). Various types of connections have been investigated in vitro.[86]

Loading of Orthodontic Forces

Application of orthodontic forces to MIs can be immediate, early (during the first 2 weeks) or delayed (later than 2 weeks). Three studies in the meta-analysis considered this[25,32,38] and indicated that delayed loading presented lower failures, but this was not statistically significant. Other studies have reported both an advantage from immediate loading[65] and a disadvantage.[62,87] Differences may reflect the type of bone used for the insertion,

with dense mature bone responding better to immediate loading. Premature loading leads to healing characterized histologically by formation of fibrous tissue between the bone and the MI (see Chapter 4).

Differences between loaded and unloaded MIs are considered to be of no clinical relevance.

Magnitude of Orthodontic Forces

No comparison was possible concerning MI failure rates and the magnitude of orthodontic forces applied to the MIs, since no such data were included in the studies of our analysis. However, a retrospective study found no difference for applied forces of 150 g and 250 g.[65] Significant MI displacements have been reported after applying immediate forces of 400 g[34] and in vitro data indicate that MI length and diameter significantly influence MI stability, but only when the applied forces exceeded 1 N.[72] Both very low and very high strains can induce bone resorption and a negative bone-remodeling balance.[88]

Method of Force Application

No correlation was found with the method of force application (e.g. power chains, super threads, Ni-Ti coil springs and ligature tiebacks) or force direction and MI failure, which agrees with previous data.[2] Torsional stress has been proposed as a significant factor, and some investigators recommend avoiding lateral, torsional and extrusive orthodontic forces, if possible.[29]

Type of Anchorage

No comparison of type of anchorage provided by the MIs (direct or indirect) could be made in the meta-analysis. One retrospective study showed no significant differences between direct and indirect anchorage,[1] while another found indirectly loaded MIs to be successful but with a slight anchorage loss observed in terms of maxillary incisor proclination and increased overjet at the end of movement.[30]

Table 49.8 Summary estimates of miniscrew implant failure rates with outcome-related factors

Factor	Studies	Heterogeneity (p value)	Event rate	95% CI	Between subgroups p value
Inflammation					
Yes	2	<0.001	48.7	3.4–96.2	0.260
No	2	0.001	10.3	2.2–36.9	
Mobility					
Yes	1	1.000	24.4	14.1–39.0	<0.001***
No	1	1.000	1.4	0.4–5.6	
Unclear	1	1.000	14.0	6.4–27.8	
MI reinstallation					
No	1	1.000	24.8	17.6–33.7	0.130
Yes	1	1.000	38.2	23.7–55.3	
MI reinstallation site					
Same	1	1.000	31.6	14.9–54.8	0.371
Adjacent	1	1.000	46.7	24.1–70.7	

MI, miniscrew implant; CI, confidence interval.
***p < 0.001.

Type of Orthodontic Tooth Movement

Several prospective studies reported failure rates of MIs during dental movements but few investigated any possible association.[6,11,37,38,44,46,48] Utilization of MIs for different types of tooth movement does not seem to be accompanied by different failure rates,[58] but en masse distalization of teeth had the lowest failure rate (1.9%) and intrusion of molars the highest (11.4%) in one study.[1] Other studies have shown higher (5.3 times) risk of failure for anchors (miniplates and MIs) used for uprighting compared with intrusion[62] and a two times higher risk of failure for retraction/protraction compared with intrusion.[66] One study found intrusion more problematic than retraction.[63]

It is clear that additional evidence is needed to clarify any association of MI failure with the type of orthodontic tooth movement.

Duration of Treatment

Higher MI failure rates were observed when treatment with MIs lasted less than 6 months (27.3%) compared with longer treatment (8.1%). After the first 6 months of treatment, anchorage loss appears to be statistically insignificant.[61] This may be because of osseointegration, but often studies do not consider a MI successful until after a minimum of 6 months of force application, and therefore a certain degree of confounding might be present.

OUTCOME-RELATED FACTORS

Outcome-related factors are summarized in Table 49.8.

Inflammation of the Peri-implant Soft Tissues

The association of inflammation with higher MI failure rates did not reach statistical significance in pooled data from two studies included in the meta-analysis.[2,47] A retrospective cohort study of MIs and miniplates[3,62] showed that, after adjusting for confounding factors, mild inflammation was associated with almost seven times more MI failures and severe inflammation with almost 36 times more failures.[47]

Mobility of Miniscrew Implants

Only one study in the meta-analysis assessed MI mobility.[2] Higher failure rates were observed for MIs that showed clinical mobility (24.4%) or unclear mobility (due to overlying soft tissues) (14.0%) compared with those that were clinically stable (1.4%). Data from animal studies indicate that MI mobility seems to be negatively associated with insertion torque and positively correlated with bone mineral density and thickness of the cortical bone,[89] but a study in rats showed that a significant decrease in mobility after 3 weeks was linked to a good prognosis for subsequent stability.[90]

Reinstallation of Miniscrew Implant

No failure penalty was observed for failed MIs that were reinstalled either at the same site or at adjacent sites in the only relevant study that was included in our analysis.[11]

CONCLUSIONS

Orthodontic MIs have a modest mean failure rate of 13.5% (or in other words a mean success rate of 86.5%), indicating their usefulness in clinical practice. Among the potential risk factors for MI failure, there is substantial evidence that patient gender and age and side of insertion were not associated with failures. In contrast, jaw of insertion and root contact seem to influence MI failures. More specifically, MI failure may be influenced by smoking, oral hygiene, skeletal sagittal relationships, clinician expertise and learning curve, cortical bone thickness, flap deflection, insertion torque values, some insertion sites, root contact, splinting of MIs, treatment duration and MI mobility. Taking these factors into consideration during treatment can lower MI failure rates to below 10%. Nevertheless, the limited number of studies in many categories can possibly provide a biased estimate or even fail to identify a significant effect that is present.

Large-scale prospective randomized or non-randomized studies under controlled conditions could further enrich our knowledge and enhance the outcome of MIs used in orthodontic treatment.

REFERENCES

1. Antoszewska J, Papadopoulos MA, Park HS, et al. Five-year experience with orthodontic miniscrew implants: a retrospective investigation of factors influencing success rates. Am J Orthod Dentofacial Orthop 2009;136:158.

2. Park HS, Jeong SH, Kwon OW. Factors affecting the clinical success of screw implants used as orthodontic anchorage. Am J Orthod Dentofacial Orthop 2006; 130:18–25.

3. Miyawaki S, Koyama I, Inoue M, et al. Factors associated with the stability of titanium screws placed in the posterior region for orthodontic anchorage. Am J Orthod Dentofacial Orthop 2003;124:373–8.

4. Moon CH, Lee DG, Lee HS, et al. Factors associated with the success rate of orthodontic miniscrews placed in the upper and lower posterior buccal region. Angle Orthod 2008;78:101–6.

5. Moon CH, Park HK, Nam JS, et al. Relationship between vertical skeletal pattern and success rate of orthodontic mini-implants. Am J Orthod Dentofacial Orthop 2010;138:51–7.

6. Lee SJ, Ahn SJ, Lee JW, et al. Survival analysis of orthodontic mini-implants. Am J Orthod Dentofacial Orthop 2010;137:194–9.

7. Wu TY, Kuang SH, Wu CH. Factors associated with the stability of mini-implants for orthodontic anchorage: a study of 414 samples in Taiwan. J Oral Maxillofac Surg 2009;67:1595–9.

8. Schätzle M, Männchen R, Zwahlen M, et al. Survival and failure rates of orthodontic temporary anchorage devices: a systematic review. Clin Oral Implants Res 2009;20:1351–9.

9. Chen Y, Kyung HM, Zhao WT, et al. Critical factors for the success of orthodontic mini-implants: a systematic review. Am J Orthod Dentofacial Orthop 2009;135:284–91.

10. Crismani AG, Bertl MH, Celar AG, et al. Miniscrews in orthodontic treatment: review and analysis of published clinical trials. Am J Orthod Dentofacial Orthop 2010;137:108–13.

11. Baek SH, Kim BM, Kyung SH, et al. Success rate and risk factors associated with mini-implants reinstalled in the maxilla. Angle Orthod 2008;78:895–901.

12. Papageorgiou SN, Zogakis IP, Papadopoulos MA. Failure rates and associated risk factors of orthodontic miniscrew implants: a meta-analysis. Am J Orthod Dentofacial Orthop 2012;142:577–95.

13. Basha AG, Shantaraj R, Mogegowda SB. Comparative study between conventional en-masse retraction (sliding mechanics) and en-masse retraction using orthodontic micro implant. Implant Dent 2010;19:128–36.

14. Liu Y, Ding W, Liu J, et al. Comparison of the differences in cephalometric parameters after active orthodontic treatment applying mini-screw implants or transpalatal arches in adult patients with bialveolar dental protrusion. J Oral Rehabil 2009;36:687–95.

15. Upadhyay M, Yadav S, Nagaraj K, et al. Treatment effects of mini-implants for en-masse retraction of anterior teeth in bialveolar dental protrusion patients: a randomized controlled trial. Am J Orthod Dentofacial Orthop 2008;134:18–29.

16. Aboul-Ela SM. Miniscrew implant-supported maxillary canine retraction with and without corticotomy-facilitated orthodontics. Am J Orthod Dentofacial Orthop 2011;139:252–9.

17. Lehnen S, McDonald F, Bourauel C, et al. Expectations, acceptance and preferences of patients in treatment with orthodontic mini-implants. J Orofac Orthop 2011;72:214–22.

18. Hedayati Z, Hashemi S, Zamiri B, et al. Anchorage value of surgical titanium screws in orthodontic tooth movement. Int J Oral Maxillofac Surg 2007;36:588–92.

19. Maddalone M, Ferrari M, Barrilà S, et al. [Intrusive mechanics in orthodontics by the use of TADs.]. Dent Cadmos 2010;78:97–106.

20. Park H, Yoon DY, Park C, et al. Treatment effects and anchorage potential of sliding mechanics with titanium screws compared with the Tweed–Merrifield technique. Am J Orthod Dentofacial Orthop 2008;133:593–600.

21. Shi YT, Ping Y, Shan LH, et al. [Stability of mini-implant during orthodontic treatment as anchorage.]. J Clin Rehabil Tissue Eng Res 2008;12:5109–12.

22. Upadhyay M, Yadav S, Patil S. Mini-implant anchorage for en-masse retraction of maxillary anterior teeth: a clinical cephalometric study. Am J Orthod Dentofacial Orthop 2008;134:803–10.

23. Wilmes B, Olthoff G, Drescher D. Comparison of skeletal and conventional anchorage methods in conjunction with pre-operative decompensation of a skeletal Class III malocclusion. J Orofac Orthop 2009;70:297–305.

24. Apel S, Apel C, Morea C, et al. Microflora associated with successful and failed orthodontic mini-implants. Clin Oral Implants Res 2009;20:1186–90.

25. Garfinkle JS, Cunningham LL Jr, Beeman CS, et al. Evaluation of orthodontic mini-implant anchorage in premolar extraction therapy in adolescents. Am J Orthod Dentofacial Orthop 2008;133:642–53.

26. Upadhyay M, Yadav S, Nagaraj K, et al. Dentoskeletal and soft tissue effects of mini-implants in Class II, division 1 patients. Angle Orthod 2009;79:240–7.

27. Blaya MG, Blaya DS, Guimarães MB, et al. [Patient's perception on mini-screws used for molar distalization.]. Rev Odonto Cienc 2010;25:266–70.

28. Brandão LBC, Mucha JN. [The mini-implants acceptance rate by patients in orthodontic treatments: a preliminary study.]. Rev Dent Press Ortodon Ortopedi Facial 2008;13:118–27.

29. Cheng SJ, Tseng IY, Lee JJ, et al. A prospective study of the risk factors associated with failure of mini-implants used for orthodontic anchorage. Int J Oral Maxillofac Implants 2004;19:100–6.

30. Gelgor IE, Buyukyilmaz T, Karaman AI, et al. Intraosseous screw-supported upper molar distalization. Angle Orthod 2004;74:838–50.

31. Herman RJ, Currier GF, Miyake A. Mini-implant anchorage for maxillary canine retraction: a pilot study. Am J Orthod Dentofacial Orthop 2006;130:228–35.

32. Justens E, de Bruyn H. Clinical outcome of mini-screws used as orthodontic anchorage. Clin Implant Dent Relat Res 2008;10:174–80.

33. Kim SH, Kang SM, Choi YS, et al. Cone-beam computed tomography evaluation of mini-implants after placement: is root proximity a major risk factor for failure? Am J Orthod Dentofacial Orthop 2010;138:264–76.

34. Liou EJW, Pai BCJ, Lin JCY. Do miniscrews remain stationary under orthodontic forces? Am J Orthod Dentofacial Orthop 2004;126:42–7.

35. Luzi C, Verna C, Melsen B. A prospective clinical investigation of the failure rate of immediately loaded mini-implants used for orthodontic anchorage. Prog Orthod 2007;8:192–201.

36. Miyazawa K, Kawaguchi M, Tabuchi M, et al. Accurate pre-surgical determination for self-drilling miniscrew implant placement using surgical guides and cone-beam computed tomography. Eur J Orthod 2010;32:735–40.

37. Motoyoshi M, Hirabayashi M, Uemura M, et al. Recommended placement torque when tightening an orthodontic mini-implant. Clin Oral Implants Res 2006;17: 109–14.

38. Motoyoshi M, Matsuoka M, Shimizu N. Application of orthodontic mini-implants in adolescents. Int J Oral Maxillofac Surg 2007;36:695–9.

39. Motoyoshi M, Yoshida T, Ono A, et al. Effect of cortical bone thickness and implant placement torque on stability of orthodontic mini-implants. Int J Oral Maxillofac Implants 2007;22:779–84.

40. Motoyoshi M, Inaba M, Ono A, et al. The effect of cortical bone thickness on the stability of orthodontic mini-implants and on the stress distribution in surrounding bone. Int J Oral Maxillofac Surg 2009;38:13–18.

41. Motoyoshi M, Uemura M, Ono A, et al. Factors affecting the long-term stability of orthodontic mini-implants. Am J Orthod Dentofacial Orthop 2010;137:588.

42. Oh YH, Park HS, Kwon TG. Treatment effects of microimplant-aided sliding mechanics on distal retraction of posterior teeth. Am J Orthod Dentofacial Orthop 2011;139: 470–81.

43. Polat-Ozsoy O, Arman-Ozcirpici A, Veziroglu F. Miniscrews for upper incisor intrusion. Eur J Orthod 2009;31:412–16.

44. Suzuki EY, Suzuki B. Placement and removal torque values of orthodontic miniscrew implants. Am J Orthod Dentofacial Orthop 2011;139:669–78.

45. Thiruvenkatachari B, Pavithranand A, Rajasigamani K, et al. Comparison and measurement of the amount of anchorage loss of the molars with and without the use of implant anchorage during canine retraction. Am J Orthod Dentofacial Orthop 2006;129:551–4.

46. Türköz C, Atac MS, Tuncer C, et al. The effect of drill-free and drilling methods on the stability of mini-implants under early orthodontic loading in adolescent patients. Eur J Orthod 2011;33:533–6.

47. Viwattanatipa N, Thanakitcharu S, Uttraravichien A, et al. Survival analyses of surgical miniscrews as orthodontic anchorage. Am J Orthod Dentofacial Orthop 2009;136:29–36.

48. Wang HN, Liu DX, Wang CL, et al. [Influence of periodontal ligament injury on initial stability for immediately loaded mini-implant.]. Hua Xi Kou Qiang Yi Xue Za Zhi 2009;27:224–6, 236.

49. Wiechmann D, Meyer U, Büchter A. Success rate of mini- and micro-implants used for orthodontic anchorage: a prospective clinical study. Clin Oral Implants Res 2007;18:263–7.

50. Alves M Jr, Baratieri C, Nojima LI. Assessment of mini-implant displacement using cone beam computed tomography. Clin Oral Implants Res 2011;22:1151–6.

51. Bayat E, Bauss O. Effect of smoking on the failure rates of orthodontic miniscrews. J Orofac Orthop 2010;71:117–24.

52. Berens A, Wiechmann D, Dempf R. Mini- and micro-screws for temporary skeletal anchorage in orthodontic therapy. J Orofac Orthop 2006;67:450–8.

53. Chaddad K, Ferreira AFH, Geurs N, et al. Influence of surface characteristics on survival rates of mini-implants. Angle Orthod 2008;78:107–13.

54. El-Beialy AR, Abou-El-Ezz AM, Attia KH, et al. Loss of anchorage of miniscrews: a 3-dimensional assessment. Am J Orthod Dentofacial Orthop 2009;136:700–7.

55. Freudenthaler JW, Bantleon HP, Haas R. Bicortical titanium screws for critical orthodontic anchorage in the mandible: a preliminary report on clinical applications. Clin Oral Implants Res 2001;12:358–63.

56. Gelgor IE, Karaman AI, Buyukyilmaz T. Comparison of 2 distalization systems supported by intraosseous screws. Am J Orthod Dentofacial Orthop 2007;131:161.

57. Fritz U, Ehmer A, Diedrich P. Clinical suitability of titanium microscrews for orthodontic anchorage: preliminary experiences. J Orofac Orthop 2004;65:410–18.

58. Kim YH, Yang SM, Kim S, et al. Midpalatal miniscrews for orthodontic anchorage: factors affecting clinical success. Am J Orthod Dentofacial Orthop 2010;137: 66–72.

59. Kuroda S, Yamada K, Deguchi T, et al. Root proximity is a major factor for screw failure in orthodontic anchorage. Am J Orthod Dentofacial Orthop 2007; 131(Suppl.):68–73.

60. Wang ZD, Li QY, Wang L, et al. [Comparative evaluation of two kinds of microimplant system with different sizes.]. Hua Xi Kou Qiang Yi Xue Za Zhi 2009;27: 150–3.

61. Papadopoulos MA, Papageorgiou SN, Zogakis IP. Clinical effectiveness of orthodontic miniscrew implants. J Dent Res 2011;90:969–76.

62. Chen YJ, Chang HH, Lin HY, et al. Stability of miniplates and miniscrews used for orthodontic anchorage: experience with 492 temporary anchorage devices. Clin Oral Implants Res 2008;19:1188–96.

63. Kuroda S, Sugawara Y, Deguchi T, et al. Clinical use of miniscrew implants as orthodontic anchorage: success rates and postoperative discomfort. Am J Orthod Dentofacial Orthop 2007;131:9–15.

64. Lim HJ, Eun CS, Cho JH, et al. Factors associated with initial stability of miniscrews for orthodontic treatment. Am J Orthod Dentofacial Orthop 2009;136:236–42.

65. Manni A, Cozzani M, Tamborrino F, et al. Factors influencing the stability of miniscrews. A retrospective study on 300 miniscrews. Eur J Orthod 2010;388–95.

66. Chen YJ, Chang HH, Huang CY, et al. A retrospective analysis of the failure rate of three different orthodontic skeletal anchorage systems. Clin Oral Implants Res 2007;18:768–75.

67. Shibli JA, Piattelli A, Iezzi G, et al. Effect of smoking on early bone healing around oxidized surfaces: a prospective, controlled study in human jaws. J Periodontol 2010;81:575–83.

68. Choi NC, Park YC, Lee HA, et al. Treatment of Class II protrusion with severe crowding using indirect miniscrew anchorage. Angle Orthod 2007;77:1109–18.

69. Ohnishi H, Yagi T, Yasuda Y, et al. A mini-implant for orthodontic anchorage in a deep overbite case. Angle Orthod 2005;75:444–52.

70. Büchter A, Wiechmann D, Koerdt S, et al. Load-related implant reaction of mini-implants used for orthodontic anchorage. Clin Oral Implants Res 2005;16:473–9.

71. Poggio P, Incorvati C, Velo S, et al. "Safe zones": a guide for miniscrew positioning in the maxillary and mandibular arch. Angle Orthod 2006;76:191–7.

72. Chatzigianni A, Keilig L, Reimann S, et al. Effect of mini-implant length and diameter on primary stability under loading with two force levels. Eur J Orthod 2011;33:381–7.

73. Chen CH, Chang CS, Hsieh CH, et al. The use of microimplants in orthodontic anchorage. J Oral Maxillofac Surg 2006;64:1209–13.

74. Tsaousidis G, Bauss O. Influence of insertion site on the failure rates of orthodontic miniscrews. J Orofac Orthop 2008;69:349–56.

75. Kim YK, Kim YJ, Yun PY, et al. Effects of the taper shape, dual-thread, and length on the mechanical properties of mini-implants. Angle Orthod 2009;79:908–14.

76. Lin CL, Yu JH, Liu HL, et al. Evaluation of contributions of orthodontic mini-screw design factors based on FE analysis and the Taguchi method. J Biomech 2010;43:2174–81.

77. Nagamatsu JBT. Bone response to orthodontic miniscrew placement: an in vivo study. St. Louis University, MO: Master Thesis; 2008.

78. Wilmes B, Rademacher C, Olthoff G, et al. Parameters affecting primary stability of orthodontic mini-implants. J Orofac Orthop 2006;67:162–74.

79. Wang Z, Zhang D, Liu Y, et al. Buccal mucosal lesions caused by the interradicular miniscrew: a preliminary report. Int J Oral Maxillofac Implants 2010;25:1183–8.

80. Wilmes B, Su YY, Drescher D. Insertion angle impact on primary stability of orthodontic mini-implants. Angle Orthod 2008;78:1065–70.

81. Stahl E, Keilig L, Abdelgader I, et al. Numerical analyses of biomechanical behavior of various orthodontic anchorage implants. J Orofac Orthop 2009;70:115–27.

82. Motoyoshi M, Ueno S, Okazaki K, et al. Bone stress for a mini-implant close to the roots of adjacent teeth: a 3D finite element analysis. Int J Oral Maxillofac Surg 2009;38:363–8.

83. Cho UH, Yu W, Kyung HM. Root contact during drilling for microimplant placement. Angle Orthod 2010;80:130–6.

84. Asscherickx K, Vannet BV, Wehrbein H, et al. Root repair after injury from miniscrew. Clin Oral Implants Res 2005;16:575–8.

85. Hwang YC, Hwang HS. Surgical repair of root perforation caused by an orthodontic miniscrew implant. Am J Orthod Dentofacial Orthop 2011;139:407–11.

86. Leung MTC, Rabie ABM, Wong RWK. Stability of connected mini-implants and miniplates for skeletal anchorage in orthodontics. Eur J Orthod 2008;30:483–9.

87. Chung KR, Kim SH, Kook YA. The C-orthodontic micro-implant. J Clin Orthod 2004;38:478–86.

88. Melsen B, Lang N. Biological reactions of alveolar bone to orthodontic loading of oral implants. Clin Oral Implants Res 2001;12:144–52.

89. Cha JY, Kil JK, Yoon TM, et al. Miniscrew stability evaluated with computerized tomography scanning. Am J Orthod Dentofacial Orthop 2010;137:73–9.

90. Uemura M, Motoyoshi M, Yano S, et al. Orthodontic mini-implant stability and the ratio of pilot hole implant diameter. Eur J Orthod 2012;34:52–6.

50 Root and bone response to proximity of miniscrew implants

Hyewon Kim and Tae-Woo Kim

INTRODUCTION

Use of miniscrew implants (MIs), particularly inter-radicularly in the alveolar bone in proximity to adjacent roots, carries certain risks and clinicians need to understand the likely response of roots and surrounding bone and the potential consequences.

ROOT CONTACT WITH MINISCREW IMPLANTS

RISK FACTORS

If injury to a tooth root occurs during MI insertion, loss of tooth vitality, osteosclerosis and dentoalveolar ankylosis may follow.[1,2] During orthodontic loading, MI failure or migration may occur[3] and soft tissue complications such as inflammation or infection may also have subsequent effects on bone and tooth roots.[1]

EXTENT OF DAMAGE AND PREVENTION METHODS

A good knowledge of the average inter-radicular space in the area of planned implant insertion is essential. Stents and guides that are placed over the adjacent teeth can help to identify the insertion position[4-7] and can be used in conjunction with radiography or CT to evaluate the inter-radicular space available and to safely insert the MIs avoiding contact with the adjacent roots.[8-10] However, radiography taken after MI insertion to verify root contact has limitations: it only provides a two-dimensional representation of a three-dimensional object, only shows lesions of a certain dimension and cannot indicate the severity of root resorption.[11] It has been suggested that the use of self-drilling and self-tapping MIs may decrease the chances of root damage as they improve tactile feedback to the operator during drilling and have less overheating, more bone-to-metal contact and possible decreased mobility.[12,13]

An experimental study intentionally damaged roots and surrounding structures during MI insertion for 42 MIs in seven beagle dogs and observed that out of the MIs that contacted the root, 7.2% caused direct damage to the periodontal ligament, 19.0% caused damage isolated to the cementum, 26.2% caused damage to the dentin, and 14.2% caused severe damage to the pulp.[14] Most of the MIs that failed or were mobile showed bone loss and necrotic tissue in the peri-implant area, which may serve as a stimulus for root resorption. The presence of inflammation increased the damage caused by the MIs.

Failure rates for MIs increase when the implants invade the adjacent roots, being as high as 79.2%, with an average retention period of 16 days.[15] Proximity of MIs to dental roots, as seen by radiography and three-dimensional CT, was a major risk factor for MI failure.[16]

MINISCREW IMPLANT DIAMETER AND CLEARANCE

MIs with a larger diameter increase pressure on the periodontal ligament and both inter-radicular space and MI diameter need to be considered when planning treatment.

Various space recommendations for inter-radicular MIs have been made: 1 mm between the periodontal ligament and the MI,[17] at least 5 mm between adjacent roots,[18] 3.5 mm between adjacent roots for MIs of maximum diameter 1.5 mm[19] and a minimum of 2.0 mm between the implant and root surfaces.[3]

ROOT RESPONSE

ROOT RESORPTION AFTER CONTACT

Root resorption during tooth movement has most often been found where there is overcompression of the periodontal ligament.[20]

The mechanism of root resorption that occurs after iatrogenic trauma to the root surface, as is the case after contact with a MI, appears to be repaired quite quickly and, when the damage is limited to the periodontal ligament, with no further consequences.[21] However, if the cementum layer is mechanically damaged with exposure of the dentin surface, the process of resorption starts. The first changes occur in the periphery of the necrotic tissue where multinuclear cells and cells staining for tartrate-resistant acid phosphatase accumulate.[22] These resorbing cells require continuous stimulation during phagocytosis, and without further stimulation the process stops spontaneously.

Repair of the affected area occurs through formation of cementum-like tissue within 2 or 3 weeks, depending on the area of the root that is injured. Three different types of root resorption response can be described:[23]

- when the MI is in proximity (<1 mm) but bone exists between MI and root (Fig. 50.1A)
- when the MI thread is away from the root but in contact with the periodontal ligament (Fig. 50.1B,C)
- when the MI thread touches the root and stays in contact with it without resorption following (Fig. 50.1D,E).

Fig. 50.2 shows a possible sequence of events after root contact with a MI.

Root resorption has been shown to occur indirectly when the MI is inserted in close proximity to the root surface even if a clear width of bone of around 1 mm exists between the root surface and the MI (Fig. 50.1A). This may be a result of pressure from the MI on the alveolar bone, causing bone compression and compression of the periodontal ligament. Damage to the periodontal ligament is known to cause root resorption. Macrophages and osteoclasts in viable periodontal ligament will initiate wound healing by removing the damaged tissue. During this activity, bone and cementum can be removed along with necrotic periodontal ligament tissue.

Pressure from bleeding into the periodontal ligament may also elicit minor areas of damage to the root surface. This type of edema has been shown to directly affect the arrangement and structure of the extracellular matrix of the periodontal ligament.[24] Mechanical stresses to a tooth root may be responsible for vascular flow alterations that trigger cellular degeneration, leading to hyalinization.[25] The first steps of root resorption can be seen as the removal of this hyalinized necrotic tissue.

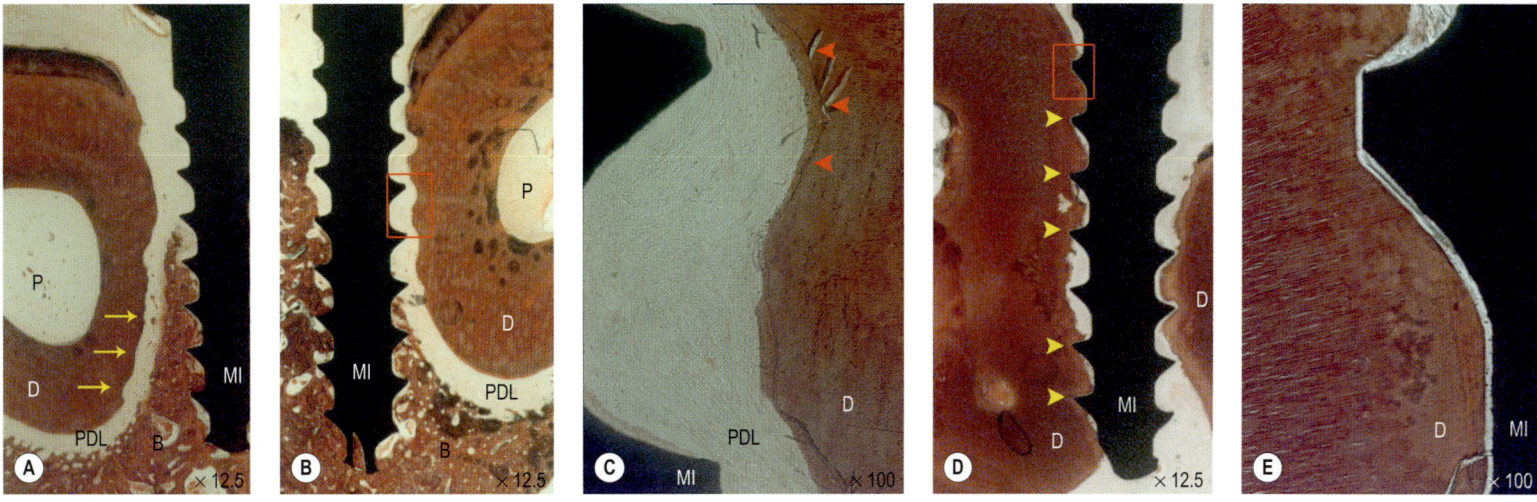

Fig. 50.1 Root resorption with miniscrew implants (MIs). (A) MI in close proximity to root causes resorption (yellow arrows) even though a clear width of bone is present between the MI and the root surface. (B) MI in contact with the periodontal ligament and dentin. (C) Close up of the area in the red box in (B) showing cementum deposition (red arrowheads) on the resorbed root surface. (D) MI thread in contact with root (yellow arrowheads). (E) Close up of red box in (D) showing no cementum repair of the root surface. D, dentin; B, bone; P, pulp; PDL, periodontal ligament.

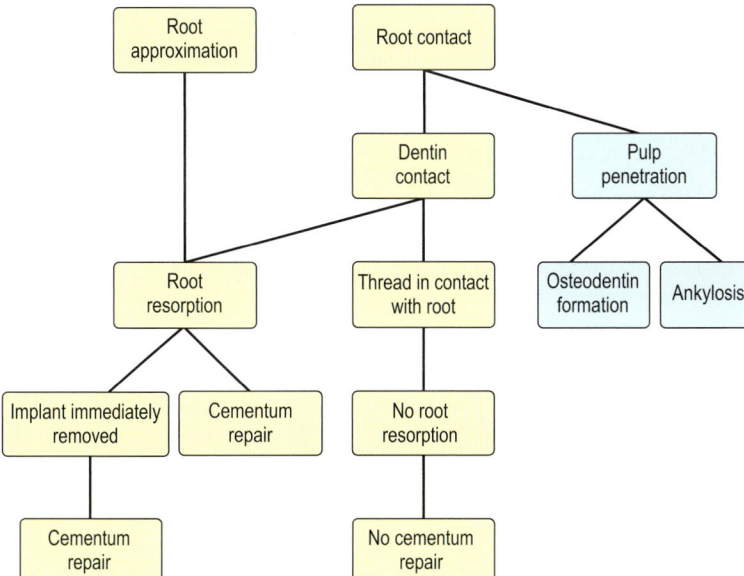

Fig. 50.2 Possible sequence of events after root contact with a miniscrew implant.

ROOT HEALING

Normal healing has been defined as formation of a cementum layer, normal periodontal ligament attachment and bone regeneration. Abnormal healing is associated with absence of periodontal ligament or bone regeneration and may lead to root ankylosis or pulp invasion.[26] The consequences of root damage may include healing without root resorption, surface root resorption that heals with cementoid tissue or replacement resorption leading to ankylosis. It is believed that a favorable environment for root resorption includes destruction of the protective surface covering the mineralized tissue, presence of vascular connective tissue or an inflammatory stimulus such as bacteria or trauma.[27] Damaged roots usually heal unless the damage extends to the pulp.[15] Deposition of cementoid tissue starts at the periphery of a damaged area and extends to cover the entire defect over time, with new cementum layers becoming thicker.[19] Healing can occur in as short a time as 4 weeks.[21] Normal healing, reattachment of the periodontal ligament, regeneration of bone and new cementum layers on exposed dentin are all evident by 6 weeks but if inflammatory infiltration or invasion of the pulp chamber occurs, the normal healing sequence could be interrupted.[26]

Healing Versus Non-healing

When any part of the MI thread was left touching the root surface, no definite cementum repair was observed on the damaged root surface (Fig. 50.1D,E).[23] After MI contact with the root surface, the possibility of healing through cementum deposition or no healing depends on whether the MI stays in contact with the root surface.

When a MI is left in contact with the root surface, minimal healing occurs in most cases. When a tooth was pushed against the MIs through orthodontic force, there was no sign of repair in the resorption lacunae, but swift repair of tooth surfaces occurred when root contact was discontinued, and abundant cellular cementum was deposited.[19,21] When a MI is drilled between two roots with large force, the implant may become lodged between the adjacent roots (Fig. 50.1D,E) and this absence of mobility would mean that the pressure between the root and the implant is maintained. Resorption is an active process that requires viable cells in the vicinity of the root surface and the first sign of it occurring is penetration of cells from the periodontal ligament into the mineralized cementum.[20] If the periodontal ligament itself is damaged or destroyed, this source of healing cells is lost. The resorbing cells also require continuous stimulation during phagocytosis and the process stops spontaneously if stimulation fails.

When a MI is removed immediately after root contact has been made, relieving pressure on the root, cementum repair occurs on the damaged root surface (Fig. 50.3).

PULP DAMAGE AND RESPONSE

When the MI goes beyond touching the root and penetrates the dentin, much more severe damage can be expected. Dentin tissue is ruptured and rapid formation of osteodentin is observed (Fig. 50.4). Osteodentin is the response of dentin to a severe attack, and consists of tertiary dentin with sparse and irregular tubular patterns with cellular inclusions. This has a similar appearance to bone. Rupturing the pulp tissue seems to have irreversible consequences and should be avoided.

ANKYLOSIS

Ankylosis may occur after severe root damage from MIs. A patent periodontal ligament space is essential to prevent contact between root and

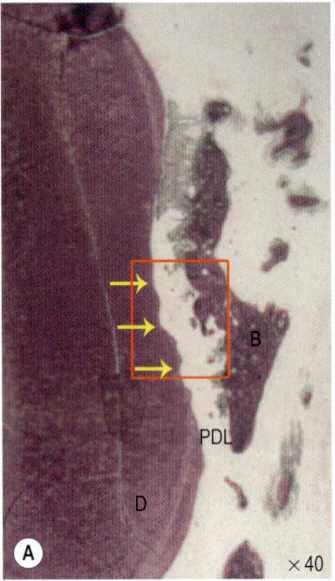
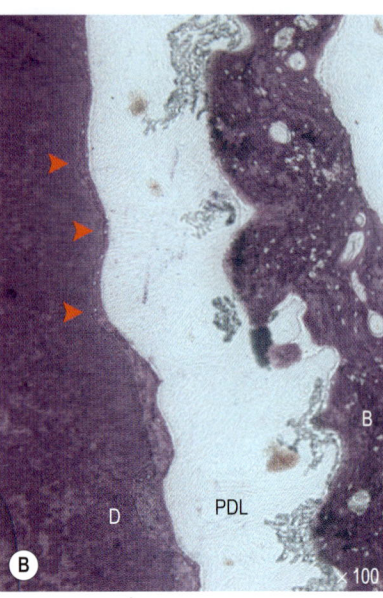

Fig. 50.3 Changes seen following immediate removal of a miniscrew implant (MI) after its insertion. (A) Mechanical damage and resorption of the root surface (long yellow arrows) where contact with the MI was made. (B) The area in the red box in (A) showing cementum repair of the resorbed root surface (short red arrows). D, dentin; PDL, periodontal ligament; B, bone.

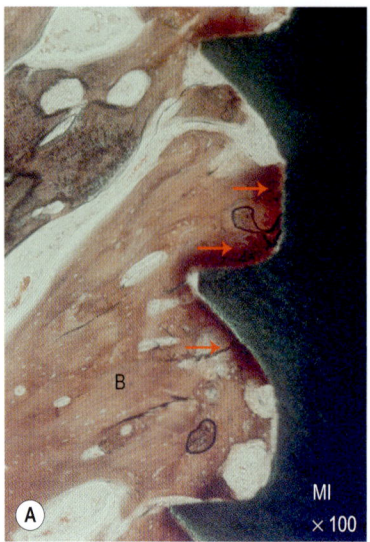
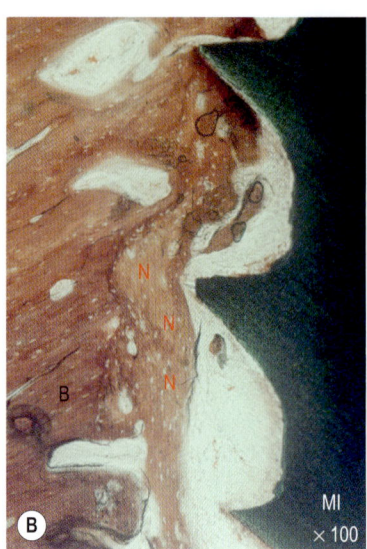

Fig. 50.5 Bone response following insertion of a miniscrew implant (MI). (A) Osseointegration of bone and MI (long red arrows). (B) New bone formation next to the MI thread (red N). B, bone.

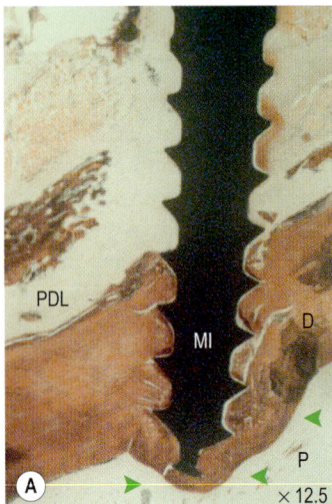
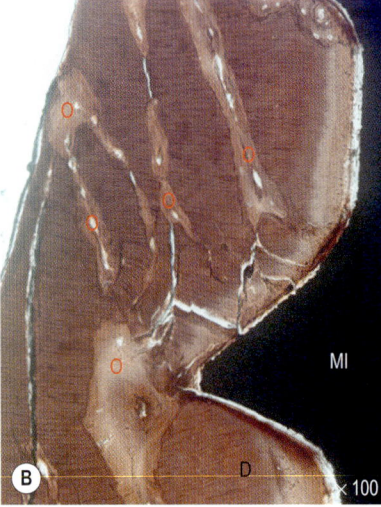

Fig. 50.4 Penetration of the miniscrew implant (MI) into the pulp space. (A) Formation of osteodentin cap (green arrows) around the MI tip. (B) Close-up view of a section showing formation of osteoids (red circles) inside the dentin tissue. P, pulp; D, dentin; PDL, periodontal ligament; B, bone.

BONE RESPONSE

BONE REMODELING AROUND IMPLANT

When a MI is inserted into the alveolar bone, there is a mismatch between the elastic moduli of the two materials at the bone–implant interface, which causes stresses in the bone surrounding the MI and leads to increased bony remodeling at the interface. Masticatory forces may also create strain at the bone surfaces. The bone responds by depositing more bone, which is then remodeled into stronger compact bone with time. However, if there is contact between the MI and the root surface, jiggling forces will be set up at the MI–root contact. It can be speculated that this may decrease mechanical retention and eventually lead to a higher failure rate.[15]

OSSEOINTEGRATION

Osseointegration can be defined as direct contact between bone and an inert object, with histological evidence suggesting that new woven bone is formed around the inert object and, for a MI, around and within the threads. This newly formed bone is relatively darker than surrounding trabecular bone (Fig. 50.5). The quality and amount of osseointegrated bone around the MIs, as well as other factors such as the degree of inflammation, possible excess orthodontic force and the proximity of the MIs to the roots, affect their stability and consequently their failure rates.[16]

CONCLUSIONS

Every effort should be made to avoid contacting root surfaces when inserting MIs inter-radicularly into alveolar bone. If contact is made, resorption of the root surface occurs, with or without cementum healing, depending on specific circumstances. Where excessive force causes penetrative injury to the pulp, irreversible damage occurs with possible ankylosis of the root with the bone. When contact between MI and root is suspected, immediate removal of the MI and reimplantation is recommended, since the removal of the contact will allow healing of the root surface. Care must also be taken when a MI is inserted closer than 1 mm to a root surface, since root resorption may occur even when a thin layer of bone and periodontal ligament exists between the MI and the root surface.

bone. If this barrier is severely damaged and bone grows towards the resorbed root, ankylosis may occur. A MI totally perforating a root caused ankylosis in beagle dogs.[28] In such severe damage, root resorption and ankylosis were observed on the opposite side to the MI insertion. This may indicate that insertion pressure on one side of the root can induce root resorption and ankylosis on the opposite side. Ankylosis has been observed only in severe injury with displacement of root fragments, and this may be caused by compression of the lamina dura causing by obliteration of the periodontal ligament space.[29]

An ankylotic response has not been seen when the periodontal ligament space was well maintained even when the pulp was penetrated.[23,30] Studies of resorption after replanting of a tooth indicate that the healing responses of the periodontal ligament depend on the extent of the damage to the ligament, with up to 2 mm of loss of periodontal ligament being repaired by new attachment without ankylosis.[19] With time, minor areas of possible ankylotic spots are expected to be resolved.

REFERENCES

1. Kravitz ND, Kusnoto B. Risks and complications of orthodontic miniscrews. Am J Orthod Dentofacial Orthop 2007;131(Suppl.):S43–51.
2. Asscherickx K, Vannet BV, Wehrbein H, et al. Root repair after injury from miniscrew. Clin Oral Implants Res 2005;16:575–8.
3. Liou EJ, Pai BC, Lin JC. Do miniscrews remain stationary under orthodontic forces? Am J Orthod Dentofacial Orthop 2004;126:42–7.
4. Choi HJ, Kim TW, Kim HW. A precise wire guide for positioning inter-radicular miniscrews. J Clin Orthod 2007;41:258–61.
5. Cousley RR, Parberry DJ. Surgical stents for accurate miniscrew insertion. J Clin Orthod 2006;40:412–17.
6. Kitai N, Yasuda Y, Takada K. A stent fabricated on a selectively colored stereolithographic model for placement of orthodontic mini-implants. Int J Adult Orthodon Orthognath Surg 2002;17:264–6.
7. Suzuki EY, Buranastidporn B. An adjustable surgical guide for miniscrew placement. J Clin Orthod 2005;39:588–90.
8. Kim SH, Choi YS, Hwang EH, et al. Surgical positioning of orthodontic mini-implants with guides fabricated on models replicated with cone-beam computed tomography. Am J Orthod Dentofacial Orthop 2007;131(Suppl.):S82–9.
9. Hernandez LC, Montoto G, Puente Rodriguez M, et al. "Bone map" for a safe placement of miniscrews generated by computed tomography. Clin Oral Implants Res 2008;19:576–81.
10. Gracco A, Lombardo L, Cozzani M, et al. Quantitative cone-beam computed tomography evaluation of palatal bone thickness for orthodontic miniscrew placement. Am J Orthod Dentofacial Orthop 2008;134:361–9.
11. Heimisdottir K, Bosshardt D, Ruf S. Can the severity of root resorption be accurately judged by means of radiographs? A case report with histology. Am J Orthod Dentofacial Orthop 2005;128:106–9.
12. Kim J, Ahn S, Chang Y. Histomorphometric and mechanical analyses of the drill-free screw as orthodontic anchorage. Am J Orthod Dentofacial Orthop 2005;128:190–4.
13. Chen Y, Shin H, Kyung H. Biomechanical and histological comparison of self-drilling and self-tapping orthodontic microimplants in dogs. Am J Orthod Dentofacial Orthop 2008;133:44–50.
14. Hembree M, Buschang PH, Carrillo R, et al. Effects of intentional damage of the roots and surrounding structures with miniscrew implants. Am J Orthod Dentofacial Orthop 2009;135:280.
15. Kang Y, Kim JY, Lee YJ, et al. Stability of mini-screws invading the dental roots and their impact on the paradental tissues in beagles. Angle Orthod 2009;79:248–55.
16. Kuroda S, Yamada K, Deguchi T, et al. Root proximity is a major factor for screw failure in orthodontic anchorage. Am J Orthod Dentofacial Orthop 2007;131(Suppl.):S68–73.
17. Schnelle MA, Beck FM, Jaynes RM, et al. A radiographic evaluation of the availability of bone for placement of miniscrews. Angle Orthod 2004;74:832–7.
18. Gautam P, Valiathan A. Implants for anchorage. Am J Orthod Dentofacial Orthop 2006;129:174; author reply 174.
19. Maino BG, Weiland F, Attanasi A, et al. Root damage and repair after contact with miniscrews. J Clin Orthod 2007;41:762–6.
20. Brudvik P, Rygh P. The initial phase of orthodontic root resorption incident to local compression of the periodontal ligament. Eur J Orthod 1993;15:249–63.
21. Kadioglu O, Buyukyilmaz T, Zachrisson BU, et al. Contact damage to root surfaces of premolars touching miniscrews during orthodontic treatment. Am J Orthod Dentofacial Orthop 2008;134:353–60.
22. Brudvik P, Rygh P. Root resorption beneath the main hyalinized zone. Eur J Orthod 1994;16:249–63.
23. Kim H, Kim TW. Histologic evaluation of root-surface healing after root contact or approximation during placement of mini-implants. Am J Orthod Dentofacial Orthop 2011;139:752–60.
24. Khow F, Goldfaber P. Changes in vasculature of the periodontium associated with tooth movement in *Rhesus* monkey and the dog. Arch Oral Biol 1970;15:1125–43.
25. Faltin R, Faltin K, Sander FG, et al. Ultrastructure of cementum and periodontal ligament after continuous intrusion in humans: a transmission electron microscopy study. Eur J Orthod 2001;23:35–49.
26. Brisceno CE, Rossouw PE, Carrillo R, et al. Healing of the roots and surrounding structures after intentional damage with miniscrew implants. Am J Orthod Dentofacial Orthop 2009;135:292–301.
27. Gold SI, Hasselgren G. Peripheral inflammatory root resorption: a review of the literature with case reports. J Clin Periodontol 1992;19:523–34.
28. Lee YK, Kim JW, Baek SH, et al. Root and bone response to the proximity of a mini-implant under orthodontic loading. Angle Orthod 2010;80:452–8.
29. Renjen RA, Maganzini AL, Rohrer MD, et al. Root and pulp response after intentional injury from miniscrew placement. Am J Orthod Dentofacial Orthop 2009;136:708–14.
30. Chen YH, Chang HH, Chen YJ, et al. Root contact during insertion of miniscrews for orthodontic anchorage increases the failure rate: an animal study. Clin Oral Implants Res 2008;19:99–106.

INTRODUCTION

The maxillary sinus (Higmoro antrum) is a natural cavity found in maxillary bone on both sides of the face. Its function is not clear, but it may serve to amplify sounds, aid olfactory and respiratory functions (heating and humidifying inhaled air) or simply may reduce the weight of the cranium.

The maxillary sinus is found at the level of the premolars and molars, between the maxillary dental arches and the eye sockets, from which it is separated by an extremely thin strip of bone (bilaterally with respect to the nasal fossae, and anteriorly with respect to the pterygomaxillary fissures).

In adults, the maxillary sinus is pyramidal in shape. Its base corresponds to the lateral wall of the nose, while its apex is located at the level of the maxillary zygomatic process. The floor of the maxillary sinus is generally convex and located approximately 1 cm below the nasal cavity, while its maximum depth is found at the level of the first molars. The sinus measures roughly 25–35 mm in depth, 36–45 mm in height and is approximately 38–45 mm long in adults, although a great anatomical variability has been noted.[1] The shape and volume of the sinus vary considerably between individuals, with irregularities in the bony floor from the protrusion of roots of the underlying teeth into the antrum and bony septa in some young adults (prevalence, 16–58%).[2,3]

The internal wall of the maxillary sinus is lined with ciliated respiratory mucosa (the Schneiderian membrane), which is a continuation of that in the nose but is normally thinner with a less extensive network of blood vessels. This ciliated respiratory epithelium transports fluids (mucus and pus) through the nasal ostium, which links the cranial portion of the sinus and the middle meatus of the nasal cavity. The pseudostratified Schneiderian membrane forms a vital barrier, protecting and defending the sinus cavities.[4] It is blue-gray in color and may be particularly thin, fragile and atrophic in smokers. Analysis of the Schneiderian membrane samples from 20 different cadavers indicated that it has a mean thickness of 90 μm (±45).[5] The membrane could be stretched to up to 132.6% of its original size in one direction and up to 124.7% if the stretching force was applied in two directions. As expected, the strain needed to break the membrane is reduced as the membrane thins; the tendency to perforation occurred at an average tension value of 7 N/mm.[5]

The maxillary sinus is supplied with blood by the greater palatine artery, the infraorbital artery and the posterior superior alveolar artery.[1] The latter two arteries have numerous anastomoses within the lateral wall of the sinus and supply the Schneiderian membrane.

The anterior wall of the sinus is made up of thin compact bone and houses the neurovascular system for the anterior dentition. The posterior teeth are supplied by neurovascular bundles from the maxillary tuberosity.

Loss of teeth may induce resorption and remodeling of the surrounding alveolar bone, resulting in formation of an atrophic bony ridge, loss of vertical bone volume and progressive pneumatization of the sinus, which, in turn, may cause craniocaudal resorption of the alveolar process.

MAXILLARY SINUS PERFORATION

Perforation of the Schneiderian membrane can occur easily during insertion of an orthodontic miniscrew implant (MI) into the zygomatic crest, a location that is considered a suitable skeletal anchorage site for a number of orthodontic procedures (Fig. 51.1).[6,7]

Zygomatic crest thickness at the level of the first molar's mesiobuccal root is suitable for the insertion of orthodontic MIs; here the presence of two cortical layers (the alveolar and the sinus cortex) helps to ensure excellent primary stability. A MI should be placed 14–16 mm above the occlusal plane with an angulation of 55–70° (Fig. 51.2),[8] which

Fig. 51.1 Miniscrew implant insertion in the zygomatic crest. (A) Insertion position. (B) Maxillary sinus perforation by an orthodontic miniscrew implant.

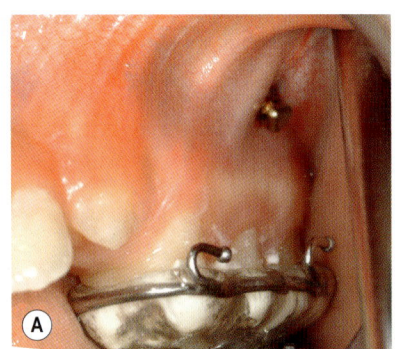

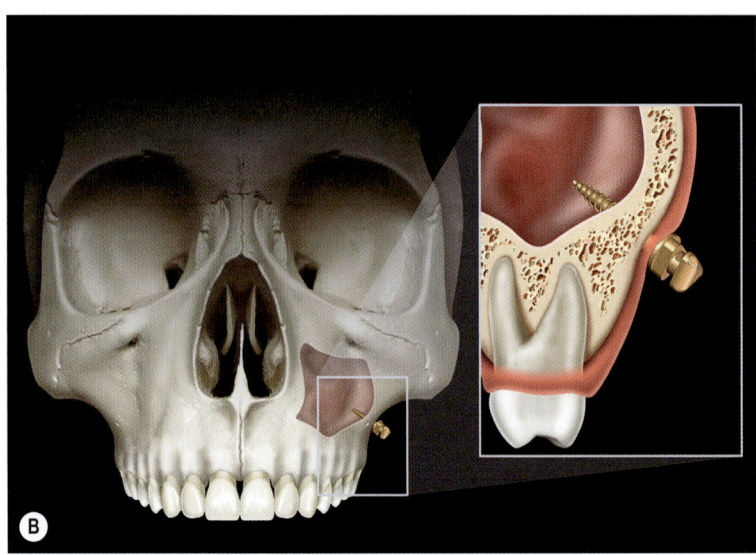

allows for considerations of individual anatomical variation in sinus pneumatization and the length and inclination of the tooth roots. The safest area for MI insertion in the maxilla in all patients (regardless of their different skeletal growth patterns) seems to be between the second premolar and the first maxillary molar (Fig. 51.3).[9] The zygomatic crest gets gradually thinner in an apical direction and the risk of sinus perforation increases.[10]

The most common cause of this type of iatrogenic damage is the insertion of graft material in the maxillary sinus in order to raise its floor and aid implantation in patients with atrophic alveolar crests.[5] Perforation is most frequent at the crestal margin, particularly in the presence of bony protrusions or septa, and may be inevitable when there is excessively thin sinus mucosa or improper surgical technique.

A small perforation that occurs where the membrane is folded over itself will heal spontaneously.[11] A perforation of the Schneider membrane of less than 2 mm in diameter is unlikely to become inflamed,[12] and upon MI removal heals completely over a short period of time. Consequently, MIs with diameters 2 mm or less should be used in the palatal area of the maxilla.[13]

An experimental and clinical study of osseointegrated titanium implants penetrating the nasal cavity and maxillary sinus showed healthy, noninflamed tissue around implants and normal bone regeneration, indicating that penetration does not have adverse effects in the maxillary sinus during the healing process.[14] Rhinoscopic investigations after perforation have also shown the presence of healthy tissue and lack of sinusitis or other pathological events (Fig. 51.4).[15] In fact, healing processes have been shown to commence spontaneously within 48 hours of a traumatic event.[16] (Videos of MI insertion into the maxillary sinus can be viewed at https://www.youtube.com/watch?v=JX5MdKbNhK8 and http://youtu.be/Lp9OPbED4GE.)

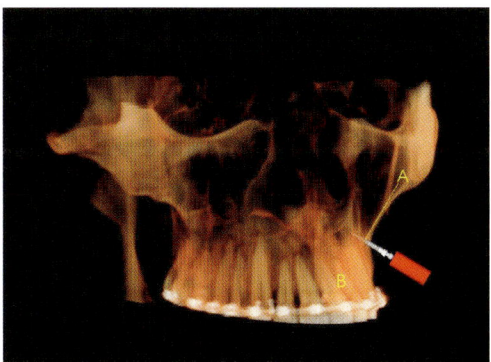

Fig. 51.2 Miniscrew implant inserted with proper angulation to avoid iatrogenic damage.

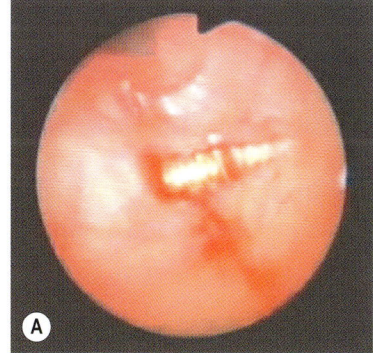 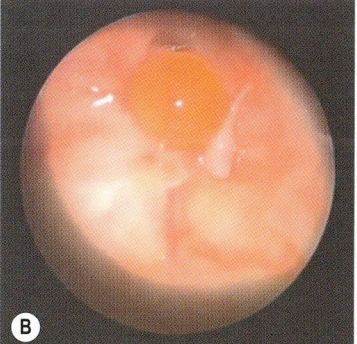

Fig. 51.4 Images taken during a sinuscopy evaluation. (A) An orthodontic miniscrew implant (MI; diameter, 2 mm; length, 10 mm) passing through the sinus cortex and mucosa. (B) Image showing a MI (diameter, 1.4 mm; length, 8 mm) passing through the sinus mucosa close to a mucosal cyst.

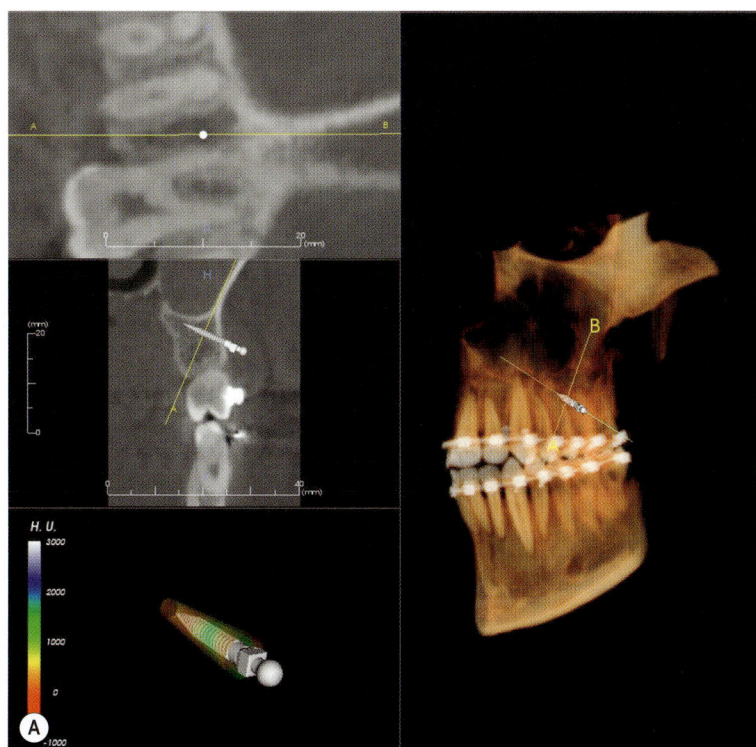 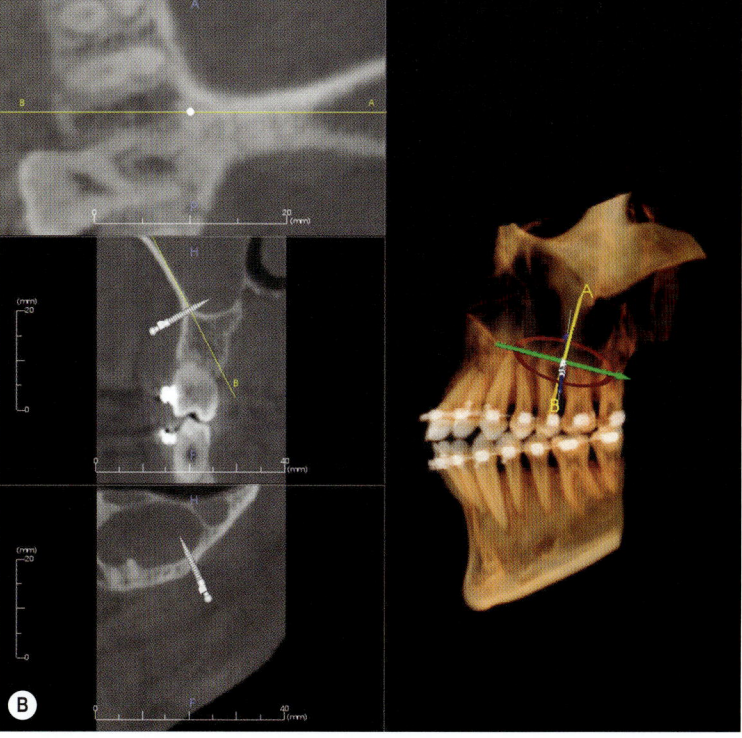

Fig. 51.3 Cone beam CT. (A) Orthodontic miniscrew implant correctly inserted in the inter-radicular space between the maxillary second premolar and first molar. (B) Sinus cortex perforation by an orthodontic MI.

Fig. 51.5 Cone beam CT. (A) Coronal section showing inflammatory hypertrophy of the left sinus mucosa, nasal septum deviation, nasal turbinate hypertrophy and radiopaque alterations located in the right sinus cavity. (B) Axial image showing the difference between a normal right sinus cavity and a pathological mucosal hypertrophy in the left one.

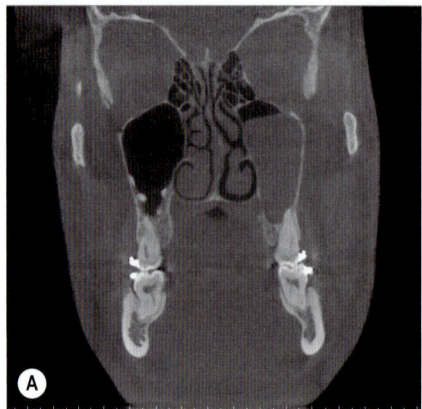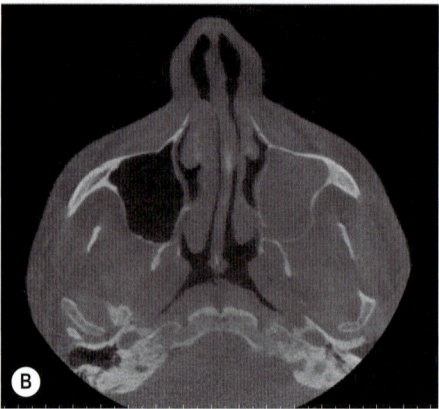

CONCLUSIONS

The maxillary sinus may have pathological alterations before any orthodontic treatment is commenced; cone beam CT carried out before treatment showed incidental pathological alterations in approximately 50%, including mucosal thinning, polyps and acute sinusitis (Fig. 51.5).[17] This would suggest that a preliminary otorhinolaryngology consultation would be useful to evaluate the condition of the sinus, detect any predisposing factors for iatrogenic damage and solve any pathological problems before initiation of orthodontic treatment.[13]

REFERENCES

1. McGowan DA, Baxter PW, James J. The maxillary sinus and its dental implications. Oxford: Wright, Butterworth-Heinemann; 1993. p. 1–125.
2. Baumgaertel S, Hans MG. Assessment of infrazygomatic bone depth for mini-screw insertion. Clin Oral Implants Res 2009;20:638–42.
3. Koymen R, Gocmen-Mas N, Karacayli U, et al. Anatomic evaluation of maxillary sinus septa: surgery and radiology. Clin Anat 2009;222:563–70.
4. Ardekian L, Efrat Oved-Peleg E, Mactei EE, et al. The clinical significance of sinus membrane perforation during augmentation of the maxillary sinus. J Oral Maxillofac Surg 2006;64:277–82.
5. Pommer B, Unger E, Sütö D, et al. Mechanical properties of the Schneiderian membrane in vitro. Clin Oral Implants Res 2009;20:633–7.
6. Poggio PM, Incorvati C, Velo S, et al. "Safe zones": a guide for miniscrew positioning in the maxillary and mandibular arch. Angle Orthod 2006;76:191–7.
7. Wang Z, Li Y, Deng F, et al. A quantitative anatomical study on posterior mandibular interradicular safe zone for miniscrew implantation in the beagle. Ann Anat 2008;190:352–7.
8. Liou EJ, Chen PH, Wang YC, et al. A computed tomographic image study on the thickness of the infrazygomatic crest of the maxilla and its clinical implications for miniscrew insertion. Am J Orthod Dentofacial Orthop 2007;131:352–6.
9. Chaimanee P, Suzuki B, Suzuki EY. "Safe zones" for miniscrew implant placement in different dentoskeletal patterns. Angle Orthod 2011;81:397–403.
10. Baumgaertel S, Hans MG. Assessment of infrazygomatic bone depth for mini-screw insertion. Clin Oral Implants Res 2009;20:638–42.
11. Pikos MA. Maxillary sinus membrane repair: update on technique for large and complete perforations. Implant Dent 2008;17:24–31.
12. Raiser GM, Rabinovitz Z, Bruno J, et al. Evaluation of maxillary sinus membrane response following elevation with the crestal osteotome technique in human cadavers. Int J Oral Maxillofac Imp 2001;16:833–40.
13. Gracco A, Tracey S, Baciliero U. Miniscrew insertion and the maxillary sinus: an endoscopic evaluation. J Clin Orthod 2010;44:439–43.
14. Branemark PI, Adell R, Albrektsson T, et al. An experimental and clinical study of osseointegrated implants penetrating the nasal cavity and maxillary sinus. J Oral Maxillofac Surg 1984;42:497–505.
15. Raghoebar GM, Batenburg RH, Timmenga NM, et al. Morbidity and complications of bone grafting of the floor of the maxillary sinus for the placement of endosseous implants. Mund Kiefer Gesichtschir 1999;3(Suppl. 1):65–9.
16. Skoglund LA, Pedersen SS, Holst E. Surgical management of 85 perforations to the maxillary sinus. Int J Oral Surg 1983;12:1–5.
17. Pazera P, Bornstein MM, Pazera A, et al. Incidental maxillary sinus findings in orthodontic patients: a radiographic analysis using cone-beam computed tomography (CBCT). Orthod Craniofac Res 2011;14:17–24.

Risk management of skeletal anchorage devices in orthodontics

52

Gudrun Lübberink and Vittorio Cacciafesta

INTRODUCTION

The availability of miniscrew implants (MIs) and miniplates has facilitated many aspects of orthopedic treatment, and in some cases actually makes such treatments possible. However, MI-based treatments, in common with all medical procedures, are not without problems, complications and risks.

A single problem or mistake during planning and insertion of a MI can have a range of consequences. Very often, a whole cascade of adverse events is triggered. Orthodontists are becoming increasingly aware of what works well, what lies in the gray area between success and failure and what is bound to fail. Because of this, it is essential that the patient is informed of the potential risks and of the availability of alternative treatments.

SUCCESS AND FAILURE RATES

Chapters 48 and 49 discuss in detail the success rates and risk factors for miniplates and MIs. Because published studies will have used different brands of MI, different MI diameters and lengths, different sites of insertion and in a variety of patients, it is difficult to draw simple straightforward conclusions on causes and effects. What is frequently not mentioned in published studies is the level of experience of the operating practitioner at the start of the study, which is also an important factor that determines outcome.

Consequently, a clinician who intends to use MIs needs to be aware of the numerous influencing factors but also have a willingness to learn, from both his/her own mistakes and those of others. The success rate, in theory, should be well above 90%, although this is unlikely to be achieved by an inexperienced practitioner starting to use MIs, and clinicians may experience a 75–80% success rate, depending on skill levels.[1] There is a demonstrable learning curve with this type of treatment, particularly with regard to the insertion procedure itself. The cause of most problems lies within this surgical procedure.

The main, or most common, problem is the loss of a MI. There is a whole range of possible causes for such a loss. These are covered in detail in Chapters 48 and 49 and only a few aspects will be discussed in this chapter.

TREATMENT PLANNING AND MINISCREW IMPLANT LOCATION

Carefully planning is undoubtedly one of the key factors to success. The documentation and information required for other maxillary orthopedic procedures are perfectly adequate and should be used also when planning treatment involving MIs. The biomechanical approach should be based on medical history, assessment findings (including possible contraindications), diagnosis and treatment outcome desired.

The main contraindications are those of implant procedures in general, such as systemic diseases associated with increased bone metabolism or negative bone balance (e.g. osteoporosis or uncontrolled diabetes), which can reduce the chances of success.[2]

The location of the insertion site appears to be the most important factor determining the success of MIs. Patients have shown significantly different success rates in different insertion areas. MIs inserted in the anterior palate present a success rate of more than 97% (see Fig. 30.1B), whereas those inserted in the mandibular lingual aspects, the retromolar areas (Fig. 52.1) and inter-radicularly between the incisors (see Fig. 39.1E) have a success rate of 60% or less.[3] The morphology of the insertion site is also significant. A MI placed in a location that has a characteristically higher success rate (e.g. between the mandibular second premolars and first molars) is more likely to fail if inserted too high or too low. The ideal insertion site is the mucogingival junction within the attached gingiva, with a slight apical angulation of the MI.[4,5] However, even MIs inserted in these well-chosen sites can be troublesome when placed by an operator with inferior skill, knowledge and experience. For example, failure rates increase significantly with incorrect MI diameter or length, when using an insertion technique that compromises primary stability or with improper loading forces and vector biomechanics (Fig. 52.2).[4,5]

MINISCREW IMPLANT INSERTION SITES

The best site for the insertion of MIs should be selected on the basis of the planned biomechanical approach. The following should be taken into consideration:

- at least 0.5 mm bone around the MI on all sides
- MI head should be positioned on inflammation-free, attached gingiva.

It is very important to determine the quantity and quality of bone at the selected site. However, radiography only provides limited information in

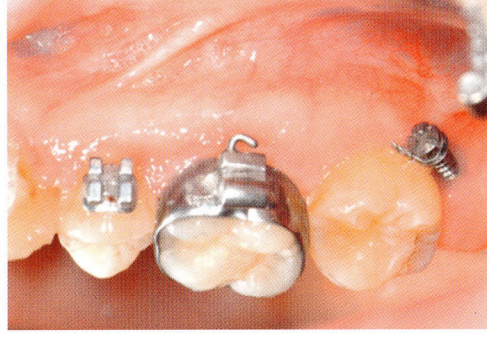

Fig. 52.1 Insertion of miniscrew implant in the retromolar area.

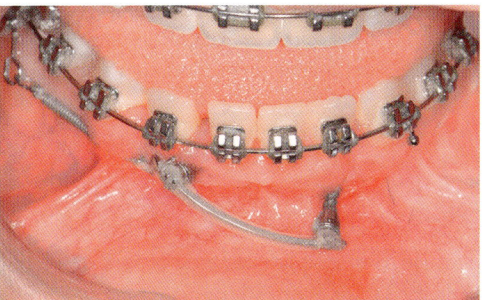

Fig. 52.2 Improper biomechanics with high loading force and wrong vector.

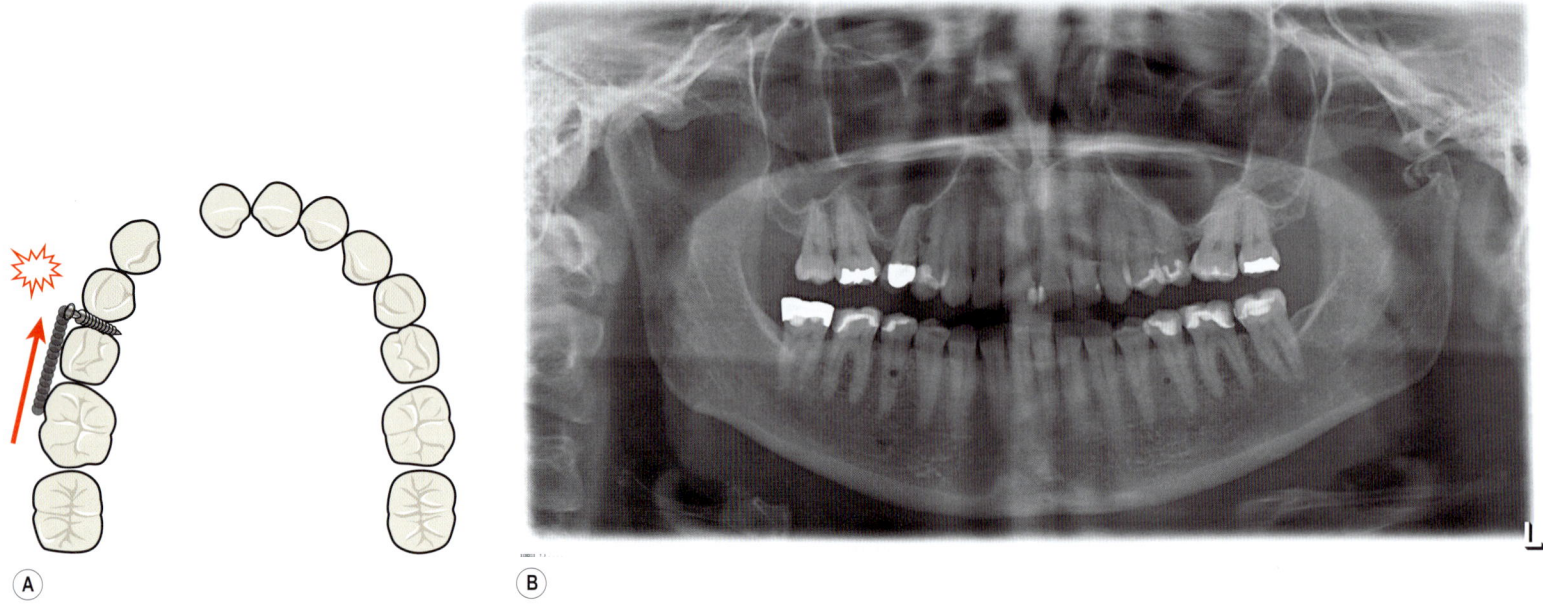

Fig. 52.3 Root injury. (A) Root approximation with a miniscrew implant (MI). (B) Panoramic radiograph depicting root injuries following insertion of MIs.

two dimensions and can have distortions arising from the direction of exposure. The spatial situation can also be assessed by reproducing the mucogingival line, the tooth axes and the roots on a cast.

The required direction of tooth movement must also be considered during planning, as the spatial arrangement of the dentition will change during the course of treatment. A MI must not interfere with or obstruct the desired movement and may need to be moved part way through the treatment course (Fig. 52.3A).

In alveolar bone, the best sites are between the first molars and second premolars, where sufficient inter-radicular space is available, while mid-palatal and retromolar pad areas have sufficient cortical bone thickness and provide excellent sites.[6] Adequacy of inter-radicular space should always be ascertained with at least a panoramic radiograph; cone beam CT is even better. If possible, it is best to place MIs in the attached gingiva to lessen the chance of inflammation, a factor associated with a higher failure rate.[6] When placement in unattached mucosa is essential, careful insertion technique (by stretching the mucosa during insertion) and careful hygiene instruction could help to achieve satisfactory stability.

INSERTION RISKS AND COMPLICATIONS

OPERATOR

There is much in favor of MI insertion being done by the orthodontist. Studies have shown that orthodontists have a far better developed sensitivity and biomechanical knowledge in this regard.[7] If the orthodontist is not the one to insert the MI, a good line of communication with the surgeon must be maintained as surgeons usually insert MIs simply where there is plenty of space, which may not be a useful place. Inappropriate insertion could cause clinical and biomechanical problems such as root injury (Fig. 52.2), obstruction of tooth movement or the wrong location for the connecting systems, which could be too short and ineffective.

OPERATOR EXPERIENCE

Many problems can arise because of inadequate training or lack of experience of the operator (see Table 49.3): for every additional group of 18 MIs inserted, a failure rate of 25% was observed for the first group of MIs,

8.8% for the second, 2.1% for the third and 4.3% for the fourth group.[8] The personal learning curve can be greatly improved by practicing on porcine bone samples to get a "feel" for bone resistance. In order to minimize potential risks, particularly during insertion, it is advisable to adopt a standardized procedure for routine use.

BONE QUALITY

It is only possible to test bone quality at the selected site immediately prior to insertion. A probe should be first inserted in the bone. If the probe penetrates deeply, the bone quality is not adequate and a different site should be selected.

ROOT INJURIES

The MI must not be in contact with the dental roots, with consequences that vary with the level of contact (see Chapter 50). The risk of injury to dental roots during placement is one of the greatest concerns with orthodontic MIs (Fig. 52.3B), particularly when they are inserted between teeth. Placement of a MI too close to a root can also result in insufficient bone remodeling around the MI and transmission of occlusal forces through the teeth to the MIs, which can lead to implant failure (Fig. 52.3A). Even though periodontal structures can heal after being injured by temporary anchorage devices, it is important to select the insertion sites carefully to avoid damage that cannot be retrieved.

FRACTURE OF MINISCREW IMPLANTS

Some MIs have depth stops that signal that screwing must stop when they touch the bone surface. However, depending on clinical factors, such as bone quality, site, angle of insertion and insertion technique, the moment of contact is not generally detectable. There is, therefore, a risk of overinsertion (Fig. 52.4A) and destruction of bone structure by the MI thread. The initial (or primary) stability of the MI appears to be good, but the MI is rapidly lost. In order to avoid this problem, it is advisable to measure the thickness of the gingiva prior to MI insertion as this gives a good indication of how far the MI can be inserted in the bone.

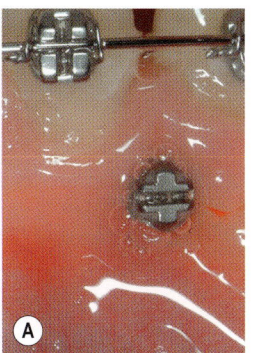 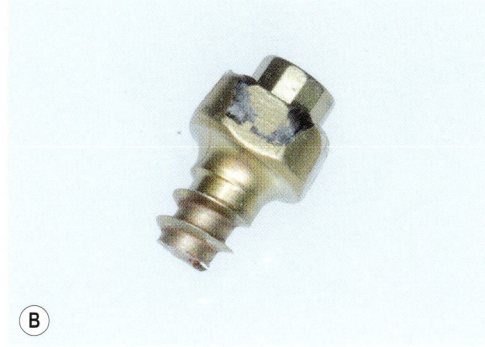

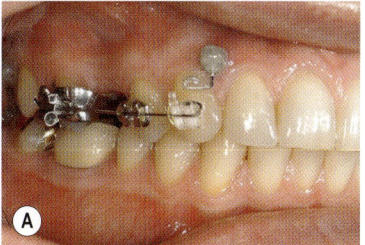 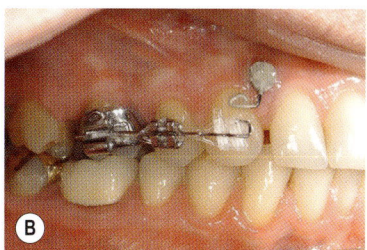

Fig. 52.5 Micromovement of a miniscrew implant. (A) Before molar mesialization. (B) After molar mesialization.

Fig. 52.4 Miniscrew implant problems. (A) Overinsertion. (B) Fracture.

Fracture of a MI is a very rare occurrence (Fig. 52.4B). The following parameters (alone or in combination) determine the risk of fracture:

- MI design: thin (diameter, <1.4 mm) and long (>10 mm) MIs tend to fracture more easily
- anatomical factors: thick cortical layer (>2 mm) without a pilot hole created prior to MI insertion
- insertion conditions: too much torque and/or inconsistent rate of insertion.

The most important way to avoid fractures is to place the MIs very gently, with a steady speed. A torque driver can be used, as the driver rotates freely if the resistance reaches the fracture limit.[9]

If a MI fractures during insertion, it is advisable to remove the fractured part of the MI from the bone immediately, raising a flap and carefully eliminating the surrounding bone.

The simple way to remove a MI at the end of treatment is by turning the manual screwdriver counterclockwise very gently. Touching the head of the MI with a round carbide bur can loosen it so that removal can be swift and safe.[10,11] A MI that is fractured during removal is better left in place, because removal involves flap opening, grinding of the surrounding bone and grasping and turning the MI with Weingart pliers. Because buccal MIs are inserted near the gingival margin, removal of marginal bone may produce periodontal breakdown. A small piece of titanium MI would not cause serious complications, and if the patient accepts leaving it in place, it is less traumatic. Another strategy that makes it easy to remove a fractured MI is to use an ultrasonic scaler to stir up the interface, then wait for 1–2 weeks and apply gentle force to remove it.[10,11]

INSERTION TECHNIQUE

Generally, a self-drilling and self-tapping technique for MI insertion is preferred, using only topical anesthetic and watching for patient discomfort, which indicates possible root contact. A continuous, non-wobbling force helps to keep the MI in a straight path. Desired force vectors should be considered carefully when choosing direct or indirect anchorage. Indirect anchorage allows the clinician to apply a force vector similar to conventional orthodontics while enhancing the stability of the MI. Direct anchorage may be more beneficial for certain types of tooth movement, such as molar intrusion or en masse anterior retraction, where it can provide an intrusive component of the force vector that will facilitate control of the vertical dimension.[10,11]

PRIMARY AND SECONDARY STABILITY

Attempts to place MIs in areas of difficult access or poor bone quality, wobbling during insertion and pilot hole drilling often result in lack of primary stability and, ultimately, in MI failure.

The quality of bone is the most important factor determining primary stability; the strain obtained by loading a MI perpendicular to the long axis with 50 cN leads to loss of primary stability when the cortex is equal to or smaller than 0.5 mm.[12] MI stability is mainly determined by the dimensions of the cortical layer, with any part of the MI within the spongiosa contributing little towards retention. The reasons for poor primary stability include:

- inadequate bone quality or quantity
- overlarge hole in bone caused by using the wrong drilling technique (e.g. repeated insertion of the drill in the hole or deviation from required axis)
- inappropriate MI thread (size and profile of the thread and the relation of the shaft to the external diameter).

To enhance primary stability, the insertion angle should be kept stable during insertion and the threaded part should be inserted totally into bone.[10,11] A MI must present primary stability immediately after insertion as it cannot be achieved subsequently. If this is not achieved, then it is best to remove the MI and select an alternative insertion site.

The regeneration of bone required for secondary stability commences shortly after insertion. Anything that inhibits this process, such as micromovements of the MI, may lead to MI failure.

The second factor determining primary stability is the actual MI insertion pressure. Moderate initiatory pressure is required to engage the first portion of the MI threads, but after that, insertion pressure should be reduced to allow the MI to draw itself in with each rotation. This will prevent stripping and hole widening. Another risk is the gradual, almost indiscernible, forward movement (away from the practitioner) of the hand and driver shaft with each turn of the MI. Not only does this change the initial trajectory of the MI, thus increasing the chance of root impingement, but more importantly, it again widens the hole around the MI.[10,11]

APPLICATION OF LOADING FORCES

Whether a MI is loaded immediately or some time later probably has no influence on failure rates. Forces should be such that no damage is caused to the teeth to be moved. When a MI is coupled to elastic chains or springs, this can result in micromovements of the MI (Fig. 52.5). While research seems to indicate maximum acceptable forces in the range 250–300 g, higher success rates can be obtained using Ni-Ti springs delivering a constant, predetermined force of 50–100 g.[10,11]

The distance between the MI and the site of force application, using springs directly attached to it, should be kept to a minimum. Otherwise, these will be ineffective.

Loading a MI perpendicular to its long axis is preferable. If the MI is used indirectly by adding a cantilever to a bracket-like head, a force generating a counterclockwise moment around the long axis should be avoided since this moment will unscrew the MI.

Fig. 52.6 Peri-implantitis. (A) Healthy palatal soft tissues. (B) Development of peri-implantitis.

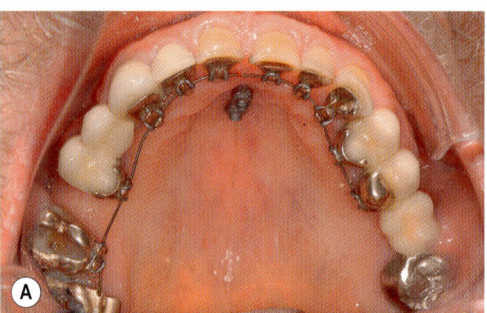
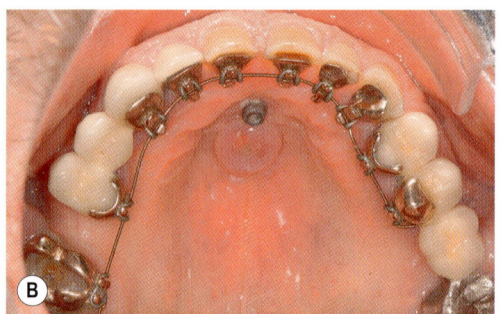

General

You have just received one or more miniscrew implant(s). Your miniscrew implant will help you greatly in achieving our treatment objectives. However, miniscrew implants are delicate and can loosen and fall out. Here are some things to consider.

Home care

Be careful with an electric toothbrush (particularly Sonicare or any vibrating brush) and do not touch the miniscrew implant with a vibrating brush head.
    Keep the area of the miniscrew implant clean by gently using an interdental brush.
    Use a salt-water rinse before bed.

Food

Please avoid eating hard, crunchy, chewy, and sticky foods. They can hit or stick to the miniscrew implant and loosen it.

Habits

There is a possibility that habits like clenching and bruxism can loosen miniscrew implants. While this may be hard for you to control, we'd like you to be aware.

Activities

Trauma to the area can loosen the miniscrew implants. Be aware that sports may involve injury to the face and can increase the risk of loosening the miniscrew implants.

Discomfort

Typically you will not need any medication for discomfort. You may take an ibuprofen only if you need it.
    Your miniscrew implant is an invaluable addition to your orthodontic treatment. Please take care of it, as it is an essential part of your specialized treatment.

POST-INSERTION RISKS AND COMPLICATIONS

INFLAMMATION

There is a high probability that a MI will fail if perimucositis or peri-implantitis develops (Fig. 52.6). It is, therefore, important to ensure that the patient is appropriately informed (including instructions for immaculate oral hygiene) and attends follow-up examinations (Box 52.1). The stability of the MI and of the condition of the surrounding tissue is assessed at each follow-up examination. Attached elements (springs, extension arms) may cause pressure sores or even ulceration of the mucosa, which needs monitoring and treating as necessary.

Infection control is essential during MI insertion (see Chapter 14). Prophylatic antibiotics (e.g. a penicillin or cephalosporin) can be prescribed to be taken 2 hours before or after surgical placement.

ORAL HYGIENE

During treatment, patients are instructed to clean the MIs carefully and not to apply intentional force with a finger or implement. A normal toothbrush or a Waterpik should be used for cleaning. There is evidence that electric toothbrushes, particularly those with rotating heads, can loosen MIs. In addition to the cleaning technique itself, the frequency and intensity of cleaning are undoubtedly also important. Very frequent cleaning that results in persistent micromovement of the MI could well be disadvantageous.

Patients are instructed to dip their toothbrush in a small bottle of 0.12% chlorhexidine solution and brush the MI twice a day. Patients must understand that they should not be afraid of the MI, as proper brushing maintains a firm, healthy gingiva around it.[10,11]

A toothbrush, if not properly used, may irritate the marginal soft tissue and aggravate inflammation. If local inflammation occurs, with signs of redness of the soft tissue margin at the neck of the MI, antibiotics are usually not prescribed. Instead, the patient is instructed to enhance the hygiene regimen, for example using a Waterpik.

LIABILITY ISSUES

In order to protect themselves if a claim for negligence is made, orthodontists should ensure that they follow certain basic rules based on the currently existing evidence.

INSURANCE

Orthodontists who wish to insert MIs themselves are frequently unsure about various aspects of indemnity insurance. Policies available cover claims ranging from 1.5 to 5 million euros. When deciding on the extent of cover required (and so the premiums), the special circumstances of the practice need to be considered. An indemnity insurance policy will cover the practice's personnel but may exclude temporary employees. If there are any changes in the activity profile of the practice, these must be covered by the policy. There are insurance companies that do not differentiate in their policies between dental and orthodontic practices (the policy specifies "with implants" or "with surgery"). Where an orthodontist is planning to personally insert MIs, this is usually automatically covered by the policy. If there is any doubt, policyholders should always contact their insurers and inform them of the extension of the range of treatments provided in the office, particularly if the policy does not specifically cover maxillary orthopedic or implant procedures. In this case, the annual premium is likely to be slightly increased.

DUTY OF INFORMATION

Prior to the initiation of any treatment procedure, the patient must be informed of the nature and effect of potential risks, of alternative treatments and of the consequences if no treatment is provided. It is a good idea to use preprinted material to gather information on medical history and provide information. These can act as an aide memoire or prompt when talking to the patient. Written material should never be used instead of a personal dialogue. Printed materials used (e.g. in the form of a note) must document that the relevant verbal information has been given to the patient. It is not enough merely to have the signature of the patient, a witness and the practitioner.

DOCUMENTATION

Good documentation is absolutely essential. Treatment records, including patient files, radiographs, casts, photographs and so on, must clearly document the course of treatment, as well as any problems and complications. Scrupulous and accurate documentation is very valuable if, for example, a legal dispute ensues. Lawsuits are often lost because documentation was incomplete.

INSURANCE CLAIMS

If a patient suffers an injury or decides to register a claim, it is advisable to get in touch with the policy provider. The insurer will supervise all the financial and legal aspects.

CONCLUSIONS

The main parameters that determine the clinical success of MIs are bone quality, the space available at the planned insertion site, the use of an insertion technique appropriate to the system employed, the use of a well-considered biomechanical concept and the avoidance of inflammation or infection around the MIs.

REFERENCES

1. Antoszewska J, Papadopoulos MA, Park HS, et al. Five-year experience with orthodontic miniscrew implants: a retrospective investigation of factors influencing success rates. Am J Orthod Dentofacial Orthop 2009;136:158, discussion 158–9.
2. Luzi C, Verna C, Melsen B. Guidelines for success in placement of orthodontic mini-implants. J Clin Orthod 2009;43:39–44.
3. Melsen B, Graham J, Baccetti T, et al. Factors contributing to the success or failure of skeletal anchorage devices: an informal JCO survey. J Clin Orthod 2010;44:714–18.
4. Cheng SJ, Tseng IY, Lee JJ, et al. A prospective study of the risk factors associated with failure of mini-implants used for orthodontic anchorage. Int J Oral Maxillofac Implants 2004;19:100–6.
5. Park HS, Jeong SH, Kwon OW. Factors affecting the clinical success of screw implants used as orthodontic anchorage. Am J Orthod Dentofacial Orthop 2006;130:18–25.
6. Park J, Cho HJ. Three-dimensional evaluation of inter-radicular spaces and cortical bone thickness for the placement and initial stability of microimplants in adults. Am J Orthod Dentofacial Orthop 2009;136:314.
7. Osterman WL. Who places miniscrews? An informal JCO survey. J Clin Orthod 2008;42:519, discussion 519–27.
8. Wiechmann D, Meyer U, Büchter A. Success rate of mini- and micro-implants used for orthodontic anchorage: a prospective clinical study. Clin Oral Implants Res 2007;18:263–7.
9. Motoyoshi M, Hirabayashi M, Uemura M, et al. Recommended placement torque when tightening an orthodontic mini-implant. Clin Oral Implants Res 2006;17:109–14.
10. Cacciafesta V, Bumann A, Cho HJ, et al. JCO round table. skeletal anchorage, Part 1. J Clin Orthod 2009;43:303–17.
11. Cacciafesta V, Bumann A, Cho HJ, et al. JCO round table. skeletal anchorage, Part 2. J Clin Orthod 2009;43:365–78.
12. Dalstra M, Cattaneo PM, Melsen B. Load transfer of miniscrews for orthodontic anchorage. Orthod 2004;1:53–62.

Index

Page numbers followed by "f" indicate figures, "t" indicate tables, and "b" indicate boxes.